AF411936

Susan MD

A bit of thought process for you to use in your surgical career.

VASCULAR GRAFT INFECTIONS

edited by

T.J. Bunt, MD, FACS

Professor of Surgery
Director of Vascular Residency
Loma Linda University Medical Center
Loma Linda, California

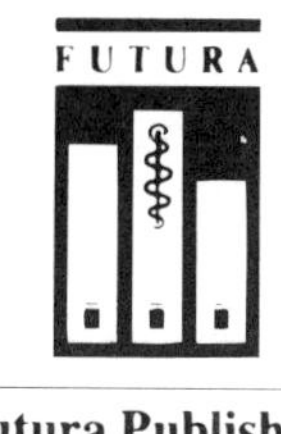

**Futura Publishing
Company, Inc.**
Armonk, NY
1994

Library of Congress Cataloging-in-Publication Data

Vascular graft infections / edited by T. J. Bunt.
    p.   cm.
  Includes bibliographical references and index.
  ISBN 0-87993-576-6
    1. Vascular grafts.   2. Blood-vessels—Infections.   3. Blood—
vessels—Transplantation—Complications.   I. Bunt, T. J.
    [DNLM: 1. Infection.   2. Blood Vessel Prosthesis.   3. Tissue
Transplantation.   4. Graft Occlusion, Vascular.   WG 170 V3288   1994]
RD598.55.V37   1994
617.4'130592—dc20
DNLM/DLC
for Library of Congress   93-44332
                                                                      CIP

Published by
Futura Publishing Company, Inc.
P.O. Box 418
135 Bedford Road
Armonk, New York 10504

L.C. No.: 93-44332
ISBN No.: 0-87993-576-6

Every effort has been made to ensure that the information in this book is as up to date
and accurate as possible at the time of publication. However, due to the constant
developments in medicine, neither the author, nor the editor, nor the publisher can
accept any legal or any other responsibility for any errors or omissions that may occur.

Printed in the United States of America on acid-free paper.

Dedication

This tretise on vascular graft infection is dedicated to **Wesley Moore,** a truly consummate academician who has produced a continuous series of essential laboratory research papers elucidating the basic principles on which our understanding of treatment modalities may be constructed, who senior-authored credible and honest analyses of the clinical work done at Arizona and UCLA, and who has pursued for 15 years the concept of the antibiotic-bonded graft as a real therapeutic intervention of the future. In all of these endeavors he has taken an unassuming yet ineffably competent and knowlegeable role not as the self-proclaimed expert but as a senior thinker and researcher. He is a mentor and academic professor in all the right senses of the word!

T. J. Bunt, MD

Contributors

Thomas M. Bergamini, MD
Assistant Professor of Surgery
University of Louisville
Louisville, Kentucky

John J. Bergan, MD
Clinical Professor of Surgery
University of California San Diego
San Diego, California
Clinical Professor of Surgery
Uniformed Services University
of Health Sciences
Bethesda, Maryland

Scott S. Berman, MD
Fellow in Vascular Surgery
Arizona Health Sciences Center
Tucson, Arizona

T.J. Bunt, MD, FACS
Professor of Surgery
Director of Vascular Residency
Loma Linda University Medical Center
Loma Linda, California

Keith D. Calligaro, MD
Section of Vascular Surgery,
Pennsylvania Hospital
Clinical Assistant Professor of Surgery
University of Pennsylvania
Philadelphia, Pennsylvania

G. Patrick Clagett, MD
Professor of Surgery and Chief of
Vascular Surgery
Southwestern Medical Center
Dallas, Texas

Michael D. Colburn, MD
Resident in General Surgery
University of California Los Angeles
Los Angeles, California

Enrique Criado, MD, FACS
Assistant Professor of Surgery
University of North Carolina at
Chapel Hill
Chapel Hill, North Carolina

Dominic A. DeLaurentis, MD
Chief, Vascular Surgery
Pennsylvania Hospital
Professor of Surgery
University of Pennsylvania
Philadelphia, Pennsylvania

Richard L. Feinberg, MD
Clinical Assistant Professor of Surgery
George Washington University
Bethesda, Maryland

A. Geroff, BS
Temple University Hospital
Philadelphia, Pennsylvania

Ralph S. Greco, MD
Professor and Chief, Division of General
Surgery, Vice Chairman, Department of
Surgery
University of Medicine and Dentistry of
New Jersey
New Brunswick, New Jersey

Richard A. Harvey, PhD
Professor of Biochemistry,
University of Medicine and Dentistry of
New Jersey
New Brunswick, New Jersey

Max C. Hutton, MD
Assistant Professor of Surgery
Case Western Reserve University
Cleveland, Ohio

Kaj Johansen, MD, PhD
Professor of Surgery
University of Washington
Director of Surgical Education
Seattle, Washington

Louis Kozloff, MD
Associate Clinical Professor
George Washington University
Bethesda, Maryland

Peter F. Lawrence, MD
Professor of Surgery
University of Utah School of Medicine
Salt Lake City, Utah

Elna M. Masuda, MD
Fellow in Vascular Surgery
Eastern Virginia Medical School
Norfolk, Virginia

Kenneth E. McIntyre, Jr, MD
Professor of Surgery, Chief of Vascular
Surgery
University of Texas Medical Branch
Galveston, Texas

Steven W. Merrell, MD
Clinical Assistant Professor of Surgery
University of Utah School of Medicine
Salt Lake City, Utah

Wesley S. Moore, MD
Professor of Surgery and Chief
Division of Vascular Surgery
University of California Los Angeles
Los Angeles, California

Bruce A. Perler, MD
Associate Professor of Surgery
The Johns Hopkins University School of
Medicine
Baltimore, Maryland

Robert J. Pitsch, MD
Chief Resident of General Surgery
University of Utah School of Medicine
Salt Lake City, Utah

Jeffrey R. Rubin, MD
Chairman, Department of Surgery
Western Reserve Care System
Professor of Surgery
Northeastern Ohio University College of
Medicine
Youngstown, Ohio

Stanley O. Snyder, MD
Associate Professor of Surgery
Eastern Virginia Medical School
Norfolk, Virginia

David L. Steed, MD
Assistant Professor of Surgery
University of Pittsburgh
Pittsburgh, Pennsylvania

Hugh H. Trout, III, MD
Clinical Professor of Surgery
George Washington University
Bethesda, Maryland

Thomas W. Wakefield, MD
Associate Professor of Surgery
University of Michigan, Ann Arbor
Veterans Administration Medical Center
Ann Arbor, Michigan

K. Whang, BA
Temple University Hospital
Philadelphia, Pennsylvania

John V. White, MD
Director of Surgical Research
Temple University Hospital
Philadelphia, Pennsylvania

Frank J. Veith, MD
Chief of Surgery
Montefiore Medical Center
Professor of Surgery
Albert Einstein College of Medicine
Bronx, New York

Richard A. Yeager, MD
Associate Professor of Surgery
Oregon Health Sciences University
Portland Veterans Affairs Medical Center
Portland, Oregon

Foreword

This is the second book I have struggled to write, one that essentially evolved from my disappointment with the current literature on this esoteric but important topic. Journal articles tended to present slanted viewpoints that were not necessarily true when held up to the perspective of other's experience, and treatment of the topic in textbooks tended to be both cursory and limited to the viewpoints of the authors.

Writing books such as this is therefore a simple pleasure, because it circumvents the purportedly all-important purview of peer review. The author does not have his thoughts and style edited into the usual monochromatic style, with all heretical thoughts deleted. More importantly, one can present the material in a manner that will allow readers to make their own conclusions, rather than having an *expert* dictate to them what the *appropriate* method of management might be. This is an important concept that is sometimes forgotten in our ongoing vascular education.

I was most impressed by and learned the most from those few courses in my higher education that presented the story as a collection of experiments and discoveries, with the conclusions the authors came to, and discussion of whether or not those conclusions were indeed valid. That is the style of this book — a recitation of the various studies that have been offered in the literature with a critique of their results and conclusions. Although I may express my opinion, you will be equally able to either agree or refute, because the facts of each study are related for you. That is the essential point of education, as opposed to catechism.

In collating this book from the hundreds of articles available, I was continually struck by two facts:

1. Too many papers were rehashes of poorly controlled multiple surgeons, multiple institutions, and multiple time frames experience collated into a mishmash of *results.*

2. In certain papers, there was at best some poetic license with the conclusions rendered, and careful analysis of that data often allowed for much different conclusions. Such *wisdom* was then recited by successive authors as a foundation for their studies.

Despite the process of peer review, there is room for reassessment of mandates for therapy even when emanating from respected institutions. This, too, is an essential credo of education.

All of this might be seen to represent a fairly downbeat assessment of the quality of either our peer review process or of our literature. To the extent that this is true, it is a sad commentary that, in our rush to be published and then to be national experts in a field, we may lose sight of the necessity for rigorous quality. Sometimes we publish so much that is not newsworthy or good science. That is not to say that there has not been quality work. Indeed, the norm is of course high quality. It is not my purpose to paint all with a broad brush of opproprium, nor am I criticizing all or even most of the people who have published in this or any other field. But I do feel that academic surgery can do better. I offer this book in that spirit.

I have personally managed many more cases of graft infection than most, and have meticulously examined everything in the literature to have some solid footing for what I do for these patients. This book is just a compendium of what I have learned about this complex and extremely challenging problem, complete with many unanswered questions that have occurred to me. I am sometimes more awed by the questions than by the knowledge so gained.

This is also the work of a number of authors who I felt had contributed significantly because they personally tried something different and carefully evaluated the results of their efforts. Their thoughts and results are tabulated, but not to tell you that there is only one answer to this complex problem. We will not tell you what to do, but we will try to tell you why we have all respectively tried what we have tried, and whether or not it seems to work.

I am proud of this book. It is the way I believe we should approach any difficult subject in surgery; thoroughly examine the facts and thoroughly reexamine the opinions from on high. I sincerely hope that you will find it equally useful in forming your own opinions.

Acknowledgment

None of my work, much less this book, would ever have been completed properly and on time without the cheerful, dedicated, and highly expert assistance of my secretary. There are secretaries, and there are individuals who far surpass that mundane, almost belittling title. Esther Thompson is an exemplar of the latter group.

Contents

Section I. Historical Review

Section II. Pathophysiology

Section III. Prevention

SECTION I

Historical Review

A thoughtful surgeon will conduct a well-thought out operation and thereby find himself well thought of.

Chapter 1

Arterial Graft Infections:
A Personal Perspective

J.J. Bergan

Introduction

In what now would be regarded as the early days of vascular surgery, R.S. Shaw of Boston opined that arterial graft infections would "lead to loss of the patient or a large part of him."[1] Shaw was a genius and innovator in vascular surgery. His perceptive description of the seriousness of arterial graft infection which was made 30 years ago has stood the test of time throughout the remaining years of the 20th century. The pragmatic observations made by Shaw and his coauthor Baue laid down the guidelines for treatment of graft infections. Their description of the obturator bypass added an important instrument to the armamentarium of arterial reconstructive surgery.

Scientific articles usually are not noted for their use of descriptive adjectives or adverbs, but these parts of speech are prominent in papers dealing with graft infections. Phrases used have an ominous ring and include such wording as "grave implications," "frightful problems," and to paraphrase Shaw's observation, " . . . in the loss of an extremity or a life."[2]

Primary Arterial Infections

In reviewing this personal perspective of the diagnosis and treatment of graft infections, clear principles, observations, and descriptions emerge that illuminate the sometimes obscure pathways which led to successful treatment of these problems.

Historically, Paré is credited with establishing the first principle of modern treatment; this was the application of ligature and excision of infected vessel and surrounding tissue. This remains a firm principle in treating infected iatrogenic arterial injury and drug abuse-related infected groin pseudoaneurysms.

Sir William Osler, an internist whose *Textbook of Medicine* went through many editions after the turn of the 20th century, coined the term, "mycotic aneurysm" which describes one of the late sequelae of arterial infections. Osler's observations carried great weight because of his prominence in medicine. However, arterial abscesses

Aided by a grant from the Vascular Center of Scripps Memorial Hospital, La Jolla, California

From Bunt, TJ: *Vascular Graft Infections.* Armonk: Futura Publishing Co., Inc.; © 1994.

had previously been described by others in spotty fashion throughout the last half of the 19th century. Koch described rupture of a superior mesenteric artery aneurysm. Tufnell and others described popliteal artery aneurysms and their mycotic cauliflowerlike excrescences. The term "embolomycotic" had even been coined by Eppinger before the turn of the century.[3] This term may well be used to describe the pathogenesis of late graft infections.

Synthetic Graft Infections

Surgical attention turned from the problems of primary infection of arteries prior to 1950 to infection of arterial reconstructions and synthetic grafts after that time. Among the significant contributions of Szilagyi to the early development of modern vascular surgery was a useful classification of arterial reconstruction infections. In general terms, Szilagyi differentiated superficial infections (type I) from deeper infections (type II) and these from those infections that involved the graft itself.(type III)[4]

Bunt further clarified the situation 10 years later, suggesting that additional information was necessary for classification of the type III infections. This would include knowledge of graft material, infecting pathogen, and whether or not proximal or distal anastomoses were involved.[5] Other clinical classifications were envisioned by Bunt and are logical. These include separation of graft or perigraft infection from graft-enteric erosions and these from graft-enteric fistulae and sepsis involving an aortic stump.

In the last quarter of the 20th century, significant advances have been made in managing patients who have problems associated with graft sepsis. Thus, mortality has been decreased and amputation prevented. Perhaps the single most important advance has been the realization that surgical nutrition is important to the care of patients with graft sepsis. Knowledge that restoration of immunocompetence by parenteral or enteral feeding prior to attack upon the infected graft is of primary importance in successful patient care. Some would argue that learning to stage the necessary surgical procedures has been the factor that has had the most favorable effect upon mortality of patients with graft infection. Probably the combination of attention to nutrition and staging of operation has acted synergistically to improve results.

Unanswered questions that remain at the end of the 20th century involve methods of arterial reconstruction. Among the many options available to the operating surgeon are in-line replacement of vascular prostheses after removal of infected graft and debridement of surrounding tissue; extra-anatomic reconstruction following treatment of the infected graft; and definitive arterial reconstruction through intracavitary, extra-anatomic routes after successful management of graft infection.

Prevention of Infection

There are five factors that are important relative to wound infection in general surgery. These are age of the patient, duration of operation, type of operation, presence of bacteria in the wound, and the presence of drains. Another factor, more difficult to quantitate, is wound surveillance itself. This makes the surgical team aware of the problem of infection. When these factors are viewed from our perspective in vascular surgery, it is clear that arterial reconstructions are disadvantaged by age of the patients, duration of the operation, and a laissez faire interest in surgical wound infections.

In 1973, a study by Peter Cruse was so well done, presented at an important surgical meeting, and published in a highly visible journal that it has become a standard for reference ever since.[6] This study did not specifically address infection in vascular surgery nor compare it to general surgery, but it did examine elements of wound infection. It concluded that wound sepsis rates varied widely between 1.8% and 8.9%, depending on whether the wounds were clean or clean-contaminated. General surgery clean wound infection rates ranged around 1.6% and vascular surgery clean wounds ranged around a 3.7% incidence, thus underscoring the importance of age and duration of procedure in contributing to wound infection. Showering and washing of the patient with a hexachlorophene soap appeared to be of value in reducing wound infection and it was surprising in 1973 to find that the unshaved patient fared better than one who was shaved. Further, plastic drapes made no difference to wound infection. Patient factors, including age, diabetes, obesity, and malnutrition were deleterious to primary wound healing.

A separate study by Davidson and Clark at about the same time identified five factors important in wound infections.[7] These included: 1) a potentially dirty procedure; 2) presence of bacteria in the wound at the end of the operation; 3) environment of the patient's ward; 4) patient's age; and 5) duration of operation. Once again, factors integral to and important to vascular surgery included the patient's age and the duration of surgery.

Clearly, experience in general surgery teaches that vascular surgery is a field that is liable to be fraught with wound infections.

Endogenous Infection

Studies of the specific problems of positive bacterial cultures relating to vascular pathology are not a standard part of general surgical studies; e.g., bacteria in the contents of an abdominal aortic aneurysm. Ernst found that 15% of aneurysm-content cultures yielded bacterial growth,[8] and others have found similar results. Further, Ernst found that the late graft sepsis rate was 10% in patients with a positive intraoperative culture, and 2% in those in cases in which the culture was negative. Despite that observation, the actual significance of a positive intraoperative bacterial culture is unclear. This is because uniform use of prophylactic antibiotics and/or topical irrigation of the wound undoubtedly affects the eventual graft sepsis rate.

The organisms found in aortic-aneurysm contents are of interest. Over 80% are Gram-positive, the majority of which are staphylococcal. Increasingly, *Staphylococcus epidermidis* is an important component of the latter percentage. McCauley, Steed, and Webster have taken this observation further, concluding that "a positive result of culture may not imply clinical infection at the time of operation and that prolonged postoperative organism-specific antibiotic therapy does not appear necessary in the patient with an asymptomatic aneurysm and no overt evidence of infection of the aneurysm at the time of operation."[9] That conclusion is very carefully worded. It rules out the finding of positive culture in aneurysm contents at the time of surgery or positive culture found at the time of aortic aneurysm rupture and emphasizes the importance of Gram-positive organisms.[10]

The importance of bacteria in the transudate recovered during aortic surgery also was emphasized by Ernst. He found organisms in 11% of such carefully done cultures. Others have concluded that prophylactic antibiotics starting before surgery can decrease the incidence of recovery of organisms from intestinal bag cultures. Russell's study from Iowa found only three positive cultures in 119 attempts.[11] Two of these were *S epidermidis* and only one was *Staphylococcus aureus*.

For many reasons, including those implied above, it seems important not to omit prophylactic antibiotics in aortic surgery. It is hard to understand now why the subject of prophylactic antibiotics was so vigorously debated in the early 1960s, near the beginning of the present era of vascular reconstruction.[12] Nevertheless, vascular surgeons were among the first to develop models for study of such prophylaxis[13] and the experimental background for clinical prophylactic antibiotics was well founded by 1970. Contrary opinions were expressed[14] and when they appeared in as prestigious a journal as the *New England Journal of Medicine*, they had to be given due respect. Ultimately, it was agreed that patients who needed a prosthetic graft should have antibiotics in their blood stream at the time of prosthetic implantation. A Nashville study[15] presented at the American Surgical Association meeting of 1978 was very influential in this regard. It was a randomized, prospective, double-blind study of cefazolin versus placebo in a large group of arterial reconstructive procedures. In the 565 arterial reconstructions, the infection rate was 6.8% for placebo recipients versus 0.9% for those receiving cefazolin. Of the 18 infections, 4 were type III and involved vascular grafts. All four of these infections occurred in the placebo group. Ever since that report, vascular surgeons have paid attention to the choice of antibiotic prophylaxis rather than whether or not to use prophylactic antibiotics. Once a choice is made, that antibiotic must be given before the surgical event commences.[16]

The duration of antibiotic administration has gradually decreased in vascular surgery. Of some influence has been a report from Sweden[17] which confirmed that prophylactic antibiotics are important, but extension of prophylaxis beyond the day of surgery offers no additional protection. That study has supported suggestions by many to use short-term prophylactic antibiotics in vascular surgery. From a practical point of view, the presence of central lines defines the duration of antibiotic administration. Most vascular teams today continue antibiotics until after central lines are removed.

Systemic versus Topical Antibiotics

There is some question regarding the use of topical antibiotic irrigation, systemic antibiotics, or perhaps both. Using the belt-and-suspenders approach, many vascular surgeons use both systemic and topical antibiotics today.[18] An early advocate of this was the pioneer vascular surgeon, Jere Lord, Jr. of New York Hospital.[19]

Today's vascular surgeons do not understand why there was such an argument about antibiotic wound irrigation; this is because they were not exposed to the teachings of William A. Altemeier of Cincinnati. Professor Altemeier was the supreme oracle of surgical infections before 1980, and was a powerful voice against the use of topical antibiotics.[20] Eventually the topic was closed forever by experience with patients who had undergone transplantation. Various transplant groups proved the value of topical antibiotic irrigation in immunocompromised patients.[21] This implied that vascular patients could also profit from the surgeon's use of antibiotic irrigation.

Mechanical Factors and Graft Infection

Harry Goldsmith's interest in the use of the omentum for various aspects of surgery led to his careful study of placing omentum as a barrier between a prosthetic graft and external bacterial contamination.[22] Such a barrier is often used now in vascular surgery, but not usually in primary aortic reconstruction.

For a long time, Dacron has been the dominant material used in prostheses; however, availability of expanded polytetrafluoroethylene (PTFE) after 1972 gradually challenged Dacron's superiority. Experimental studies suggested that PTFE was resistant to surgical wound contamination[23,24] and that such resistance was related to decreased bacterial adherence. Polytetrafluoroethylene seemed to be advantageous when compared to either woven or knitted Dacron.[25]

An early tenet of management of graft infections was that the infection would stay localized if a graft were patent but would propagate if a graft were thrombosed.[1] Experimental and clinical observations later challenged that dogma. Now, it is generally assumed that propagation of infection is intraluminal and that total graft excision is necessary to prevent proximal suture line sepsis even in patent grafts.[26]

The importance of arterial wall microbiology became generally appreciated after the mid-80s. Bioassays allowed determination of the active antibiotic level within the aortic wall, and it was found that cefazolin and cefoxitin attained satisfactory aortic wall tissue levels while clindamycin did not. Interestingly, blood levels did not correlate well with tissue levels in early studies.[27] Those studies preceded interest of Malone's group in arterial microbiology; his group found *S epidermidis* in a very high percentage (43%) of arterial wall biopsies taken at surgery.[28] Fallibility of intraoperative Gram stains in detecting such infections has been proven.[29]

Emphasis in the early days of vascular surgery was on *S aureus* in graft infection. It is to the credit of the Milwaukee group and Jon Towne that *S epidermidis* has been increasingly recognized as a source of overt graft infection. This group has linked *S epidermidis* to occult development of pseudoaneurysms especially at the groin suture line.[30]

Clinical experience with Gram-negative bacteria and graft infections had shown that these were particularly virulent and dangerous types of infection. As is often true in vascular surgery, clinical observations were subsequently confirmed by experimental study.[31] Thus, it is now well known that Gram-negative infections can be lethal in the presence of a vascular graft.

While much experimental work has been done on bonding of antibiotics to vascular prostheses, clinical application of observations has simply not occurred. Perhaps the future will see antibiotic bonding assuming a more important place in the prevention of graft infection.

Diagnosis

Acknowledging that the true prosthetic graft infection rate is somewhat higher than the ideal clean wound infection rate suggests that there is a risk of considerable morbidity and even mortality in patients receiving prostheses that might become infected. Clearly, early diagnosis is of paramount importance in decreasing morbidity and mortality. Early diagnosis allows excision of the septic focus prior to depletion of immune mechanisms and prior to the state of cachexia seen in patients harboring long-standing graft infections.

Even after the postoperative period and safe implantation of a graft has occurred, the prosthesis is still susceptible to secondary infection from blood-borne bacteria–the embolomycotic phenomenon. Actual incidence of such bacteremic infections in well-incorporated prostheses in humans is unknown but is thought to be less than 1%; considering the number of prostheses implanted, this still represents a considerable number of patients at risk. Similarly, the late infectious complications caused by the risk of bacteremic infection decreases with incorporation of a prosthesis into host tissue; it is unreasonable to expect that this occurs in a totally satisfactory fashion in humans. Even variations of construction of the graft, such as knitted versus woven textiles, are of more theoretic than actual importance. The true endothelial lining does not completely cover human prostheses; instead, the layers adjacent to the prosthesis consist of fibrous connective tissue which penetrate graft interstices and loosely bind the inner layer to the prosthesis. This mainly fibrin, flattened layer has occasional polymorphonuclear leukocytes, monocytes, and fibroblasts within it.

Methods of detection of graft infection include ultrasonography, computerized tomography (CT), magnetic resonance imaging (MRI), and use of a variety of labeled isotopes as well as sinus tract injections (Fig. 1).

Ultrasound generation of analogue and digital B-mode images of grafts can be obtained, especially using low-frequency (3.5 to 5 mHz) transducers. Ultrasound is partic-

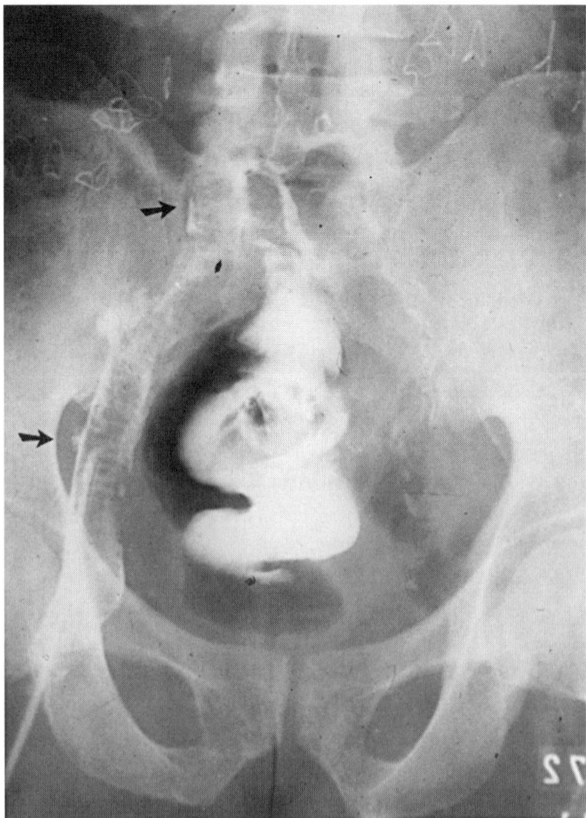

Figure 1. Contrast media injected through a sinus tract in cases of suspected graft infection can be very informative. This sinogram shows an unexpected communication between the periaortic graft infection and the sigmoid colon. Clearly, an unusual form of graft-enteric erosion had developed.

ularly useful in identifying failures in healing of graft to artery as occurs in anastomotic false aneurysms. However, perigraft fluid accumulations and hematomas can also be identified as sonolucent areas; these can be complex collections in some instances. Ultrasound is not as useful as arteriography to delineate intraluminal abnormalities but finds its place in detection of perigraft fluid collections or thrombus within grafts.[33]

Computerized tomographic assessment of graft healing and detection of graft infection has been in use for more than 10 years. The normal progression of healing following aortic graft implantation as seen on CT scans has been well defined. Early postoperative findings include areas of increased perigraft tissue density that do not opacify with intravenous contrast material; these are found chiefly in the region of the proximal anastomosis and are interpreted as hematoma. This hematoma resolves within the first 2 to 3 weeks of surgery. Distal anastomoses show a similar picture. When the graft has been implanted for aortic aneurysm, the initial examinations show the body and proximal limbs of the graft to be surrounded by the original aneurysm wall with hematoma present between the graft and the aneurysm wall. Perigraft air will be seen occasionally in such early views. These air collections are small, multiple, and may be located anteriorly and posteriorly. However, they uniformly disappear between 2 to 6 weeks.[34]

Computerized tomographic scans suspected of showing graft infection or infection of the perigraft fluid usually demonstrate a thickened graft wall or increased perigraft soft tissue. Perigraft fluid may also be identified and anastomotic pseudoaneurysms may or may not be present. Bubbles of gas collected in the graft bed, in the thickened graft wall, or in the perigraft fluid are pathognomonic of graft infection (Fig. 2). If such fluid collection is present without gas, fine needle aspiration for smear and culture can be performed.

Computerized tomographic scans performed to detect graft infection should include the abdomen, pelvis, and the proximal thigh to insure that imaging is obtained at the groin anastomoses. Computerized tomographic scans performed to detect graft infection occasionally will show other causes of fever and abdominal pain such as acute cholecystitis. It is in the diagnosis of retroperitoneal graft sepsis that CT findings are of most importance.

The clinical diagnosis of retroperitoneal graft infection is often difficult because the signs and symptoms such as fever, leukocytosis, and abdominal pain are actually nonspecific. Furthermore, since these subtle clinical findings of graft infection may be manifested early after surgery or even many months after surgery, the importance of imaging becomes better understood. When purulence appears at the groin in conjunction with failure of healing of a groin wound, the diagnosis is obvious and sonograms performed may show extensive involvement of the prosthesis and occasion-

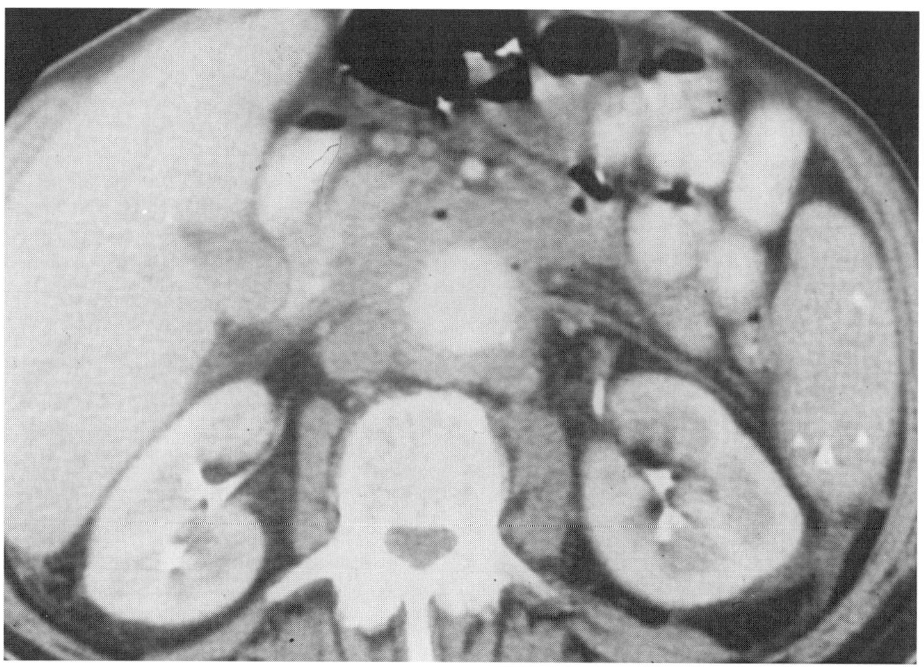

Figure 2. Computerized tomographic scanning has added a dimension of certainty to the diagnosis of perigraft infection. When perigraft fluid is present, it can be aspirated for culture but when perigraft gas is present at a time remote from operation the diagnosis is virtually certain. This is the finding shown in this illustration.

ally demonstrate the source of the infection to be the small bowel in situations of graft-enteric erosion. However, because of the excellent spatial and contrast resolutions of CT, delineation of normal and abnormal graft morphology is easy. Experience shows a sensitivity approaching 100% when CT is used. Unfortunately, some of the CT features of graft infection are actually nonspecific. In particular, perigraft hematoma is difficult to separate from abscess, and even the hallmark of infection–perigraft air–has been disputed by some.[35]

Because of the suspected failures of CT, isotope studies have been performed to detect graft infection in the retroperitoneum. Various materials have been labeled, including immunoglobulin G (IgG) labeled with indium 111, leukocytes labeled with technetium Tc 99m, and leukocytes labeled with indium 111.[36,37] Such scans are of less value in the early postoperative period due to expected inflammation, but achieve greater usefulness later in the course. Positive scans obtained late after graft implantation are highly sensitive and specific.

On the other hand, false-negative scans have been a problem when the infection is relatively quiescent. Also, the labeling of leukocytes is flawed by unintentional cross-labeling of platelets which adhere to graft surfaces giving false-positive results. Thus, the labeling of immunoglobulin has some advantages over labeling of leukocytes. The scans do not require removal of leukocytes from the patient. The IgG has a long shelf-life and a higher concentration of indium 111 can be safely administered since the IgG is not sequestered in the spleen. As with all scans, if active inflammation is not present in the area of infection at the time of the scan, there will be a false-negative report. Because antibiotics often have been given in shotgun fashion, this finding of subdued inflammation is frequently a problem, The antibiotics silenced the infectious process for a short time. It should also be remembered that the scanning techniques are not accurate in delineating the extent of prosthetic involvement.

Magnetic resonance imaging of perigraft fluids has become increasingly important in the detection of perigraft infection. Edema or fluid collections can be well visualized along the course of bypass grafts at any location. There was an initial prejudice against MRI due to its perceived nonspecificity; however, as MRI has improved and capture times have been shortened, the modality is becoming increasingly important in the diagnosis of graft infection.

Treatment

In general terms, once the diagnosis of graft infection is made, strong consideration must be given to total excision of the infected prosthesis. However, more conservative treatments have worked in selected instances. Local antibiotic irrigation has been reported to succeed in selected instances, but a broad experience of success with such modality is lacking.[38]

Localized infections of graft at the groin often are satisfactorily treated with debridement of infected tissue and antibiotic or povidine-iodine irrigations. After such debridement and relative sterilization of the perigraft tissues and granulation tissue, it is possible to swing muscle flaps to cover the graft and its anastomosis.[39] However, there always remains the danger of subsequent anastomotic hemorrhage should such flaps fail to sterilize the infection.

The general principles of operative management of established graft infections consist of two phases: revascularization and infected graft excision. Graft excision alone is rarely feasible; such cases are those in which the graft has been chronically occluded and the patient's extremities have retained viability postgraft occlusion. Similarly, when the patient has had an aortic graft placed for chronic occlusion of the aortoiliac arterial segment, a graft excision may be feasible. After excision of the graft, the aortotomy may be closed with autogenous tissue derived from endarterectomized occluded distal arteries or other source. In most situations, revascularization generally consists of axillofemoral or axillopopliteal reconstruction as necessary. Staging the revascularization procedure and subsequent graft excision is recommended in order to reduce physiologic stress, but a decision for a staging is best made in individual circumstances. Patients chronically infected and metabolically depleted should, of course, be treated by stage procedures. Otherwise healthy and fit individuals harboring a chronic subacute graft infection may safely undergo a one-stage procedure.

One advantage of performing the revascularization operation first is that the surgical team can focus on complete debridement of infected tissue in the retroperitoneum as the infected prosthesis is removed. This can be done without concern for progressive lower extremity ischemia when the limbs have already been revascularized. Careful intra-abdominal surgery can be done and adequate retroperitoneal drainage can be placed. Experience has shown that the incidence of subsequent extra-anatomic bypass infection is the same whether revascularization is performed before or after the excision of an infected aortic graft. Patients with graft-enteric erosions who are undergoing active gastrointestinal bleeding, of course, will require emergency aortic graft excision as a primary procedure. Secondary revascularization will follow.

The Portland experience of one-stage graft excision and revascularization is an outstanding example of success of that simplified approach.[40] Much of the modern success of one-stage surgery can be attributed to meticulous intensive care management of patients, however. The subsequent axillofemoral or axillopopliteal graft infection rate has been reported in the neighborhood of 20%, showing the dangers of vascular reconstruction in patients harboring sepsis. Increasing experience with PTFE grafts as

the axillofemoral reconstruction material of choice suggests that the external reinforcement of PTFE favors this material.

The most serious problem in terms of fatal complications with excision of infected prosthesis is closure of the aortic stump. The aortic stump is subject to recurrent infections and, therefore, radical debridement of infected tissues is absolutely mandatory. Furthermore, if possible, the aortic stump closure should be a secure, two-layer closure. Aortic wall tissue should be sent for culture. When such arterial wall cultures are positive, suture line disruption occurs at least 50% of the time. If cultures are negative, however, healing is to be expected. Rarely, renal revascularization from a supraceliac origin can be used to allow debridement of aortic tissue and closure of the stump through uninfected aortic wall. In this situation, omentum can be used as vascularized tissue to cover the aortic stump. If an extensive perigraft abscess is present at the proximal suture line, posterior drainage of that area is of greatest importance.[40]

Aortic stump blowout can also be prevented by an in situ reconstruction after removal of infected graft and debridement of infected tissues. The cardiovascular system is unique in that a prosthesis can be safely placed after removal of an infected prosthesis if organism-specific antibiotics can be given for coverage. The situation arises in aortic valve replacement when the prosthesis must be removed for infection and yet a patient will not survive wide open aortic insufficiency. Since the early days of reconstructive aortic surgery, there has been a school of thought that in situ replacement was a feasible option if the infected prosthesis was removed and debridement was adequate. Now it is clear that the option does exist if and when specialized circumstances arise, for example, when the infecting organism is less virulent and less active, as when the organism is *Staphylococcus*-negative surviving within a biofilm. Certainly, in properly selected patients, the in situ aortic graft replacement may be a rational treatment.[41,42]

An intriguing possibility exists for the use of allogenic aortic graft material to treat infectious graft complications.[43] Now that organ harvest is routine for transplantation purposes, a reconsideration of aortic homografting may come about especially in situations of repair of aortic reconstructions after removing infected grafts. As indicated above, these are solutions to aortic stump blowout and may be found to be effective with increased experience in the future.

Throughout the modern experience with arterial reconstruction, a minority opinion has held that simple suture closure of aortoenteric fistulae or in situ replacement of infected grafts can achieve success.[44] Certainly, if the cases are very carefully selected, noninfected grafts can be preserved by the direct suture technique. Grossly infected grafts present a more difficult problem and removal is probably mandatory. Most surgeons have taken the conservative approach to graft infections and have not used the in situ technique. It seems clear that late deaths are related to the original infection, whether or not a graft-enteric erosion has been present.[45] Most of those late deaths occur within 6 months of the graft excision (75%) and nearly all within a year of that time.

Delayed intracavitary reconstruction of the aortic segment can be performed safely within 12 months. After 12 months, removal of the infected graft is necessary; such reconstruction is best performed by the thoracofemoral route.[46–48]

References

1. Shaw RS, Baue AE. Management of sepsis complicating arterial reconstructive surgery. *Surgery.* 1962;53:75–86.
2. Fry WJ. Vascular prosthesis infections. *Surg Clin North Am.* 1972;52:1419–1424.
3. Wilson SE, Van Wagenen P, Passaro E Jr. Arterial infection. In: Bergan JJ, Yao JST, eds. *Year Book of Vascular Surgery.* St. Louis: Mosby Year Book Inc; 1978;6–49.
4. Szilagyi DE, Smith RF, Elliott JP, Vrandecic MP. Infection in arterial reconstruction with synthetic grafts. *Ann Surg.* 1972;176:321–333.
5. Bunt TJ. Synthetic vascular graft infections. *Surgery.* 1983;93:733–746.
6. Cruse PJE, Foord R. A five-year prospective study of 23,649 surgical wounds. *Arch Surg.* 1973;107:206–210.
7. Davidson AIG, Clark C, Smith G. Postoperative wound infection: a computer analysis. *Br J Surg.* 1971;58:333–337.
8. Ernst CB, Campbell HC, Daugherty ME, Sachatello CR, Griffen WO. Incidence and significance of intraoperative bacterial cultures during abdominal aortic aneurysmectomy. *Ann Surg.* 1977;185:626–633.
9. McAuley CE, Steed DL, Webster MW. Bacterial presence in aortic thrombus at elective aneurysm resection: is it clinically significant? *Am J Surg.* 1984;147:322–324.
10. Buckels JAC, Fielding JWL, Black J, Ashton F, Slaney G. Significance of positive bacterial cultures from aortic aneurysm contents. *Br J Surg.* 1985;72:440–442.
11. Russell HE, Barnes RW, Baker WH. Sterility of intestinal transudate during aortic reconstructive procedures. *Arch Surg.* 1975;110:402–404.
12. Bernard HR, Cole WR. The prophylaxis of surgical infection: the effect of prophylactic antimicrobial drugs on the incidence of infection following potentially contaminated operations. *Surgery.* 1964;56:151–157.
13. Lindenauer SM, Fry WJ, Schaub G, Wild D. The use of antibiotics in the prevention of vascular graft infection. *Surgery.* 1967;62:487–492.
14. Karl RC, Mertz JJ, Vieth FJ, Dineen P. Prophylactic antimicrobial drugs in surgery. *N Eng J Med.* 1966;275:305–308.
15. Kaiser AB, Clayson KR, Mulherin JL Jr, et al. Antibiotic prophylaxis in vascular surgery. *Ann Surg.* 1978;188:283–288.
16. Classen DC, Evans RS, Pestotnik SL, et al. The timing of prophylactic administration of antibiotics and the risk of surgical wound infection. *N Eng J Med.* 1992;326:281–286.
17. Hasselgren PO, Ivarsson L, Risberg B, Seeman T. Effects of prophylactic antibiotics in vascular surgery: a prospective, randomized, double-blind study. *Ann Surg.* 1984;200:86–92.
18. Pitt HA, Postier RG, MacGowan WAL, et al. Prophylactic antibiotics in vascular surgery. *Ann Surg.* 1980;192:356–364.
19. Lord JW Jr. Intraoperative antibiotic wound irrigation. *Surg Gynecol Obstet.* 1983;157:357–360.
20. Altemeier WA. Comment on: Lord JW Jr, Rossi G, Daliana M. Intraoperative antibiotic

wound lavage: an attempt to eliminate postoperative infection in arterial and clean general surgical procedures. *Ann Surg.* 1977;185:634–641.

21. Belzer FO, Salvatierra O, Schweizer RT, Kountz SL. Prevention of wound infections by topical antibiotics in high-risk patients. *Am J Surg.* 1973;126:180–183.

22. Goldsmith HS, de los Santos R, Vanamee P, Beattie EJ Jr. Experimental protection of vascular prosthesis by omentum. *Arch Surg.* 1968;97:872–878.

23. Stone SK, Walshaw R, Suglyama GT, Dean RE, Dunstan RW. Polytetrafluoroethylene versus autogenous vein grafts for vascular reconstruction in contaminated wounds. *Am J Surg.* 1984;147:692–695.

24. Shah PM, Ito K, Clauss RH, Babu SC, Reynolds BM, Stahl WM. Expanded microporous polytetrafluoroethylene (PTFE) graft in contaminated wounds: experimental and clinical study. *J Trauma.* 1983;23:1030–1033.

25. Schmitt DD, Bandyk DF, Pequet AJ, Towne JB. Bacterial adherence to vascular prostheses: a determinant of graft infectivity. *J Vasc Surg.* 1986;3:732–740.

26. Kron IL, Georgitis JW, Holmes P, Britton RC. Propagation of sepsis in vascular grafts. *Arch Surg.* 1980;115:878–879.

27. Mutch D, Richards C, Brown RA, Mulder DS. Bioactive antibiotic levels in the human aorta. *Surgery.* 1982;92:1068–1071.

28. Macbeth GA, Rubin JR, McIntyre KE Jr, Goldstone J, Malone JM. The relevance of arterial wall microbiology to the treatment of prosthetic graft infections: graft infection vs. arterial infection. *J Vasc Surg.* 1984;6:750–756.

29. Samson RH, Gupta SK, Scher LA, Veith FJ. Fallibility of intraoperative Gram stain in the diagnosis of vascular infection. *Angiology.* 1982;680–684.

30. Bandyk DF, Berni GA, Theile BL, Towne JB. Aortofemoral graft infection due to *Staphylococcus epidermidis. Arch Surg.* 1984;119:102–107.

31. Geary KJ, Tomkiewicz ZJ, Harrison HN, et al. Differential effects of a Gram-negative and a Gram-positive infection on autogenous and prosthetic grafts. *J Vasc Surg.* 1990;11:339–347.

32. Wilson SE, Bennion RS, Serota AI, et al. Bacteriological implications in the pathogenesis of secondary aortoenteric fistulas. *Br J Surg.* 1982;69:545–548.

33. Gooding GAW, Effeney DJ, Goldstone J. The aortofemoral graft: detection and identification of healing complications by ultrasonography. *Surgery.* 1981;89:94–101.

34. Qvarfordt PF, Reilly LM, Mark AS, et al. Computerized tomographic assessment of graft incorporation after aortic reconstruction. *Am J Surg.* 1985;150:227–231.

35. Johnson KK, Russ PD, Bair JH, Friefeld GD. Diagnosis of synthetic vascular graft infection: comparison of CT and gallium scans. *Am J Radiol.* 1990;154:405–409.

36. LaMuraglia GM, Fischman AJ, Strauss W, et al. Utility of the indium 111-labeled human immunoglobulin G scan for the detection of focal vascular graft infection. *J Vasc Surg.* 1989;10:20–28.

37. Vorne M, Laitinen R, Lantto T, et al. Chronic prosthetic vascular graft infection visualized with technitium-99m- hexamethylprophyleneamine oxime-labeled leukocytes. *J Nucl Med.* 1991;32:1425–1428.

38. Almgren B, Eriksson I. Local antibiotic irrigation in the treatment of arterial graft infections. *Acta Chir Scand.* 1981;147:33–36.

39. Dacey LJ, Miett, TOC, Huntsman WT, et al. Efficacy of muscle flaps in the treatment of prosthetic vascular graft infections. *J Surg Res.* 1988;44:566–572.

40. Yeager RA, Moneta GL, Taylor LM, et al. Improving survival and limb salvage in patients with aortic graft infection. *Am J Surg.* 1990;159:466–469.

41. Robinson JA, Johansen K. Aortic sepsis: is there a role for in situ graft reconstruction? *J Vasc Surg.* 1991;13:677–684.

42. Bandyk DF, Bergamini TM, Kinney EV, et al. In situ replacement of vascular prostheses infected by bacterial biofilms. *J Vasc Surg.* 1991;13:575–583.

43. Bahnini A, Ruotolo C, Koskas F, Kieffer E. In situ fresh allograft replacement of an infected aortic prosthetic graft: eighteen month followup. *J Vasc Surg.* 1991;14:98–102.

44. Thomas WEG, Baird RN. Secondary aortoenteric fistulae: towards a more conservative approach. *Br J Surg.* 1986;73:875–878.

45. Reilly ML, Ehrenfeld WK, Stoney RJ. Delayed aortic prosthetic reconstruction after removal of an infected graft. *Am J Surg.* 1984;148:234–239.

46. O'Brien DP, Waldron RP, McCabe JP, Courtney DF. Descending thoracic aortobifemoral bypass graft: a safe alternative in the high-risk patients. *Irish Med J* 1991;84:58–59.

47. McCartney WJ, Rubin JR, Flinn WR, Williams LR, Bergan JJ, Yao JST. Descending thoracic aorta to femoral artery bypass. *Arch Surg.* 1986;121:681–688.

48. Criado E, Keagy BA. Descending thoracic aorta to femoral artery bypass. *Contemp Surg.* 1991;39(5):15–19.

SECTION II

Pathophysiology

One must thoroughly understand anatomy and physiology to understand pathophysiology, which then leads naturally to a logical basis for therapeusis . . .

Chapter 2

Laboratory Models

T.J. Bunt

In a remarkably short period of time, vascular surgery has developed so that much of the accepted doctrine of clinical intervention is based more on anecdotal and/or institutional clinical experience than on well-conceived and thoroughly performed basic bench research. This is no truer a statement than for synthetic vascular graft infections, as this chapter will demonstrate. Most of the decisions for therapy are based on reported experience over 10 or 15 years at one institution by many different surgeons. What is sadly lacking in the field is a truly concrete examination of the underlying pathophysiology. Questions that should be addressed include the following:

1. How do grafts become infected? By one, ten, a hundred bacteria? Are there differences between bacterial species, and for each type of graft or even each implantation situation? Does external inoculation require specific substrates? Is there a difference in the number of bacteria required at each site?

2. Is there a differential infectability between grafts? If so, is it true for all grafts at all sites, or is the site an equal determinant factor? Can the difference (if any) be modulated by impregnation, by surface agents, etc.?

3. Are there controllable factors in graft infection? Does control of lymphatic drainage decrease infection rates, and if so, is this true only for certain situations?

4. Is there a difference between bacteria? Are Gram-positive and Gram-negative infections equivalently dangerous, or conversely, is arterial secondary infection/disruption more frequent with some species? What factors make a given agent more virulent, and how does the presence of the graft itself modify this?

5. In wound infection studies, abdominal incisions become infected more often than groin incisions; and in peripheral operations, the more distal incisions have higher wound complications than the inguinal incisions. Yet the highest rate of graft infection is seen at the groin. Why?

6. Are graft infections a function of the time that a wound is exposed at initial operation, and if so, is this equally true at all sites?

7. What is the role of prophylactic antibiotics in reducing both wound and graft infection?

8. Is bacterial invasion of grafts possible from the external surface once a graft is well incorporated? What about invasion intraluminally—by bacteremias alone? Or does it require secondary infection of adherent

---

thrombus. Does bacteremic invasion require an exposed graft matrix, or can it occur via intact pseudointima? If bacteremias occur, how many bacteria are necessary for successful graft colonization?

9. Once a graft is locally colonized, can the infection spread along the graft if the graft is patent but incorporated? Is there secondary dissolution of incorporation by certain bacteria or within certain time frames? Is a nonincorporated graft (graft infection) therefore a primary or secondary event?

The supposed answers to some of these questions are not based on hard research data. Rather, they are usually statements of dogmatic fact by the purported experts in this field even though they are based on anecdotal observations only. This chapter will examine the remarkably few bench studies that have been done to present the known facts. Extrapolation from these predominantly canine studies to the human situation is at best uncertain, yet it is the only model that we have.

Literature Review

Harrison[1] published the first model of graft infection in a paper seeking to show how synthetic grafts fared in a contaminated field. He implanted 5-cm segments of 6–8-mm woven Teflon and homograft tube grafts at the infrarenal aorta of dogs. His group noted anecdotally that they could not produce a reliable graft infection with a variety of solutions of streptococci and staphylococci, so they settled on direct graft inoculation with 1 cc of a 10% solution of canine feces strained through gauze to remove particulate matter. Utilization of this inoculum produced retroperitoneal abscesses of 15- to 20-cc size in 80% to 90% of animals.

In group I animals (No. 20), a retroperitoneal abscess was first produced then drained, and a graft was implanted in the infected bed; streptomycin and penicillin were not given until 24 hours later and were continued for 3 weeks. Group II animals underwent primary graft placement with simultaneous inoculation of the graft; antibiotics were delayed for 24 hours.

Group I animals with homografts had five early deaths—three from graft rupture and exsanguination and two from aortic thrombosis. In six other animals the infections resolved. Group I animals with Teflon grafts had three early deaths—two by anastomotic disruption and one by graft thrombosis. Two more animals had graft infections, one with a thrombosed graft. The remaining five experienced resolution of their infections.

Group II animals with homografts had 5 early deaths—3 by graft rupture, and two by thrombosis; one other animal had a graft infection with lysis of the graft but no frank rupture at the time of harvest at 42 days. Three others had resolution of their infections. Three early deaths occurred in group II animals with Teflon grafts, all by sepsis with graft infection and one with thrombosis. Four additional dogs survived with graft infections, all with thrombosed grafts and three with small pseudoaneurysms. Four others had resolution of their infections, but the grafts were noted to have dense fibrous reactions.

This first study established a number of observations which would be duplicated by other researchers as well as by clinical experience.

1. Infected homografts tended to frankly disrupt (6/20); infected synthetic grafts remained intact but had one of three additional complications: anastomotic disruption (6/20), graft thrombosis (7/20), or clinical sepsis (10/20).

2. Inoculation of a graft at time of surgery (10/21) was equivalently effective at producing a graft infection (GIF) as was in situ placement into an infected field (13/20).

3. Even with gross fecal contamination of a graft, not all grafts became infected; 16/41 grafts did not show infection; however, the incidence of GIF may well have been

higher, since the diagnosis of GIF was made on gross clinical inspection only, and the dogs were followed only for an average of 30 days.

4. Grafts tend to become thrombosed when infected (12/41).

Harrison theorized that homograft disruption occurred due to proteolysis from the enzymes released from leukocytes, and postulated that even if immediate rupture did not occur, elastic fiber degradation would lead to later aneurysm formation. Demonstration of the tendency for homografts to frankly lyse and disrupt in the face of infection was noted clinically by a number of subsequent researchers and, in part, led to the abandonment of that graft in favor of synthetic grafts.

Foster[2] also used direct inoculation of 1 cc of canine feces into a retroperitoneal pocket and infrarenal aortic graft placement; the dogs were then returned to surgery 48 hours later, the resultant abscess drained (cultures *Escherichia coli*, *Proteus*, and *Aerobacter*), and infrarenal aortic grafting with either woven nylon or homograft performed in the infected field. Initially, all animals died within 4 to 5 days; subsequent institution of parenteral antibiotics allowed the study of 140 dogs.

Phase I: Twenty control dogs were not inoculated and no infections occurred, but two thromboses occurred. Ten dogs were then inoculated without antibiotics, and all died within 5 days, four—by hemorrhage and six by sepsis. The hemorrhage occurred by anastomotic disruption of the suture line from the aorta for nylon grafts, but by disruption of the suture line from the deteriorated graft itself for homografts.

Phase II: Twenty animals were then inoculated and bypasses were done under antibiotic coverage for 1 week. Nine of 10 homograft animals died, 8 of hemorrhage, and in the final animal, thrombosis of the graft occurred; all 10 animals with prosthetic grafts also died, 3 by hemorrhage and the other 7 by sepsis—the mode of exsanguination from the nylon graft was again by anastomotic disruption, while suture pullout of the graft or frank graft disruption occurred equivalently in the homografts.

Phase III: In 30 animals, graft implantation after inoculation was performed under antibiotic coverage. Forty-five percent of the dogs with nylon prosthesis survived with one additional graft thrombosis, whereas only 7% of the dogs with homografts survived, and that was with an additionally thrombosed graft. Eighty percent of the dogs with homografts exsanguinated versus 27% of the nylon grafts; the disruption was of the homograft itself in five dogs or by suture pullout in seven, while nylon failures were again by aortic anastomotic disruption.

Phase IV: Inoculation in the above groups was done 48 hours prior to formal graft implant. In 40 dogs, graft implantation and inoculation were carried out simultaneously (under 1 week parenteral antibiotic coverage as well as topical neomycin irrigation of the para-aortic tissues postimplantation). Forty-five percent of the dogs with nylon prostheses survived—one with additional graft thrombosis versus only 25% of the homograft group; one with additional graft thrombosis. Seventy percent of the dogs with homografts, but only 10% of the dogs with prosthetic grafts, died from exsanguination, with the same etiology for hemorrhage.

Phase V: In 20 animals, antibiotic coverage was changed from penicillin and streptomycin to chloramphenicol based on the notation of bacterial resistance to the usual organisms cultured. The penicillin and streptomycin were for 14 dogs, chloramphenicol added in for 5 days, and a neomycin topical irrigant again used. This led to 90% (9/10) survival in both homograft and prosthetic implants, with each loss being by exsanguination.

A final part of the study involved long-term follow-up of all surviving dogs. Deaths occurred within 2 weeks of operation; survivors were sacrificed at intervals from 6 to 18 months. In 16 survivors with homografts, there was no evidence of persistent infection; in 25 survivors with nylon grafts, five had clinically persistent graft infection, with two of these grafts secondarily thrombosed. Histologic examination revealed true pseudointima that never progressed more than 1 cm from the anastomosis, and fibrous encasement measurement of the graft. This lengthy series of experiments led the researchers to conclude:

1. That homografts were particularly vulnerable to disruption or suture line disruption in the face of infection; conversely that the synthetic graft was more durable.
2. That there was residual infection in 20% of the nylon prostheses followed long-term, indicating the capacity for occult residual infection.
3. That prolonged antibiotic therapy could eradicate infection in 90% of cases, whereas shorter term (6 days) therapy resulted in no survival in dogs with homografts, and in only 40% of dogs with nylon grafts.

This lengthy series reiterated the basic principles of graft infection outlined by Harrison. It indicated a clear superiority of the newer synthetic grafts over homografts in the face of subsequent infection, and demonstrated that the homograft collagen tube simply disintegrated with catastrophic hemorrhage once infected. It also established thrombosis as a major complication of the infected graft, and established the potential for synthetic grafts to harbor latent infections for prolonged time frames. The model itself is a rigorous one, resulting not only in 100% graft infection but animal death in most cases without surgical abscess drainage and/or antibiotics; and it clearly represents a situation that is analogous only to in situ replacement of a fresh aortic graft into a clearly contaminated field—e.g., in situ repair of graft-enteric fistula or infected aneurysm/pseudoaneurysm. It is more difficult to extrapolate the model results to standard clean revascularization.

Lindenauer[3] looked at the potential role of antibiotics in decreasing GIF. His group performed four types of operations in dogs, sham controls in which the femoral artery was exposed only; a second group in which femoral arteriotomies were closed with Tevdek sutures; a third in which femoral arteriotomies were closed with knitted Teflon patch angioplasties; and a fourth in which the femoral arteriotomy was closed with autologous jugular vein. All wounds were inoculated at closure with 0.5 cc solution containing 1×10^4 to 1.75×10^5 *Staphylococcus aureus* which was phage-typed for tracking purposes. Wounds were reopened under sterile conditions at 4 days and cultures obtained. Nine control animals received no antibiotics, while 15 study animals received 4 days of perioperative antibiotics.

The results were mixed. Seventeen of 18 wound sites became infected; 15 animals received 4-day perioperative antibiotics; 0/5 arteriotomy dogs, 0/1 vein patches, and 0/5 Teflon patches, 0/12 sites for delayed retrieval from 7 to 14 days.

This study was primarily designed to show the efficacy of perioperative antibiotics in reducing wound infections, which it certainly does. As a model for graft infection, it is of interest for demonstrating that autologous tissue repairs and small synthetic patch angioplasties can be expected to heal in the face of contamination if adequate perioperative antibiotic coverage is instituted.

Goldsmith[4] looked at the potential benefit of wrapping an aortic prosthesis in autologous tissue to aid in preventing GIF. He used the canine infrarenal Dacron aortic replacement model under 10 days of antibiotic coverage. In group I, 10 dogs underwent graft placement followed by inoculation with 1 cc of liquid feces; in group II, the graft was wrapped with an omental flap, and the feces inoculated on the omental pedicle. In group III and IV, an initial retroperitoneal abscess was formed, drained at 48 hours, and in situ Dacron graft implantation then performed with and without omental protection. Fourteen of 19 group-nonprotected dogs died, seven each of sepsis or anastomotic disruption; the other 5 survived; 3 of these were culture negative at graft explantation although 2 grafts thrombosed at 1 year. Nineteen omentum-protected dogs had 5 deaths, 2 by sepsis and 3 by hemorrhage; 11 of 14 survivors had culture-negative grafts at 1 year; 1 had a pseudoaneurysm and 4 had perianastomotic fibrotic stenosis. As a final corollary study, 5 dogs had a devascularized free omental flap applied to their grafts, and all 5 died of sepsis. Histologic examination of all explanted grafts at 1 year was said to show infiltration of the omentum into the graft fabric and formation of an "endothelial lining within the lumen."

This seminal work in the prophylaxis of vascular graft infection used the then standard model of fecal inoculation in the canine aortic replacement situation. The marked reduction in graft sepsis was attributed to the omental pedicle; I would point out however, that this was true for the second half of the study only in which in situ replacement in an infected field was performed; in the first half of the study, the fecal inoculum was placed onto the graft. It is of interest that three of nine dogs (30%) had GIFs in this model.

Bricker[5] attempted a variation on the canine model, implanting 6-mm-knitted Dacron grafts in either the iliac or femoral artery and autologous vein grafts in the contralateral iliac vessels under 2 weeks of penicillin coverage. Study animals had local inoculation with 1×10^5 *S aureus.* In the control noninfected group, 3 of 10 vein, and 8 of 10 Dacron grafts occluded; in the infected group, 3 of 18 vein grafts occluded and two disrupted, while 11 of 18 Dacron grafts occluded. The researchers concluded that infection did not adversely affect the thrombosis rate, and that vein grafts generically had better patency in the face of infection than Dacron. However, they did also note the tendency for autologous vein grafts to

disrupt when infected, and noted that this was probably the result of ischemia due to lack of incorporation into surrounding tissue with formation of neovascularization. I would note that the high rate (80%) of thrombosis of Dacron grafts in the control limb makes any conclusions about thrombosis as an indicator of tolerance to infection tenuous at best; the rate of thrombosis was essentially unchanged for either vein or Dacron from control to infected model, but the Dacron rate is too high to make valid conclusions.

Humpert[6] introduced a new concept for graft infection models, suggesting that incorporated Dacron grafts could become secondarily infected by bacteremias. They placed Dacron aortic grafts in dogs and then subjected the dogs to prolonged *Staphylococcus* septicemia induced by ligation of the left ureter with concomitant intravenous *Staphylococcus* infusion (producing a renal abscess). They found that 3 dogs died of sepsis, all with graft thrombosis; 2 other dogs died of sepsis prior to explantation, and 7 of 10 surviving animals showed graft infections despite no clinical stigmata of infection. Histologic examination showed that areas of localized purulence corresponded to area of "neointimal disruption" where the graft matrix was exposed. This study introduced the bacteremic model for graft infection which would then be used by most researchers in the field. The study also reiterated the concept (introduced by Moore[7]) that a graft could be infected at areas of matrix nonincorporation, e.g., at exposed graft fabric.

Dr. Moore's group, at Arizona and then at UCLA, first introduced the concept of the bacteremic model for GIF in a series of laboratory studies. The first of these was in 1969; 3-cm infrarenal aortic Dacron grafts were placed in dogs and 1×10^7 *S aureus* infused with production of 100% (12/12) graft infection. Bacterial infusions were then administered at intervals postimplantation; at 2 weeks there was 100% infection, at 3 months this fell to 57%, and at 12 months it fell to

30%. Furthermore, they correlated the finding of clinical graft infection with the presence or absence of a complete pseudointima infusion There were no infections in 26 dogs with complete pseudointimas, but 95% of incidence in 57 dogs with incomplete coverage.

Variations on the basic canine bacteremic infusion model were then reported. Moore[8] noted that 5-day perioperative cephalothin prophylaxis was studied; the infusion was begun intravenously prior to surgery and continued to 30 minutes postincisional closure and supplanted by intramuscular doses thereafter. A simultaneous intravenous bacteremia with 1×10^7 S aureus was infused at a second I.V. site 30 minutes prior to operation. The presence of graft infection was determined at graft explantation 3 weeks later. Seventy-two percent (18/25) of placebo-treated dogs developed graft infections, compared to 24% (6/25) of antibiotic-treated dogs.

This study is interesting for the fact that there was such a high rate of GIF noted even though the bacteremia had occurred at least 60 to 90 minutes prior to graft placement; no confirmation of the level of persistent bacteremia was provided. Conversely, a simultaneously administered dose of appropriately sensitive antibiotic could reduce the infection rate to one third; presumably there was a concomitant reduction in the levels of bacteremia due to immediate bactericidal activity. Thus, the set of studies shows that bacteremias at any point from graft implant to 1 year will reliably infect a percentage of grafts, the rate of infection is directly related to the amount of pseudointimal coverage, and perioperative antibiotics may reduce but cannot eliminate graft infections.

Moore[9] reexamined the question of autologous versus synthetic conduits in an infected field, and used the same model as Bricker had in 1970. Canine femoral artery segments were exposed and the tissues inoculated with S aureus to produce a wound infection. Three days later, the arterial segment was resected and interposition grafts placed. In 12 dogs, the contralateral femoral artery was used; in 12 a femoral allograft was used, and in 12 continuity was restored with a 4-mm knitted Dacron graft. All dogs were covered with perioperative cephalothin. Grafts were harvested at 3 months and cultures taken. Eleven out of 12 arterial autografts were sterile with 4 of these thrombosed; 10/12 allografts were sterile with 1 of these thrombosed. In contrast, 7 of 8 Dacron grafts were infected. All infected autografts and allografts disrupted, and 3 of the 7 infected Dacron grafts had anastomotic disruption. Curiously, there was no histologic evidence of allograft rejection in this canine model, despite no immunosuppressive therapy.

The researchers specifically noted that the success of the allograft model was due to it being a nonpreserved fresh transplant, something not clinically or ethically permissible in humans. Although this study was specifically designed to address the question of differential resistance to secondary infection for conduits placed into a contaminated field, it also provides a different laboratory situation for producing a synthetic graft infection, and in so doing provides information as to how synthetic grafts will function when placed in situ.

A succession of articles was then reported on variations of the bacteremic infection model first noted in the 1969 paper.

Malone[10] reported a similar model for bacteremic infection, using infrarenal knitted Dacron aortic replacement followed with 1×10^7 S aureus infection at intervals of 3 days, 7 days, 14 days, 30 days and 3, 4, 5, and 12 months. At graft explantation 3 weeks later, 100% (10/10, 2/2, 4/4) of dogs infused at 3, 7, or 14 days became infected; this fell to 93% (14/15) at 1 month, 57% (8/14) at 3 months, 75% (9/12) at 4 months, 38% (3/8) at 5 months, 13% (1/8) at 6 months, and 30% (3/10) at 1 year. This was correlated with pseudointimal coverage; none of 26 completely covered grafts became infected, versus 95% (45/57) of incompletely covered grafts ($P < .05$).

Swanson, in 1976, then looked at the time frame in which grafts were vulnerable to bacteremias; the now standard infrarenal aortic replacement model was used with 1×10^7 intravenous *S aureus* infused at 3 days, and at 1, 3, and 4 months postimplantation. Grafts were explanted 3 to 5 weeks later. One hundred percent (10/10) at 3-day and 1-month-old grafts became infected; this fell to 70% (7/10) at 3 months and 62% (5/8) for 4-month grafts. They theorized that this relative resistance to infection resulted from more complete pseudointimal lining, but did not make definitive histologic comparisons.

Roon[11] extended the study to look at other graft types. The infrarenal aortic model was again used; ultra-lightweight Dacron (ULWD) woven, external, velour-knit Dacron (EVD), and PTFE grafts were used; 15 dogs with each graft type were explanted at either 3 or 6 months; 3 weeks prior to explant, an I.V. infusion of 1×10^8 *S aureus* was given. Ultra-lightweight Dacron grafts showed 80% (8/10) 3-month and 60% (6/10) 6-month infectability rates; EVD showed 50% (5/10) early and 40% (4/10) late infections; and PTFE showed 50% (5/10) early and 20% (2/10) late infections. This was correlated with the degree of pseudointimal lining, which at 3 months was 29%, 60%, and 30% respectively; and at 6 months was 40%, 87% and 87% ($P < .05$). They concluded that all grafts showed a more complete pseudointima with increasing time of implantation, and that the infectability rate seemed to be correlated with this, although they noted that these were trends only and not of statistical significance. I would reemphasize that point; due to the multipronged nature of the study, there are insufficient numbers of dogs in any one group to attain significance. It would be equally reasonable to suggest that synthetic grafts subjected to major bacteremias will fairly reliably (20% to 60%) become infected even at delayed time intervals.

Cheek[12] also prepared an infrarenal canine aortic replacement model with inoculation of 0.5 cc of liquid feces. Various autologous preparations were compared to knitted Dacron grafts which were soaked for 60 minutes in a 1% cephalothin solution; grafts were explanted at 30 days. Thirty percent of the Dacron grafts became grossly infected with a retroperitoneal abscess. There was no additional information about less than grossly evident infection in the remaining grafts. Basically, although this study purported to show that synthetic grafts fared better than autologous in an infected field, the data provided are less than complete.

Wilson's group at UCLA provided a series of articles looking at graft infection; within these were models for producing a GIF. Wilson[13] looked at the bovine graft as compared to woven Dacron; his group used the canine infrarenal replacement model with an intravenous infusion of 1×10^8 *S aureus* perioperatively; grafts were explanted at 6 weeks. One hundred percent of (15/15) Dacron grafts became infected, with five dogs dying of sepsis and anastomotic rupture; 100% (15/15) of bovine grafts also became infected, 14 of which ruptured at the anastomosis with dissolution of the graft itself.

This initial study was followed up by Parsa[14] to look at the effect of prophylactic antibiotics. In addition, he sought to more accurately characterize the physiology of the common model by analysis of the time course of bacteremias. They found that all blood cultures were positive for 2 hours following infusion and became negative thereafter. However, four of five dogs showed delayed (3 to 5 days) positive cultures that correlated at autopsy with positive spleen and liver cultures. Concomitant infusion of an appropriate susceptibility antibiotic markedly decreased the absolute levels of bacteria, with cultures being negative by 1 hour. Overall, 92% (15/16) of control grafts became infected, with 31% of dogs dying; for antibiotic-treated dogs, the infection rate dropped to 8% (1/16).

The researchers postulated that in the canine bacteremic model, bacteria could be cleared by the reticuloendothelial system within 2 hours; however, they also noted a delayed repeat bacteremia occurring days later. Simultaneously administered antibiotics cleared this bacteremia and eradicated the secondary bacteremias; this was correlated by a reduced incidence of graft infection by culture. Wilson used the data to suggest intraoperative dosing and redosing.

Bennion[15] then followed up with a study indicating that there was a varying degree of success in obtaining graft infection dependent on the absolute dose of bacteria.

Weber[16] looked specifically at the question of how the dose of bacterial inoculum and the type of implanted graft might affect graft infectability. He studied a unilateral aortofemoral bypass model, using woven Dacron, knitted Dacron, and knitted velour Dacron prostheses; bacteremias of 1×10^5 or 1×10^6 S aureus were then induced at operation or at 2 or 4 weeks postoperatively; these were introduced percutaneously onto the palpated prosthesis at its inguinal ligament midportion. Grafts were then examined at 1 week. Positive graft cultures were obtained at 1 month in this model in 83% (10/12) of woven grafts at 10^5 and 58% (7/12) at 10^6 organisms. At 2 weeks, the respective rates were 50% (6/12) for all grafts at 10^5, and 58% to 67% (6 to 8/12) at 10^6 organisms; and at 1 day, the respective rates were 67% to 100% (9 to 12/12) at 10^5 and 92% to 100% (11 to 12/12) at 10^6 organisms. This data was interpreted to show that there was no real difference in initial graft infectability, but that knitted and velour Dacron grafts demonstrated a higher resistance to infection at 1-month implantation as compared to immediately postoperatively, presumably due to better incorporation.

One obvious problem with this study is the lack of certainty that the grafts were actually being "inoculated," particularly at the later dates; percutaneous introduction of the bacteria may well have been producing only a subcutaneous abscess not actually in contact with the graft. Secondly, there was no difference noted between the two sizes of inocula because both are excessively large (as demonstrated in Bennion's data). On the other hand, this very different model of infection would best mimic the effect of a postoperative wound infection at the groin and its potential for producing clinical graft infections.

Weiss[17] extended the canine bacteremic aortic replacement model to include both Dacron and PTFE grafts. Eight out of 11 (72%%) PTFE grafts became infected with 3 deaths and 3 thromboses; 90% (9/10) of Dacron grafts became infected, with 2 deaths and 1 thrombosis. Histologic examination was remarkable for demonstrating cocci within the graft matrices for each graft; Weiss also noted a correlation with absence of neointimal formation. The researchers also noted persistent positive blood cultures for weeks following implantation in dogs with infected grafts.

Kron[18] developed a new model using the pig and specifically looked at whether an introduced graft infection would propagate along the graft. He inserted two infrarenal aortic 6-mm knitted Dacron grafts at the infrarenal position, using end to side aortic and iliac anastomoses for each; one of these dual implanted grafts was then ligated. A disk containing 1×10^6 S aureus was then sutured to the combined proximal suture lines. Four of the 11 pigs died of peritonitis prior to graft culture/explantation at 5 days; cultures of the internal aspect of the proximal, midportion, and distal portions of each graft were taken after in vivo formalin preservation of the en bloc specimen; 7/8 proximal, 6/8 midportion, and 5/8 distal cultures were positive for patent, and 6/8 thrombosed grafts.

The researchers used the data to state that bacteria will readily propagate along a thrombosed or a patent graft and, therefore, limited graft excision is not reassurable. As much as I agree with the premise, the study does not appropriately afford the data on which to make that conclusion. This model does not test the clinical situation of propagation along the presumed virginal planes from a primary source of sepsis (e.g., the groin) and, in particular, does not test the model of such propagation along a well-incorporated but currently thrombosed graft, which is the clinical situation of delayed occult graft infection. The model is simply a refined variation of the local retroperitoneal inoculation model, with the predictable result of overwhelming sepsis—such that graft explants had to be done at the very early interval of 5 days because all animals died within 1 week! One would expect all graft cultures at all sites to be culture positive in that situation. The model does not test for propagation, but rather for overwhelming local contamination. A more appropriate model would be production of sepsis in the groin of aortofemoral grafts, both acutely and with chronically implanted grafts, and then see if infection indeed can be localized or does it ascend along the graft. Such a model has not been tested.

Akhondzadeh[19] tested four different grafts, using the canine infrarenal aortic replacement model and woven Dacron, bovine, PTFE, and human umbilical vein (HUV) grafts. Five $\times$ 10^7 S $aureus$ bacteremias were then induced at the conclusion of the procedure, or at an interval of 3 weeks following implantation; graft explantation was performed 6 weeks later. For perioperative infusions, infections occurred in 100% (10/10) of Dacron grafts with five anastomotic disruptions; in 100% (18/18) bovine grafts with nine anastomotic and one graft disruption; in 100% (10/10) PTFE grafts with one anastomotic disruption; and 100% (5/5) HUV grafts with one anastomotic disruption. A delayed infusion however resulted in a different spectrum; 54% (6/13) Dacron; 28% (4/14) bovine with two anastomotic disruptions and three thromboses; 60% (6/10) PTFE, all with minimal gross changes but culture positive; and 20% (1/5) HUV grafts. The researcher interpreted the data to show a decrease in absolute infection rates with increasing incorporation of the graft. It more specifically tests for the direct infectability of various grafts by a high-dose perioperative bacteremia, and that all grafts were equally susceptible at that high level. The frequency of infection with delayed bacteremia was indeed decreased, presumably due to intraluminal matrix coverage by fibrin which may be a function of incorporation. It is also noteworthy that PTFE grafts tended to be occultly infected, a topic taken up elsewhere in this chapter.

Knott[20] revived the canine femoral artery replacement model, looking at PTFE, Dacron, and autologous vein grafts exposed to a local inoculum of 4×10^7 S $aureus$, under cephalothin prophylaxis. Dacron grafts became infected in 100% (5/5), with anastomotic disruption in 60% (3/5); PTFE also showed a 100% (5/5) and 80% disruption rate, while vein grafts disrupted in 80% of cases (4/5). The primary etiology for the disruptions was arterial edema and friability for the synthetic grafts, and for vein grafts it was equally arterial or vein graft dissolution.

Shah[21] performed a similar model, placing PTFE or vein grafts in the canine femoral artery and then inoculating the wound with both 1×10^7 $E.$ $coli$ and S $aureus$ with and without cefoxitin prophylaxis. At 3 weeks, 100% of the wounds without antibiotic coverage became infected, with culture positive for $E.$ $coli,$ S $aureus,$ and an additional 6 with $Pseudomonas.$ Institution of antibiotics reduced the gross wound infection rate to zero with both grafts; however, 100% (5/5) of PTFE and 80% (4/5) vein grafts were positive for both inoculated bacteria. This paper emphasized the tendency for PTFE to be occultly infected despite clinical wound healing. Both papers demonstrate that neither synthetic nor autologous grafts fare well in a grossly contaminated field, despite perioperative antibiotic coverage; the mode of graft failure is just different.

Fletcher[22] devised a variation of the inoculation model for producing GIF, using increasing doses of *aureus* from 1×10^2 through 1×10^8 CFU locally introduced onto protein-sealed Dacron or PTFE graft used as carotid replacements in sheep. Grafts were harvested and cultured at 3 weeks. No infections occurred with 1×10^2; at 1×10^4 1 of 3 had no Dacron grafts become infected; at 1×10^6 and 1×10^8, 11 of 12 grafts became infected. It was further noted that whereas it required 1×10^8 CFU to produce a wound infection in this model, the presence of a graft reduced the necessary inoculum to 10^4 for PTFE and 10^6 for Dacron. In the sheep model, infection reliably resulted in thrombosis of the graft, whereas anastomotic disruptions were not seen.

Geary[23] used the canine femoral artery replacement model to study the influence of bacterial virulence on the production of GIF. Polytetrafluoroethylene grafts were implanted in one groin and autologous veins in the contralateral groin, followed by direct local inoculation of either 1×10^8 *Staphylococcus epidermidis* or *Pseudomonas aeruginosa*; grafts were harvested at 7 to 10 days. *S epidermidis* inoculations resulted in no clinically apparent infections; veins and PTFE were, however, culture or histologically positive for bacteria. In addition, one vein and one PTFE graft thrombosed. In contrast, all vein and PTFE grafts inoculated with *Pseudomonas* were infected; all five vein grafts and three of five PTFE grafts disrupted. The researchers observed that *S epidermidis* had the ability to occultly persist in tissues or graft matrix, while *Pseudomonas* resulted in gross arterial disruptions, and noted that the graft material was less important than the virulence of the bacteria.

Mehran[24] presented a multipronged trial of various modalities for treatment of a *S aureus* locally inoculated infection of an infrarenal PTFE graft in pigs. This resulted in a 100% clinical graft infection. After 1 week to establish an infection, the pigs were reexplored and six methods of graft treatment were used. All animals were treated with 7 days of culture-specific antibiotics

and reoperation performed at 21 days to determine graft thrombosis, clinical infection, and bacterial cultures of the graft and perigraft tissues.

Ten animals undergoing simple drainage of the abscess showed 100% thrombosis and 70% infection rates. Replacement with an in situ PTFE graft resulted in 40% infection and thrombosis rates. Addition of either a jejunal seromuscular wrap or an anterior rectus muscle flap wrap significantly decreased infection levels to 1/6 and 2/6, but all 12 grafts thrombosed. If the PTFE grafts were replaced and wrapped in autologous tissue, infection rates were significantly reduced ($P < .05$) to 1/10 and 1/10 while thrombosis rates also were significantly reduced to 2/10 and 1/10 ($P < .05$).

The rationale for the improved control of infection with either type of autologous perigraft tissue is that the local graft environment is changed positively for host immunocompetence. A healed synthetic graft is surrounded by a thick relatively acellular outer capsule; in the retroperitoneum, the surrounding tissues are fatty and also relatively avascular. Hypoxia is known to increase susceptibility to infection as a function of impaired leukocyte function. A seromuscular or muscle flap provides increased oxygen delivery and wound oxygen tension. Histologic examination of the grafts showed dense incorporation where the muscle was adherent as opposed to a loose poorly cellular granulation tissue on the posterior aspect away from the graft.

The paper gives solid laboratory evidence for the role of autologous vascularized tissue coverage of grafts to prevent graft infection, both at initial implant and potentially for in situ replacement of a contaminated graft. A criticism may be leveled in that the follow-up of 21 days may not be sufficient to conclusively state that no infection has occurred—the dense incorporation at the muscular pedicle was not present posteriorly in the bed, and one can theorize that infected granulation tissue here might result in (delayed recognition) graft infection at a later date. It is also of curious interest that by their criteria, simple incision and drainage allowed a 30% healing and incision and drainage with in situ replacement resulted in 60% healing; this would again lead to a question of whether or not the model accurately assesses infection or is hampered by the early (21 day) follow-up. The converse of these figures is also worthy of note; that local therapy resulted in a 70% failure rate, and in situ replacement a 40% failure rate.

Discussion

Production of a synthetic vascular graft infection in the laboratory is done in basically three models:

a. canine infrarenal aortic replacement with local inoculation.
b. canine infrarenal aortic replacement with bacteremia
c. canine femoral artery replacement with local inoculation.

There are a number of variations on this theme with different animals, whether or not antibiotics are used, and what types of grafts are used.

All three models rely on heavy (1×10^6 or greater) bacterial inocula to obtain the GIF; for the most part a 90% to 100% GIF rate will result. This makes them useful as baseline laboratory control on which to study the effects of various prevention measures (antibiotics, impregnations, etc). However, the first two models do not reasonably reproduce any clinical situation save the development of a retroperitoneal abscess in continuity with the graft, and perhaps major graft-enteric erosions/fistulae with major and/or uncontrolled local sepsis. Conversely, the femoral artery model reasonably reproduces the situation of an acute postoperative (grossly purulent) wound infection at the groin. It is unlikely that such large inocula are present in any other clinical situation; this is particularly

true for the bacteremic model, since clinical bacteremias without frank sepsis generally involve less than 10^5 organisms.

This means that the models cannot answer many of the questions raised about the basic pathophysiology of clinical graft infections. In particular, only 30% to 40% of graft infections in the literature have presented as acute postoperative problems of groin sepsis; the next most common presentation is that of delayed recognition (months to years) and is usually due to *S epidermidis*, presenting as limb thrombosis or pseudoaneurysm. There is no model to help study this common problem.

Furthermore, the logical choice of the various treatment regimens should be based on solid laboratory and/or clinical evidence for the principles that are inherent; yet, the models do not provide a wealth of that necessary basic data.

For example, does infection that starts in one groin remain localized, or does it ascend? Is this as true for an acute nonincorporated graft as it is for a chronic well-incorporated graft? Is infection more or less likely to ascend along a thrombosed as opposed to a patent graft? The models do not provide an answer to these questions.

One can therefore summarize the laboratory model data as follows:

a. acute (groin) wound infection involving a freshly implanted graft
b. the rare case of retroperitoneal abscess (e.g., ischemic colitis/perforation) in continuity with a freshly implanted graft

The models may, however, provide some experimental basis for the management principles outlined in Section V. For example:

a. the foreign body concept as a potentiator of infection
b. propagation concept
c. tendency for intraluminal fibrin to be infected

However, it is not a good model for explaining or understanding:

a. *S epidermidis* infections
b. delayed bacteremias, because most clinical bacteremias are of much lower (10^2 to 10^3) levels
c. secondary infection of a previously noninfected graft at redo surgery; e.g., a well-incorporated graft with a new direct (small) local inoculation
d. lymphatic effluent bathing the graft externally with bacteria rather than intraluminal bacterial contamination
e. GEF/GEE without massive local abscess/sepsis—e.g., where the process stays very well localized.

Things that the model does tell us, once a graft infection is present:

a. Patch angioplasties tend to fare fairly well; the internal surface probably reendothelializes quickly, and the external surface is small enough to afford success with local therapy. Conversely, one can question why the size of the foreign body involved in the infection should have any effect on its role as a foreign body potentiator.

b. Autologous grafts (vein or artery; homograft, allograft, autogenous) tend to dissolve with most virulent infections (although only *E. coli*, *S aureus*, and *Pseudomonas* have been tested) causing exsanguination in 20% to 30% of cases. The significance of this point was recognized long ago for homografts, which were abandoned; it is a very real concern for the current practice of freeze-dried allografts and autologous superficial femoral artery grafts being used for in situ reconstructions in infected beds.

c. Synthetic grafts remain intact when in an infected field, but appear to exacerbate the inflammatory response at the artery resulting in a 30% rate of anastomotic disruption. This results in acute exsanguinations and chronic pseudoaneurysms.

d. Infected grafts of all types tend to thrombose when infected or when traversing an infected field. This laboratory finding has been recognized clinically by acute thromboses of grafts with postoperative infections and by the tendency for chronic smoldering (*S epidermidis*) GIFs to present thromboses. What triggers this thrombotic response is not clearly understood.

e. Grossly infected grafts may be clinically recognized by a denser inflammatory reaction in the perigraft space, as well as by nonincorporation of the matrix to the immediate perigraft sheath. They also tend to cause strictures in the artery to which they are anastomosed (if end to end). This has correlated to the clinical maxim that an unincorporated graft or graft segment is infected, unless it can be clearly demonstrated that encystment has occurred; defined as a clearly delineated cystic cavity, lined with a membrane that looks like pleura or peritoneum, and is filled with a clear fluid with no histologic bacteria and very few,if any, leukocytes.

f. Polytetrafluoroethylene is notorious for the capability to appear clinically "healed" (e.g., partially incorporated, no gross perigraft fluid) yet demonstrate culture positivity. This frequently observed laboratory finding has been noted clinically as well. It has great import for the purported success with local therapy of grafts that appear to heal but may remain culture positive. It also is important in the initial determination of whether or not an infection is actively "localized." The long-term evolution of this culture-positive state is unknown, but presumably would lead to subsequent thrombosis and/or formation of a delayed pseudoaneurysm; whether there is clinical bacteremic seeding of such a culture-positive matrix is also unknown. All of these are major questions requiring answers!

g. Bacteremic infection is a factor of the degree of complete neointimal formation; fibrin, fibronectin, thrombus, and exposed graft matrix are all reliable traps for bacteria and sites for infection. This factor may or may not be ameliorated by antibiotic graft impregnations. It has great import for the initial choice of graft; certainly any graft placed at the groin (highest incidence site for GIF) and redo operations at the groin should entail consideration for utilization of a graft that attains and maintains excellent neointimal coverage. (knitted velour, with PTFE a close second choice).

h. Gram-negative infections are generically more virulent than Gram-positive, with higher incidences of arterial and/or autologous graft dissolution. This has translated directly into caveats on the use of local, in situ, and partial resection regimens for treatment of GIF.

i. Autologous tissue pedicles must be well vascularized to provide their intended role, and they must entirely encircle the graft for maximal effectiveness; simply laying the pedicle down on the exposed surface will not reliably eradicate the infection, unless the posterior aspect of the graft is also incorporated. The question of whether or not grafts so treated remain culture positive, and the long-term import of that, remains unknown.

j. Concomitant administration of antibiotics during a bacteremic episode will *reduce* but not eliminate the bacteremia. Grafts can still be shown to entrap bacteria and become infected. This a fairly disheartening finding. Whether prophylactic antibiotics are sufficient to eradicate the presumably smaller inocula of local contamination in a clean wound is an unstudied point.

The most vexing problem with all the graft models is that they do not present data on which to assess treatment modalities. They provide a reliable model for GIF production, but leave unanswered questions, as for example:

Local therapy: Will such treatment totally eradicate bacteria from the graft matrix? Is there a difference for acutely infected versus chronically infected grafts? Is there a difference for the type of infecting bacteria? Can bacteria be eradicated from the fibrous

tunnel surrounding a graft, and if not, are these then a source for ascending infection?

Partial excision: Is the tunnel sterilized, and if not, can bacteria persist/migrate up the tunnel? Does the dissection interrupt lymphatics, and if so, can these reinfect the presumably clean proximal graft stump by bathing it in bacteria-laden effluent?

Excision only, or excision and extra-anatomic bypass (EAB): Does the surrounding infected bed remain culture positive and is this differentially true for various bacteria? Is it, therefore, truly safe to do an in situ reconstruction? How long does it take for the bed to become sterilized and, therefore, when is it safe to perform tertiary reconstruction? What are the actual levels of bacteremia encountered at graft excision, and are these sufficiently high to cause secondary EAB infection? How much tissue needs to be interposed between the newly placed EAB and the infected field to insure that no cross-contamination will occur? How long do bacteria persist in the aortic stump or femoral/iliac arteriotomy wall, and what mechanisms allow their persistence there?

In situ: Recognizing that placing the new synthetic graft in a grossly contaminated field will reliably lead to secondary GIF—how much is gross, or conversely how little is safe to allow in situ? Does the surrounding infected bed remain culture positive and is this differentially true for various bacteria? Is it, therefore, safe to do an in situ reconstruction? How long does it take for the bed to become sterilized, and when is it safe to perform tertiary reconstruction? As with local, does this graft become culture positive despite clinical healing. Does this lead to secondary PA and thrombosis, and if so over what time (how long a surveillance?).

We make very broad assumptions about the management of graft infections, assumptions that quite frankly are not as solidly grounded in a laboratory model as they need to be.

References

1. Harrison JH. Influence of infection on homografts and synthetic (Teflon) grafts. *Arch Surg.* 1958;76:1:67–73.
2. Foster JH, Berzins T, Scott HW. An experimental study of arterial replacement in the presence of bacterial infection. *Surg Gynecol Obstet.* 1959;108:2:141–148.
3. Lindenauer SM, Fry WJ, Schaub G, et al. The use of antibiotics in the prevention of vascular graft infections. *Surgery.* 1967;62:3:487–492.
4. Goldsmith HS, de los Santos R, Vanamee P, et al. Experimental protection of vascular prostheses by omentum. *Arch Surg.* 1968;97:6:872–878.
5. Bricker DL, Beall AC, DeBakey ME. The differential response to infection of autogenous vein vs. Dacron arterial prosthesis. *Chest.* 1970;58:6:566.
6. Humpert EL, Quinn EL, Dienst SG, et al. Infection of the well-incorporated Dacron graft caused by septicemia. *Surg Forum.* 1972;23:234.
7. Moore WS, Rosson CT, Hall AD, et al. Transient bacteremia: a cause of infection in prosthetic vascular grafts. *Am J Surg .* 1969;117:342.
8. Moore WS, Rosson CT, Hall AD. Effect of prophylactic antibiotics in preventing bacteremic infection of vascular prostheses. *Surgery.* 1971;69:6:825–828.
9. Moore WS, Swanson RJ, Campagna G, et al. The use of fresh arterial substitutes in infected fields. *J Surg Res.* 1975;18:229–233.
10. Malone SE, Hermosillo CX, Parsa F, et al. Experimental infection of Dacron and bovine grafts. *J Surg Res.* 1975;18:221–227.
11. Roon AJ, Malone JM, Moore WS, et al. Bacteremic infectability: a function of vascular graft material and design. *J Surg Res.* 1977;22:489–498.
12. Cheek RC, Cole FH, Smith HF. Comparison of Dacron and aortic autografts in wounds contaminated with fecal matter. *Am Surg.* 1974;40:8:439–442.
13. Wilson SE. Experimental infection of Dacron and bovine grafts. *J Surg Res.* 1975;18:221–227.
14. Parsa F, Gordon HE, Wilson SE. Intraoperative antibiotics in the prevention of experimental Dacron graft infection. *Vasc Surg.* 1976;10:64–71.
15. Bennion RS, Williams RA, Wilson SE. Comparison of infectability of vascular prosthetic material by quantitation of median infective dose. *Surgery.* 1984;95:1:22–25.
16. Weber TR, Lindenauer SM, Miller TA, et al. Focal infection of aortofemoral prostheses. *Surgery.* 1976;79:3:310–312.
17. Weiss JP, Lorenzo FV, Campbell CD, et al. The behavior of infected arterial prostheses of expanded polytetrafluoroethylene (Goretex). *J Thorac Cardiovasc Surg.* 1977;73:4:630–636.
18. Kron IL, Georgitis JW, Holmes P, et al. Propagation of sepsis in vascular grafts. *Arch Surg.* 1980;115:1:878–879.
19. Akhondzadeh L, Wilson SE, William RA, et al. Infection of materials used in vascular access surgery: an evaluation of Dacron, bovine heterograft, Teflon, and human umbilical vein. *Dial Transplant.* 1980;9:7:697–700.
20. Knott LH, Crawford FA, Grogan JB. Comparison of autogenous vein, Dacron, and Goretex in infected wounds. *J Surg Res.* 1978;24:288–293.
21. Shah PM, Katsuki I, Clauss RH, et al. Expanded microporous PTFE grafts in contaminated wounds: experimental and clinical study. *J Trauma.* 1983;23:12:1030–1033.
22. Fletcher JP, Dryden M, Monro R, et al. Establishment of a vascular graft infection model in the sheep carotid model. *Aust NZ J Surg.* 1990;60:801–803.
23. Geary KJ, Tomkiewicz ZM, Harrison HN, et al. Differential effect of a gram negative and a gram positive infection in aortic prosthetic infection. *J Vasc Surg.* 1990;11:2:339–346.
24. Mehran KT, Jewell ER. Local antiseptic treatment of infected grafts in the groin. *Br J Surg.* 1988;75:1037–1038.

Chapter 3

Natural History of Graft Infections

R.J. Pitsch
P.F. Lawrence

Introduction

Infection of a vascular prosthetic graft is one of the most uncommon and difficult complications that a vascular surgeon must manage. The incidence of graft infection has been reported in the literature to range from 0.8% to 4.1%.[1,2] Clear symptoms and signs of graft infection are often absent. High morbidity and mortality rates are also associated with this complication; amputation rates range from 8% to 60%,[3,4] and mortality rates range from 6% to 47% with treatment and as high as 100% without treatment.[5,6] The mean duration of hospitalization following graft infection was found to be 90 days by Lorentzen and 114 days by Johnson et al.[7,8] The large variation in incidence of complications and death rates is in turn due to variations in time of onset, types of infecting organisms, and the location of graft infections.

The interval between prosthetic graft implantation and the development of graft infection varies greatly and may be as brief as only a few days to as long as 173 months.[9] When considering graft infections, it is helpful to divide them into early and late infections.

Early Graft Infections

Many earlier series reporting on graft infections documented a higher incidence of early rather than late graft infections predominantly associated with *Staphylococcus aureus* and often presenting with obvious signs of infection. Reporting on 40 patients with graft infections in 1972, Szylagyi noted that 65% of the cases presented in less than 30 days.[10] Fletcher found that 90.9% (10/11) of graft infections occurred in less than 30 days also.[11] Liekweg noted that 80% of groin infections were detected within 5 weeks of the date of operation.[5] The most common organism isolated in these three series was *S aureus*, with Szylagyi reporting 41% (9/22), Liekweg 50%, and Fletcher 90.9% (10/11).[5,10,11] Goldstone noted that *S aureus* was the most common organism in his series, with 69% (9/13) of patients presenting with graft infections within 3.5 months of operation.[1]

Although *S aureus* is the most common organism isolated in early graft infections, many other organisms including Gram-negative bacilli and anaerobes may be identified less frequently (Table 1). Occasion-

Table 1
Pathogens in Early Graft Infections

Pathogen	Cherry	Liekweg	Fletcher
Staphylococcus aureus	30.8%	50%	64%
S epidermidis	10.3%	3.6%	27%
Group D Streptococcus	12%	—	—
Gram-negative bacilli not Pseudomonas	28.2%	—	—
Citrobacter	—	—	—
Escherichia coli	—	13.4%	9%
Klebsiella	—	5.4%	—
Proteus	—	4.8%	9%
Pseudomonas	7.7%	6.1%	—
Fungal pathogens	7.7%	—	—
Anaerobes	7.7%	—	—

ally, graft infections may also be polymicrobial.[5,12]

Early infections usually appear first in the subcutaneous positions and become apparent by the discharge of pus.[13] Szylagyi noted that acute graft sepsis usually involves a wound infection, and that in aortofemoral grafts it is commonly manifested as a purulent draining wound.[10] Goldstone noted that of all *S aureus* infections, 64% (9/14) occurred in the groin and that 10 out of 14 early infections occurred in the groin.[1] The incidence of graft infection is higher in patients with groin incisions after either aortofemoral bypass or femoropopliteal bypass than after aortoiliac graft placement (Table 2). Thus, early graft infections are frequently associated with *S. aureus* and with grafts at the femoral level.

However, early graft infections may present in many ways. Cherry et al. reviewed 39 infected femorodistal bypasses which had a median time from graft placement to initial symptoms of graft infection of 48 days. The most frequent presentation was an abscess adjacent to the graft (51.3%) followed by an infected sinus tract (38.5%), cellulitis (28.2%), systemic sepsis (20.5%), hemorrhage (10.3%), pseudoaneurysm (10.3%), graft exposure (10.3%), poor tissue incorporation (5.1%), acute arterial ischemia with graft thrombosis (2.6%), and septic emboli (2.6%).[14] Most early graft infections present with obvious signs or symptoms (Table 3).

The administration of systemic antibiotics is effective in reducing the incidence of early infection, especially due to *S aureus*

Table 2
Incidence of Wound Infection by Level of Prosthetic Graft

Level	Fletcher	Szylagyi	Goldstone
ABI	2.9%	0.7%	1.2%
ABF	6.5%	1.6%	3.0%
Axillofemoral	5.0%	0.9%	5.3%
Femorofemoral			7.7%
Iliofemoral			—
Femoropopliteal	3.4%	3.0%	2.3%

Table 3
Symptoms in Early Graft Infections

Symptoms	Bandyk ≤ 30 mo.	Cherry	Liekweg	Fletcher
Local infection	75%	28.2%	48.2%	91%
Systemic signs of sepsis	50%	20.5%	11.7%	64%
Graft occlusion	—	—	4.6%	45%
Sinus	—	38.5%	9.2%	36%
Hemorrhage	—	10.3%	9.8%	18%
Pseudoaneurysm	—	10.3%	9.8%	9%
UGI bleed	—	—	6.5%	—
Abscess adjacent to graft	—	51.3%	—	—
Graft exposure	—	10.3%	—	—
Poor tissue incorporation	—	5.1%	—	—
Acute ischemia and graft thrombosis	—	2.6%	—	—
Septic emboli	—	2.6%	—	—
Graft-enteric fistula	—	—	—	—
Groin swelling only	—	—	—	—

(UGI = upper gastrointestinal).

and Gram-negative bacteria.[15-17] Reviewing the incidence of graft infection prior to 1965 when antibiotic prophylaxis was used postoperatively only, Goldstone and Moore found a 4.1% incidence of graft infection. In 1965, they began to use preoperative, intraoperative, and postoperative antibiotics; this resulted in a 1.5% incidence of graft infections.[1] In a later article Bandyk reported on 30 cases of aortofemoral graft infection; only 10% 3/30 presented in less than 4 months. The incidence of early graft infections has declined with the routine use of preoperative and postoperative antibiotics.[18]

Late Graft Infections

Late vascular prosthesis infections may not be recognizable clinically for months to years after graft implantation.[1,10,18-20] Clinical signs of late graft infections are commonly associated with graft healing-complications including cutaneous sinus tracts, lack of graft incorporation by surrounding tissue, anastomotic aneurysm, and graft-enteric fistula formation.[21-23] However, late graft infections can present in many different ways. Edwards reviewed 18 patients with infected aortic prosthetic grafts which occurred an average of 45 months after graft implantation. The most common presenting manifestation was a draining sinus in a groin wound (8/18), localized groin abscess (3/18), groin swelling only (4/18), gastrointestinal hemorrhage (2/18), and femoral pseudoaneurysm (1/18).[19] Goldstone and Moore reported a higher incidence of pseudoaneurysm, finding that 13 of 27 infections presented as a false aneurysm. Other signs of graft infections in that series included local hemorrhage (5/27) and sepsis (5/27) of which two out of the five patients with sepsis also had evidence of septic emboli.[1] Bandyk's review of aortofemoral graft infections presenting at a mean interval of 41 months from prosthesis implantation also included the findings of aortoduodenal fistula (2/30), multiple anastomotic aneurysms (11/18), perigraft exudate (16/18), and poor graft incorporation (16/18) (Table 4). Bandyk contrasted these presenting symptoms with those of patients presenting prior to 30 months with graft infections; earlier infections presented with leukocytosis,

Table 4
Symptoms in Late Graft Infections

| | Series | | |
| | Average time interval | | |
Symptoms	Goldstone 15 mo.	Bandyk 41 mo.	Edwards 45 mo.
Local infection	51.8%	0	0
Systemic signs of sepsis	18.5%	0	0
Graft occlusion	29.6%	0	0
Sinus	51.8%	27.7%	44.4%
Hemorrhage	25.9%	0	0
Pseudoaneurysm	48.1%	61.1%	5.5%
UGI bleed	0	11.1%	11.1%
Abscess adjacent to graft	0	0	16.6%
Graft exposure	0	0	0
Poor tissue incorporation	0	88.8%	0
Acute ischemia and graft thrombosis	0	0	0
Septic emboli	0	0	0
Graft-enteric fistula	0	11.1%	0
Groin swelling only	0	0	22.2%

(UGI = upper gastrointestinal).

fever, bacteremia, and were culture-positive for *S aureus* (3/12), Gram-negative organisms (7/12), and streptococci (2/12). Later infections were, however, strongly associated with *Staphylococcus epidermidis* (18/30).[18]

Evidence of sepsis occurs more frequently with early graft infections, but is relatively uncommon in cases of late graft infections. While late graft infections may be evident clinically as described above, there is growing evidence that many graft infections are occult.

Graft colonization may lead to the development of late graft-healing complications such as cutaneous sinus tracts, lack of graft incorporation, anastomotic aneurysms, graft-enteric erosions, and graft-enteric fistulae.[16,24] Patients presenting with these late graft complications may not be diagnosed correctly until well beyond the initial examination (Table 5).

Failure of Graft Incorporation

The use of double velour Dacron grafts to improve graft adherence to perigraft tissues was reported by Cooley et al. in 1978.[25] However, late graft healing can still be complicated by poor graft incorporation associated with graft infection. Bandyk noted a circumferential absence of tissue ingrowth in 16/18 grafts at the time of surgical exploration.[18] Seabrook, while studying pseudoaneurysms, noted 6/27 grafts had either a perigraft capsule, exudate, or purulent fluid surrounding the anastomotic site at the time of surgery.[9] When perigraft fluid is found, it is often mucoid. Gram stains of

Table 5
Healing Complications of Late Graft Infections

Cutaneous sinus formation
Failure of graft incorporation
Anastomotic aneurysms
Graft-enteric erosions
Graft-enteric fistulas

this perigraft fluid identified many PMNs but did not identify any bacteria; however, *S epidermidis* was the most common bacteria isolated in cultures.[18]

Anastomotic Aneurysms

Many late graft infections present without clinical signs or symptoms of infection. Kaebnick et al. reported on 44 patients presenting with femoral anastomotic aneurysms (n = 21) or thrombosis (n = 26). None of the patients had prior treatment of graft infection or preoperative signs of graft sepsis, i.e., fever or leukocytosis. At operation, clinical signs of graft infection such as perigraft inflammation, perigraft exudate, or absence of graft incorporation, were absent. Explanted graft material, which grossly appeared to be free of infection, was placed in tryptic soy broth and ultrasonically oscillated (20 mHz for 10 minutes to disrupt the adherent graft surface biofilm). Bacteria were isolated from 90% (19/21) of the grafts associated with psuedoaneurysms and 69% (18/20) of thrombosed grafts. *S epidermidis* was the organism most commonly isolated, being present in 69% of the isolates.[26] Seabrook also demonstrated that graft material is frequently colonized with bacteria in the absence of clinical signs of graft infection. Upon review of 45 femoral pseudoaneurysms with no clinical evidence of infection at a mean of 45 months after prosthetic graft placement, bacterial isolates were recovered from 60% of the specimens, with coagulase-negative staphylococci accounting for 24/27 of the recovered species.[9]

Late graft infections are most commonly associated with coagulase-negative staphylococci and *S epidermidis* is the most common isolated organism. In patients presenting with graft infections more than 3.5 months from implantation, Goldstone reported isolating coagulase-negative *Staphylococcus* in seven patients and *S aureus* in two patients.[1] Bandyk found that 90% of aortofemoral graft infections presented be-

yond 4 months from the time of graft implantation and that *S epidermidis* was documented as the infecting organism in 18 cases (66%).[18]

At the opposite end of the clinical spectrum, infected pseudoaneurysms may present clinically with life- or limb-threatening complications.[27] Pseudoaneurysms usually present without major symptoms; however, there are several ways in which they may present symptomatically[12]: painful discomfort related to a palpable mass (51/81), simple painful discomfort (29/81), signs of local or systemic infection (11/81), hemorrhage (8/81), and ischemic pain secondary to embolization or thrombosis (5/81).[28]

Infected pseudoaneurysms are associated with increased complications.[29] Pseudoaneurysms have a tendency to expand and may range in size from 2 to 15 cm at presentation. Almost one third presented with life- or limb-threatening emergencies. Amputations were required in 5/81 cases, while no amputations were necessary in patients without infected false aneurysms. There was a significantly increased incidence of hemorrhage, emergency operation, and recurrent pseudoaneurysms in patients with infected pseudoaneurysms. The mortality rate is also higher in patients with infected pseudoaneurysms, (33%) compared to (2%) in patients with noninfected pseudoaneurysms.[28]

The pathogenesis of pseudoaneurysms is varied; however, graft infection has been reported to present as a false aneurysm in 10% to 13.5% of patients.[5,30] The overall incidence of false aneurysms appears to be decreasing, possibly reflecting an increased awareness of the technical factors that predispose to pseudoaneurysm formation.[31] Sedwitz et al. reported an 8% incidence of infected pseudoaneurysms before 1977, whereas 30% of pseudoaneurysms treated in the following 10 years were infected. This may suggest that infection as a cause of pseudoaneurysm is increasing or it may reflect improved culture techniques of explanted graft specimens.[28]

Graft-Enteric Erosions

Graft-enteric erosions (GEE) result when the graft has eroded through the bowel wall and into the lumen of the bowel. Consequently, there is direct communication between the bowel lumen and the prosthetic graft material. Graft-enteric erosions are not as common as the more dramatic graft-enteric fistula (GEF). Bunt's extensive review (1983) noted 38 documented cases of GEE compared with 256 cases of GEF reported in the literature.[22] However, the true incidence is not known.

The interval between graft placement and development of GEE may range from 2 days to 156 months, but on average, erosions tend to develop in 2 to 3 years. Graft-enteric erosions, like GEF tend to develop most often between the aortic graft and the third or fourth portion of the duodenum. The cause of GEE development is believed to be due to the development of adhesions between graft and bowel followed by mechanical erosion. The most common presentation of GEE was sepsis (57%) and abdominal pain (20%). Graft-enteric erosions are associated with high mortality, being 100% fatal without treatment, but as low as 18% with aggressive management.[13,22]

Graft-Enteric Fistula

Graft-enteric fistula (GEF) may be either primary, occurring without graft material being present, or secondary, occurring after a prosthetic graft has been placed.[32] Secondary GEFs are either type 1 or type 2. Type 1 occurs at the anastomotic suture line. Type 2 is a periprosthetic or paraprosthetic fistulous formation where infection, as a result of erosion of the intestinal wall, reaches the suture line after invasion of the paraprosthetic tissue.[33]

The frequency of aortoenteric fistula was almost seven times greater than the frequency of GEE in Bunt's 1983 review (256 GEF/38 GEE). Paaske reported on eight patients with GEF and one with GEE. The incidence of GEF after aortic graft placement was 0.5%, which appears to be less than earlier reports of 2% to 4%.[22,33] The majority of GEFs occur in the aortoduodenal location; however, they also occur less frequently in the aortojejunal, aortoiliac, and aortosigmoid locations.

More often, GEFs tend to present as delayed complications rather than early complications. Paaske noted a mean of 36 months with a range of 2 weeks to 58 months.[33] Patients may present with a wide range of symptoms which vary from subtle to life threatening complications. Reilly studied 39 patients with GEF and found gastrointestinal bleeding occurred in 61.5% compared to a 9.4% occurrence in patients with periaortic graft infection and 0% incidence in patients with peripheral graft infections. In the past, much emphasis has been placed on *herald bleeding,* which is a self-limited gastrointestinal tract bleed occurring before a massive hemorrhage. Reilly noted that 38% of patients with GEF had no evidence of bleeding at any time. Acute bleeding tends to be associated with an anastomotic (type 1) fistula while paraprosthetic fistulae often did not bleed or bled subacutely.[30] Gastrointestinal tract bleeds can present with hematemesis, melena, or hematochezia.[22] Other findings associated with GEFs included systemic signs with fever, leukocytosis, bacteremia, hypotension, sepsis, septic joint, septic emboli, graft occlusion, abdominal pain, and localized hypertrophic osteoarthropathy.[22,30,34]

Reilly noted that the incidence of sepsis in patients with GEF (21%), was significantly higher than among patients with perigraft infections (3.0%) involving aortoiliac or aortofemoral grafts. While late perigraft infections are frequently related to *S epidermidis,* GEE and GEF are frequently positive for enteric bacteria. Positive cultures from patients with GEFs and GEEs have included *Escherichia coli, Enterococcus, Bacteroides,* and *Streptococcus faecalis.*[35,36] These organisms are more virulent than *S epidermidis,* and may be the cause of the higher incidence of sepsis.

Voiriot reported a case of a man presenting with recurrent episodes of bacteremia and hypertrophic osteoarthropathy. Joint cultures were positive for *Fusobacterium, Peptostreptococcus*, and *E coli*. Blood cultures were positive for *S faecalis, Klebsiella oxytoca, S epidermidis*, and *E coli*. Subsequently, this man was diagnosed with a GEF.[34]

Bunt noted that the factors that predispose to graft infection (GIF) also predispose to GEF. Risk factors include emergency operations, revisionary operations, inadequate peritoneal revascularization, pseudoaneurysms, systemic sepsis, and mycotic aneurysms. The outcome of GEF, if no treatment is provided, is a 100% mortality.[22,33,37]

Late Infections and Staphylococcus Epidermidis

Late graft infections appear to be associated with colonization of the graft material by organisms with low virulence, many of which can produce an environmentally protective surface biofilm. The microorganisms most frequently cultured are coagulase-negative staphylococcal species. *S epidermidis* is the organism most frequently identified.[38] *S epidermidis* has been known for some time to be the prevalent organism associated with infections of indwelling prosthetic devices in humans. It has been identified in infected vascular catheters, heart valves, and total joints. The surface biofilm increases the bacteria's ability to adhere to the graft surface, assists in protecting the bacteria from natural host immune responses and antibacterial drugs, and allows nutrients to reach the bacterial colonies. The biofilm is produced by the bacteria and consists of microcolonies of bacteria and a surrounding fibrous anionic matrix of exopolysaccharide glycocalyx.[21,26] It is becoming clear that the absence of early infec-

tion does not assure graft sterility. Because of the nonvirulent nature of *S epidermidis*, it is difficult to detect early phases of infection. Infection may occur at the time of implantation, during the postoperative recovery phase, or possibly even during bacteremic events well after discharge from the hospital.

There is little if any host inflammatory response during the initial colonization of the graft by *S epidermidis*. Clinical infection may not appear for years. During this time, autolysis and suture-line tension strength may diminish, resulting in graft-healing complications such as loss of graft incorporation, pseudoaneurysm, and sinus tract formation.[21,26] Bacteria sequestered within a surface biofilm may not always be identified by routine culture techniques. Tollefson reported on seven patients with femoral anastomotic pseudoaneurysms. Explanted graft material was sent for routine culture studies and also cultures after ultrasonic oscillation of graft material. Only one out of four cultured on agar plates was positive; three out of seven broth cultures were positive; however, all seven cultures were positive after ultrasonic oscillation. All seven grafts grew *S epidermidis*, occurring from 5 to 13 years after graft implantation.[21] This demonstrates that routine culture techniques may result in no growth, but if the same specimen is subjected to ultrasonic disruption of the graft biofilm, then cultures may actually be positive.

Using ultrasonic oscillation to disrupt surface biofilm or *slime* in explanted prosthetic graft from patients undergoing graft revision for femoral pseudoaneurysm or thrombosed grafts without clinical evidence of graft infection, Kaebnick found the overall incidence of colonization of vascular prosthesis was 79%. The subgroup of patients with pseudoaneurysms had a 90% positive culture rate while those presenting with graft thrombosis had a 69% positive culture rate.[26] This suggests that graft colonization with low-virulence *S epidermidis* plays a role in the development of anastomotic aneurysms.

Slime production, that ability to produce a surface biofilm, is a characteristic of many of the *S epidermidis* cultures isolated from prosthetic grafts and has been implicated as a pathogenic characteristic.[39] Seabrook noted 42% of coagulase-negative staphylococcal isolates from anastomotic aneurysms exhibited the ability to produce an exopolysaccharide slime.[9]

Tollefson found 75% and Kaebnick found that 87% of the *S epidermidis* recovered from anastomotic aneurysms produced slime. Kaebnick also noted that 33% of the *S epidermidis* isolated from thrombosed grafts produced slime.[21,26] The recovery rate of slime-producing *S epidermidis* appears to be highest with anastomotic aneurysms suggesting that the growth characteristics of bacteria able to produce a biofilm may be associated with late graft complications, such as anastomotic aneurysms and lack of graft incorporation. This is particularly impressive since these organisms are generally considered to be associated with low virulence.

Many patients present with clinically silent late graft infections. Even when purulent material and poor graft incorporation is observed at the time of surgery, it is difficult to identify the infecting organism by routine cultures.[18] Culture techniques may be the cause of significant discrepancy. The actual incidence of graft infections may vary depending on the methods used. Sonication of graft specimens to disrupt surface biofilms has significantly increased the number of positive cultures compared to routine culture results.[21]

Using sonication techniques to investigate bacterial adherence to graft material has produced some conflicting reports. Schmitt reported that bacterial adherence to expanded polytetrafluoroethylene (ePTFE) is decreased compared to woven or knitted Dacron graft for both Gram-positive and Gram-negative organisms.[40,41] Tollefson, working with a canine model, reported no statistical difference in the incidence of microorganism recovery from contaminated knitted Dacron grafts (80%) compared with PTFE grafts (64%).[21] Similarly, there was no statistical difference demonstrated in the incidence of colonization of Dacron (82%) or PTFE (69%) by Kaebnick while studying explanted graft material from 44 patients.[26] Polterauer et al. compared Dacron and PTFE grafts in a prospective, randomized trial and failed to confirm any advantage of PTFE over Dacron in aortoiliac surgery.[42] Based on culture results using sonication techniques, there does not appear to be a significant difference in infectability between PTFE and Dacron grafts.

Risk

Graft infection may occur during the intraoperative, perioperative, or posthospitalization periods. There are many opportunities for the sterile graft to become contaminated. Possible breaks in sterile technique in the operating room, skin contamination, unrecognized violation of the gastrointestinal tract, contamination by mycotic aneurysms, culture-positive aneurysmal wall and thrombic wound infections, bacteremia, and lymphatic spread may all be factors in establishing colonization of the prosthetic graft and subsequent complications both early and late (Table 6).

Table 6
Risk Factors of Graft Contamination

Sterile technique
Skin contamination
GI tract violation
Periaortic tissues
Arterial wall
Bacteremia
Lymphatic spread
Wound complications
Emergency surgery
Secondary procedures
Additional procedures

(GI = gastrointestinal).

Contamination of the graft by skin flora was investigated by Wooster in a prospective trial. Although no gross breaks in sterile technique were identified, grafts became contaminated in 56% of cases using standard sterile techniques. The graft contamination rate was lowered to 35% when the surgeon changed gloves before preclotting the graft. Subsequent positive graft cultures correlated with the patients' skin cultures. Despite the high rate of contamination, only one patient (1.3%) developed a graft infection.[43]

Seeding of the graft from an infected site during a bacteremic episode has also been implicated. Occasionally, patients have been noted to have urinary tract infections, pneumonia, and soft tissue infection at the time of surgery. Samson et al. noted that of 34 patients with a major graft infection, 16 had soft tissue infections of the foot or toe at the time of their last vascular graft placement.[6] Liekweg and Greenfield reported that ipsilateral inguinal infections occurred proximal to open foot infections in 33% (20/60) of cases. However, Bouhoutsos noted no significant increase in graft infections in patients with foot infections.[44]

The association of graft infection and groin incision appears to be clearer. This may be related to the fact that the concentration of staphylococcal species in the axilla and groin is quite high. It is also difficult to keep the groin dry postoperatively, and skin can easily macerate in these areas. Szylagyi found that 23 out of 40 graft infections occurred at inguinal incisions.[10] Goldstone found that 77% of graft infections occurred at the inguinal incision.[1] Cherry noted 64.1% (25/39) of patients with infected lower extremity grafts had previous groin operations.[14] Fletcher commented that the groin was the most common site of infection, occurring in 45% (5/11).[11] Jamieson reported that there was only a 2% (6/293) incidence of graft infection when the inguinal incision healed without complication; however, when there was a complication, defined as swelling, drainage of blood, or ser-

ous fluid, then the incidence of graft infection 18% (4/22) was significantly higher.[45] Yashar noted that 33% of wound hematomas were associated with graft infection.[46] Thus, it appears that wound complications are associated with an increased risk of prosthetic graft infection.

Lymphatic transport of bacteria has also been implicated in graft contamination. Bunt and Mohr found 27% (8/30) of inguinal lymph nodes harvested from normal legs were positive for *S epidermidis*. Two other patients with distal extremity infection had cultures that grew out cephalothin-resistant bacteria identical to bacteria at the other site.[47] Rubin performed lymphatic transection in dogs and found the incidence of graft infection was only 20% in the group undergoing excision and ligation of lymphatics compared to an 87.5% rate in the transection group and preservation group.[48] White obtained preoperative and postoperative lymphangiograms on canines. Major lymphatic channels with numerous interconnections about the aorta were documented. Immediate postoperative lymphangiograms revealed a significant lymphatic leak and contrast pooling in the area of dissection. By postoperative day 7, leakage was no longer present.[49] It appears that intact lymphatics probably contribute to hematogenous contamination of prosthetic grafts while disrupted lymphatics may result in pooling of contaminated lymph fluid in the dissected field.

The arterial wall and perianeurysmal contents are also suspected in the pathogenesis of graft infection. Schwartz cultured tissue from abdominal aortic aneurysms finding positive cultures in 10.4% (22/211). *S epidermidis* was the most common organism recovered 54% (12/22).[50] Ernst found 15% (12/78) positive aneurysm wall cultures, isolating *S epidermidis* in 56%.[51]

Emergency surgery is also considered a risk factor for repair of abdominal aortic aneurysms (AAA). Positive intraoperative culture rates for ruptured AAA range from 7.5% to 38%, symptomatic aneurysms 6.2%

to 13%, and for elective cases 0.8% to 9.4%.[11,45,50,51] In Ernst's series, if operative cultures were positive, the late graft sepsis rate was 10%; however, if operative cultures were negative, the late graft sepsis rate was only 2%. It appears that late graft infection is more likely to develop after emergency surgery and when positive operative cultures are identified.[15,51]

Another risk factor for prosthetic graft infection is revisionary or secondary procedures.[5,52] Goldstone and Moore noted that 46% of infections occurred after surgical revision.[1] While studying patients with pseudoaneurysms, Seabrook noted cultures identifying bacteria in 76% (13/17) of patients' grafts who had previous secondary operative procedures in the groin compared to only 50% (14/28) positive cultures in explanted grafts when no prior secondary groin procedure was performed.[9]

Additional procedures that are performed at the same time as the graft placement have also been investigated as a potential source of contamination. Goldstone and Moore noted that 2 of 14 graft infections were associated with an incidental appendectomy at the time of vascular reconstruction.[1] Edwards et al. identified risk factors for infection in 19 patients (79%). In three cases, other operations were added which included lumbar sympathectomy, inguinal hernia repair, and cholecystectomy.[53] In another series by Edwards et al., 3 out of 18 patients with graft infection had a tube gastrostomy; 2 of the 3 also underwent a vagotomy, pyloroplasty, and cholecystectomy.[19] Ameli et al. retrospectively reviewed 56 patients who underwent cholecystectomy at the same time as aortic aneurysm repair or aortofemoral bypass. Although one patient developed a graft infection, this was unrelated to the cholecystectomy. Ameli concluded that concomitant cholecystectomy can be performed without increased risk if the vascular procedure has been uncomplicated and if the cholecystectomy appears straightforward.[54] The actual risk of graft infection secondary to concomitant procedures is unknown; however, prior to performing additional procedures, the potential risks and benefits must be carefully considered.

Summary

Early and late prosthetic graft infections present with various clinical signs and symptoms. While early infections are usually associated with purulent wounds, late graft infections often are occult with no symptoms or are associated with late graft complications, which may or may not be clinically evident, such as anastomotic aneurysms, graft-enteric erosions, graft-enteric fistulae, and cutaneous sinus tracts. Clinical presentation may even be misleading such as in the patient on multiple medications with upper or lower gastrointestinal tract bleeding or in patients with other associated nonspecific problems, such as fever or leukocytosis. Without a high degree of suspicion and knowledge of the natural history of graft infections, the diagnosis could easily be delayed or missed. Early graft infections more frequently grow out *S aureus*, while late graft infections more often are associated with *S epidermidis*. Antibiotic prophylaxis in the perioperative period has significantly reduced the number of early graft infections. In recent years, there has been an increase in the number of late graft infections, yet many of these are occult infections. In part, this increase probably reflects new microbiologic culture techniques and improved handling. This may also reflect increased clinical awareness and recognition of late graft infections. The complications of graft infections both early and late are associated with significant morbidity and mortality. Risk of graft infection appears to be associated with emergency operations, groin incisions with a history of subsequent complications, and a history of secondary procedures. Along with these risk factors, there are several other factors implicated in the pathogenesis of graft infections.

References

1. Goldstone J, Moore WS. Infection in vascular prostheses. *Am J Surg.* 1974;128:225–233.
2. Macbeth GA, Rubin JR, McIntyre KE, et al. The relevance of arterial wall microbiology to the treatment of prosthetic graft infections: graft infection vs. arterial infection. *J Vasc Surg.* 1984;1:750–756.
3. DeRose G, Provan JL. Infected arterial grafts: clinical manifestations and surgical management. *J Card Surg.* 1984;25:51–57.
4. Satiani B. False aneurysms following arterial reconstruction. *Surg Gynecol Obstet.* 1981;152:357–363.
5. Liekweg WG, Greenfield LJ. Vascular prosthetic infections: collected experience and results of treatment. *Surgery.* 1977;81:335–342.
6. Samson RH, Veith FJ, Janko GS, et al. A modified classification and approach to the management of infections involving peripheral arterial prosthetic grafts. *J Vasc Surg.* 1988;8:147–153.
7. Johnson JA, Cogbill TH, Strutt PJ, et al. Wound complications after infrainguinal bypass. *Arch Surg.* 1988;123:859–862.
8. Lorentzen JE. Graft infection: introduction. *Acta Chir Scand.* 1987;538:70–71.
9. Seabrook GR, Schmitt DD, Bandyk DF, et al. Anastomotic femoral pseudoaneurysm: an investigation of occult infection as an etiologic factor. *J Vasc Surg.* 1990;11:629–634.
10. Szylagyi DE, Smith RF, Elliott JP. Infection in arterial reconstruction with synthetic grafts. *Ann Surg.* 1972;176:321–333.
11. Fletcher JP, Dryden M, Sorrell TC. Infection of vascular prostheses. *Aust NZ J Surg.* 1991;61:432–435.
12. Bandyk DF, Bergamini TM, Kinney EV, et al. In situ replacement of vascular prostheses infected by bacterial biofilms. *J Vasc Surg.* 1991;13:575–583.
13. Brand EJ, Sivak MV, Sullivan BH. Aortoduodenal fistula endoscopic diagnosis. *Dig Dis Sci.* 1979;24:940–944.
14. Cherry KV, Roland CF, Pairolero PC, et al. Infected femorodistal bypass: is a graft removal mandatory? *J Vasc Surg.* 1992;15:295–305.
15. Buckels JA, Fielding JW, Black J, et al. Significance of positive bacterial cultures from aortic aneurysm contents. *Br J Surg.* 1985;72:440–442.
16. Bunt TJ. Synthetic vascular graft infections I: graft infections. *Surgery.* 1983;93:733–746.
17. Kaiser AB, et al. Antibiotic prophylaxis in vascular surgery. *Ann Surg.* 1979;188:283–289.
18. Bandyk DF, Berni GA, Thiele BL, et al. Aorto-femoral graft infection due to *Staphylocccus epidermidis*. *Arch Surg.* 1984;119:102–108.
19. Edwards MJ, Richardson JD, Klamer TW. Management of aortic prosthetic infections. *Am Surg.* 1988;155:327–330.
20. Satiani B, Kazmers M, Evans WE. Anastomotic arterial aneurysms: a continuing challenge. *Ann Surg.* 1980;192:674–682.
21. Tollefson DF, Bandyk DF, Kaebnick HW, et al. Surface biofilm disruption. *Arch Surg.* 1987;122:38–43.
22. Bunt TJ. Synthetic vascular graft infections II: graft enteric erosions and graft enteric fistulas. *Surgery* 1983;94:1–9.
23. Gutman H, Zelikovski A, Reiss R. Ruptured anastomotic pseudoaneurysms after prosthetic vascular graft bypass procedures. *Isr J Med Sci.* 1984;20:613–617.
24. Haiart DC, Callam MJ, Ruckley CV, et al. Reoperations for late complications following abdominal aortic operation. *Br J Surg.* 1991;78:204–206.
25. Cooley DA, Wukasch DC, Bennett JG, et al. Double velour knitted Dacron grafts for aortic vascular replacement. In: Sawer PN, Kaplitt MJ, eds. *Vascular Grafts.* New York: Appleton-Century-Crofts; 1978;197.
26. Kaebnick HW, Bandyk DF, Bergamini TW, et al. The microbiology of explanted vascular prostheses. *Surgery.* 1987;102:756–762.
27. Berridge DC, Earnshaw JJ, Makin GS, et al. A 10-year review of false aneurysms in Nottingham. *Ann R Coll Surg.* 1988;70:253–256.
28. Sedwitz MM, Hye RJ, Stabile BE. The changing epidemiology of pseudoaneurysm. *Arch Surg.* 1988;123:473–476.
29. Welch GH, Reid DB, Pollock JG. Infected false aneurysms in the groin of intravenous drug abusers. *Br J Surg.* 1990;77:330–333.
30. Reilly LM, Ehrenfeld WK, Goldstone J, et al. Gastrointestinal tract involvement by prosthetic graft infection. *Ann Surg.* 1985;302:342–348.
31. Szylagyi DE, Smith RF, Elliott JP, et al. Anastomotic aneurysms after vascular reconstruction: problems of incidence, etiology, and treatment. *Surgery.* 1975;78:800–816.
32. Wheeler WE, Hanks J, Raman VK. Primary aortoenteric fistulas. *Am Surg.* 1992;58:53–54.
33. Paaske WP, Hansen HJ. Graft enteric fistulas and erosions. *Surg Gynecol Obstet.* 1985;161:161–164.
34. Voiriot P, Duperval R, Teijeira J, et al. Localized hypertrophic osteoarthropathy due to arterial graft sepsis from an enteroprosthetic fistula. *Rev Infect Dis.* 1987;9:376–381.
35. Becker RM, Blundell PE. Infected aortic bi-

furcation grafts: with 14 patients. *Surgery.* 1976;80:544–549.

36. Busuttil RW, Rees WR, Baker JD, et al. Pathogenesis of aortoduodenal fistula: experimental and clinical correlates. *Surgery.* 1979;85:1–13.

37. Corson JD, Baraniewski HM, Shah DM. Large diameter expanded polytetrafluoroethylene grafts for infrarenal aortic aneurysm surgery. *J Card Surg.* 1990;31:702–705.

38. Vinard E, Eloy R, Descotes J, et al. Human vascular graft failure and frequency of infection. *J Biomed Mater Res.* 1991;25: 499–513.

39. Lalka SG, Malone JM, Fisher DF, et al. Efficacy of prophylactic antibiotics in vascular surgery: an arterial wall microbiologic and pharmacokinetic perspective. *J Vasc Surg.* 1989;10:501–510.

40. Schmitt DD, Bandyk DF, Pequet AJ, et al. Mucin production by *Staphylococcus epidermidis. Arch Surg.* 1986;121:89–95.

41. Schmitt DD, Bandyk DF, Pequet AJ, et al. Bacterial adherence to vascular prostheses. *Vasc Surg.* 1986;3:732–740.

42. Polterauer P, Prager M, Holzenbein T, et al. Dacron versus polytetrafluoroethylene for Y-aortic bifurcation grafts: a six-year prospective, randomized trial. *Surgery.* 1992;111: 626–633.

43. Wooster DL, Louch RE, Krajden S. Intraoperative bacterial contamination of vascular grafts: a prospective study. *Can J Surg.* 1985; 28:407–409.

44. Bouhoutsos J, Chavatzas D, Martin P, et al. Infected synthetic arterial grafts. *Br J Surg.* 1974;61:108–111.

45. Jamieson GG, DeWeese JA, Rob CG. Infected arterial grafts. *Ann Surg.* 1975;181:850–852.

46. Yashar JJ, Weyman AK, Burnard RJ, et al. Survival and limb salvage in patients with infected arterial prostheses. *Am J Surg.* 1978; 135:499–504.

47. Bunt TJ, Mohr JD. Incidence of positive inguinal lymph node culture during peripheral revascularization. *Am Surg.* 1984;10: 522–523.

48. Rubin JR, Malone JM, Goldstone J. The role of the lymphatic system in acute arterial prosthetic graft infections. *J Vasc Surg.* 1985; 2:92–98.

49. White JV, Freda J, Kozar R, et al. Does bacteremia pose a direct threat to synthetic vascular grafts? *Surgery.* 1987;102:402–408.

50. Schwartz JA, Powell TW, Burnham SJ, et al. Culture of abdominal aortic aneurysm contents. *Arch Surg.* 1987;122:777–780.

51. Ernst CB, Campbell HC, Daughtery ME, et al. Incidence and significance of intraoperative bacterial cultures during abdominal aortic aneurysmectomy. *Ann Surg.* 1977;185: 626–633.

52. Reifsnyder T, Bandyk DF, Seabrook G. Wound complications of the in situ saphenous vein bypass technique. *J Vasc Surg.* 1992;15:843–850.

53. Edwards WH, Martin RS III, Jenkins JM, et al. Primary graft infections. *J Vasc Surg.* 1987; 6:235–239.

54. Ameli FM, Weiss M, Provan JL, et al. Safety of cholecystectomy with abdominal aortic surgery. *Can J Surg.* 1987;30:170–173.

Chapter 4.1

Epidemiology: Immunocompetence

T.J. Bunt

Introduction

Prophylaxis of both wound and graft infections may be initiated at three fronts:

1. Eradication or control of potential pathogens by prophylactic antibiotics.
2. Minimal destruction of the body's intact defensive environment; that is, good surgical technique to minimize wound problems (hematomas, lymphatic leaks, undue tissue injury, dead space) and less well-recognized conditions as iatrogenic vascular injury, for which the reader is referred to a previous text.[1]
3. Preservation or augmentation of the host's immunologic and related defense mechanisms.

The role of host defense mechanisms has been elucidated by a number of surgical researchers who have demonstrated that anergic patients have higher septic complications and eventual mortality rates than patients demonstrating immunoreactive systems.

The potential for surgical induction of immunosuppression developed out of the recognition of immunosuppression after major burns or trauma, and was based on the concept of major surgery as a "controlled trauma." Immunosuppression was noted to be profound but of short duration after cholecystectomy , and to be more prolonged in duration after major trauma. This led a number of researchers to study the possibility of an equivalent immunosuppression following major vascular surgery, with the view toward this being a potential etiologic factor in the development of vascular graft infections.

Literature Review

The groundwork was laid by Meakins et al. in several publications from 1975 to 1979. They demonstrated that cutaneous anergy was a marker for sepsis and mortality in surgical patients, and that anergy was associated with age greater than 80, carcinoma, malnutrition, shock, sepsis, and major trauma. In a study of 1332 patients, those with normal skin testing had a 7% major sepsis and 2% mortality rate versus 52% sepsis and 36% mortality rates for anergic patients. Anergy could be reversed by successful correction of the underlying general surgical condition in 84% of patients. Total parenteral nutrition could also reverse the anergic state; levamisole appeared to also be beneficial.[2–4]

Specific application ot the vascular situation then appeared. Christou in 1986 studied 64 elective and nine emergency peripheral vascular surgical patients, excluding for study those who died within 24 hours of admission. Five recall antigens were tested and reported as a mean score of induration (not erythema); a positive test was 8 mm or greater induration at 24 hours. Anergy was defined as no response to any test, and reactivity if two or more responses were positive. Additional measures of immunocompetence included whole blood neutrophil adherence and neutrophil chemotaxis. The study included 58 men and 15 women, average age 63.2 ± 9.8 years, undergoing 37 aortic aneurysmorrhaphies, 22 aortic reconstructions, and 7 infected aortic graft resections.

Eighty-nine percent of patients undergoing elective cases were reactive, 5% relatively anergic, and 6% anergic. The mortality for the reactive group was 4%, none with septic etiology. However, three of the four anergic patients suffered major bacteremic sepsis, two from pneumonitis and the third from a central line; two of the three died of septic complications.

Two patients for ruptured abdominal aortic aneurysmorrhaphy arrived relatively anergic, became totally anergic within 24 hours, and died of sepsis. Only one of seven patients with infected aortic grafts was reactive at admission; all seven had further septic complications; the only reactive patient survived, whereas two of the remaining six died of sepsis. The four who recovered had lesser degrees of infection and converted to positive reactivity within 1 week of admission. Thus, the researchers were able to convincingly relate immunocompetence to the incidence and mortaltiy of postoperative septic complications. A pessimistic note was, however, added; attempt to correct the immunosuppression by postoperative nutritional manipulation did not reverse the defects. Presumably, preoperative manipulation would have been more useful, but no data was presented.[5]

Casey, speaking for the Northwestern group in 1983, studied the role of nutritional depletion/malnutrition in inducing failure of immunocompetence in 79 patients. Markers of competence included height, weight, mid-arm circumference, triceps skin fold; serum albumin, zinc, transferrin, and lymphocyte counts, and cutaneous anergy panel. Patients were then observed postoperatively for wound problems indicating delayed healing or infection. Significant variables identified were a serum albumin less than 3 gm/dL and transferrin levels less than 150 mg/dL ($P < .0001$). Only 29% of anergic patients had normal wound healing, while 56% with normal cutaneus reactivity had normal healing. Anthropometric measurements were not, per se, predictive. The patients studied included 15 cases of aortic reconstructions, 52 cases of femorodistal bypasses, and 4 cases of extra-anatomic bypasses. All were 70 years of age or older and were felt to be high risk due to medical illness, repetitive surgery, and ischemic or nonhealing wound problems.

The study thus indicates that there is a high incidence of malnutrition in a largely nursing-home-aged population which requires predominantly distal revascularization for ischemic ulcer or gangrene, and that serum albumin and transferrin are more selective predictors of wound problems than cutaneous anergy or anthropometric parameters. One can also note the high incidence (30% to 49%) of wound problems in normal patients at this age and debility.[6]

Keane, speaking in 1982 for the Hopkins group, studied 13 patients for aortic revascularization under nonimmunosuppressive anethesia. Procedures averaged 40 minutes in patients whose average age was 60 years (51 to 72); anesthesia was thiopental-nitrous oxide-enflurane. Immunocompetence was assayed as lymphocyte responsiveness to streptodornase, mumps, phytohemagglutinin, and concanavalin A. All 13 patients showed postoperative depression from normal preoperative states; pooled results were used. Response to streptodornase fell from 10.447 ± 3842 CPM (mean ± SEM) to 1441 ± 600 at 1 to 4 days ($P < .05$), 1967 ± 497 at 5 to 8 days and 637 ± 173 (NS) at 9 to 11 days ($P < .05$). Response to mumps fell from 13.251 ± 3803 to 2079 ± 1360 ($P < .05$), 3699 ± 1515 ($P < .05$), and 400 ± 103; to phytohemaglobin from 79.601 ± 7.33 to 44.136 ± 6310 ($P < .001$), 52.380 ± 7414 ($P < .05$); and 50.287 ± 13.193; and to concanavalin A from 21, 502 ± 2984 to 5823 ± 1603 ($P < .001$), 11.829 ± 3329 ($P < .05$), and 8235 ± 2958 ($P < .05$). Despite the observed immunosuppression and its persistence through the second postoperative week, the patients' courses were uncomplicated and none showed serious postoperative sepsis, which the researchers attributed to concomitant continuous antibiotic usage.[7]

Kwaan, in 1984, studied 12 patients with established "advanced and fulminating" graft infections and noted critical deficiencies in immunocompetence in all 12. Graft infections (GIFs) were aortic in 8, and axillofemoral and femoropopliteal in 4 each, respectively; all grafts were Dacron; 6 were with *Pseudomonas*, 4 *Staphylococcus aureus*, and 2 *Escherichia coli*. Four patients with aortic GIF recieved no specific immunologic support; 2 died of aortic stump sepsis, and 2 survived stormy courses with major amputations. Conversely, 8 patients receiving total parenteral coverage had shorter hospital stays (mean 6 weeks) with fewer complications; 6 of the 8 reverted to normal cutaneus responses.[8]

Although this paper echoes the previous ones on the high incidence of anergy in patients who develop septic or GIF complications, and suggests a beneficial effect of total parenteral nutrition (TPN) in decreasing the morbidity and mortality of subsequent GIF management, it must be addressed with some caution. The groups are not comparable even at face value—four aortic versus four aortic plus four peripheral GIFs; the treatment modalities for each are not detailed nor are the bacteria correlated with either success or failure of therapy. All of the pertinent individual facts are lost in the summary presentation. Furthermore, it is not clearly stated *when* anergic conversion occurred, and whether this represented the expected cause of events after successful surgical removal of the septic source, or whether successful conversion obtained *prior* to graft removal allowed it to be done successfully. And finally, the positive effect of TPN on outcome may be entirely due to restoration of adequate nutritional balance in patients who were clearly stated to be *emaciated* at admission; and therefore *not* candidates for operation until weight gain was restored. Anergic conversion may have been an unrelated and incidental phenomenon. Be that as it may, the paper does at least suggest a beneficial effect of TPN in the treatment of GIF, in part by restoration of weight and nutritional status and potentially in part by reversal of cutaneous anergy.

Discussion

One can summarize the limited literature on immunocompetence in vascular surgery by stating that in general the principles of surgical nutrition should be equally applicable to major vascular surgery. The longer and larger the case, the more likely profound immunosuppression will occur and the longer it is likely to last postoperatively. A higher frequency of septic complications is to be expected with immunosuppression; however, an actual increase in the incidence of subsequent graft infection has not been proven, in large part due to the small series evaluated to date.

Significant immunosuppression would not be expected in a reasonably healthy, well-nourished individual undergoing lesser degrees of invasive vascular surgery (femoropopliteal, carotid, or perhaps extra-anatomic bypass) but might be a significant contributing factor if there is evidence of the established risk factors (age, cancer, malnutrition), if aortic surgery is contemplated, or when emergency surgery (risk factor of shock) is involved. In all of these situations, preoperative anergy testing might well be indicated. Detection of significant immunosuppression might then be a valid if relative contraindication of the contemplated surgery, pending its correction with hyperalimentation, etc.

References

1. Bunt T.J. *Iatrogenic Vascular Injury: a Discourse on Surgical Technique.* Mt. Kisco: Futura Pub Co, Inc; 1990.
2. Meakins JL, Christou NV, Shizgal HM, et al. Therapeutic approaches to anergy in surgical patients: surgery and levamisole. *Ann Surg.* 1979;190:3:286–295.
3. Meakins JL, MacLean APH, Kelly R, et al. Delayed hypersensitivity and chemotaxis: effect of trauma. *J Trauma.* 1978;18:240–243.
4. Meakins JL, Pietsch JB, Bubenik O, et al. Delayed hypersensitivity: indicator of acquired failure of host defenses in sepsis and trauma. *Ann Surg.* 1977:186:241–246.
5. Christou NV, Morin JE. Host defense mechanisms in elective and emergency vascular surgery: predicting septic-related mortality. *J Vasc Surg.* 1986;3:2:338–343.
6. Casey J, Flinn WR, Yao JST, et al. Correlation of immune and nutritional status with wound complications in patients undergoing vascular operations. *Surgery.* 1983;93:822–827.
7. Keane RM, Munster AM, Birmingham W, et al. Suppression of lymphocyte function after aortic reconstruction: use of nonimmunosuppressive anesthesia. *Arch Surg.* 1982;117:9:1133–1135.
8. Kwaan JHM, Dahe RK, Connolly J. Immunocompetence in patients with prosthetic graft infection. *J Vasc Surg.* 1984;1:1:45–51.

Chapter 4.2

Pathobiology of the Graft Surface Bacterial Biofilm

T.M. Bergamini

Introduction

In recent years, it has become widely recognized that delayed vascular prosthesis infections in humans are often secondary to *Staphylococcus epidermidis*; for example, Bandyk et al.[1] identified *S epidermidis* as the pathogen in 60% of cases of aortofemoral graft infection. Emphasis has also been placed on the difficulty in diagnosing the graft infection caused by these low-virulent organisms that present late, without the classic signs of graft sepsis; this is due to their survival in a surface biofilm. Bacterial biofilm infections have been shown to affect a wide variety of biomaterials and devices that are routinely implanted in humans including hip prostheses, prosthetic heart valves, peritoneal dialysis catheters, intravenous catheters, cerebrospinal fluid shunts, as well as vascular grafts.[2] Despite great differences in the surface characteristics of the biomaterials and the anatomic site of implantation, the underlying pathobiology of the biomaterial surface bacterial biofilm is strikingly similar. The low-virulent organisms colonize, adhere, and harbor in a graft surface biofilm, a very complex structure that provides the optimal environment for persistent growth of *S epidermidis*. The graft surface bacterial biofilm is composed of coalescing microcolonies of bacteria which are enclosed in an extracellular nutrient glycocalyx produced by the organisms, also known as "slime." The bacteria are present only in very low concentration along the prosthetic surface and have a stationary mode of growth. The slime layer provides nutrients and protection from host defenses, permitting bacterial growth on the prosthetic surface.

Initially, the graft surface bacterial biofilm results in a symbiotic infection, with no clinically apparent signs or symptoms. After a dormant period, a poorly understood event triggers an interaction between the graft surface bacterial biofilm and the patient's immune system. Host recognition of the bacterial biofilm provokes a chronic inflammatory process, resulting in a perigraft abscess, anastomotic pseudoaneurysm, or a graft-cutaneous sinus tract (Fig. 1). Clinical recognition of these rare but curious graft infections is late, typically months to years following implantation.[1,3,4]

The two most important factors in the

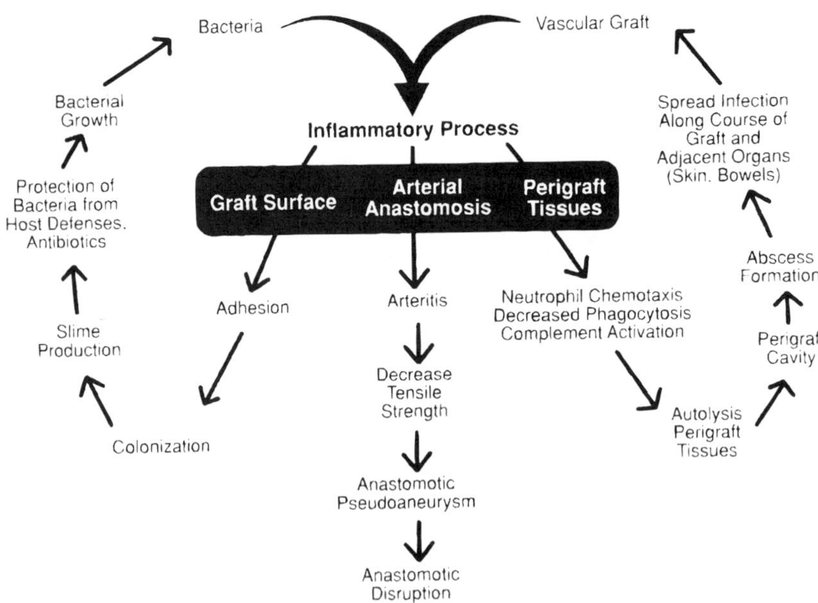

Figure 1. Diagram of the pathobiology of the inflammatory process created by the graft surface bacterial biofilm.

pathobiology of the bacterial biofilm graft infections are the mechanisms of bacterial adherence and immune regulation of the surface biofilm. Only in the past decade have these two factors been studied. If the incidence and treatment of graft infections are to be improved, it will be the result of a better understanding of the interactions between the bacteria, adherence on the prosthetic surface, and regulation of the immune response. This chapter will focus on the recent investigations into the adherence and immune regulation of the graft surface bacterial biofilm, with the goal of decreasing the incidence and improving the outcome of these dreaded infections.

Adherence

Adhesion of bacteria to the surface of the prosthesis is a fundamental initial step in the pathogenesis of graft infection. The relative adhesiveness of bacteria to vascular grafts,[5] cardiac valves,[6] cerebrospinal fluid shunts,[7] and intravascular catheters[8] has been shown to correlate with the occurrence of clinical infection. Adherence is dependent upon the bacterial species and the physical and chemical properties of graft surface. The cell wall structure and substances produced by the bacteria can affect adherence. There is a wide strain-to-strain variation in the adherence of *S epidermidis*, *Staphylococcus aureus*, and *Escherichia coli* to biomaterials. *S aureus* adheres to suture and vascular grafts at rates as high as two logs greater than *E. coli*.[5,9] *S epidermidis* (RP-12) adheres more tenaciously to graft material than *S epidermidis* (SP-2).[5] To further complicate the problem of determining bacterial adherence, *S epidermidis* has many recognized strains and is just one of more than 25 recognized species of coagulase-negative staphylococci that have been recovered from clinical specimens.[10]

The predilection of these organisms for foreign body infection is not well understood, but pathogenic strains, those that characteristically have an increased quantitative adherence to prosthetic surfaces, produce slime. Slime-producing organisms adhere significantly better to a variety of biomaterials than do nonslime producing strains.[8,11,12] Slime-producing strains of *S epidermidis* adhered 10 to 100 times greater to vascular grafts than nonslime-producing strains.[13] Slime production is therefore a commonly recognized virulence factor for clinically significant *S epidermidis* infections of biomaterials. Eighty-seven percent of *S epidermidis* recovered from infected vascular grafts with anastomotic pseudoaneurysm demonstrate the capability to produce slime.

The actual mechanisms that lead to the production of the tenacious bacterial surface biofilm known as slime is not known. The slime is a viscus, mucoid substance made up of an exopolysaccharide glycocalyx that provides protection and nutrients for bacterial growth. Bacterial adhesion and formation of microcolonies are mediated by this maze of polysaccharide fibers that extends from the bacterial cell(s) surface to biomaterial surface. Specific mediators of adhesion to biomaterial surfaces are now being identified within the exopolysaccharide glycocalyx. Peters et al.[14] have identified a mannose-rich material from *S epidermidis* (KH-11) which they have named extracellular slime substance (ESS). The ESS was identified from both slime and nonslime-producing strains of *S epidermidis*, and thus was not specific for slime production. Christensen et al.[15] has isolated an antigenic marker specific for slime production called slime-associated antigen (SAA). Pier et al. has characterized exopolysaccharides from *S epidermidis*,[16] *Pseudomonas aeruginosa*,[17] and *S aureus*.[18] The galactose-rich substance isolated from *S epidermidis* (RP-62A) is called capsular polysaccharide adhesin (CPA). Pier has demonstrated that purified CPA produced by *S epidermidis* strains will adhere to silastic tubing, that coating the catheter with CPA will prevent bacterial adherence, and that antibody to CPA from RP-62A will inhibit bacterial adherence.

The further identification and characterization of specific adhesins and receptors for adhesion of bacteria to biomaterial surfaces may lead to the development of methods for the prevention of bacterial adherence and prosthetic infections. Slime promotes adherence to the prostheses but also impedes the identification of the organisms by routine culture. Investigations into the mechanisms of bacterial adherence and slime production began with the development of innovative methods for processing explanted biomaterial for culture. Routine microbiologic techniques will frequently not recover the microorganism from the graft or surrounding tissues.[1,19-21] We have demonstrated in vitro, in a canine model and from human graft specimens, that identification of *S epidermidis* is not accurate with routine culture techniques because the bacteria are sequestered in the graft surface biofilm. In addition, because these low-virulence organisms do not invade the perigraft tissues, culture of the blood or fluid/tissue surrounding the graft will be negative. Mechanical disruption of the surface biofilm from the graft is therefore a necessary and optimal method for identifying the pathogen. (Fig. 2). Disruption of the surface biofilm, by either ultrasonic oscillation or tissue grinding, permits dispersion of the bacteria into the broth media for optimal growth and subsequent identification.[17] Quantitative determination of bacterial adherence to the graft surface can be performed with serial dilutions of the effluent following mechanical biofilm disruption.[13]

Results of microbiologic studies of biomaterial infections due to surface bacterial biofilms have demonstrated, however, that nonslime-producing *S epidermidis* can result in clinically significant infections as well. Therefore, other factors besides slime must also be important in the mediation of bacterial adherence and growth. For example, the surface composition and construction of the biomaterial has been shown to affect bacterial adherence. *S epidermidis*, *E. coli*, and *S aureus* adhere to Dacron vascular grafts in

Microbiology Recovery Techniques

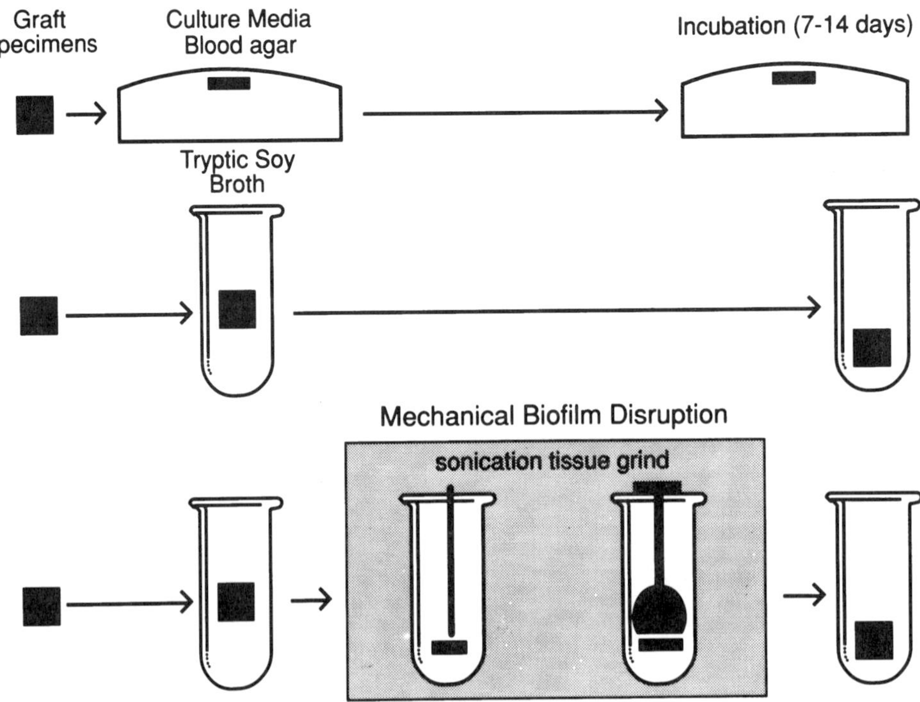

Figure 2. Microbiology recovery techniques. Mechanical biofilm disruption with broth culture of the graft is the most sensitive microbiologic technique for recovering *Staphylococcus epidermidis* when compared to agar or broth culture alone.

greater numbers than polytetrafluroethylene (PTFE). These organisms adhere to velour knitted Dacron fibers in significantly higher numbers than woven Dacron.[5] The surface area may partially explain the difference in bacterial adherence, as PTFE is relatively nonporous compared to Dacron. The chemical structure of the graft is also important, as PTFE is more hydrophobic than Dacron and less likely to form bonds with bacteria whose cell walls also have hydrophobic properties. Decreasing the hydrophobicity of the biomaterial surface by coating it with albumin has been shown to decrease bacterial adherence to intravascular catheters[22] and Dacron grafts.[23] Other studies, however, have shown no correlation between hydrophobicity and bacterial

adherence, mandating the need for further investigations.[24]

The determination of bacterial adherence to clean biomaterials however, may not correlate to the mechanism following implantation if not viable tissue. The bioprostheses are immediately coated with serum, proteins, platelets, neutrophils, and fibrin in vivo, all of which can significantly alter adherence of bacteria; thus, there may be very little vascular graft matrix actually exposed following preclotting with blood. Serum coating of catheters has resulted in marked reduction of bacterial adherence.[24] By contrast, fibronectin has been shown to enhance bacterial adherence to intravascular catheters.[22,25] Bacterial adherence was not altered by fibronectin for all strains of staphylococci, however. A clearer understanding of the differential adherence of bacteria to biomaterials is undoubtedly of importance in the development of methods of prevention and treatment of prostheses infections.

Immune Regulation

The ability of *S epidermidis* to adhere, colonize, and produce a bacterial biofilm infection is also dependent upon the patient's immune response. Immune regulation is dependent upon slime and other factors produced by the bacteria and the competence of the patient's neutrophil and lymphocyte function. *S epidermidis* is a well-recognized pathogen in the immunocompromised patient.[26–28] Alterations of host defenses are felt to be important determinants of *S epidermidis* infections of vascular grafts,[2] intravascular catheters,[29] and peritoneal dialysis catheters.[30,31] Recent investigations on patients undergoing major arterial reconstructions have shown a significant depression of lymphocyte function.[32] Experiments using multiple in vitro assays have demonstrated a significant depression in the postoperative responses to concanavalin A, mumps antigen, and phytohemagglutinin and streptokinase/streptodornase for approximately 1 week after major arterial reconstruction. This suppression of lymphocyte function may predispose to adherence, colonization, and bacterial biofilm infection by the low-virulent *S epidermidis*.

Defects in both humoral and cellular defense mechanisms have been shown in patients prone to *S epidermidis* continuous ambulatory peritoneal dialysis (CAPD) catheter infections.[30] Patients with CAPD catheters with a high incidence of peritonitis had a lower peritoneal fluid IgG concentration and lower opsonic activity, as well as a decreased bactericidal capacity of the macrophage believed to be related to low levels of Il-1 and interferon-γ production. Treatment of these patients with highly purified IgG into the peritoneal dialysis solution has been shown to result in a threefold increase in opsonic capacity of peritoneal fluid for *S epidermidis*, and to significantly decrease the peritonitis rate. Treatment of these patients with interferon-γ has also increased the bactericidal activity of the macrophage and decreased the peritonitis rate.

The deficiency in opsonic capacity and bactericidal activity is due, in part, to slime production by *S epidermidis*. Slime greatly reduces the human cellular immune response.[28,29] Slime results in a decreased opsonic capacity, phagocytosis, bacterial killing, and B- and T-cell function. The depressed immunologic response due to slime does not occur immediately, but takes several days and is related to the amount of slime production. Slime, however, is likely one of many products of *S epidermidis* that alters the immune response. Toxins, DNAase, and protease produced by *S epidermidis* can also affect the pathogenicity and phagocytic killing.[28] In addition, a factor produced by neutrophils from patients with *S epidermidis* has been identified and recovered in their blood. The factor inhibits bactericidal activity.[33]

The immune deficits that result in a biomaterial infection are not well defined. Attempts at developing chronic animal models of *S epidermidis* have shown that suppression of the animals' immune response is necessary to permit continued bacterial growth. Immunocompetent mice will clear the bacteria from a graft adherent biofilm over 8 to 10 weeks. We have shown that bacterial clearance in these animals is related to normal phagocytic and lysozyme activity. Persistence of bacterial growth can be achieved by immunosuppressive agents that result in neutropenia and suppression in lymphocyte antigen presentation capacity (unpublished data). Further studies are needed to clarify the immune regulation of these infections.

Even though immunosuppression is felt to be important in permitting the initial adherence, biofilm formation, and growth

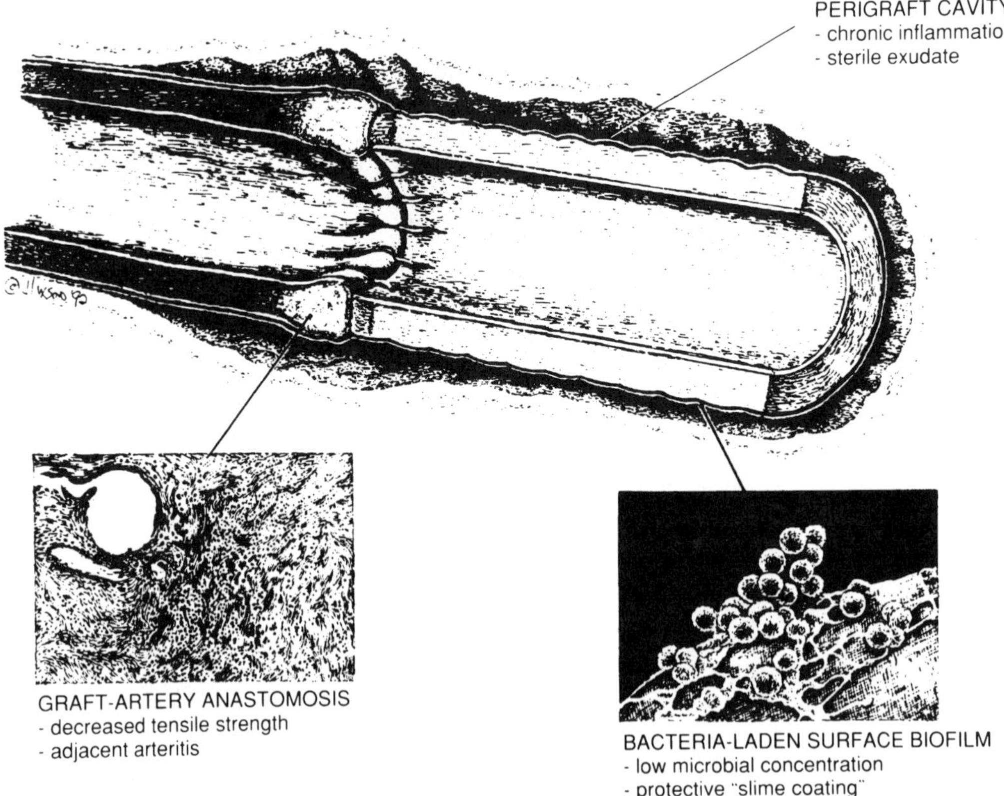

Figure 3. The graft surface bacterial biofilm results in a chronic inflammatory process with the formation of a perigraft cavity and decreased strength of the anastomosis, recognized clinically as a perigraft abscess and pseudoaneurysm, respectively.

of this low-virulence organism, the delayed recognition and activation of the chronic bacterial biofilm by the patient's immune system is equally important. The chronic inflammatory process is mediated by the host's immune response, producing autolysis of the periprosthetic tissues. For vascular grafts, the triggering of the patient's immune system against the bacterial biofilm results in the late appearance of anatomic signs and symptoms of a graft infection.[2] The immune response results in poor graft incorporation with surrounding tissue inflammation and a perigraft cavity, containing an exudate of many polymorphonuclear leukocytes. Further progression of the inflammation in the perigraft tissues can result in a graft-cutaneous sinus tract or a graft-enteric fistula, depending on the site of the graft. The chronic inflammation mediated by the host's immune system can also result in an adjacent arteritis, producing a decreased anastomotic tensile strength and subsequent pseudoaneurysm formation (Fig. 3). Animal experiments have demonstrated that *S epidermidis* graft infections do result in decreased anastomotic tensile strength[34] and the formation of a perigraft cavity and graft-cutaneous sinus tract (unpublished data), but the immune mechanisms are poorly understood and will be the subject of future investigations.

References

1. Bandyk DF, Berni GA, Thiele BL, Towne JB. Aortofemoral graft infection due to *Staphylo-*

coccus epidermidis. Arch Surg. 1984;119: 102–108.

2. Bergamini TM. Vascular prostheses infection caused by bacterial biofilms. *Semin Vasc Surg.* 1990;3:101–109.

3. Goldstone J, Moore WS. Infection in vascular prostheses. clinical manifestations and surgical management. *Am J Surg.* 1974;128: 225–233.

4. Edwards MJ, Richardson JD, Klamer TW. Management of aortic prosthetic infections. *Am J Surg.* 1988;155:327–330.

5. Schmitt DD, Bandyk DF, Pequet AJ, Towne JB. Bacterial adhrence to vascular prostheses: a determinant of graft infectivity. *Vasc Surg.* 1986;3:732–740.

6. Slaughter L, Morris JE, Starr A. Prosthetic valvular endocarditis: a 12 year review. *Circulation.* 1973;47:1319–1325.

7. Schoenbaum SC, Gardner P, Shillito J. Infection of cerebrospinal fluid shunts: epidemilogy, clinical manifestation, and therapy. *J Infect Dis.* 1975;131:543–551.

8. Peters G, Locci R, Pulverer G. Adherence and growth of coagulase-negative staphylococci on surfaces of intravenous catheters. *J Invest Dis* 1982;146:479–482.

9. Chih-Chang C, Williams DF. Effects of physical configuration and chemical structure of materials on bacterial adhesion. *Am J Surg.* 1984;147:197–204.

10. Edminston CE, Schmitt DD, Seabrook GR. Coagulase-negative staphylococci infections in vascular surgery: epidemiology and pathogenesis. *Infect Control Hosp Epidemiol.* 1989; 10:111–117.

11. Christenson GD, Simpson WA, Bisno AL. Adherence of slime-producing strains of *Staphylococcus epidermidis* to smooth surfaces. *Infect Immun.* 1982;37:318–326.

12. Franson TR, Sheth NK, Rose HD. Scanning electron microscopy of bacteria adherent to intravascular catheters. *J Clin Microbiol.* 1984; 20:500–505.

13. Schmitt DD, Bandyk DF, Pequet AJ, Malangoni MA, Towne JB. Mucin production by *Staphylococcus epidermidis*: a virulence factor promoting adherence to vascular grafts. *Arch Surg.* 1986;121:89–95.

14. Peters G, Schumacher-Perdreau F, Jansen B, Bey M, Pulverer G. Biology of *Staphylococcus epidermidis* extracellular slime. *Zentralbl Bakteriol Suppl Mikrobiol Hyg Abt* (suppl 1)1987; 16:15–32.

15. Christensen GD, Barker LP, Mawhinney TP, Baddour LM, Simpson WA. Idenfification of an antigenic marker of slime production for *Staphylococcus epidermidis. Infect Immun.* 1990;58:2906–2911.

16. Tojo M, Yamashita N, Golmann D, Pier GB. Isolation and characterization of a capsular polysaccharide adhesin from *Staphylococcus epidermidis. J Infect Dis.* 1988;157:713–722.

17. Pier GM, Matthews WJ Jr, Eardley DD. Immunochemical characterization of the mucoid exopolysaccharide *Pseudomonas aeruginosa. J Infect Dis.* 1983;147:484–503.

18. Lee JC, Michon F, Perez NE, Hopkins CA, Pier GB. Chemical characterization and immunogenicity of capsular polysaccharide isolated from a mucoid *Staphylococcus aureus. Infect Immun.* 1987;55:2191–2197.

19. Tollefson DF, Bandyk DF, Kaebnick HW, Seabrook GR, Towne JB. Surface biofilm disruption: enhanced recovery of microorganisms from vasular prostheses. 1987;122: 38–43.

20. Bergamini TM, Bandyk DF, Govostis D, Vetsch R, Towne JB. Identification of *Staphylococcus epidermidis* vascular graft infections: a comparison of culture techniques. *J Vasc Surg.* 1989;9:665–670.

21. Bergamini TM, Bandyk DF, Govostis D, Kaebnick HW, Towne JB. Infection of vascular prostheses caused by bacterial biofilms. *J Vasc Surg.* 1988;7:21–30.

22. Vaudauz P, Pittet D, Haeberli A, et al. Host factors selectively increase staphylococcal adherence on inserted catheters: a role of fibronectin and fibrinogen or fibrin. *J Infect Dis* 1989;160:865–874.

23. Siverhus DJ, Schmitt DD, Edmiston CE, Bandyk DF, Seabrook GR, Towne JB. Adherence of mucin and non-mucin producing staphylococci to preclotted and albumin coated velour knitted vascular grafts. *Surgery.* 1990; 107(6):613–619.

24. Kristinsson KG. Adherence of staphylococci to intravascular catheters. *J Med Microbiol.* 1989;28:249–257.

25. Russell PB, Kline J, Yoder MC, Polin RA. Staphylococcal adherence to polyvinyl chloride and heparin-bonded polyurethane catheters is species dependent and enhanced by fibronectin. *J Clin Microbiol.* 1987;25: 1083–1087.

26. Wade JC, Schimpff SC, Newman KA, Wiernik PH. *Staphylococcus epidermidis*: an increasing cause of infeciton in patients with granulocytopenia. *Ann Intern Med.* 1982;97: 503–508.

27. Forse RA, Dixon C, Bernard K, Martinez L, McLean PH, Meakins JL. *Staphylococcus epidermidis*: an important pathogen. *Surgery.* 1979;86:507–514.

28. Gemmell CG. Pathogenicity of coagulase-negative staphylococci with respect to the

nature of the host response. *Zentralbl Bakteriol Hyg A.* 1987;266:52–59.

29. Gray ED, Peters G, Verstegen M, Regelmann WE. Effect of extracellular slime substance from *Staphylococcus epidermidis* on the human cellular immune response. *Lancet.* 1984; 1365–1367.

30. Lamperi S, Carozzi S. Immunologic defenses in CAPD. *Curr Concepts CAPD Blood Pur.* 1989;7:125–143.

31. Dasgupta MK, Costerton JW. Significance of biofilm-adherent bacterial microcolonies on tenckhoff catheters of CAPD patients. *Curr Concepts CAPD Blood Pur.* 1989;7:144–155.

32. Keane RM, Munster AM, Birmingham W, Winchurch RA, Gadacz TR, Ernst CB. Suppression of lymphocyte function after aortic reconstruction: use of nonimmunosuppressive anesthesia. *Arch Surg.* 1982;117: 1133–1135.

33. Noble MA, Grant SK, Hajen E. Characterization of a neutrophil-inhibitory factor from clinically significant *Staphylococcus epidermidis. J Infect Dis.* 1990;162:909–913.

34. Vetsch R, Bandyk DF, Schmitt DD, Bergamini TM, Storey JD, Towne JB. Anastomotic tensile strength following in situ replacement of an infected abdominal aortic graft. *Arch Surg.* 1989;124:425–428.

Chapter 4.3

Aneurysm Cultures

D.L. Steed

Introduction

Infections in prosthetic grafts used in repair of abdominal aortic aneurysms are devastating complications with extensive morbidity and mortality. Multiple risk factors predispose to prosthetic infections including improper sterile technique, skin infections or contamination, emergency aneurysm repair, perigraft hematoma, multiple previous abdominal vascular operations, transient bacteremia in the perioperative period, and complications in the groin wound.[1]

Infected aneurysms have been recognized for more than 100 years as described by Koch in 1851.[2] The term mycotic aneurysm refers in general to infection in an aneurysm caused by any microorganism, although some more rigorously reserve the term mycotic to infections caused by fungi.

True mycotic aneurysms are quite uncommon. Although, there is one report of six cases of primary infection (3.3%) in 178 atherosclerotic aneurysms,[3] the incidence of mycotic aneurysms among atherosclerotic aneurysms is probably much lower. Most reports of mycotic aneurysms are for a handful of cases only or are isolated case reports without the total number of repaired aneurysms being reported.[4-25] A variety of different microorganisms causing infection have been reported. *Staphylococcus*[9,24,26] and *Salmonella*[5,7,8,11,12,14,16,24] are particularly common. However, a variety of other microorganisms have been reported including *Streptococcus*,[11,24,25] *Escherichia coli*,[24] *Campylobacter*,[23] *Bacteroides*,[13,22] *Pseudomonas*,[24] *Proteus*,[24] *Klebsiella*,[24] *Mycobacterium*,[15,24] and *Clostridium*.[4,6,20] Aneurysms infected with *Bacille billié Calmette-Guérin* have been reported[18] as have infections from fungi.[27]

Mycotic aneurysms occurring as a primary infection are more common than ones that become secondarily infected from bacterial endocarditis or direct inoculation from another infectious focus or trauma. Since the advent of antibiotics, bacterial endocarditis occurs less frequently and thus is less likely to cause a mycotic aneurysm.[28] The diagnosis should be suspected in any patient with a clinically evident aneurysm associated with pain, fever, and leukocytosis. Other factors suggesting an infected aneurysm include positive blood cultures, erosion of lumbar vertebrae, or prolonged bacteremia.[24]

Literature Review

In 1977, Ernst identified two potential sources of late graft sepsis, which had heretofore not been widely recognized; aneurysm contents and intestinal bag fluid. Routine cultures were performed from the aneurysm contents and fluid transuded into the bowel bag in 80 patients undergoing aneurysm repair (Table 1). None of the patients was suspected of having an infected aneurysm. Prophylactic antibiotics were given in the perioperative period. Fifteen percent of aneurysm cultures and 11% of intestinal bag fluid cultures were positive. Bacterial growth occurred from cultures of the aneurysm contents, intestinal bag fluid, or both in 20% of patients. Eighty-one percent of the cultures were Gram-positive organisms, most commonly, *Staphylococcus epidermidis* or *Staphylococcus aureus.* The Gram-negative cultures (19% of cases) were *Enterobacter, E. coli,* or *Bacteroides.* A higher incidence of positive cultures (38%) were found in patients with ruptured aneurysms. Although 20% of patients in this series were considered to be at increased risk for graft sepsis because of a "positive" culture, graft infection occurred in 2.5% of patients only. Comparing those who survived and were

Table 1
Outcome of Patients with Cultures from Aneurysm

Author/Year	No. Pts.	Positive Cultures (%)	Graft Infection With Positive Cultures (%)	Graft Infection With Negative Cultures (%)	Antibiotics Given
Ernst (1977)[26]	78	12 (15.4%)	1 (8.3%)	1 (1.6%)	Preop and 4–5 days postop
Williams (1977)[29]	68	7 (10.0%)	0 (0%)	NG	Preop and 8–14 days postop
Scobie (1979)[30]	31	7 (22.6%)	0 (0%)	0 (0%)	Preop and 8 days postop
Eriksson (1983)[31]	85	12 (14.1%)	0 (0%)	0 (0%)	47 patients preop and 1–3 days postop. 38 patients none.
McAuley (1984)[32]	64	9 (14.1%)	0 (0%)	0 (0%)	Preop and 2 days postop.
Macbeth (1984)[38]	11	3 (27%)			
Buckels (1985)[33]	275	22 (8.0%)	7 (31.8%)	6 (2.4%)	Preop and 5–7 days postop.
Schwartz (1987)[34]	211	22 (10.4%)	0 (0%)	1 (0.05%)	Preop and 1 day postop.
Ilgenfritz (1988)[35]	56	11 (19.6%)	0 (0%)	0 (0%)	Preop and 2 days postop.
Brandimarte (1989)[36]	90	28 (31.1%)	0 (0%)	1 (1.6%)	
Higgins (1990)[37]	116	6 (5%)	0 (0%)	0 (0%)	Preop and 2 days postop
Total	1085	139(12.8%)	8(5.8%)	9(1.0%)	

NG = not given

followed for more than 6 months, late graft sepsis occurred in 10% of the positive culture group and 2% of the negative culture group. Except for this, the significance of the positive cultures form the aneurysm contents or intestinal bag fluid was unclear. The reason for the graft sepsis rate being only 2.5% despite a 20% positive culture rate may have been related to host resistance, virulence of the organism, or the use of perioperative antibiotics. Also, a number of the positive cultures were microorganisms felt to be contaminants and thus were not significant.

Furthermore, during most aneurysm repairs, all the thrombus and a portion of the aortic wall may be removed; thus, the potentially infectious source may have been debrided. The researchers thus recommended a routine culture of aneurysms and their contents as well as intestinal bag contents; upon identifying bacterial growth from those sources, antibiotic therapy was recommended.[26]

In the same year, Williams reported the results of 68 cultures taken from abdominal aortic aneurysms. Cultures were taken from nonblood fluids, thrombus, aneurysm wall, or atheromatous plaques. Ten percent of the cultures were positive, and most microorganisms identified were not sensitive to the standard perioperative antibiotics. The patients with positive cultures but no other evidence of infection were treated with short courses of high-dose antibiotics and none developed a graft infection.[29]

Those findings were refuted by Scobie who found 22.6% of aneurysm wall cultures grew bacteria as did 14.2% of bowel bag cultures. Perioperative antibiotics were given to the patients undergoing aneurysm repair. However, only 11 graft infections occurred in 517 abdominal aortic grafts inserted over a 10-year period. Six of these 10 patients had infection present at the time of aneurysm repair of a developed paraprosthetic enteric fistula. In the other five patients with graft infection, the cultures were negative. This study, then, failed to demonstrate any value for routine culture of the aneurysm contents or intestinal bag fluid.[30]

Eriksson sampled and cultured the aortic wall of 85 patients undergoing abdominal aortic aneurysm repair. Half of the patients received no antibiotics and the other half received perioperative antibiotics only. Fourteen percent had positive cultures. Thirteen strains of bacteria were isolated, but most of these were present only in low colony counts and were considered contaminants. Many of the bacteria cultured were normal skin flora. The only one of these patients who developed a graft infection had ischemic colitis. Thus, it was concluded that the aneurysm wall did not represent a significant source of graft infection.[31]

McAuley reported the results of cultures of intraluminal thrombus in 64 patients undergoing repair of abdominal aortic aneurysm. Eight of nine patients received no antibiotic therapy other than routine prophylaxis in the perioperative period. Bacteria were isolated in 14% of the cases; this report was strikingly similar in incidence to the reports of Ernst[26] and Williams.[29] There were no early or late prosthetic graft infections in a mean follow-up of 25 months. Interestingly, in six cases, the microorganisms were sensitive to the prophylactic antibiotic regimen.[32]

Buckels cultured the contents of 275 patients undergoing aneurysm repair. Eight percent of cultures were positive. This was more likely to be the case in patients undergoing emergency aneurysm repair. Not surprisingly, the incidence of positive cultures fell when they began to give prophylactic antibiotics prior to operation. The incidence of graft sepsis was higher in patients with positive versus negative cultures, 31.8% versus 2.43%. Of course, the incidence of graft sepsis was also higher in patients undergoing emergency repair. Only six of the patients had a primary graft infection while the other seven had a graft-enteric fistula or a graft-enteric erosion. He recommended routine surveillance cultures of all aneurysms at the time of repair and prolonged microorganism-specific therapy for patients with a positive culture.[33]

Schwartz performed aerobic and anaerobic cultures of nonblood fluid, laminated thrombus, or ulcerated plaque in 211 patients undergoing aortic aneurysm repair. Antibiotics were given in the perioperative period only. Positive cultures occurred in 10.4% of patients. The most common organism was *S epidermidis*, and the largest percentage of positive cultures occurred in patients operated upon for ruptured aneurysm. This was in agreement with what other researchers had found. Only one patient had a prosthetic graft infection and that occurred with a negative culture.[34]

Ilgenfritz[35] took cultures from 56 patients undergoing aortic aneurysm repair. Prophylactic antibiotics were given preoperatively and for 2 days following the operation. Eleven patients (19.6%) had positive cultures. The most common organism isolated was *S epidermidis*. During a 2-year follow-up, graft infections were not found in patients with either a positive or a negative culture.

Brandimarte cultured the aneurysm walls of 90 patients undergoing vascular grafting for aortic aneurysm. One graft infection occurred in 62 patients with a negative culture and graft infection did not occur in the 28 patients with a positive culture. This review reported two patients with inflammatory aneurysms who had negative cultures. He concluded that a positive culture at the time of operation did not imply clinical infection and postoperative organism-specific antibiotic therapy was not needed.[36]

Higgins found that only six cultures of intraluminal thrombus (5%) were positive in 116 patients undergoing aneurysm repair. Antibiotics were used just prior to the operation and for 2 days after the operation. Of these six positive cultures, five were considered to be contaminants. Thus, the incidence of *positive* cultures was less than 1%. There were no graft infections in any of these patients with positive cultures. The true incidence of positive cultures in this series was lower than had been reported previously. He concluded that the positive cultures were either not clinically significant or were adequately covered by the prophylactic antibiotics given in the perioperative period. Routine culture of aneurysm thrombus in the absence of clinical evidence of infection was judged not to be cost effective.[37]

Seventy-nine percent of the microorganisms isolated in the series presented were Gram-positive and thus should be sensitive to prophylactic antibiotics given in the perioperative period (Table 2). Of the Gram-positive organisms found by culture, the most commonly reported bacterium was *S epidermidis*, which is commonly found as a contaminant. In fact, 50% of the organisms isolated from aneurysm cultures are commonly considered contaminants. Thus, many of the positive cultures reported may not represent true infection, and most organisms found are sensitive to the antibiotics used in the perioperative period.

In summary, results of cultures in over 1000 patients have demonstrated an incidence of positive cultures of 12.8% with a range of 5.0% to 31.1%) (Table 1). However, it does appear as though many of these *positive* cultures are contaminants. In addition, many microorganisms cultured are sensitive to the perioperative antibiotic regimen used routinely in abdominal aortic aneurysm repair. There is little evidence to suggest that graft sepsis is more likely to occur in patients with positive cultures. Rather, graft infection is more likely related to other factors such as breaks in sterile technique, emergency aneurysm repair, perigraft hematoma, or complications occurring in the groin wound.

It, therefore, seems prudent and cost effective to culture the intraluminal thrombus, atherosclerotic plaque, aneurysm wall, or nonblood fluids in any case where infection is clinically suspected. Antibiotics should be used in these cases and chosen based on sensitivity reports. Although peri-

Table 2
Microorganisms Cultured from Aneurysm Thrombus

Author/Year	No. Pts.	% Gram-Positive	Gram-Positive Organisms (No. of Cultures)	Gram-Negative Organisms (No. of Cultures)
Ernst (1977)[26]	12	83%	(7)† *S epidermidis* (1) *S aureus* (1)† *Micrococcus* (1)† *Bacillus*	(1) *Enterobacter* (1) *E. coli*
Williams (1977)[29]	7	71%	(4) *Staphylococcus* (1) *Streptococcus*	(1) *E. coli* (1) *Pseudomonas*
Scobie (1979)[30]	7	75%	(5)† *S epidermidis* (1) *Streptococcus*	(1)* *Klebsiella pneumoniae* (1)* *Enterobacter aerogenes*
Eriksson (1983)[31]	12	83%	(4)† *S epidermidis* (2) *Streptococcus* (3)† *Propionibacterium* sp. (1) anerobic rod	(1)* *Enterobacter* (1) *Hemophilus influenzae*
McAuley (1984)[32]	9	73%	(4) *Staphylococcus* (2)* *Streptococcus* (1)† *Propionibacterium* (1)† diphtheroids	(1)* *E. coli* neisseria flora (1) *Pseudomonas*
Macbeth (1984)[38]	3		(1)*† *S epidermidis* (1)* *Streptococcus* (only cases reported)	
Buckels (1985)[33]	22	71%	(7)† *Micrococcus* (5) *S aureus* (3) *Streptococcus* (2) *Pneumococcus* (1 patient with multiple organisms)	(3) *E. coli* (2) *Proteus* (1) *Salmonella* (1)† *Acinetobacter*
Schwertz (1987)[34]	22	86%	(12)† *S epidermidis* (3)† *Micrococcus* (2)† diphtheroids *S aureus*	(2) *Salmonella* (1) *Hemophilus influenzae*
Higgins (1990)[37]	6	100%	(4)* *Staphylococcus* (1)† *Bacillus* (1)* *Streptococcus* (1) *Clostidia perfringens*	
Total	100	79%		

S = Staphylococcus.
† Commonly a contaminant when isolated.
* Multiple organisms isolated in the same patient.

operative prophylactic antibiotics should be used in aortic aneurysm repair, prolonged antibiotic therapy seems to be of little benefit in patients with positive cultures from the aneurysm contents without other clinical or intraoperative signs of infection. In addition, long-term antibiotic therapy is expensive and not without risk.

References

1. Moore WS, Malone JM. Vascular infection. In: Simmons RL, Howard RJ, eds. *Surgical Infectious Diseases, 2nd ed.* Norwalk: Appleton & Lange; 1988;585–605.
2. Koch L. *Ueber das Aneurysma der Anteria Meseraica,* Dissertation. Erlangen: JJ Barfies;1851.
3. Sommerville RL, Allen EV, Edwards JE.

Bland and infected arterosclerotic abdominal aortic aneurysms: a clinicopathologic study. *Medicine* 1959;38:207–211.

4. Skipper D, Birch HA, Fallowfield ME, Taylor RS. Clostridial mycotic aneurysm of the suprarenal abdominal aorta. *J Cardiovasc Surg.* 1991;32:4:472–474.

5. Purnell RA. Ruptured myocotic aneurysm of the internal iliac artery and septic arthritis complicating salmonella infection. *Br J Clin Prac* 1990;44:11:497–499.

6. Brahan RB, Kahler RC. Clostridium septicum as a cause of pericarditis and mycotic aneurysm. *J Clin Microbiol.* 1990;28:10: 2377–2378.

7. Jagjivan B, Nakielny RA. Salmonella aortitis and aneurysm formation: the role of CT in management. *Clin Radiol.* 1990;42:1:55–56.

8. Gabbi E, Rossi G, Ghidoni I. *Salmonella typhimurium* infection of a thoracic aortic aneurysm in an immunocompetent subject: case report and literature review. *Infection.* 1989; 17:5:306–308.

9. Borris LC, Petersen K. Rapid growth and early rupture of a primary mycotic aneurysm of the abdominal aorta. *Europ J Vasc Surg.* 1989;3:5:461–463.

10. Willing SJ, Fanizza-Orphanos A, Thomas HA. Mycotic aneurysm of the abdominal aorta: diagnosis by duplex sonography. *J Ultrasound Med.* 1989;8:9:527–529.

11. Baird RN. Mycotic aortic aneurysms. *Europ J Vasc Surg.* 1989;3:2:95–96.

12. Mestres CA, Ninot S, de Lacy AM, et al. AIDS and samonella: infected abdominal aortic aneurysm. *Aust NZ J Surg.* 1990;60:3: 225–226.

13. Jewkes AJ, Black J. Infection of an abdominal aortic aneurysm from an apppendix abscess. *J Cardiovasc Surg.* 1989;30:5:870–872.

14. Chan P, Lan CK, Wan YL. *Salmonella cholerasius* bactermia and mycotic aneurysm of the abdominal aorta: report of five cases. *Hsueh-Chang Gung Med J* 1989;12:2:115–120.

15. Ringswald M, Roy TM. Synchronous mycotic aneurysms secondary to tuberculosis. *J Kentucky Med Assoc.* 1989;87:7:320–324.

16. Barthel J, Bosschaerts T, Locufier JL, Delwarte D, Barroy JP. Consecutive infected aneurysms caused by salmonella. *Ann Vasc Surg.* 1988;2:1:79–81.

17. Abet D, Pietri J. So-called "primary" infected aneurysms of the subrenal abdominal aorta: five observations. *J Des Maladies Vasculaires.* 1988;13:4:321–327.

18. Woods JM, Schellack J, Stewart MT, Murray DR, Schwartzman SW. Mycotic abdominal aortic aneurysm induced by immunotherapy with bacille Calmette-Guérin vaccine for malignancy. *J Vasc Surg.* 1988;7:6:808–810.

19. Tran-Minh VA, Le Gall C, Pasquier JM, et al. Mycotic aneurysm of the abdominal aorta in the neonate. *J Clin Ultrasound.* 1989;17:1: 37–39.

20. Hurley L, Howe K. Mycotic aortic aneurysm infected by clostridium septicum: a case history. *Angiology.* 1991;42:7:585–589.

21. Cave C, Longaker MT, Merrick S, Teitel DF, Goldstone J, Verrier ED. Infective endocarditis and an embolomycotic aneurysm. *J Cardiovasc Surg.* 1990;31:6:805–808.

22. Reddy DJ, Lee RE, Oh HK. Surprarenal mycotic aortic aneurysms: surgical management and followup. *J Vasc Surg.* 1986;3:6: 917–920.

23. Rutherford EJ, Eakins JW, Maxwell G, Tackett AD. Abdominal aortic aneurysm infected with *Campylobacter fetus* subspecies fetus. *J Vasc Surg.* 1989;10:2.193–197.

24. Jarrett F, Darling RC, Mundth ED, Austen WG. Experience with infected aneurysms of the abdominal aorta. *Arch Surg.* 1975;110: 1281–1287.

25. Mundth ED, Darling RC, Alvarado RH, Buckley MJ, Linton RR, Austen WG. Surgical management of mycotic aneurysms and the complications of infection in vascular reconstructive surgery. *Am J Surg.* 1969;117: 460–469.

26. Ernst CB, Campbell HC, Daugherty ME, Sachatello CR, Griffen WO. Incidence and significance of intraoperative bacterial cultures during abdominal aortic aneurysmectomy. *Ann Surg.* 1977;185:6:626–629.

27. Deulofeu F, Barbeta S, Bernet V, Sentis C, Pujol F. Massive hemoptysis secondary to mycotic aortic aneurysm. *Anales de Medicina Interna.* 1989;6:7:373–375.

28. Bennett DE, Cherry JK. Bacterial infection of aortic aneurysms: a clinicopathology study. *Am J Surg.* 1967;113:321–325.

29. Williams RD, Fisher FW. Aneurysm contents as a source of graft infection. *Arch Surg.* 1977; 112:415–416.

30. Scobie K, McPhail N, Barber G, Elder R. Bacteriologic monitoring in abdominal aortic surgery. *Can J Surg.* 1979;22:4:368–371.

31. Eriksson I, Forsbert O, Lundquist B, Schwan A. Significance of positive bacterial cultures from aortic aneurysms. *Acta Chir Scand.* 1983; 149:33–35.

32. McAuley CE, Steed DL, Webster MW. Bacterial presence in aortic thrombus at elective aneurysm resection: is it clinically significant? *Am J Surg.* 1984;147:322–324.

33. Buckels JA, Fielding JW, Black J, Ashton F,

Slaney G. Significance of postive bacterial cultures from aortic aneurysm contents. *Br J Surg.* 1985;72:440–442.

34. Schwartz JA, Powell TW, Burnham SJ, Johnson G. Culture of abdominal aortic aneurysm contents. *Arch Surg.* 1987;122:780–785.

35. Ilgenfritz FM, Jordan FT. Microbiological monitoring of aortic aneurysm wall and content during aneurysmectomy. *Arch Surg.* 1988;123:4:506–508.

36. Brandimarte C, Santini C, Venditti M, et al. Clinical significance of intraoperative cultures of aneurysm walls and contents in elective abdominal aortic aneurysmectomy. *Eur J Epidemiol.* 1989;5:4:521–525.

37. Higgins RS, Steed DL, Dummer JS, Webster MW. Culture of intraluminal thrombus during abdominal aortic aneurysm resection: significant contamination is rare. *Proceedings of the Eastern Vascular Society,* May 1990. Abstract.

Chapter 4.4

Lymphatic Contribution to Graft Infection

J.R. Rubin

Introduction

The lymphatic system has been implicated as a potential source of bacterial transfection from a distal septic focus, such as a pedal infection, to the systemic circulation and to a freshly implanted prosthetic graft.[1-5] Logically, when one considers the anatomic and histologic structure of arterial and venous capillaries and that of the lymphatic system, the latter would be the logical conduit for absorption and transportation of bacteria.

Histology and Function

The lymphatic system consists of an extensive network of interconnecting superficial and deep, thin-walled vascular conduits which communicate with regional lymph node groupings via small connecting channels. The lymphatics of the superficial dermis are valveless while the majority of lymph vessels contain unicuspid or bicuspid valves. The lymphatics have been classified according to their functional anatomy into initial and collecting systems.[6] The initial lymphatics function by absorbing and removing material from tissues, whereas the collecting system transports the absorbed material proximally. The lymphatic network is found in the fascial planes but most noticeably in the perivascular and adventitial tissues in close proximity to the major blood supply of a specific region.

Lymphatic functions include the absorption, filtration, transportation and return to systemic circulation of fluids, proteins, and particulate material from soft tissue spaces.

Approximately 10% of extracellular fluid is not reabsorbed in the venous capillary system and this is mediated by the presence of macromolecules, most importantly, proteins.[7] Larger molecules, such as proteins, cannot gain access into the post-capillary venous system due to the limited size of their openings. Venous capillaries generally have a diameter of about 8 millimicrons, although the slit pores, which regulate what is absorbed, measure 80 to 90 A.[8] Although the venous capillary openings may dilate to larger sizes, the absorption of large molecules is impeded. Fluids will generally shift with the movement of macro-

From Bunt, TJ: *Vascular Graft Infections*. Armonk: Futura Publishing Co., Inc.; © 1994.

molecules; therefore, this material is absorbed into the specialized terminal lymphatic capillaries (initial lymphatics) which have wide, overlapping intracellular junctions that may open to 10 millimicrons.[9-11] This system favors the entry of fluid and macromolecules into the lymphatics and prevents egress back into the interstitial spaces. It has therefore been established that there is a preferential movement of macromolecules, such as proteins, and particulate matter into the lymphatic circulation as opposed to the venous capillary system.

The initial lymphatics coalesce to form collecting channels which pass through lymph nodes and empty into the systemic circulation through peripheral lymphatic-venous communications, lymph-node venous channels or via the thoracic duct-jugular/subclavian vein. Material absorbed directly by lymphatics may reach the systemic circulation directly or after filtering through lymph nodes. Given the average size of bacteria, which measure 0.5 to 2.5 millimicrons,[12] and which are larger than the venous capillary openings, it is only reasonable to assume that bacteria will generally gain access to the systemic circulation via the lymphatic system. In addition, when this is considered in the context of prosthetic arterial reconstruction, graft infections should theoretically be eliminated if the surgeon is able to both disrupt lymphatic-to-systemic circulation flow and avoid direct contact between contaminated lymph and the implanted graft.

Experimental Lymphatic-Handling Techniques

Experimentation with a canine model was carried out in order to evaluate theories regarding the lymphatic contribution to prosthetic graft infection, when grafts are implanted in the presence of a septic focus.[4] In this study, bilateral interpositional femoral artery graft (polytetrafluoroethylene PTFE) replacements were performed in 21 greyhounds, accompanied by unilateral limb ischemia-rendering operations and ipsilateral bacterial inoculations with standardized inocula of *Escherichia coli*, and *Staphylococcus aureus*. Inguinal lymphatics in the ischemic limb were either simply transected (group I), carefully preserved (group II), or excised and ligated (group III) at the time of graft implantation. Animals were observed for 48 hours after which grafts were harvested and appropriate cultures were taken.

There was an 87.5% incidence of positive blood cultures in groups I and II with both organisms being cultured more commonly in group II than group I. The incidence of positive graft cultures with two organisms was highest in group II animals, followed by group I, and the overall incidence of one or two organism-positive cultures was similar for both of these groups. Group III had positive graft cultures in 20% of the animals which was significantly less than the 87.5% and 100% incidence in groups I and II.

The results of this study suggested that lymphatics probably contribute to the development of acute prosthetic graft infection by facilitating bacteria absorption from the distal septic focus, and by providing access to the systemic circulation via lymphatic-venous communications when the lymphatics are intact causing hematogenous contamination of the graft, or by directly bathing the implanted prosthesis when the lymphatics are disrupted above the distal septic focus.

Unfortunately, with extensive regional lymphatic isolation, division, and ligation during graft implantation one would expect a significant amount of postoperative lymphedema which would be an unacceptable operative complication.

Regional Lymph-Flow Patterns

To better define the results of the previous study and in order to quantify lymphatic flow changes that may occur during and as a consequence of inguinal lymphatic manipulation, further laboratory studies were undertaken.[13]

Thirty-five greyhounds underwent popliteal lymph node dissection and microvascular silastic tube cannulation of the node. Through this infusion setup, 2.5% patent blue-violet dye was injected to illuminate the inguinal lymph vessels and verify efferent lymphatic integrity during subsequent inguinal dissection (Fig. 1). Through the same catheter, technetium 99m labeled human serum albumin (HSA) was injected and radioactivity was measured in several fixed locations including the popliteal, inguinal, and iliac regions, before and after inguinal dissection. Radioactivity measurements were taken with an isotope localization monitor and scintillation counter before and after the following operative procedures were carried out. Inguinal dissection was performed and lymphatic handling was divided into three groups which included: no inguinal lymphatic manipulation, (group I); local perivascular lymphatic ligation (group II); and radical inguinal lymphatic excision and ligation (group III). Lymphatic flow was calculated by technetium 99m HSA clearance (counts per minute).

The results of this study demonstrated a statistically significant reduction in lymph flow for groups II and III, compared to group I ($P < 0.001$), while there was no significant difference between groups II and III. This project verified that lymph flow was similarly reduced when lymphatics were locally ligated and when they were radically excised and ligated proving that the more obliterative techniques did not result in a more significant flow reduction than local perivascular lymphatic ligation. In the study, the quantity of lymph flow re-

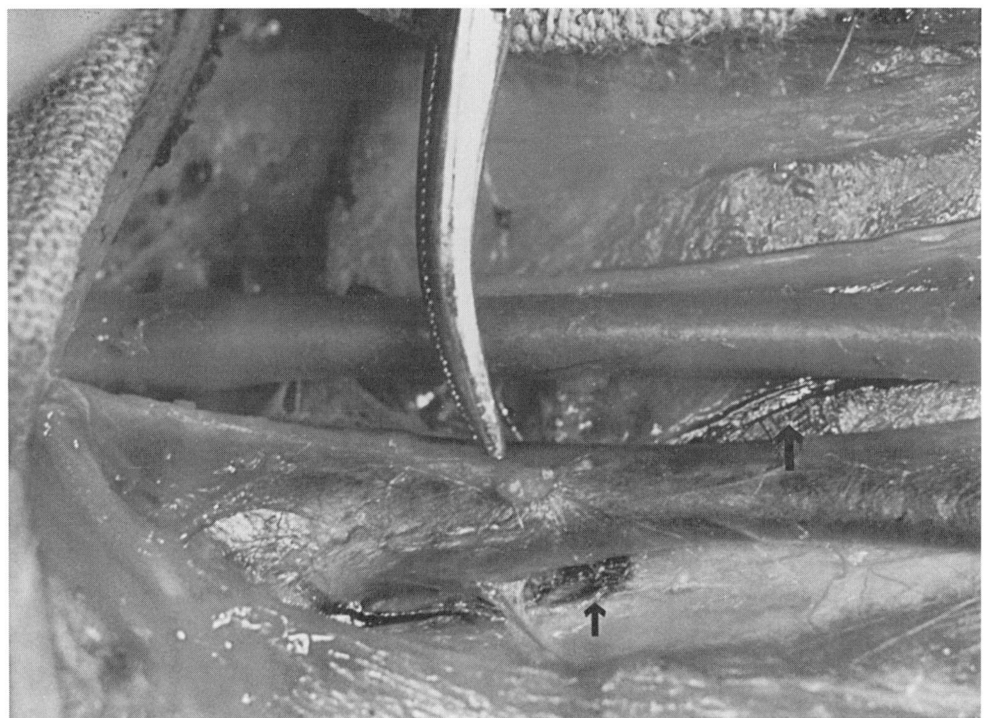

Figure 1. Perivascular lymphatics enhanced with 2.5% patent violet-blue dye.

duction that will result in a significant incidence of lymphedema was not determined.

Translymphatic Antibiotic Delivery

In an attempt to reduce the incidence of acute prosthetic graft infection, while at the same time avoiding inguinal lymphatic manipulation during graft implantation, a new technique for antibiotic administration was attempted experimentally.[14]

Twenty greyhounds underwent bilateral femoral artery prosthetic interpositional grafting after ipsilateral hind-paw septic foci was established. The animals were divided into three experimental cohorts. Group I animals were the control; group II were given intravenous antibiotic therapy, and group III were given transpopliteal lymph node intralymphatic antibiotic therapy. The latter was delivered through a microvascular silastic catheter inserted transcutaneously into the popliteal lymph node (Fig. 2). Efferent flow was verified using 2.5% patent blue-violet dye. Appropriate bacteria-specific antibiotics in groups II and III were initiated prior to graft placement, were continued at regular intervals following graft insertion, and the amount given was calculated in the same manner for both cohorts.

The incidence of graft infection was significantly reduced with intralymphatic antibiotic therapy compared to intravenous therapy and controls. In addition, the incidence of positive blood and tissue cultures was significantly lower with intralymphatic antibiotic therapy (group III) compared to the controls, and although lower than group II, the latter was not statistically significant. It was concluded that intralymphatic antibiotic infusion techniques were superior to intravenous antibiotic therapy for preventing acute prosthetic graft infection, when grafts are placed in the presence of a distal septic focus.

Conclusion

In conclusion, the role of the lymphatic system in the absorption, transportation, and delivery of bacteria from the septic focus to the systemic circulation has been well documented. In addition, we have described experimental work which demonstrates the relationship between various lymphatic-handling techniques and the incidence of acute prosthetic graft infection, when fresh grafts are implanted in the presence of a distal septic focus. Due to the unacceptable clinical morbidity associated with inguinal lymphatic ablation, we currently feel that intralymphatic antibiotic infusion offers the most promise for eliminating acute graft infection when prosthetics are placed in the presence of a distal septic focus.

References

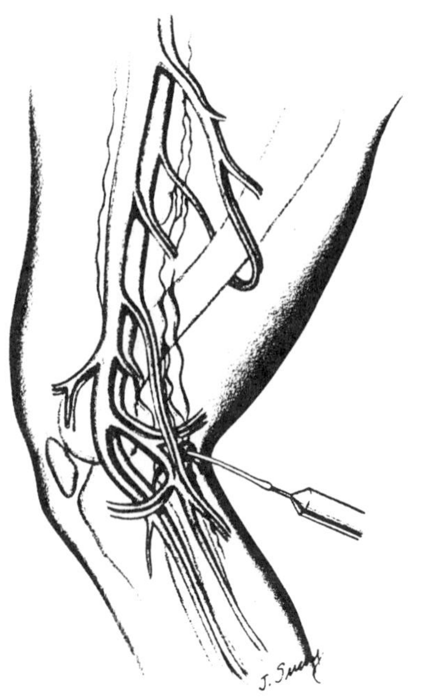

Figure 2. Canine hind-limb anatomy with site of popliteal node cannulation for intralymphatic antibiotic infusion.

1. Conn JH, Hardy JO, Chavez CM, Fain WR. Infected arterial grafts: experience in 22 cases

with emphasis on unusual bacteria and techniques. *Ann Surg.* 1970;171:704–714.

2. Bunt TJ. Synthetic vascular graft infections. *Surgery.* 1983;93:733–746.

3. Bouhoutsos J, Chavatzas D, Martin P, Morris T. Infected synthetic arterial grafts. *Br J Surg.* 1974;61:108–111.

4. Rubin JR, Malone JM, Goldstone J. The role of the lymphatic system in acute arterial prosthetic graft infections. *J Vasc Surg.* 1985; 2:92–98.

5. Rubin JR, Folsom D. Management of lower extremity graft infections. *Semin Vasc Surg.* 1990; 3:114–121.

6. Casley-Smith JR. Progress in lymphology II. In: Viamonte M, Witte C, Witte MH, Koehler PR, eds. New York: Intercontinental Medical Book Corp; 1970:51–54.

7. Guyton AC. The lymphatic system, intestinal fluid dynamics, edema, and pulmonary fluid. In: *Textbook of Medical Physiology.* Philadelphia: WB Saunders Co; 1976:387–413.

8. Rhodin JAG. Ultrastructure of mammalian venous capillaries, venules, and small collecting veins. *J Ultrastruct Res* 1968;25: 452–500.

9. Casley-Smith JR. An electron microscopic study of injured and abnormally permeable lymphatics. *Ann NY Acad Sci.* 1964;116: 803–830.

10. Casley-Smith JR. The fine structure, properties, and permeabilities of the lymphatic endothelium. In: Collette JM, Jantet G, Schonffeniels E, eds. *New Trends in Basic Lymphology.* Stuttgart: Experientia Supplementum; 1967:124:19–39.

11. Casley-Smith JR, Florey HW. The structure of normal small lymphatics. *QJ Exp Physiol.* 1961;46:101–106.

12. Burrows W. *Textbook of Microbiology, 12th ed.* Philadelphia: WB Saunders Co; 1973:16–17.

13. Rubin JR, Eberlin LB. The effect of inguinal lymphatic manipulation on regional lymph flow patterns. *J Vasc Surg.* 1993; 17:896–901.

14. Folsom D, Franceschi D, Rubin JR. Intralymphatic antibiotic delivery for reducing acute prosthetic graft infection. *J Cardiovasc Surg.* 1992;33:660–663.

Chapter 4.5

Role of the Perigraft Space

J.V. White
K. Whang
A. Geroff

Introduction

Despite the use of perioperative antibiotics, vascular graft infection continues to affect 2% to 6% of patients undergoing vascular reconstruction.[1,2] Patients so afflicted suffer a high incidence of limb loss (22% to 57%) and death (33% to 36%), despite appropriate intervention at the time of diagnosis.[3-5] As increasing lengths of the arterial tree are replaced with prosthetic material, it is likely that the morbidity and mortality of graft infection will rise. To reduce the likelihood of this catastrophic complication, pertinent bacterial characteristics, the impact of graft placement upon host defenses, and the interaction between graft and host must be understood.

The bacteriology of vascular graft infections is quite simple. The majority of synthetic vascular graft infections are caused by *Staphylococcus aureus* and *Staphylococcus epidermidis*, both common skin flora. To minimize the risks of such infections, perioperative antibiotics have been used in virtually all vascular procedures for the past decade. This has clearly reduced the overall number of vascular graft infections.[6] However, the incidence of staphylococcal vascular graft infection has actually increased from 48% prior to the routine use of antibiotics to 74% since perioperative antibiotics have become an established part of vascular reconstructive surgery (Table 1).[7,8] It is unclear whether this increase in staphylococcal infections has resulted from an increase in virulence of these organisms or a decrease in the perfusion of distal tissues with antibiotics as more ischemic extremities are salvaged.

Though contamination usually occurs at the time of surgery, the appearance of signs and symptoms of graft infection is usually delayed well beyond the immediate postoperative period. The average time from graft placement to overt infection for grafts contaminated with *S aureus* is 15 months and for grafts contaminated with *S epidermidis* is 41 months.[9,10] Upon presentation, the infection is rarely easily cured. Organism-specific antibiotic therapy administered at the time of diagnosis is usually insufficient for successful treatment of these infections frequently necessitating graft removal.[11,12]

From Bunt, TJ: *Vascular Graft Infections.* Armonk: Futura Publishing Co., Inc.; © 1994.

Table 1
Microbiology of Graft Infection

Organism	1952–1971 (%)	1978–1981 (%)
Bacteroides	2.5	8.1
Corynebacterium	2.5	1.6
E. coli	22.5	11.3
Proteus	7.5	3.2
Pseudomonas	2.5	1.6
S epidermidis	**15.0**	**27.4**
S aureus	**32.5**	**46.8**
Streptococcus	5.0	14.5
Klebsiella	—	6.5
Other	10.0	10.0

S = Staphylococcus; E = Escherichia.

These features of synthetic vascular graft infection appear to result from the process of graft implantation and alteration of the periarterial environment. Similar infections rarely occur in native arteries in the absence of trauma. Thus, intact arterial wall defenses provide significant protection against infection, even in the presence of severe atherosclerosis. An understanding of these native arterial wall defenses and their modification by graft placement provides a clearer insight into the puzzle of graft infection.

Defense of the Arterial Wall and the Periarterial Environment

In the native arterial tree, an intimate relationship exists between the luminal surface of the artery and the periarterial environment. The maintenance of thisrelationship is critical to the defense of the vasculature against bacterial invasion of the arterial wall and the periarterial environment. The benefit of this relationship is proven by the observation that, unlike synthetic vascular grafts, native arteries seldom become primarily infected without aneurysm or trauma.[13] The defense of the vasculature stems from the interaction of blood circulating within the lumen, the endothelial lining, the medial smooth muscle cells, the vasa vasorum, and the perivascular lymphatics. An examination of these defenses not only reveals the mechanism by which the native artery resists bacterial invasion, but also provides insight into the susceptibility of synthetic vascular graft to infection.

Blood, the most ubiquitous of the host defenses, contains numerous important components, such as white blood cells, antibodies, and complement and coagulation proteins, which participate in arterial wall defense against infection. Circulating white blood cells are able to marginate and adhere to endothelial cell surfaces. These marginated white blood cells can then migrate through the interendothelial junctions and gain access to the subintimal space and media where they can exhibit their phagocytic capabilities.[14] Blood-borne complement components may also pass through endothelial gaps and opsonize bacteria to enhance phagocytosis. Products of the complement and coagulation cascades contribute by stimulating chemotactic activity for white blood cells and by increasing capillary permeability.[14] Plasma proteins reversibly bind to antibiotics and aid in the delivery and distribution of antibiotics to various tissues, including the blood vessel walls.[15] All of these blood components are found in the systemic vessels as well as in the vasa vasorum to ensure protection of the entire arterial wall and the periarterial surroundings.

Endothelial cells establish the next line of arterial wall defense by providing surface resistance to bacterial adherence and by regulating the passage of molecules into the subendothelial space. The endothelial barrier is effective in repelling most Gram-positive and Gram-negative organisms with the exception of a few strains of *S aureus* and groups A and G streptococci which possess endothelial cell receptors.[16–19] Thus, the transient bacteremia which accompanies manipulation of mucous membranes such as dental work, cystoscopy, and sigmoidoscopy[20,21] rarely results in infection of the native artery. The endothelium determines the permeability of substances, such as antibiotics, into the subendothelial space. Smaller molecules may passively enter into the intercellular spaces due to concentration gradients, unlike larger molecules, such as fibrinogen, which appear to be actively transported beyond the endothelial barrier into the subendothelial space.[22] Though the exact mechanism of endothelial selectivity is unclear, this property distinctly affects the therapeutic benefits of many antibiotics. Recent studies have demonstrated that penetration of common antibiotics, such as cephalosporins, into the arterial wall varies widely.[23] Antibiotic penetration of the arterial wall occurs not only through endothelial permeability but also from the vasa vasorum.

The media also display intrinsic antibacterial defenses. Composed of alternating layers of elastin and smooth muscle cells, the media provides anatomic barriers to the rapid migration of bacteria through the arterial wall. In addition, a subset of these smooth muscle cells are capable of phagocytic activity. In cell culture, smooth muscle cells harvested from the aorta have been shown to phagocytize yeast cells (Fig. 1).[24] In vivo, a subset of medial smooth muscle cells has been found to behave as tissue histiocytes, engulfing necrotic cellular debris and foreign proteins within the arterial wall.[25] These properties further inhibit the likelihood that bacteria entering from either the luminal or abluminal surfaces can migrate unharmed through the vessel wall.

On the abluminal surface, the vasa vasorum are responsible for meeting the metabolic and immunologic needs of the adventitia and outer half of the media. The nutrient branches of this network penetrate into the midportion of the media and provide metabolic substrate, white blood cells, and antibiotics for protection of these outer layers of the arterial wall.[26] This microvascular system works in conjunction with luminal blood flow to form immunologic barriers to infection. The vasa vasorum have a

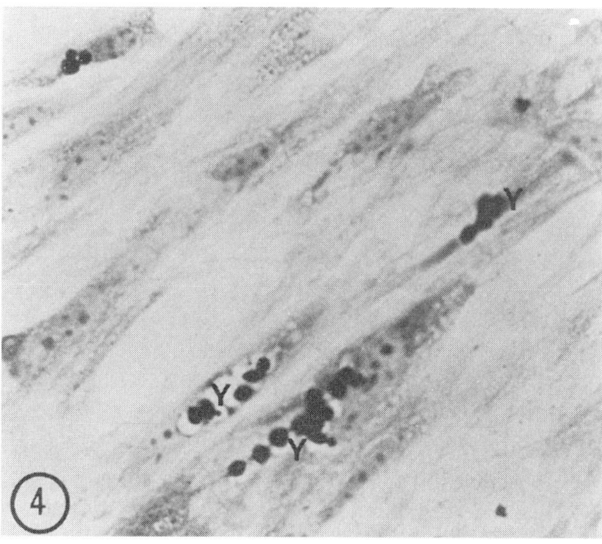

Figure 1. Smooth muscle cells from the media of guinea pig aorta demonstrating completed phagocytosis with engulfed yeast cells.

special functional relationship with the intramural and periarterial lymphatics; while the vasa vasorum imports nutrients, antibiotics, and immunocompetent cells into the arterial wall, the lymphatics export bacteria to keep the arterial wall free from infection.

Intramural lymphatic channels begin at the junction of the media and adventitia[27] and are responsible for the transport of fluid, proteins, and bacteria into the periarterial lymphatics. The flow through these intramural lymphatics appears to be driven by the movement of fluid through the lymphatic pores of the intima and inner portion of the media. Lymphatic pores are present within the internal elastic membrane (Fig. 2). These pores allow substances to pass through the intima and the inner portion of the media in a spongelike manner. Within the central portion of the media, channels begin to coalesce and take the form of lymphatics which travel through the outer media and adventitia along with the vessels of the vasa vasorum. Thus, both bacteria and large antibiotic molecules which are deposited into the subendothelial space are transported together through the arterial wall. The periarterial lymphatics empty into the lymphatic chain within the surrounding tissue and eventually drain into larger periarterial lymphatic channels (Fig.3).

The periarterial lymphatic system consists of an extensive network of connecting lymphatic channels with interspersed lymph nodes for efficient transport of fluid and filtration of bacteria. Lymphatic capillaries found in the soft tissues are blind-ended vessels which consist of a single layer of endothelium.[28] Unlike blood capillaries, lymphatic capillaries lack fenestrations in their endothelial cells and also lack a continuous basal lamina; this allows for easy passage of large particles into the lymph. Backflow of lymph is prevented by the overlapping arrangement of endothelial cells. Lymphatic capillaries are held open by mi-

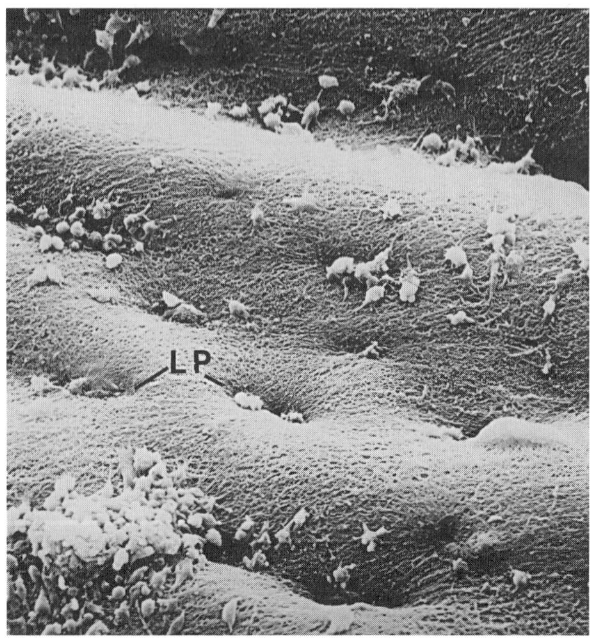

Figure 2. Thermally exposed subendothelial collagen. Note the pores (LP) penetrating the basement membrane and internal elastic lamella to permit egress of fluid and plasma constituents.

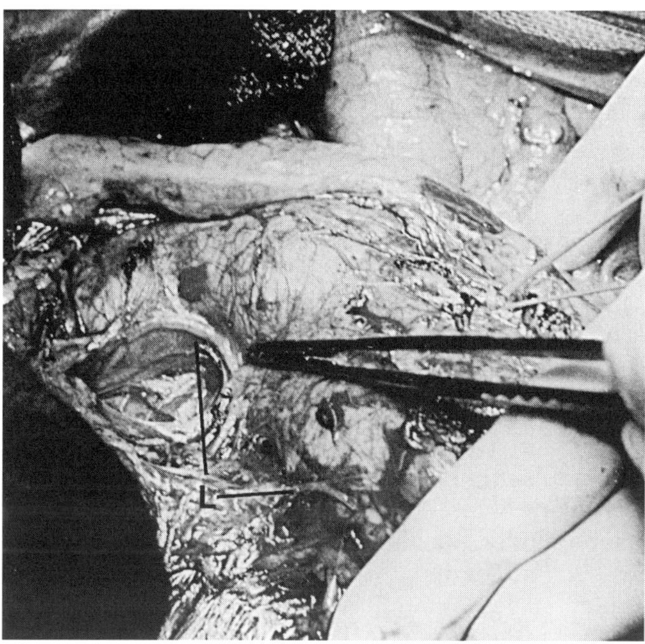

Figure 3. Periaortic lymphatics (L) adjacent to an infrarenal abdominal aortic aneurysm. Note the rather large number and close apposition of these periarterial lymphatics to the vessel wall.

crofibrils, called anchoring filaments, which bind the lymphatics to the surrounding soft tissue. As the connective tissues become distended with fluid or inflamed from infection, they exert pressure onto the anchoring filaments separating the endothelial cells and permitting an increase in flow of interstitial fluid and bacteria into the lymphatic network.

Lymphatic vessels beyond the arterial wall greater than 1 mm in diameter take on layered histologic characteristics that are similar to those of blood vessels.[29] These larger lymphatic vessels possess valves composed of thin layers of connective tissue covered by an endothelium system that restricts flow in one direction. The lymph is propelled to smaller vessels by contraction or compression of surrounding structures, while in larger lymphatic vessels there is synchronized smooth muscle contraction of vessel walls. Lymphatic channels inter-

rupted only by groups of lymph nodes ultimately drain into the thoracic duct and the right lymphatic duct, which return fluid to the systemic circulation.

The lymph node provides the body with an opportunity to screen fluid for foreign organisms or antigens prior to return to the venous circulation.[26] This occurs within the lymph node by exposing lymph to a high concentration of immunocompetent cells which can process foreign antigens in order to stimulate an adequate immune response. Lymph enters the lymph node through afferent vessels which penetrate the capsule of the lymph node at various places and open into an endothelium-lined sinus containing macrophages. This structure gives rise to several other sinuses that direct the lymph through the outer cortex and inner medullary regions of the node before it exits the node and returns to its passage through the lymphatic system. The complicated structure of the lymph node slows the passage of the lymph, allowing maximal exposure of the returning fluid to the immunocompetent cells which then have the opportunity to attack and phagocytize any foreign organisms.

Impact of Graft Placement on the Periarterial Environment

The integrity of the periarterial defense system is completely disrupted and permanently altered by the placement of a synthetic vascular graft. Simple surgical dissection and isolation of an artery from its surrounding tissue profoundly alters its intrinsic arterial wall and periarterial defenses. Communication of the intramural-lymphatic channels with the periarterial lymphatic network is severed, thus inhibiting the transport of fluid, proteins, and entrapped bacteria through the arterial wall.

Additionally, the vasa vasorum are frequently injured in the process of surgical dissection, further reducing the arterial wall defenses by limiting the flow of nutrients, immunocompetent cells, and antibiotics to the adventitia and media in the area of surgical dissection and anastomosis.

After an arterial segment is resected and replaced with a synthetic vascular graft, the process of local immunity throughout the area of grafting is remarkably altered. Shortly after blood contact, the luminal surface of the graft becomes coated with a layer of fibrin which begins pseudointima formation (Fig. 4).[30] Over a period of time, the pseudointima gradually grows representing layers of compacted fibrin interspersed with cells consisting of smooth muscle cells, fibroblasts and macrophages, and an incomplete endothelial covering found to be somewhat protective against bacterial invasion.[31] The initial layers of fibrin which become densely compacted into

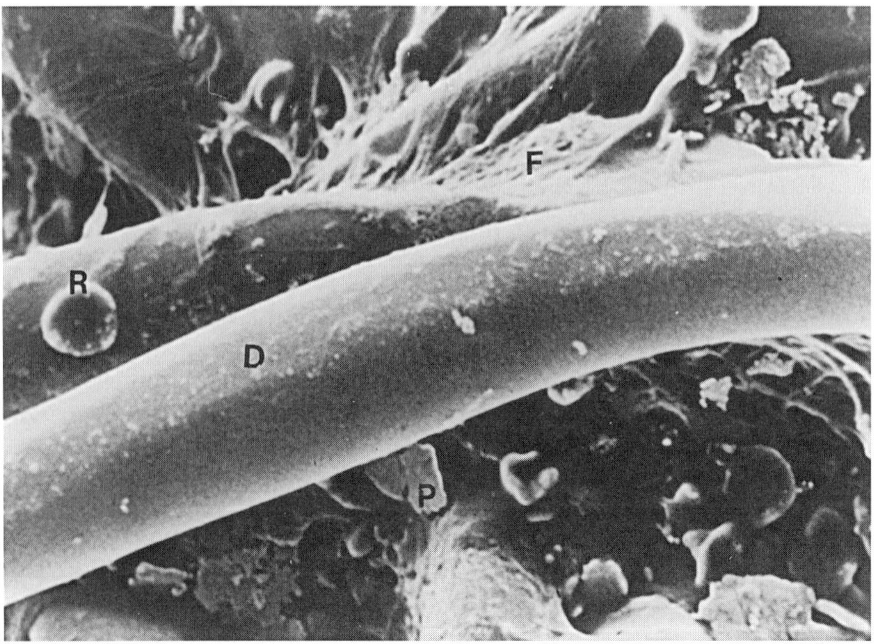

Figure 4. The flow surface of a knitted Dacron graft 5 minutes after blood contact. The Dacron fibers (D) have been coated and linked by strands and sheets of fibrin (F). This fibrin coating serves to entrap red blood cells (R) and platelet plaques (P).

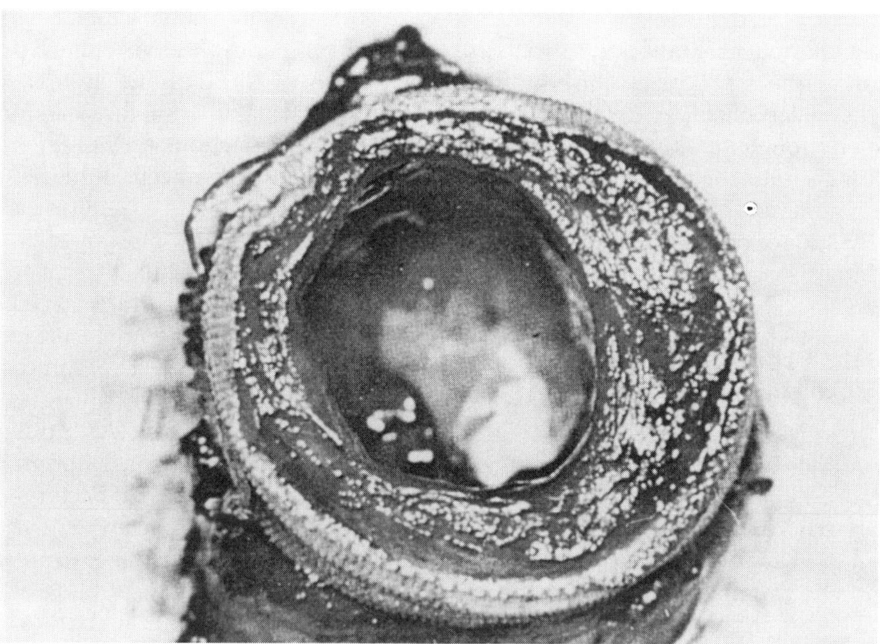

Figure 5. The appearance of a segment of knitted Dacron aortobifemoral graft explanted from a patient after 4 years. Note the exuberant pseudointima eccentrically lining the lumen of the graft. It is of note that the external surface of the graft appears pristine without evidence of collagen and capillary ingrowth through the graft interstices.

the interstices and across the weave of the Dacron or PTFE graft persist for extended periods of time (Fig. 5).[32] This hypocellular lining to the graft does not represent the incorporation of the graft by the host, but rather a process of isolation of the graft from the host. There is some metabolic exchange in the pseudointima closest to the flowing blood. The pseudointima, however, never becomes reconfigured to resemble the native arterial wall. There is no evidence for active or passive transfer of substances below the flow surface into the pseudointima and beyond. Thus, bacteria gaining access to the deeper layers of the pseudointima have few host immune defenses to overcome.

Similarly, the outer surface of the graft becomes isolated from the surrounding tissues. Immediately upon placement of the graft, there is leakage of lymph from the disrupted lymphatics throughout the course of

graft placement.[33] This thin layer of fluid completely surrounds the graft. The injury induced by placement of the graft into the soft tissues results in activation of fibroblasts and a healing response consistent with soft tissue trauma. There is macrophage and fibroblast migration into the area, deposition of fibrous tissue, and the establishment of a graft capsule. The capsule is composed of fibrous tissue which forms slowly over a period of weeks. This graft capsule serves to isolate the abluminal surface of the graft from the surrounding tissues. The fluid surrounding the graft is entrapped by the capsule and is only slowly exchanged.[34] This region between the outer surface of the graft and the inner surface of the capsule is defined as the perigraft environment. Because the pseudointima on the luminal surface of the graft isolates the graft wall, there is little interaction between the blood flowing within the lumen and the outer surface of the graft. The abluminal surface is no longer connected to the vasa vasorum or the major or minor lymphatic networks which normally defend the periarterial environment. Therefore, there is essentially a complete absence of defenses within the perigraft environment, making the outer surface of the graft most susceptible to infection.

The Process of Synthetic Vascular Graft Infection

Complete protection of the synthetic graft requires antibacterial defense of the perigraft environment. Because this environment is virtually isolated, protection of the synthetic vascular graft through the use of intravenous antibiotics is minimally efficacious. Though lymph that leaks around the graft at the time of graft placement may contain antibiotics, the presence of an antibiotic in lymph is quite variable and often transient.[35] These very same lymphatics that are leaking into the perigraft environment eventually become scarred during the deposition of fibrous tissue. Until then, they continue to clear peripheral bacteria and transport them proximally, allowing them to leak out at points of transection which are usually within the field of graft placement. Unlike the luminal surface, which can still be protected by blood-borne antibiotics and white blood cells, the perigraft environment represents a protected haven for those bacteria that can then proliferate in a slow and progressive fashion without triggering a significant immune response. Only the occasional polymorphonuclear leukocyte and macrophage are present in the perigraft space to provide graft protection.[34]

Graft infection results from lymphatic-borne bacteria which leak out into the perigraft environment during or shortly after the time of graft placement.[36] Because this environment is isolated, the bacteria can multiply without eliciting a host reaction. During this phase of bacterial growth, there are few systemic manifestations. The isolation of the perigraft environment prevents activation of the immune system, the release of interleukins, and the systemic manifestations of infection, such as fever or elevation in white blood cell count. After a period of proliferation, the bacteria can begin to invade the graft. This usually occurs along suture lines, but may also occur within the body of the graft. Once bacteria gain access to the luminal surface, they begin to stimulate a systemic immune response. Low-grade fever, myalgias, distal petechiae, and disseminated intravascular coagulation may occur in response to the transmural migration of bacteria. Thus, when graft infections become evident, there is already a large bacterial load in the isolated perigraft environment. Cure of this infection with intravenous antibiotics alone is unlikely. Treatment most often requires removal of the graft and debridement of the perigraft tissues to reduce the bacterial inoculum. At the very least, instillation of antibiotics into the perigraft environment in conjunction with systemic antibiotics is required.[37]

Some bacteria possess specific qualities which make them particularly suitable for surviving within the perigraft environment therefore increasing the likelihood of infection. Interestingly, coagulase-negative *S epidermidis* is now recognized as the most common organism responsible for synthetic graft infection.[38,39] Certain virulent strains of *S epidermidis* have demonstrated the ability to produce slime which makes the organism adhere to the graft and also protects the organism from host immune defenses.[40-42] This slime-producing capability makes *S epidermidis* particularly effective in proliferating in the perigraft space and may thus account for the delayed manifestation of infection compared to other organisms.

Though specific analysis of the periarterial defenses has not been undertaken, there is a growing body of information which supports the concept that graft infection most frequently occurs initially in the

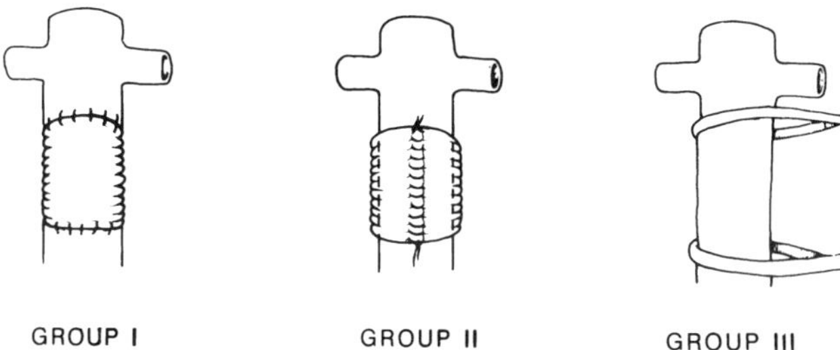

Figure 6. Experimental groups studied to determine the site of bacterial adherence to vascular grafts after bacteremia. Group I animals were the only ones to have a graft in direct contact with the blood stream. Group II animals had the graft wrapped around the intact aorta and Group III animals had aortic isolation only, without the placement of any graft material.

perigraft environment, despite the mode of bacterial entry. To document this, a synthetic Dacron tube graft was interposed into (group I) or wrapped around the intact (group II) infrarenal aortae of dogs.[36] In group III animals, the aorta was simply mobilized (Fig. 6). After closure of incisions, the animals were given an intravenous injection of 1×10^7 S. aureus. Grafts were harvested on day 1 or day 21. At the time of harvest, selective cultures of the periaortic tissues, the external surface of the grafts and aorta, and the luminal surface of the grafts and aorta were taken to distinguish infections of the luminal and abluminal surfaces (Fig. 7). Overall, 85% of the grafts in group I, 67% of the grafts in group II, and 85% of the aortae in group III were infected (Table 2). This is especially striking in light of the fact that no graft material was present in group III animals. Analysis of selective cultures demonstrated that the majority of the infections were located in the perigraft environment. The difference between perigraft and graft lumen cultures was statistically significant in all groups. All of the aortic lumen cultures in groups II and III were negative. Lymphangiography performed

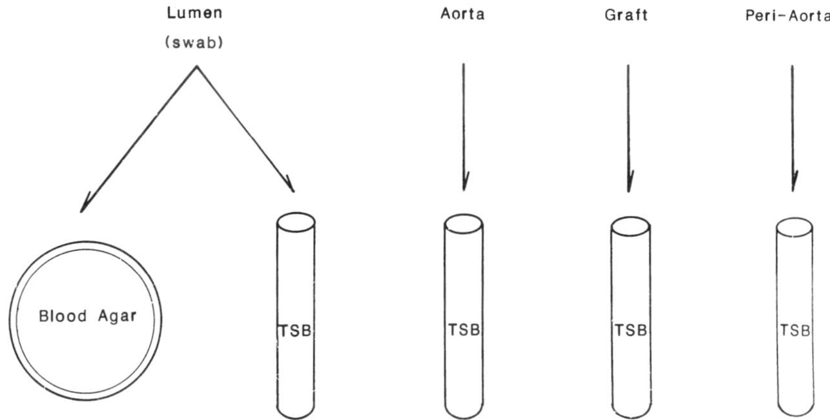

Figure 7. The selective culturing process used to differentiate luminal versus abluminal bacterial contamination.

Table 2
Cumulative Infection Rate

| Group | Positive Culture | |
	Lumen (%)	Periaorta (%)
I	4/17 (24)	14/17 (82)
II	0/9 (0)	6/9 (67)
III	0/13 (0)	11/13 (85)

through the inguinal lymphatics in these animals demonstrated lymphatic leaks in the immediate area of graft placement (Figs. 8A,B).

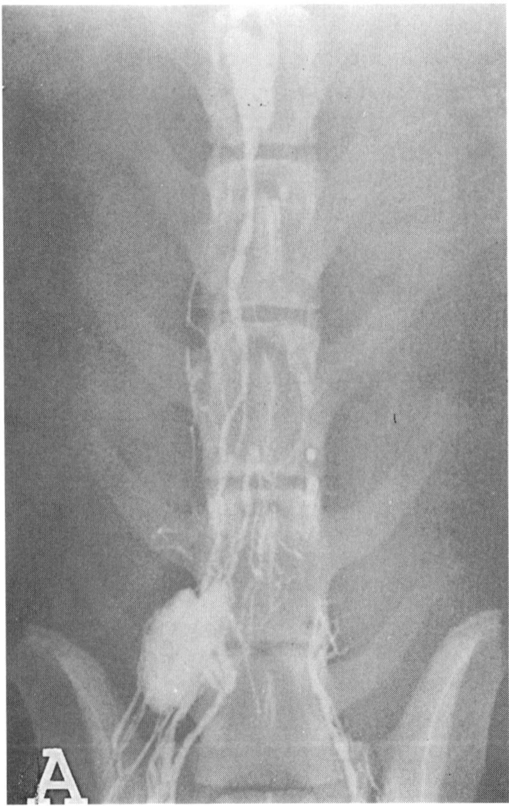

Figure 8A. A lymphangiogram of the periaortic lymphatics in the dog. There are large continuous chains which travel close to the adventitial surface of the aorta linking the aortic wall to the periarterial environment. The lymphatic chains are similar to those seen in humans (Fig. 3).

Similar results were obtained by Rubin and colleagues who evaluated the impact of bacteria-laden lymphatics upon synthetic vascular graft infection.[43] Bilateral canine femoral artery grafts were placed and were challenged with an inoculum of *E. coli* and *S aureus* into the foot pad of one of the limbs. Not surprisingly, both grafts became infected. This represents yet another demonstration that grafts are susceptible even to distant infections because of the breach of the periarterial defenses.

Minimizing the Risks of Synthetic Graft Infection

Clearly, every effort must be made to protect and preserve the periarterial and perigraft environment. The first step is to minimize dissection of the artery both proximally and distally. Technically proficient surgeons have long recognized the value of this approach in arterial reconstructive surgery.

There has also been considerable effort expended on the development of a bacteria-resistant prosthesis. Most approaches, however, have focused on limiting the luminal attachment of bacteria. Both antibiotic binding as well as endothelial seeding have been proposed as methods to reduce the likelihood of synthetic graft infection.[44,45] However, neither of these approaches adequately addresses the perigraft environment. Graft exteriors coated with antibiotic or the deposition or insulation of antibiotic in the perigraft environment should serve to reduce the likelihood of bacterial contamination and colonization of the perigraft tissues. This can be accomplished in several ways. First, preclotting the graft in blood containing high levels of dissolved powder will serve to put an outer layer of fibrin and antibiotic along the exterior surface of the graft[46]; this has been shown to be an effective method for reducing the likelihood of graft infection. Other, more traditional methods include antibiotic irrigation of the perigraft

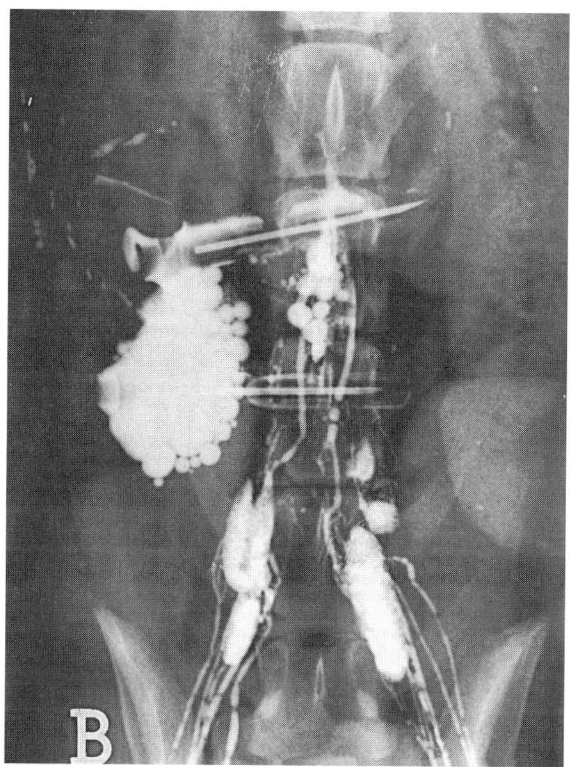

Figure 8B. A lymphangiogram of the periaortic lymphatics of the dog after careful surgical dissection and isolation of the infrarenal aorta and placement of an aortic graft. Note that the lymphangiography contrast material is diffusely leaking into the periaortic environment, spilling any transported bacteria onto the freshly placed graft.

tissues.[47] Similarly, the use of antibiotics that achieve high levels within the lymphatics can be helpful in protecting the perigraft environment through the lymphatic leaks that occur during graft placement.[48]

As increasing amounts of the human arterial tree are replaced with synthetic grafts, greater efforts to reduce the incidence of synthetic vascular graft infection must be made. These efforts must be based on a clear understanding of the mechanisms of graft infection. Recognizing the importance of the perigraft and periarterial environment in the process of graft infection provides critical insight into changes that must be made during graft placement. Me-

ticulous dissection, minimal disruption of the periarterial bed, choosing perioperative antibiotics with high levels of lymphatic penetration, and continuing the search for bacteria-resistant grafts containing antibiotics on the abluminal as well as the luminal surface will help to protect the outstanding technical achievements that have been gained in vascular reconstructive surgery over the past 4 decades.

References

1. Liekweg WG Jr, Greenfield LJ. Vascular prosthetic infections: collected experience

and results of treatment. *Surgery.* 1977;81: 335–342.

2. Bunt TJ. Synthetic vascular graft infections. I. Graft infections. *Surgery.* 1983;93:733–746.

3. Kikta MJ, Goodson SF, Bishara RA, et al. Mortality and limb loss with infected infrainguinal bypass grafts. *J Vasc Surg.* 1987;5: 566–571.

4. O'Hara PJ, Hertzer NR, Beven EG, et al. Surgical management of infected abdominal aortic grafts: review of a 25-year experience. *J Vasc Surg.* 1986;3:725–731.

5. Quinones-Baldrich WJ, Hernandez JJ, Moore WS. Long-term results following surgical management of aortic graft infection. *Arch Surg.* 1991;126:507–511.

6. Kaiser AB, Clayson KR Mulherin JL Jr, et al. Antibiotic prophylaxis in vascular surgery. *Ann Surg.* 1979;188:283–289.

7. Szilagyi DE, Smith RF, Elliott JP, et al. Infection in arterial reconstruction with synthetic grafts. *Ann Surg.* 1972;176:321–333.

8. Lorentzen JE, Nielsen OM, Arendrup H, et al. Vascular graft infection: an analysis of 62 graft infections in 2411 consecutively implanted synthetic vascular grafts. *Surgery.* 1985;98:81–86.

9. Goldstone J, Moore WS. Infection in vascular prostheses: clinical manifestations and surgical management. *Am J Surg.* 1974;128: 225–233.

10. Bandyk DF, Berni GA, Theile BL, et al. Aortofemoral graft infection due to *Staphylococcus epidermidis. Arch Surg.* 1984;119:102–108.

11. Freischlag JA, Moore WS. Infection in prosthetic vascular grafts. In: Rutherford RB, ed. *Vascular Surgery.* Philadelphia: WB Saunders Co; 1989;510–521.

12. Bernhard VM, Parent FN. Treatment of aortic graft infection. In: Ernst CB, Stanley JC, eds. *Current Therapy in Vascular Surgery.* Philadelphia: BC Decker Inc; 1991;435–440.

13. Moore WS, Malone JM. Vascular infection. In: Howard RJ, Simmons RL, eds. *Surgical Infectious Diseases.* Norwalk: Appleton & Lange; 1988;585–600.

14. Cotran RS, Kumar V, Robbins SL. *Pathologic Basis of Disease, 4th ed.* Philadelphia: WB Saunders; 1989;45–47.

15. Wise R. Protein binding of β-lactams: the effects on activity and pharmacology particularly tissue penetration. II. *J Antimicrob Chemother.* 1983;12:105–118.

16. Vercellotti GM. Lussenhop D, Peterson, PK, et al. Bacterial adherence to fibronectin and endothelial cells: a possible mechanism for bacterial tissue tropism. *J Lab Clin Med.* 1984; 103:34–43.

17. Ogawa SK, Yurberg EM, Hatcher VB, et al. Bacterial adherence to human endothelial cells in vitro. *Infect Immunol.* 1985;50: 218–224.

18. Thomas PD, Hampson FW, Hunninghake GW. Bacterial adherence to human endothelial cells. *Amer Phys Soc.* 1988;1372–1376.

19. Valentin-Weigand P, Grulich-Henn J, Chatwal GS, et al. Mediation of adherence of streptococci to human endothelial cells by complement S protein (vitronectin). *Infect Immun.* 1988;56:2851–2855.

20. LeFrock JL, Ellis CA, Turchik JB, et al. Transient bacteremia associated with sigmoidoscopy. *N Engl J Med.* 1973;289:467–469.

21. Felix JE, Rosen S, App GR. Detection of bacteremia after the use of an oral irrigation device in subjects with peridontitis. *J Peridontal.* 1971;42:785–787.

22. Jellinek H, Detre Z. Role of the altered transmural permeability in the pathomechanism of arteriosclerosis. *Path Res Pract.* 1986; 181:693–712.

23. Fradet G, Brister S, Richards GK, et al. Antibiotic prophylaxis in vascular surgery: pharmacokinetic study of four commonly used cephalosporins. *J Vasc Surg.* 1986;3:535–539.

24. Garfield RE, Chako S, Blose S. Phagocytosis by muscle cells. *Lab Invest.* 1975;33:418–427.

25. Wolfbauer G, Glick JM, Minor LK, et al. Development of the smooth muscle foam cell: uptake of macrophage lipid inclusions. *Proc Natl Acad Sci USA.* 1986;83:7760–7764.

26. Clemente CD. *Gray's Anatomy.* Philadelphia: Lea & Febinger; 1985;852,873.

27. Takacs E, Jellinek H. Lymphatics in the aorta of rats treated with a soy bean oil extract (lipofundin). *Lymphology.* 1986;19:161–166.

28. Ryan TJ. Structure and function of lymphatics. *J Invest Dermatol.* 1989;93:18S–24S.

29. Junqueira LC, Carneiro J, Kelly RO. *Basic Histology, 6th ed.* Norwalk: Appleton & Lange; 1989;214–215.

30. Pasquinelli G, Freyrie A, Preda P, et al. Healing of prosthetic arterial grafts. *Scan Micros.* 1990;4:351–362.

31. Sauvage LR, Berger KE, Wood SJ, et al. Interspecies healing of porous arterial prostheses. *Arch Surg.* 1974;109:698–705.

32. Santini C, Speziale F, Massimi GJ, et al. Preliminary results of a complete study protocol on synthetic vascular graft healing and its complications. *Int Angiol.* 1992;11:211–217.

33. Pricolo VE, Potenti F, Soderberg CH. Effect of perigraft seroma fluid on fibroblast proliferation in vitro. *Ann Vasc Surg.* 1991;5: 462–466.

34. Sedwitz MM, Davies RJ, Pretorius HT, et al.

Indium 111-labeled white blood cell scans after vascular prosthetic reconstruction. *J Vasc Surg.* 1987;6:476–481.

35. Roberts TL, Futrell JW, Sande MA. Antibiotic penetration into normal and inflamed tissues as reflected by peripheral lymph. *Ann Surg.* 1979;189;395–402.

36. White JV, Freda BA, Kozar R, et al. Does bacteremia pose a direct threat to synthetic vascular graft? *Surgery.* 1987;102:402–408.

37. Calligaro KD, Veith FJ, Gupta SK, et al. A modified method for management of prosthetic graft infections involving an anastomosis to the common femoral artery. *J Vasc Surg.* 1990;11:485–492.

38. Macbeth GA, Rubin JR, McIntyre KE, et al. The relevance of arterial wall microbiology to the treatment of prosthetic graft infections: graft infection vs. arterial infection. *J Vasc Surg.* 1984;1:750–754.

39. Kaebnick HW, Bandyk DF, Bergamini TW. The microbiology of explanted vascular prostheses. *Surgery.* 1987;102:756–762.

40. Bergamini TM, Bandyk DF, Govosois D, et al. Infection of vascular prostheses caused by bacterial biofilms. *J Vasc Surg .* 1988;7:21–30.

41. Martin LF, Harris JM, Fehr DM, et al. Vascular prosthetic infection with *Staphylococcus epidermidis*: experimentai study of pathogenesis and therapy. *J Vasc Surg.* 1989;9:464–471.

42. Edmiston CE Jr, Schmitt DD, Seabrook GR. Coagulase-negative staphylococcal infections in vascular surgery: epidemiology and pathogenesis. *Infect Control Hosp Epidemiol.* 1989;10(3):111–117.

43. Rubin JR, Malone JM, Goldstone J. The role of the lymphatic system in acute arterial prosthetic graft infections. *J Vasc Surg.* 1985;2:92–98.

44. Rosenmann JE, Kempczinski RF, Berlatzky Y, et al. Bacterial adherence to endothelial-seeded polytetrafluoroethylene grafts. *Surgery.* 1985;98:816–823.

45. Birinyi L, Douville C, Lewis SA, et al. Increased resistance to bacteremic graft infection after endothelial cell seeding. *J Vasc Surg.* 1987;5:193–197.

46. White JV, Benvenisty AI, Reemtsma K, et al. Simple methods for direct antibiotic protection of synthetic vascular grafts. *J Vasc Surg.* 1984;1:372–380.

47. Pitt HA, Postier RG, MacGowan WAL, et al. Prophylactic antiobiotics in vascular surgery: topical, systemic, or both? *Ann Surg* 1980;192:356–364.

48. Folsom DL, Franceschi D, Rubin JR. Intralymphatic antibiotic delivery for reducing acute prosthetic graft infection. *J Cardiovasc Surg.* 1992;33:660–663.

SECTION III

Prevention

It is the patient's responsibility to get well and the surgeon's responsibility to create the optimal situation for that recovery. Neither can succeed without the other.

Chapter 5

Overview of Prevention Measures

T.J. Bunt

Introduction

"An ounce of prevention is worth a pound of cure" has less situations more applicable than graft infection (GIF). Although there has been a steady decrease in absolute mortality rates for both aortic and peripheral graft infections, the amputation rate remains significant; and there has *not* been a corresponding or at least proportional decrease in the mortality from graft-enteric fistula (GEF). Clearly, prevention of these major life- and limb-threatening complications remains a first order priority.

Furthermore, prevention ultimately is the personal responsibility of the operating surgeon; the measures outlined in this chapter are, for the large part, directly a function of the dedication and finesse each vascular surgeon brings to every operation. Ham-handed surgeons get sloppy results, as do surgeons who place all too much emphasis on operative times rather than perfection in technique. Time may be money to the mercenary-motivated surgeons, but extra time taken is invaluable to his patient; obviously, I have little sympathy for the former.

It is of interest that while the incidence of aortic GIF is decreasing, the incidence of peripheral or lower extremity GIF appears to have remained stable over 30 years—probably because most are associated with wound-healing problems, particularly when lengthy incisions are made for harvesting of the saphenous vein. Breakdown of the thigh portion of these is just as frequent a problem now as it was for vascular pioneers. The incidence of aortic or other inflow graft infection seems, however, to have decreased, although admittedly there are fewer single institution longitudinal studies on which to presuppose an exact overall incidence. However, there are several recently published series and even more paper discussions indicating series of hundreds of aortic procedures without the authors noting (recognizing?) a GIF.

General Measures

Curiously, the incidence of GEF does *not* seem to be decreasing, with 301 cases noted from 1955 to 1980, and 323 from 1980 to 1992; however, the incidence or at least differential recognition of graft-enteric erosion (GEE) is increasing. All of this would seem to indicate that the generic measures of prevention that are outlined herein and which were generally promulgated during

---

From Bunt, TJ: *Vascular Graft Infections.* Armonk: Futura Publishing Co., Inc.; © 1994.

the 1970 to 1980 time frame, now may be proven effective.[1,2]

Conversely, if surgeons ignore these simple precepts or brashly decide that there is no need for such precautions, then GIF and GEF may reasonably be expected for their patients, whether the surgeons recognize their (sometimes delayed) occurrence themselves, or whether it takes the astute acuity of their peers to recognize them. Nasty as this comment might seem, it comes from a surgeon who has operated on more than 75 patients with graft infections, most of whom had complications caused by someone else![3,4]

Mechanical Prevention Methods

Graft Infections

Prevention of GIF is theoretically based on avoiding situations that may lead to contamination of the graft with bacteria either at operation or at some delayed interval; it is therefore heavily based on conclusions derived from laboratory models for either inducing or preventing GIF (See Section II), or on the logical extension of generally accepted principles for the prophylaxis of wound infections and bacteremias that might lead to GIF.

Philosophy

A treatise on GIF prevention from this author cannot omit some reference to the initial choice of patient and operation. Proponents of routine aortic reconstruction (AR) for all patients with inflow problems base that preference heavily on the higher 5- and 10-year patencies of AR over competing inflow reconstructions such as axillofemoral (AXF), crossfemoral (CF), or iliacofemoral (IF) bypasses. Proponents of the latter extra-anatomic bypasses (EAB) note that such procedures take less toll on the elderly or medically compromised patient, and some (this author included) specifically note a distinct reduction in operative mortality for EAB procedures. Equally important is a comparison of the major long-term complications of AR and EAB and the comparative ease or difficulty of handling such complications when they do occur. As I pointed out in 1983, well-documented, if seldom advertised long-term major complications of AR occur in roughly 5% to 8% of patients, and include pseudoaneurysms (PA), GIF/GEF, and limb thromboses.[5] Conversely, spontaneous (as opposed to infection of EAB placed for treatment of a GIF) GIF of an EAB is as yet a seldom reported event (five cases); the major long-term problem with EAB is its higher thrombosis rate (patency).

Philosophically, the surgeon needs to consider these long-term effects in the initial decision to offer AR versus EAB. Aortic GIF and GEF still carry significant mortality and morbidity rates and weighing the long-term morbidity and mortality for a given patency might sway one to a decide on an initial EAB.

Since multiple researchers have noted increased infection rates when an inguinal incision is used, strong consideration should be given to avoidance of the inguinal incision entirely. Performance of either tube or aortoiliac grafting for aneurysmorrhaphy procedures should always be preferred; extension to the groins with aortobifemoral bypass invites a higher risk of GIF; surgeons who routinely use tube grafting unless specific symptoms require aortobifemoral bypass (ABFB), have noted prolonged patencies of grafts anastomosed more proximally, despite an accepted 50% incidences of iliac aneurysmal extension and distal subclinical stenoses.

Primary AR, however, obviously requires the inguinal approach due to expected progression of occlusive disease in currently seemingly patent/unaffected external iliac systems.

A related philosophic judgment point

would be the consideration for providing either retroperitoneal supracoeliac or formal thoracofemoral grafting for patients with either potentially hostile abdomens (multiple previous surgeries) or major intra-abdominal infection within the past several years.

Read has presented two patients with aortic graft infections incurred during operation within 1 year of a previous episode of peritonitis and suggested that intervals greater than 1 year be instituted.[6] I have personally seen the same situation twice. In both cases, the patients were clinically well and gave no overt evidence of persistent intra-abdominal sepsis, yet at interval laparotomy for aortic grafting they were found to have seemingly innocuous 2- to 5-cc pockets of intermesenteric abscess. In one patient, fatal *Pseudomonas* aortic shaft GIF resulted, which was also cultured from the seemingly innocuous 2-cc sterile abscess. Edwards has also noted in his series of GIFs that two followed prior episodes of peritonitis, one of appendicitis and one of cholecystitis.[7] Such limited anecdotal experience should lead to caution in using the standard transperitoneal approach within 1 year of established prior peritonitis.

A similar thought process should enter into the decision for autologous versus synthetic conduits in lower extremity revascularization. This complex problem usually centers on the decision for a short-term benefit (quicker operation) with a 20% to 30% chance of needing a secondary autologous below knee or tibial bypass being balanced against a single if longer operation that uses the vein first, thus making secondary revascularization more difficult, if possibly less frequently indicated. The threat of subsequent GIF incurred with synthetic GIF should be added to this judgment decision based on patency rates, particularly if there is active pedal sepsis or other nosocomial infection complicating the picture, since these are factors that increase the risk for both wound and graft infection.

Table 1
General Preoperative Principles for Prophylaxis of Wound Infection

1. Limit the preoperative hospital stay.
2. Obtain elective angiography more than 1 week preoperatively.
3. Use antiseptic showers twice a day during the 24 h preoperatively.
4. Avoid elective operations if other major infection is present.
5. Immediately depilate preoperatively in the holding area.
6. Maintain a hospital surveillance for unusual or antibiotic resistant organisms.
7. Obtain local control of pedal sepsis preoperatively.

Preoperative Preparation

Prevention of Wound Infection

General principles of wound infection prophylaxis may be quite cogently applied here, and are based heavily on longitudinal hospital-wide studies from the general surgical literature (Tables 1,2,3).

Cruse (1973) studied 23,649 wounds, noting an overall 4.75% incidence of wound infection at 30 days; this varied from 1.81% with clean wounds to 8.9% for clean-contaminated wounds. Potential etiologies for

Table 2
General Intraoperative Principles for Prophylaxis of Graft Infection

1. Use perioperative antibiotics.
2. Ligate or avoid lymphatics/lymph nodes, rather than transecting them.
3. Obtain careful multilayer wound closure and skin approximation.
4. Avoid unnecessary skin contact by synthetic grafts.

Optional

Use wound irrigations with topical antibiotics.
Consider antibiotic graft impregnation.

Table 3
Overall Antibiotic-Antiseptic Measures

Preoperative
Antiseptic showers-scrubs.
Minimize preoperative time frames

Intraoperative
Initial antibiotic dose in holding area.
Redose at usual half-life of dose duration curve.
Redose prior to wound closure if time frame extends beyond half-life of drug from the initial or redose times.
Additional wound protection with topical antibiotic solution dressings.
Topical irrigation of graft in its bed at completion of case.
Topical irrigation of wounds that become dry, potentially contaminated, or are open for > 1 h.

Postoperative
Continued antibiotics for:
  nosocomial infection.
  distal pedal infection.
  until invasive lines removed if they are present > 5 total d.
  positive arterial, aneurysm, or other operative culture.

the development of wound infections were addressed. Puncture of a surgical glove during a clean case raised the rate to 5.3% (29/548). Diabetes increased it to 10.7%, obesity to 13.5%, and malnutrition to 16.6%; steroids in this study had no deleterious effect. Increased rates were also seen if there was no preoperative antiseptic shower (2.3% versus 1.3%), and a virtual doubling of rates was seen for each successive hour spent in surgery. If there was a prolonged preoperative hospital stay, the rate increased from 1.1% for 1 day to 2.0% for 1 week to 4.3% for 2 weeks. Use of intraoperative diathermy doubled the infection rate for all categories except neurosurgery (where it was, of course, used routinely!).[8]

Although Cruse's study still represents the gold-standard study for wound infection, a stateside national operative wound infection study had been carried out in 1964, which noted adverse effects on wound in-

fection rates from advanced age, obesity, steroids, prolonged preoperative stay, and curiously, from the use of prophylactic antibiotics (however, with various milieus and few in what would now be recognized as an appropriate fashion). The rate of wound infection increased from 6.7% to 18.4% if a remote infection was present. Similarly, Birkenstock (1973) had reported an even higher association due to a remote infectious site, with an increased incidence from 6.0% to 31.6%. Edwards (1976) had also studied 40,923 operations over 4 years, noting 1966 wound infections in 1865 patients; 61.3% of wound infections were associated with antecedent remote infections. Obviously such studies from general surgery can be extrapolated to the vascular situation, and their significance compounded by the usual presence of an implanted foreign body.[8–11]

One epidemiologic study was confined to vascular surgery. Hammarsten (1977) retrospectively looked at the specific incidence of wound infection occurring in a series of 326 patients undergoing a variety of vascular procedures over 5 years; 75% of cases were elective, 50% were done under prophylactic antibiotic coverage. The overall wound infection rate was 12% (37/326) and increased the mean hospital stay from 11.9 to 31.3 days. Sixty percent of the infections were due to *Staphylococcus aureus*. Factors increasing the incidence ($P < 0.5$) included diabetes, pedal gangrene, a preoperative stay of more than 2 days, surgical times greater than 2 hours, postoperative hematoma, multiple incisions, and anticoagulation.[12]

The findings of these generic surgical studies have direct relevance to GIF prevention. Obviously, some of these associated risk factors cannot be adequately controlled, for example, age, steroids, and malnutrition. However, the preoperative stay can be minimized; the rationale being a decrease in the incidence of skin and orifice colonization by hospital-acquired resistant bacteria. Even if a prolonged stay is necessary, liberal use of preoperative antiseptic showers/shampoos should aid in decreasing these deleterious flora. Depilation is best obtained with depilatory creams; if shaving is performed, it should be performed in the holding area and with a very gentle technique to avoid skin breaks. Furthermore, an antiseptic cream may be adjunctively used. These generic findings are summarized in Tables 1 and 2.

Long-Term Prophylaxis

Postoperative infection initiating or at least initially recognized at the inguinal incision may 1) involve already, or 2) may subsequently ascend to involve the more proximal graft. The accepted and multiply reported etiologies of this infection involve local contamination of the graft at the groin in the vast majority of cases. Once the incisions are healed and presumably graft incorporation is complete (roughly 6 to 8 weeks), the chances of local seeding are remote. An exception to this general rule might be with peripheral or EAB grafts, where local skin erosion with secondary direct infection may occur at any time; such problems, however, tend to be sharply defined locally and their management correspondingly easy (simple excision of the local segment with extra-anatomic rerouting is nearly uniformly successful).

The major theoretic risk (excluding GEE and GEF, whose etiology is covered elsewhere) for long-term seeding of a graft is from secondary bacteremias. Sources for these include septicemias from other infections (furuncles, diabetic pedal sepsis, pneumonia, urosepsis) and at least the theoretic risk for bacteremias during dental or visceral manipulations. Theoretic rationale for bacteremic graft infection is based heavily on the standard canine model for inducing GIF which is *not* necessarily a relevant model to the human clinical situation. First of all, the lab model of a freshly implanted graft with luminal thrombus is not the same as the clinical graft chronically in place with its luminal surface covered with pseudointima, which seems to offer resistance; and secondly, the bacteremias involved in dental or proctologic-prostate manipulations appear to occur at magnitudes of order lower than those of either clinical sepsis or those necessary for GIF production in the lab model.

The risk of graft seeding from late bacteremias remains confused. Bacteremia following dental manipulation was demonstrated by Paquin (1941), who described the clinical syndrome as clearly apparent to the dentist; fever, chills, weakness, and positive blood cultures for *Streptococcus viridans.* He pointed out that bacteria could be cultured from 92% of normal appearing teeth. He recommended prophylactic sulfa drugs to control these frequently noted bacteremias.[1]

Lindemann (1982)[2] updated the issue for the dental profession, and suggested that all patients with known synthetic vascular grafts should routinely receive antibiotic prophylaxis before any dental procedure. The review article provided no new information about risk, but based the recommendations on the bacteremia models of Moore (as below).[13,14]

A similar confusion has arisen regarding the possibility of bacteremic seeding following proctoscopy. Lefrock (1973)[3] noted on routine blood cultures of 200 patients undergoing routine sigmoidoscopy that, although no patient demonstrated any clinical stigmata of bacteremia, 9.5% had positive blood cultures; half of these had evidence of active colonic disease but the other half did not. All bacteremias were transient with cultures being negative at 30 minutes. The bacteria recovered included Enterococcus in 11, *Escherichia coli* in 4, *Klebsiella* in 3, and *Bacteroides* in 1; the colony counts were, however, quite small, ranging from 2 to 34 colony counts per cc. Lefrock noted that these small bacteremic episodes might well not be of clinical significance, particularly since seeding would be into the portal reticuloendothelial system with expected rapid clearance prior to actual arterial exposure.[2]

The bottom line is that although bacteremias have been noted with urologic, proctologic, dental, and irritative focus stimulation, the exact risk of these for causing a graft infection is quite unclear. The episodes are transient and of very low order of magnitude unless a clinical septic episode is noted. Laboratory models for bacteremic graft infection require much higher inoculate infusions to reliably attain graft sepsis.

Control or prevention resides in two arenas—usage of prophylactic antibiotics:

1. in the postoperative period until all monitoring and drainage catheters capable of stimulating bacteremias have been removed
2. prophylactic use in patients undergoing dental, urologic, or proctologic manipulations.

The biologic control rests with formation and preservation of an intact pseudointima.

Differential Infectability

There has been a recurrent myth that polytetrafluoroethylene (PTFE) has a lower differential infectability than Dacron. Let me destroy that myth.

Adherence Models

Sugerman[1] (1982) studied the in vitro adherence of thymidine-labeled 1×10^8 solutions of *S aureus* and *Enterobacter* to 12-mm woven and knitted Dacron and PTFE graft segments after a 60-minute incubation in 10 cc of bacterial suspensions. *Enterobacter* adhered to Dacron at a rate 10 to 100 times higher than it did to PTFE ($P < .05$); velour provided an even higher bacterial adherence. *Staphylococcus aureus* adherence was equivalent for both Dacron and PTFE. There was only nominal attachment if the grafts were exposed briefly and immediately rinsed; attachment increased in a nonlinear manner proportional to the time of exposure, with 70% total adherence at 30 minutes, regardless of bacteria or graft type. The researchers theorized that the greater total surface area afforded by Dacron (particularly velour) over PTFE might account for the differential adherence of *Enterobacter*, but could not explain the lack of increased adherence for *S aureus*. The intense negative change of PTFE was, however, invoked as a potential repellent to adherence.[1]

This study demonstrated an incompletely explained increased adherence of Gram-negative to Dacron versus PTFE, but is of questionable relevance to the clinical situation since the grafts were not implanted, not exposed to either blood or tissue fluid, and not subject to antibiotic inhibition. As further studies will elucidate, intraluminal fibrin, thrombus, and fibronectin are the key elements to bacterial adherence, and these were not present. This study provides a look at what the integral graft matrix itself offers as bacterial attraction.

Goeau-Brissoniere (1983) performed an elegant series of experiments detailing the bacterial adherence to previously implanted grafts[2]. An inoculum of 1×10^7 *S aureus* within an isotonic medium circulated through nonimplanted Dacron grafts resulted in adherence of roughly one in every 10,000 bacteria. The work was then extended to acutely (2 hours) or chronically (2 months) implanted grafts that were resected and exposed to *S aureus* in the perfusion model. In the acute model, grafts were exposed to extracorporeal circulation for 2 hours to allow deposition of a thrombus matrix on the luminal surface. The chronic model involved canine thoracoabdominal bypass grafting under gentamycin 5-day prophylaxis.

At a 2-hour exposure, PTFE grafts showed no visible thrombus on the luminal surface; at 2 months, over 50% of the lumen still remained uncovered. Dacron velour grafts showed initial thrombus, which was histologically amorphous and grossly limited to the graft weave concavities, with the convexities remaining bare. At 2 months, the luminal surface was uniformly covered with a clear fibrin mat, but many bare Dacron fibers still projected into the lumen. Bovine grafts showed scattered thin fibrin deposits at 2 hours, and a uniform confluent layer of endothelial-like cells with small areas of fibrin deposits over flow-surface defects.

Normal canine aorta entrapped an average eight (3 to 30 range) colony forming unit (CFU)/cm^2 (one in every 10^6 organisms). Polytetrafluoroethylene entrapped an average 23 (0 to 200) cells/cm^2; bovine grafts 607 (20 to 5000) ($P < .001$) and Dacron 2801 (25 to 10,000) ($P < .001$) at 2 hours. At 2 months, PTFE entrapped 19,122 (100 to 200,000) ($P < .001$), bovine 863 (30 to 40,000) and Dacron 3500 (10 to 10,000). The addition of cefazolin at 10 to 25 times the minimum inhibitory concentration (MIC) of S $aureus$ to the perfusate did not materially affect bacterial adherence rates.

There was a significantly increased bacterial adherence to both bovine and Dacron grafts compared to PTFE at 2 hours; only PTFE showed significantly increased adherence at 2 months. The entrapped bacteria were noted histologically to be on irregular fibrin strands or on surface defects. For PTFE, this occurred primarily at the midportion of the grafts where the graft matrix was either exposed or had, at most, a fragile fibrin layer; bacteria were noted to adhere to bare surfaces of Dacron grafts or to fibrin strands over the pseudointimal surface. Bovine grafts characteristically showed large surface areas devoid of fibrin strands, and only showed colonization at flow-surface defects where fibrin had collected.[2]

This extensive study emphasizes the role of intraluminal graft surface fibrin in allowing bacterial colonization of the flow surface of grafts, relating bacterial adherence to the degree of fibrin deposition. It also introduced the pessimistic note that concomitant antibiotics did not affect the rate of bacterial deposition, thus raising distinct questions about any positive role of prophylactic antibiotics in this regard.

Bennion et al. (1984) specifically addressed the accepted laboratory model of testing for infectability with sublethal bacterial inocula, and suggested that graded inocula might demonstrate a differential infectability for graft materials. They suggested that the term *median infective dose* (MID) be used, defined as the inoculum at which half of exposed grafts become infected. Prostheses were implanted in the standard canine infrarenal aortic model and an intravenous dose given at closure; grafts were explanted 6 weeks later and assessed for clinically or culture-positive infection. Human umbilical vein (HUV) grafts became culture-positive at all inocula of S $aureus$ from 1×10^2 to 1×10^5 organism/cc; silver-impregnated HUV grafts were resistant (0/4) to 1×10^2, but became infected at all higher inocula from 1×10^3 through 1×10^8; double velour Dacron grafts showed low infection rates (1/5, 2/5) at 1×10^2 and 1×10^3 ($P < .05$), but showed reliable infection (4/5) from 1×10^4 through 1×10^7 (8/8) inocula (Fig. 1). The plotted/calculated MID for the three grafts was $< 10^2$, $10^{2.8}$, and $10^{3.2}$, respectively. The study underscores the potential for very small (100 to 10,000) inocula of immediate postoperative bacteremias to cause GIF.[3]

Rosenmann (1985) speaking for Kempczinski's group, studied 4-mm grafts of knitted Dacron, HUV, and thin-walled PTFE placed in a pulsatile perfusion system in which the grafts were then exposed to 4.7 $\times 10^6$ indium-labeled S $aureus$ for 30 minutes. Bacteria were noted to be fixed to the Dacron at 9.63×10^5 bacteria/cm; to HUV at 1.04×10^5, and PTFE 2.15×10^4 ($P < .05$). Addition of a suture line in the middle of the graft increased adherence by 50%. On standard electron microscopic (SEM) and autoradiograph studies, there was uniform distribution of the bacteria in low quantity except for the suture line where there was a dense concentration.[4]

This study did not per se address the

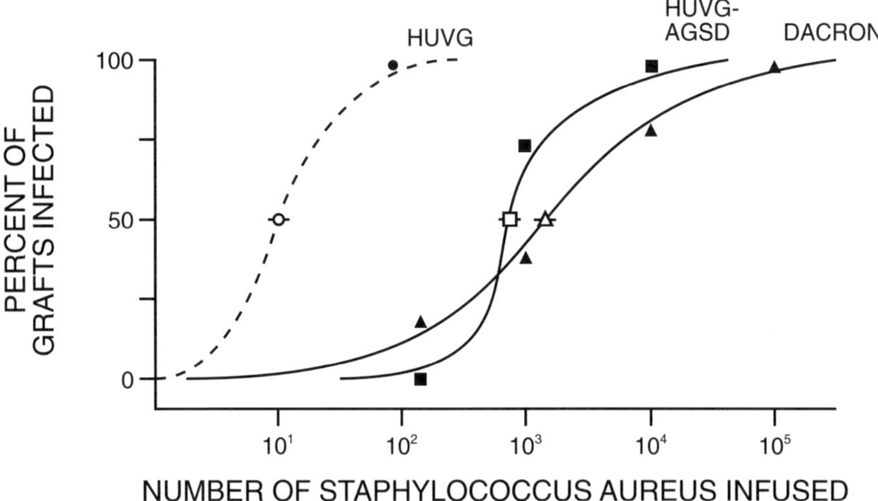

Figure 1. Curves demonstrating the rate of infection of several types of grafts exposed to increasing levels of *S aureus*. HUVG = human umbilical vein graft; HUVG-AGSD = silver-impregnated human umbilical vein graft. (From Bennion RS, et al. *Surgery*. 1984;5:1:22–25.)

degree of thrombus formation, but it is evident that there would be more thrombus/fibrin in Dacron grafts than either HUV or PTFE (at least at this early juncture), and bacteria are noted to adhere at sites of thrombus or fibrin formation. The study therefore would indicate that initially Dacron has greater bacterial adherence as a function of its thrombogenic surface.

Schmitt (1986) noted differential bacterial adherence of the three most common GIF pathogens to PTFE as opposed to either knitted or velour Dacron. Graft segments were inoculated with 1×10^7 organisms, washed repeatedly, sonicated, and then analyzed for residual bacterial adherence. The results showed significantly ($P < .01$ to $.025$) less adherence of *S epidermidis* RP-12, *S epidermidis* SP-2, *S aureus*, or *E coli* to the PTFE grafts as compared to Dacron.

Follow-up studies for the group were reported by Bergamini (1988). In this model, established *S epidermidis* RP-12 aortic graft infections in dogs were excised and replaced under antibiotic coverage with either Dacron or PTFE implants. Although the Da-

cron grafts at 1-month reexploration showed a higher (33% versus none) clinical reinfection (perigraft fluid, inflammation), biofilm cultures were higher for RP-13 in the PTFE group than the Dacron (44% versus 22%). Interestingly, standard broth cultures were all negative.[5,6] This study underscored the fact that clinically healed PTFE grafts were frequently occultly infected.

Contaminated Field Models

There is also varied clinical experience with the placement of grafts into an infected/contaminated field that is often used to indicate a presumptive differential infectability.

Bricker (1970) studied autologous vein versus Dacron interposition grafts in a canine model. Iliac or femoral arterial segments were replaced with jugular vein or 6-mm knitted Dacron under 2-week perioperative penicillin prophylaxis, and then exposed to 0.1 to 1 cc (sic) of a 1×10^5/cc culture of *S aureus*. Three of five control grafts and two of five Dacron grafts were patent at 4 to 5 weeks, none with infection. In the model, 15 of 18 vein grafts remained patent, but two animals exsanguinated after vein graft dissolution. Only seven of 18 Dacron grafts remained patent. Five of 40 grafts were culture-positive; however, all grafts showed marked perigraft fibrosis in contrast to all control wounds, suggesting a healed infection.[7]

Shah (1983) performed a similar canine study, looking at vein graft versus PTFE. Autologous jugular vein or 6-mm PTFE femoral artery interposition grafts were placed and then inoculated locally with 1×10^7 *S aureus* and *E. coli*; half were additionally covered with 5-day perioperative cefoxitin prophylaxis. All control grafts healed without incident. Local inoculation resulted in uniformly positive cultures for both organisms, as well as six for an additional *Pseudomonas*; the addition of antibiotics resulted in sterilization of one of 10 sites only. Inoculated PTFE grafts thrombosed within 2 weeks; three vein grafts caused exsanguination after dissolution.[8]

Akhondzadeh (1980) studied differential infectability in a canine model of infrarenal replacement with 6-mm woven Dacron, 8-mm bovine, 6-mm PTFE, and 6-mm HUV grafts, followed by 15-minute intravenous infusion of 5×10^7 *S aureus*, either immediately or 3 weeks postoperatively. Control Dacron and PTFE segments were noted to be contained within a variably well-developed fibrous tissue envelope; bovine and umbilical vein grafts became densely incorporated into surrounding tissue. The prosthetic materials demonstrated no resistance to immediate bacteremia. All 16 Dacron grafts were grossly infected, 15 with positive cultures and five with anastomotic disruption; all 19 bovine grafts were grossly infected, 18 with positive cultures and 9 with disruptions; 5 of 5 human umbilical vein grafts were infected, all with positive cultures, and 1 with disruption; and 10 of 10 PTFEs were grossly infected, all with positive cultures and 1 with disruption. In-

fected grafts were surrounded by a marked fibrotic inflammatory reaction with some perivascular abscesses.

Delaying the bacteremia to 3 weeks resulted in a significant reduction in clinical infection; disruption was unusual (one bovine graft), but resultant fibrosis was much denser. Dacron showed a clinical infection in 6 of 13 and a positive culture also on 6; bovine showed clinical infection (2 disruptions, 3 thromboses) in 5 and positive cultures in 4; PTFE showed minimal inflammatory changes in 5 of 10, but positive cultures in 6; and HUV had only 1 of 5 clinically and culture-positive.[9]

This study showed a clear difference between immediate and late bacteremias occurring without antibiotic coverage. Of interest was a clear description of the varying types of normal graft incorporation, the uniform appearance of clinical infection, and the distinct tendency for PTFE grafts to appear minimally infected yet be culture-positive.

Stone (1984) studied autologous jugular vein versus 6-mm PTFE used as femoral arteriovenous shunts in a canine model with local inoculation of 1×10^3 *S aureus*; half of the dogs received 5 days of cephalothin therapy. All antibiotic-treated dogs remained clinically normal and at 6-week explantation, had patent- and culture-negative grafts. Untreated dogs developed clinical wound sepsis; six of seven vein grafts disrupted (86%) versus two of seven (28%) of PTFE grafts ($P < .05$). Histologic exam of the PTFE showed spotty neointima formation only. Although the PTFE infection results parallel those of other authors, the interesting sidelight of this study was the apparent sterilization of infection with parenteral antibiotics; to a large degree, this may be due to the small inoculum (10^3 organism) used. However, since no graft cultures were obtained of the PTFE grafts in this group, the known propensity for PTFE to harbor clinically occult infection could well have been missed.[10]

Discussion

In summary, data to support a differential rate of infectability for PTFE versus Dacron is at best theoretic, with conflicting experimental findings. Dacron appears more susceptible to immediate bacterial adherence, particularly for *S epidermidis* RP-12 species; and PTFE can be shown to "heal" in situ even though it remains culture-positive and therefore occultly infected. Since all published studies are of the standard canine GIF model and short-term, and since in humans persistent *S epidermidis* infections show up in delayed fashion as graft complications, it is difficult to come down solidly for PTFE or against Dacron.

Putting these papers together, one can theorize that bacteremias must be of the 10^4 or higher magnitude to reliably cause a clinically recognizable infection of a freshly implanted graft; it is unknown whether that same level or a higher number is required for infection of chronically implanted grafts. Secondly, lower inocula of bacteria may well be successful in matrix penetration that results in an occult infection whose clinical recognition is delayed to the later onset (by a presently unknown mechanism) of an immunologic response. Thirdly, infection of the freshly implanted graft is related to intraluminal-infected thrombus, which would suggest that PTFE enjoys an initial advantage over Dacron; however, the addition of collagen impregnation to cover the luminal Dacron surface, and particularly if antibiotics are bonded to the collagen, will probably obviate this small advantage. The response to initial infection is also different; HUV and bovine graft fare poorly with early infection, tending to disrupt with secondary exsanguination.

Long term, the ability to obtain and maintain a stable and complete pseudointimal coverage of the intraluminal graft is probably the dominant factor observed for resistance to secondary bacteremias. In this respect, the data is not conclusive, but would again suggest that both Dacron and PTFE grafts have incomplete pseudointimal coverage and that fibrin laid down on areas of exposed graft is the mediator of secondary bacteremic adherence. A well-incorporated HUV or bovine graft does well in the face of late bacteremias, unless there are focal flow defects with fibrin accumulation to facilitate bacterial adherence.

The role of prophylactic antibiotics seems intellectually straightforward, yet the extensive series by Goeau-Brissoniere's group could not show any reduction in bacterial adherence when suitable antibiotics at adequate MIC levels were specifically added to the model. It is intellectually difficult to conceive how and why the addition of such antibiotics to a solution of bacteria could not reduce bacterial adherence and/ or death, yet that was clearly the experimental finding. Antibiotic usage in other models reduced the clinical evidence of GIF, but not the actual culture positivity, particularly with PTFE; this tends to corroborate the clinical concept that the bacteria are able to adhere to implanted grafts and initiate infections, since once adherent they are resistant even to appropriate antibiotics.

If indeed this is the case, then short-term prophylaxis versus bacteremia can theoretically be afforded only by direct graft matrix impregnation, and will not be obtained with standard antibiotic regimens. Protection versus late bacteremias is strictly a function of the degree of pseudointimal coverage, and also is relatively unaffected by antibiotic usage. This would place tremendous importance on the utilization of a graft that obtains excellent ingrowth, for example, velour or other knitted Dacron and/or the newer high porosity (60 to 90 micron pore) PTFE graft based on the observed neocapillary-sustained, stable, and more complete pseudointima seen with these grafts. Conversely, as will be discussed below, it is doubtful that an intravenous antibiotic dose administered at the time of delayed bacteremia will have any reliable theoretical effect on preventing bacterial adherence.

Intraoperative Measures

Graft-Enteric Fistula and Erosion

Mechanical prevention of GEE and GEF is based on the physical concept that the pulsatile and noncompliant foreign body represented by the aortic graft may mechanically erode into viscera that adhere to its surface. For GEE, the concept is straightforward. By definition, such cases involve a highly limited local infection not involving an anastomosis and must therefore involve direct mechanical enteric wall erosion. For GEF, the mechanical concept has additional competition from the concept that a primary GIF causes localized disruption (minimal pseudoaneurysm) at the (usually aortic) anastomosis, with primary or secondary erosion of the infected PA into the adjacent viscera (90% duodenum). Of course, invoking infection as primary etiology only shifts the physics of visceral erosion one step further, since there still has to be erosion into the bowel lumen via either graft or the resultant aortic pseudoaneurysm; local infection/ inflammation simply serve as catalysts and accelerating factors.

There is actually no definitive proof for either theory. The only laboratory study that attempts to delineate the role of either mechanical or infection etiologies was by Busuttil (1979). He postulated that the pathogenesis of ADF was not mechanical, but due to infection and pseudoaneurysm formation. This statement was made at the beginning of his article and purported to be due to a review of the literature. My own review hardly supports that claim of literature support (See Section VII). Be that as it may, he then devised a canine model to prove his point. Infrarenal aortic Dacron grafts were placed in 24 animals, six in each group. Group 1 dogs had suture fixation of the duodenum to the proximal anastomosis; no ADFs occurred at 6-weeks explantation. In Group 2, duodenal graft plication was followed by 1×10^8 S aureus bacteremia; two dogs developed ADF. In Group 3, the duodenum was incorporated into the anterior anastomotic line to create a false aneurysm; three of these developed ADF. In Group 4, that model was supplemented with S aureus bacteremia, with five animals developing ADF.

Busuttil correlated this experimental evidence with clinical data on 11 patients with ADF; graft infection was said to be present in 7, and 5 had proximal pseudoaneurysms. He put all of this together to come to the conclusion that ADF results from low-grade infection resulting in pseudoaneurysms, resulting in enteric erosion.[11]

However, I would note that the clinical evidence he quotes is suspect. By the time one has clinically diagnosed GEF, visceral erosion by definition has occurred and some degree of graft matrix contamination has occurred. One would expect all grafts to be culture-positive. The clinical observations to be made here are whether:

1. A GEF is seen as a localized phenomenon without aortic shaft infection or widespread inflammation indicating a GIF. The answer is yes because this is the clinical picture in roughly one third of GEFs.

2. Erosions alone are seen without evidence of GIF or anastomotic pseudoaneurysm? The answer is yes because this is the definition of a GEE and some 135 cases have been so described. Similarly, a primary aortoduodenal fistula associated with aortic aneurysm is clearly a local erosion problem and not due to infection.

The clinical evidence breaks down into a spectrum of presentations from simple GEE, in which there is no GIF and mechanical erosion is clearly etiologic; through localized GEF, where a limited local graft contamination occurs with direct nonaneurysmal connection between aortic suture line and duodenum; to the dense inflammatory mass of a clearly infected aortic shaft GIF with pseudoaneurysm and secondary GEF.

Busuttil's laboratory data represent an interesting attempt to create an ADF in a short time, and are clearly suspect for actually representing the situation as it occurs in humans. Suturing the duodenum to the graft most clearly mimics the clinical situation, in which the duodenum comes to lie in close approximation to the proximal anastomosis as the narrow apex of the retroperitoneal incision is closed; yet, this close clinical approximation model resulted in no GEFs in Busuttil's model. However, his model allowed only 6 weeks for development of the GEF, when the average time frame for GEF presentation clinically is 2.5 to 3 years. One cannot discount the purely mechanical model on such a short-changed model! Addition of bacteremic infection at time of implantation results in an acutely (and in the dog model, grossly) infected aortic shaft, with the known natural history of proximal disruption in 10% to 40%. This is not the same situation as delayed infection in an incorporated graft, as must be clearly the case for standard clinical GEF noted for their delayed presentations; acute postoperative aortic shaft infections present early with clinical sepsis. Thus, the model is actually testing a known entity, that is, acute gross aortic GIF with its complication of aortic disruption (with some 36 clearly described cases in the literature). The only new twist is that so many visceral disruptions were also produced, a phenomenon not described in countless other identical canine experiments. (See Lab Models) And finally, the Group 3 and 4 method of actually suturing the duodenal wall into the aortic anastomosis seems to predispose to acute duodenal wall infarction and immediate ADF; the authors considered this to be a "perianastomotic hematoma of which the duodenal wall was an integral part." How this is felt to represent a model for pseudoaneurysms escapes me. It rather seems to indicate that acute visceral disruption will rapidly infect the graft and result in aortic pseudoaneurysm as a consequence of GIF.

Technical Measures

Preventive measures for GEF are thus those that avoid the juxtaposition of the junction of the fourth portion of the duodenum/proximal jejunum to the proximal aortic anastomosis; and, to a lesser extent, subsequent adhesion of other visceral structures (ureter, ileum) to the remainder of the graft. A number of such measures to protect the proximal anastomosis have been devised.

Deweese (1962) described the necessity for double layer closure of the retroperitoneum to provide a thicker tissue interposition between the duodenum and the aorta.[12] Hertzer similarly described closure of the aneurysmal sac to exclude the graft[1,2] (Fig. 2).

Robiscek (1972) noted that reinforcement of the proximal anastomosis could be obtained with a cuffed graft which was then turned back over the suture line to exclude it from visceral contact; the cuff was a 2- to 3-cm segment of the graft divided lengthwise and sutured to both the graft (prior to insertion) and at the aorta. A variation of this technique could be used for standard aneurysmorrhaphy usng the posterior aneurysm wall.[14]

Miller (1979) pointed out that closure of the standard retroperitoneal incision involved replacement of the distal duodenum in anatomically close proximity to the aortic anastomosis, and suggested leaving the duodenum reflected to the right, with closure of the left peritoneal reflection to the aneurysm wall and/or right para-aortic tissues.[15]

Consideration should also be given to the technique of actual anastomosis, whether end-to-side (ETS) or end-to-end (ETE); as well as the exact technique of the latter. An ETE anastomosis for an abdominal aortic aneurysmorrhaphy (AAA) places the graft in the same anatomic plane as the original aorta (plus closure of the AAA wall). However, ETE for AR must include actual resection of a short segment of the aorta distal to the anastomosis and above the inferior mesenteric artery orifice to allow the best plane. Otherwise, the implanted graft tends to buckle upward and push against the first portion of the je-

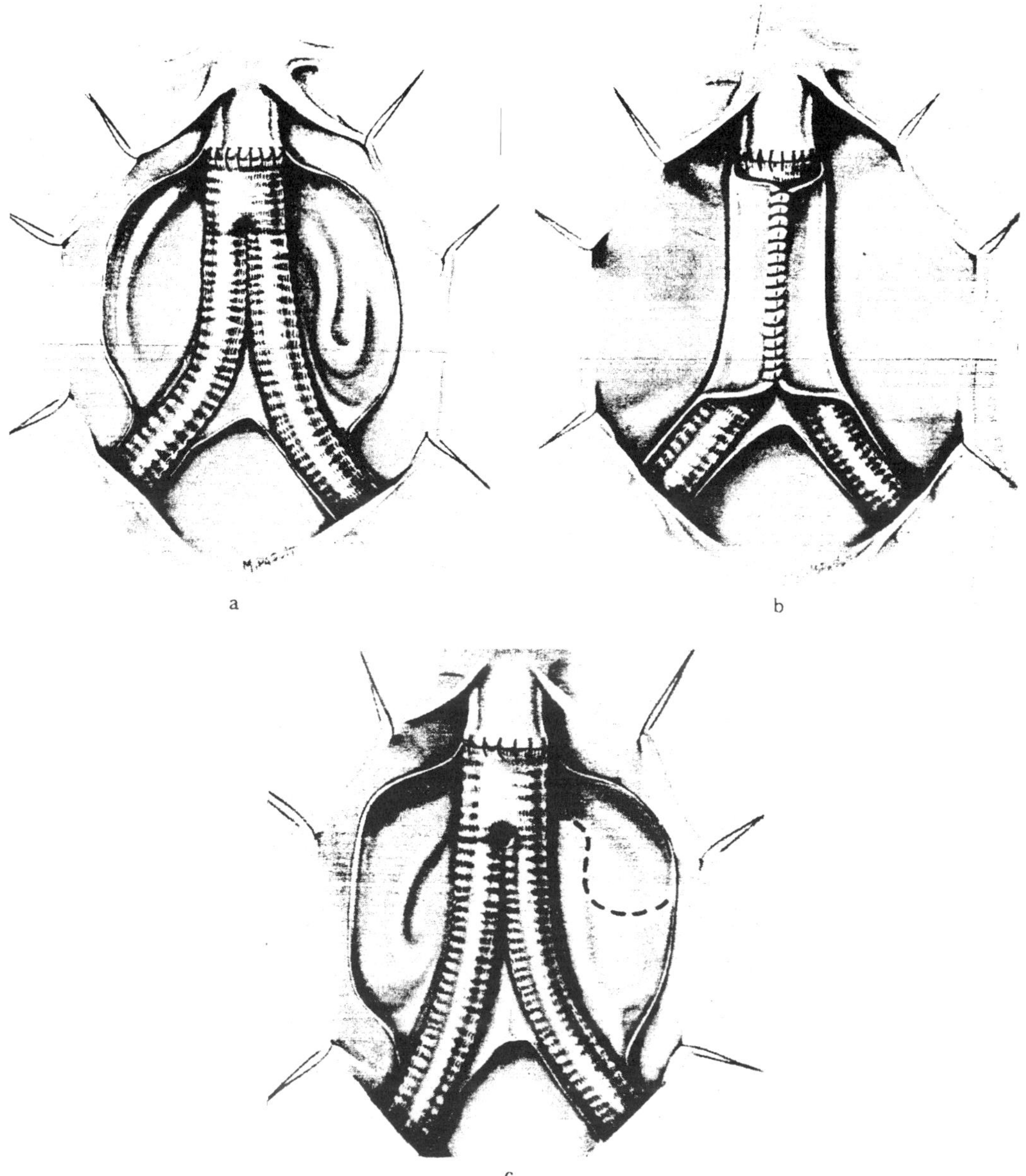

Figure 2. A rotated cuff of the aneurysm wall may be used to exclude the anastamosis. (From Hertzer NR. A rotated aneurysm cuff for separation of aortic graft and duodenum. *Surg Gynecol Obstet.* 1978;147:84–85.)

junum. An ETS or onlay anastomosis should also be performed in the technique well described by Sauvage (1979); a short aortic shaft quickly bifurcating into the limbs; otherwise, the elongated aortic shaft tends to buckle and project upward versus the jejunum.[16]

In addition, as a philosophical note, the prevention of GEF should be another factor in the original decision for ETE versus ETS for AR. We adhere to the generic principle that ETS is always preferable to 1) preserve any collateral circulation that emanates from the native aorta; 2) minimize proximity of the duodenum to the aortic anastomosis to prevent GEF; and 3) allow an easier management of GIF if it does occur postoperatively.

Review of the 416 cases of GEF and 130 GEE are of interest for the specific notation by some authors of possible etiologies. Included are multiple instances of lack of retroperitonealization, or of too large a graft, as well as seven specific instances of aneurysmal cuffs, and 36 of pseudoaneurysm formation. There were, in addition, 39 instances of clinical GIF that seemed to initiate the GEF or GEE.

Aortic Stump Sepsis Prophylaxis

Aortic Stump Closure Standardly accepted measures to close the aortic stump after aortic graft resection involve a two layer closure with monofilament suture. However, repeated experience with aortic stump sepsis (ASS) and blowout led several authors to advocate additional measures to buttress this closure.

Fry and Lindenauer (1967) recognized that the aortic stump after graft resection could be friable and its closure somewhat tenuous. They recommended buttressing of the closure with flaps fashioned from the paravertebral fascia to either side of the aorta. Siedenberg (1965) advocated using strips of harvested fascia lata as being more readily available with less dissection.[17,18]

Buchbinder (1980) described a jejunal serosal patch to reinforce the aortic stump. This was developed in a canine model and then clinically tested in three patients. The mucosa was carefully removed from a vascularized pedicle of jejunum, leaving a seromuscular flap which was then used to cover the aortic stump after removal of an infected graft (Fig. 3). In the clinical trial, graft infections in three patients were managed by total excision, EAB, and patching. Two of these patients died of cardiopulmonary complications, providing the ability to show histologic and gross confirmation that the jejunal pedicle was firmly adherent to the aortic stump, that the pedicle was viable, and that there was direct healing from the jejunum to the aorta, without demonstrable bacteria in the latter.[19]

This limited experience provides

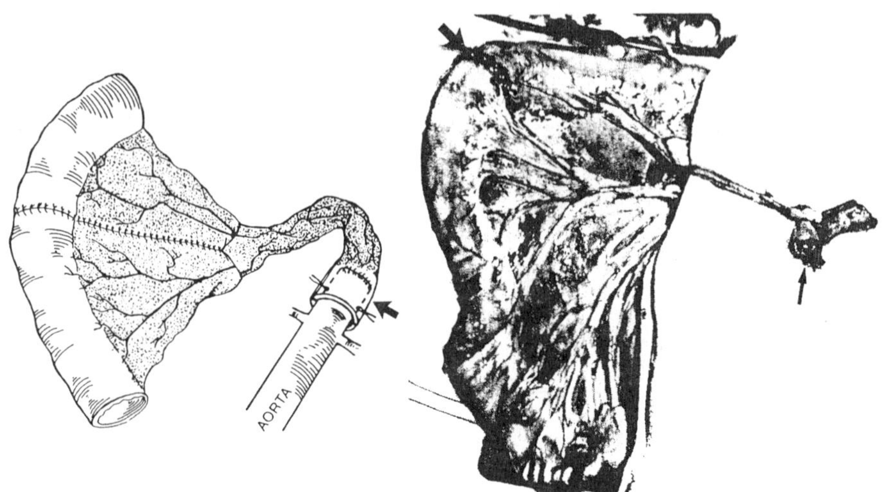

Figure 3. A pedicle of jejunal serosa may be laid over the aortic stump suture line to provide vascular tissue coverage. (From Buchbinder D, Leather R, Shah D, et al. Pathologic interactions between prosthetic aortic grafts and the gastrointestinal tract. *Am J Surg.* 1980;140:8:192–195.)

equally limited but suggestive proof that the method could be used to provide further bacterial clearance from the aortic stump. Of course, it requires that the bowel be opened, which at least theoretically limits its use to the management of GEF; and it is a technically demanding and time-consuming procedure.

Ray (1983) described a fairly complex (and to my mind a potentially dangerous) method of closure that involved splitting the aortic stump into two separately closed tubes. The rationale was that aortic stump blowout was potentiated by the increased wall tension of the single lumen-end closure, as per derivation of Laplace's law. The vector of blood pressure force versus this single closure was felt to be theoretically decreased into two smaller and partially laterally reflected pressure waves (Fig. 4). No supporting engineering texts nor clinical results were presented in this brief paper.[20] My personal experience is that one is seldom inclined to incur any more dissection at the juxtarenal proximal cuff than is absolutely necessary to allow safe aortic cuff debridement and closure. Splitting the already tenuous aortic cuff to allow closure seems risky; and if the technique requires that "the two renal arteries be connected to the aorta so as to mimic the natural bifurcation configuration," then, presumably, additional renal artery mobilization and suprarenal aortic clamping are also necessary. I have not found this method necessary in 36 consecutive aortic graft resections; perhaps, however, on occasion, the technique would be useful if the aortic cuff was very short. An easier solution would be to abandon closure of the diseased infrarenal cuff, and move to below the level of the superior mesenteric artery closure where there was normal aortic tissue, combining this with hepaticorenal and splenorenal bypasses.

Cogbill (1984) noted that although synthetic pledgets would obviously potentiate local infection and subsequent ASS, similar pledgets could be fashioned from autologous material; they used saphenous vein

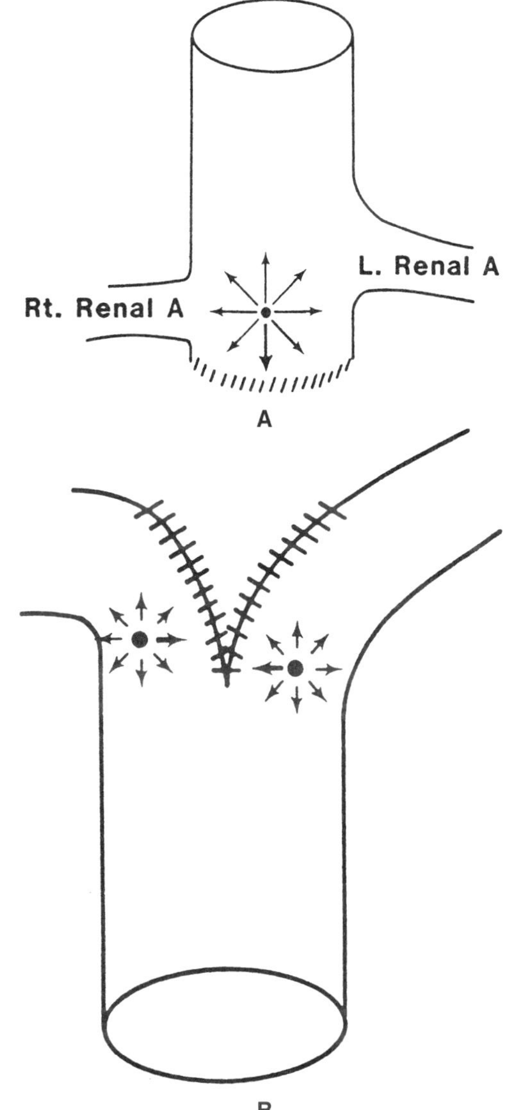

Figure 4. Aortic stump closure by a vertical rather than horizontal suture line, to deflect the flow from the closure and into the renal arteries. (From Roy A, Hayes DF. Closure of an aortic stump: a new method. *Am Surg.* 1983;145: 403–404.)

pledgets (Fig. 5) as a buttress for interrupted horizontal mattress sutures.[21]

Bacourt (1986) updated the concept first addressed by Roy and suggested that the standard cul-de-sac aortic closure be changed to an anterior-posterior suture line

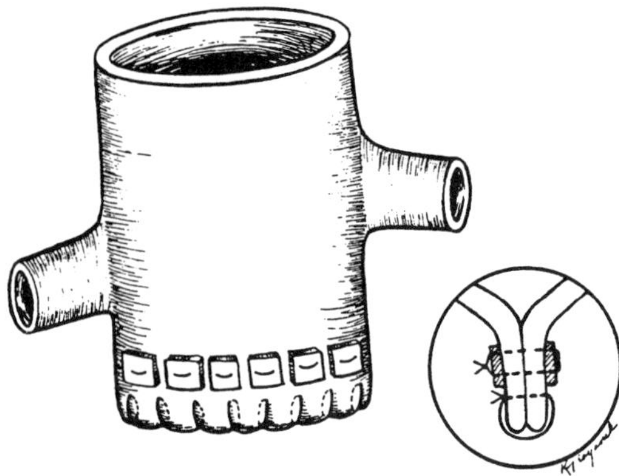

Figure 5. Aortic stump closure may be facilitated by bolsters of autogenous vein. (From Cogbill TH. Secure aortic stump closure with autogenous vein pledgets. *Surgery.* 1984;96:5:940–942.)

that essentially creates a midline strut to split the pressure wave and deflect the flow into the renal arteries. They conceived that the more proximal closure be placed in arcuate fashion (Fig. 6) to create this interrenal bifurcation.[22] I would have the same reservations about routinely applying this closure to the aortic stump as I did for Ray's concept.

Discussion In most situations, standard two-layer aortic stump closure will be possible after reasonable aortic debridement. In addition, one-layer vascular staple or monofilament closures have been noted to be successful in numerous operations. However, there are occasions to consider each of these additional measures when the aortic stump lends itself to such closure, or when local infection seems to require better control with either the omental or seromuscular pedicle techniques.

More important than such mechanical tricks is recognition of the necessity for absolute control of the local infection by thorough debridement of local tissue; thorough debridement of the aortic stump back to normal (e.g., nonfriable) tissue, which may necessitate suprarenal clamping and hepatosplenorenal grafting to allow an adequate stump; and consideration of long-term antibiotics if aortic cultures (which should be routinely obtained) are positive. Prevention of ASS is clearly dependent on the degree

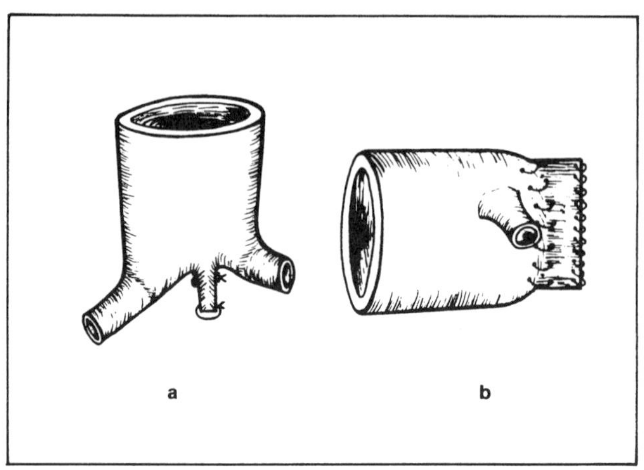

Figure 6. An alternative closure of the aortic stump. See text for critique. (From Bacourt F, Goeau-Brisseniere O, Keskas F. Aortic stump closure: a new technique. *Ann Vasc Surg.* 1986;1:271–272.)

to which the surgeon is willing to take the extra time and perspiration to provide as clean a field as possible for aortic healing to proceed, and as a seemingly nasty but obvious corollary, the incidence of ASS is going to be dependent on the surgeon's willingness to do the right thing and not try to "get out" or "get away with it."

Omental Pedicles Goldsmith (1968) described a modification of the omental pedicle as an adjunct to treatment of a graft infection. Infrarenal aortic replacement with Dacron grafts was performed in the standard canine model. Local inoculation was then obtained with 1 cc of liquid feces. All dogs received 10 days of penicillin/streptomycin treatment, and study dogs had the graft wrapped in an omental pedicle. A second group had formation of an initial retroperitoneal abscess by direct inoculation with a 1/2 cc of feces. Forty-eight hours later, the resultant 5- to 10-cc abscess was drained and infrarenal Dacron grafts were placed in situ under penicillin/ streptomycin coverage. Study dogs again underwent complete prosthesis wrapping with omentum; otherwise, there was no retroperitoneal closure in either group. Nineteen dogs were entered into the two models of local sepsis, 14 died, seven of sepsis and seven of anastomotic disruptions. At 1-year autopsies, three of the remaining five dogs had clinical and culture-proven graft infections. Of the 19 dogs with omental protection, only five died, two by sepsis and three by anastomotic hemorrhage. At 1-year explantation, two additional grafts were clinically infected.

On histologic examination, Goldsmith noted that the omental pedicle was incorporated into the graft matrix. He theorized that use of an omental pedicle for routine aortic surgery, and particularly for ruptured aortic aneurysmorrhaphy, might materially decrease subsequent GEF/GIF development by interposing viable, vascularized tissue between the aorta and the duodenum.[23]

The model Goldsmith used is quite harsh, and best approximates the situation of in situ replacement of a new Dacron graft into a local grossly contaminated field. It is of interest to realize that 30% of dogs survived in the model without omental wrapping, and that half of them were alive with demonstrably and clinically infected grafts! Omental wrapping reversed the overall incidence, with 70% of dogs surviving and only one of these with a GIF. This would indicate a real potential for using an omental pedicle in such select clinical situations as in situ reconstructions for GEF, Gram-positive mycotic aneurysm, or infected pseudoaneurysms.

This model did not test the long-term ability of an omental pedicle to prevent GEF when used either routinely or selectively in aortic surgery. I have come to use omental pedicles routinely when the retroperitoneal tissues are flimsy, preferring to use the bulkier omental flap as a palpable tissue plane between the aorta and the duodenum. In addition, we use a transmesocolic route to facilitate approximation of the pedicle over the proximal anastomosis (Fig. 7)[24] There may not be proof for the usefulness of this, but it makes intellectual sense. We have had the opportunity to reexplore several patients at intervals from 4 months to several years and have found the retroperitoneal pedicle to be a thick and persistent cushion over the graft. However, on a more pessimistic note, Moveton (1986) noted complete failure of omental pedicles in preventing ASS in five patients undergoing GIF treatment—-a disconcerting concept![25]

Antibiotic Prophylaxis

Literature Review

Routine institution of prophylactic antibiotics in major peripheral vascular surgery has become a virtual axiom based on the perception that a small risk of untoward reactions from the antibiotics is more than balanced by the major morbidity and mor-

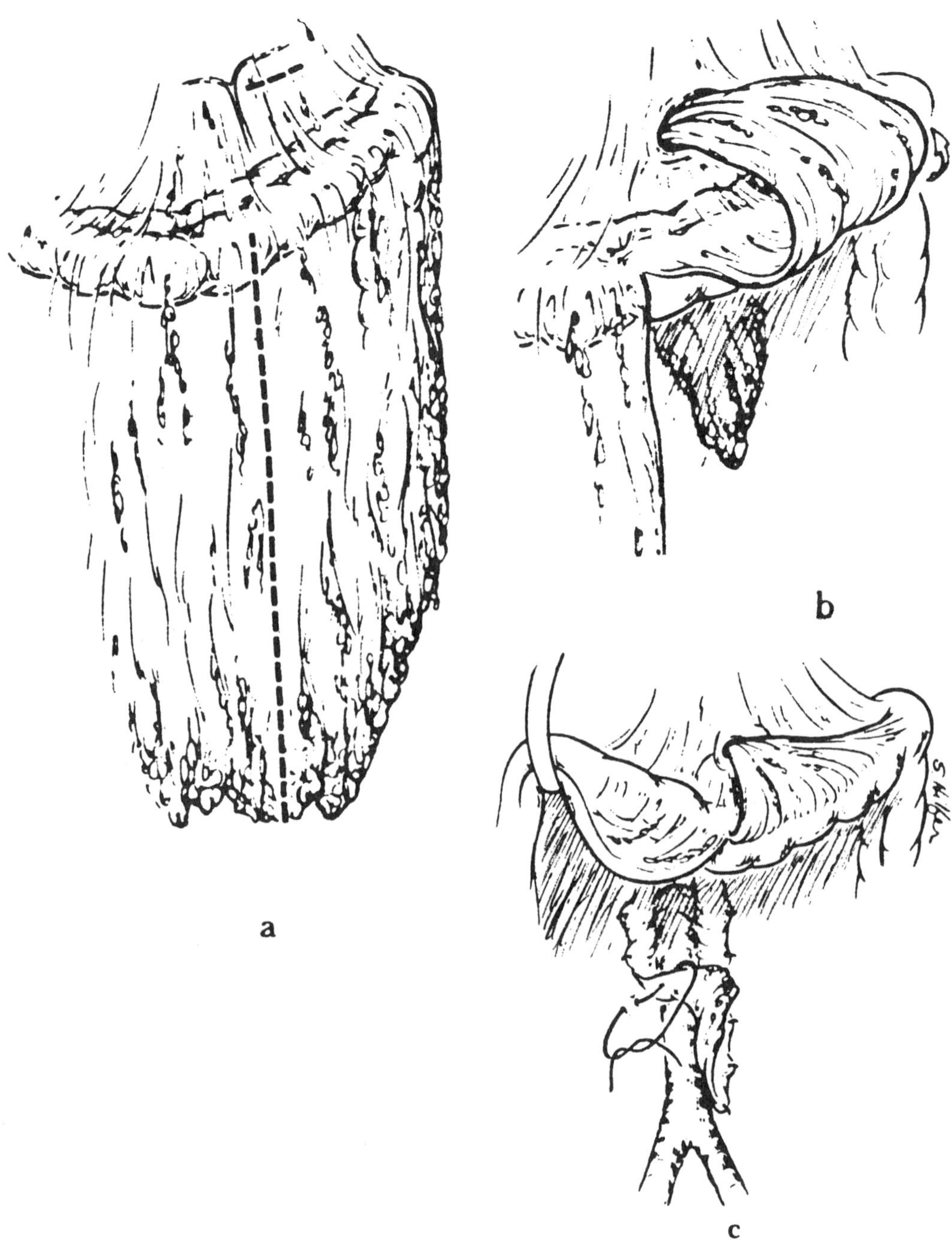

Figure 7. The omentum may be fashioned into a vascularized pedicle laid down over not only the aortic stump but also the bed of the resected graft; or it may be used prophylactically as depicted here. (From Bunt TJ, Doerhoff CR, Haynes JL. Retrocolic omental pedicle flap for routine plication of abdominal aortic grafts. *Surg Gynecol Obstet.* 1984;158:6:591–592.)

tality of a graft infection should it occur. As a result, all major series on GIF and GEF have noted routine use of antibiotics for the last 30 years.

The only major literature objection was lodged by Szylagyi (1962), who noted a 1.9% incidence of GIF in 3347 vascular cases at Henry Ford Hospital—an incidence not only comparable to but actually lower than concurrent series in which antibiotics were routinely used. He decried their use, suspecting both an increase in more resistant organisms and suppression of what might otherwise have been earlier clinical presentations. His warnings went unheeded, however, and all other authors then and now have advocated their use.[26]

A number of authors then published series of GIFs, and retrospectively noted a trend toward a reduction in GIF incidence with routine antibiotic usage. Jamieson (1975) reported a reduction from 7.3% (15/664) to 2.2% (11/510) (NSS).[27] In 1979, Goldstone and Moore noted a decrease at Arizona from 4.1% (9/222) to 1.5% (5/344) (NSS).[28] Lord (1977) noted a reduction in wound or graft infections from 1.5% (6/400) to 0.23% (1/434) when using routine topical cephalothin and kanamycin; however, the control series was historical.[29]

The next step was to perform prospective randomized trials. Pitt (1980) studied 231 inguinal incisions in 205 patients undergoing procedures that required inguinal exploration. The operations were femoral thromboendarterectomy in 48, varicose vein procedures in 55, profundoplasty in 13, and cross-femoral grafts in 10. Only one quarter of the procedures actually involved synthetic graft placement, and patients with concomitant distal pedal sepsis were excluded. The patients were observed for infectious complications 4 weeks postoperatively. Fifty-three placebo patients had 13 wound infections; 46 receiving intravenous cephradine had 3 wound infections; topical cephradine and both regimens together had no infections. All treatment groups were significantly better ($P < .01$) than placebo.

The rate of groin infection overall was the same for those with (7.7% of 52 at risk wounds) or without (7.8% of 153) synthetic grafts. There were no GIFs in the entire study. Wound infections were due to *S aureus* in 10 of 16 cases.[30]

Although widely quoted in GIF literature by proponents of prophylactic antibiotics, the difficulty with the Pitt study is that it is essentially a study demonstrating a reduction in wound infection only. It shows that this may be obtained by either topical or intravenous cephradine prophylaxis, but that there is no additional synergism to their combination. It does not address the question of GIF prevention, in large part due to the small number of synthetic grafts actually used in the series. One is also struck by the fact that most wound infections were caused by a bacteria that should have been adequately controlled by the antibiotic chosen. Thus, although widely quoted as a justification for antibiotic usage to prevent GIF, the study really gives no valid information in that regard.

Kaiser (1978) performed a randomized double-blind study of cefazolin versus placebo in 565 vascular operations. One hundred and three of these were brachiocephalic procedures in which no infections occurred, leading to the early recommendation (and subsequent vascular maxim) that prophylactic antibiotics were not necessary for these operations. Cefazolin was used as a 1-gram dose preoperatively, with redosing at 4 hours if the case lasted to that interval. Wound infections were significantly ($P < .001$) reduced from 6.8% to 0.9%, with four graft infections in the placebo group ($P = 0.62$). However, the rates were highest with abdominal incisions rather than inguinal incisions (4.9% versus 0.6%); highest rates were for abdominal incision for aneurysms, 11.8% (6/51) versus 2.6% (1/39); and lowest for aortofemoral grafting, 2.1% (1/47) versus (0/47). Three of the four GIFs occurred with placement of femoropopliteal grafts.[31]

Therefore, as much as this paper is also touted as indicating that prophylactic antibiotics will reduce graft infection, I share Szylagyi's critical viewpoint as given in the paper's discussion.

1. The crucial end point of a significant reduction in GIF is not made.
2. The GIFs that did occur were of (synthetic? autologous?) distal grafts and not of aortic grafts.
3. The reversal of usual statistics on the incidence of abdominal versus groin infection and the fact that there were no infections with cefazolin-treated ABFBs strongly suggests errors of sampling.

I would submit that the paper shows only that an inordinately high rate of abdominal incisional wound infection was decreased to acceptable levels by cefazolin. There is no hard evidence for preventing either groin infections or the deeper implication of graft infections.

A sidelight of the paper indicated that the choice of skin preparation could be a significant factor. Hexachlorophene ethanol followed by ethanol paint resulted in a 10.3% rate that soared to 18.9% if concomitant antibiotics were not used. Povidone-iodine (PVI) or hexachlorophene with PVI combinations had a significantly ($P < .01$) lower wound infection rate at 2.8%. This is the only paper in the vascular literature that addresses the commonly used differential choices of skin prep, and its conclusion strongly favors PVI over hexachlorophene combinations.

Salzmann (1982) studied 300 reconstructive procedures using either cefuroximine or cefotaxime as the agent versus placebo. The wound infection rate was significantly decreased ($P < .001$) from 15.1% to 3% and the GIF rate nonsignificantly decreased from 2.4% to 0.8%. Infections were most commonly due to *S aureus* or *S epidermidis*, despite an appropriate antibiotic spectrum for these. Infections could not be correlated with the presence of distal infection by Fontaine classification. Operative risks and operations were similar in both

groups and included aortoiliac in a third, femoropopliteal or crural in half, with the reminder being extra-anatomic; only half of all cases actually involved synthetic grafts. Again, the study is most useful as a demonstration of the efficacy of prophylactic antibiotics in reducing wound infection rates; although one can certainly question a baseline wound infection rate of 15%. It furthermore suggests a reduction in the GIF rate, but does not show statistical significance, in large part due to the fact that only half the procedures involved grafts, which is itself a distinct failing of the paper's methods![32]

Hasselgren (1984) studied two regimens of intravenous cefuroximine versus placebo in 211 patients. The procedures included 82 femoral or iliac thromboendarterectomies or thrombectomies, 13 EABs, and 83 femoropopliteal procedures, most done with autologous vein. Synthetic grafts were used only in 70 of the 211 procedures. The author incidentally noted the highest rates of wound infection in graft placement cases. The wound infection rate was 16.7% (11/66) with one GIF for placebo, with the wound but not GIF rate being significantly reduced ($P < .05$) to 3.8% (2/52) or 4.3% (3/69) for 1- and 3-day courses of antibiotic. No GIFs were seen in these latter arms of the study.[33] The study thus provides further evidence for the efficacy of antibiotics in reducing wound infection rates without providing meaningful information about GIF; and had they done so, information would have to be tempered by the fact that the grafts used were seldom synthetic and mostly peripheral in location.

Edwards (1992) looked at the kinetic profile of cefuroximine versus cefazolin, both given preoperatively, redosed through the operation, and continued for 24 hours postoperatively. Wound infections occurred in 7/272 (2.6%) cefuroximine and 3/287 (1.0%) cefazolin ($P = 0.2$). Furthermore, despite a more frequent intraoperative dosing regimen, lower trough serum levels were seen with cefuroximine. The authors concluded that superior β-lactamase resistance was not as useful for prophylaxis as superior pharmacokinetics, and therefore recommended cefazolin.[34]

Discussion

We can make some generic assessments about the efficacy of prophylactic antibiotics in vascular surgery. First and foremost, we all accept the wisdom of using them, but quite frankly, the concept simply has not been proven yet. Most studies do not focus on the situation we need to understand, namely, the synthetic (particularly aortic) graft placed at the inguinal incision. All focus on short-term evidence on infection, completely neglecting the reality that 30% to 60% of GIFs present as late manifestations, and that those typically involve *S epidermidis*. We have no meaningful information as to whether our current regimens offer adequate prophylaxis versus this seemingly ubiquitous etiologic agent! They furthermore fail to focus on the recognized risk situations such as distal infection, postoperative wound problems, lymphocoele, hematoma, redo surgery, etc. As an ultimately pertinent criticism, all involve antibiotic dosage regimens that neglect to include an intraoperative booster dose. These oversights in methodology may explain the rather high incidence of placebo or baseline wound infections—rates that exceed, in most series, the recommended CDC guidelines for clean class I wounds.

Thus, a realistic and worthwhile study has not been done yet. To do one properly:

1. would require 1000 patients to uncover significant differences in prevention rates for an occurrence that averages only 1.5% to 2.5%.
2. would focus on the inguinal incision of synthetic, particularly aortic grafts.
3. would include intraoperative dosing as a variable.
4. and would require at least a 4-year follow-up to adequately monitor for

S epidermidis complications heralding an otherwise unrecognized infection.

Such a study is highly unlikely to ever be completed. However, should prophylactic antibiotics be routinely used? The answer is yes, although we cannot prove this. The literature on the subject is often misquoted and poorly understood.

Topical Antibiotics

Many authors have indicated that they use topical antibiotics on a routine adjunctive basis, both as a periodic wound irrigant and as the solution used to moisten laparotomy pads left in wounds after preliminary dissection. Most use systemic antibiotics as well. Few authors have relied on topical antibiotics alone. However, as was the case with systemic antibiotic usage, there is a paucity of solid information on which to base the practice.

Lord presented three series within one 1977 article, indicating a total decrease in the wound infection rate from 1.5% in 400 cases to 0.23% in 434.[35] However, few of the cases involved synthetic grafts, and many involved varicose vein surgery. Furthermore, the study used historical controls, which are not truly valid for statistical comparison. The data are thus indicative of potential value but hardly adequate proof of same.

Better data is obtained from Pitt, as detailed above, who noted an equivalent reduction in wound infection rates with either systemic or topical cephradine.

There are a number of relevant laboratory studies to examine. Richardson (1970) implanted 0.5-cm by 0.5-cm patches of Dacron in the subcutaneous tissues of guinea pigs. The pocket was then inoculated with 5×10^6 *S aureus* or *E. coli* at closure. At harvest 8 days later, all control patches were infected. Saline-irrigated wounds showed infection rates of 93% for *S aureus* and 67% *E. coli*. However, the addition of antibiotics to the patch decreased infection rates, with 10% cephalothin-soaked patches showing 15% and 16% rates ($P < .001$).[36] Although used to illustrate the potential for topical antibiotics to decrease graft infection rates, the model leaves much to be challenged. It does not reproduce the clinical situation, being essentially a grossly contaminated field with an in situ foreign body. Therefore, high rates of wound infection would be expected. Exposure to a topical irrigant decreased the rates, but the residual wound infection rate was still excessive. If anything, it underscores the repeated finding in laboratory models that bacteria sensitive to an antibiotic seem able to survive exposure to same in nearly a third of cases. The clinical implications of this common laboratory finding are obvious.

Digiglia (1970) presented a canine study of Dacron 1.5-cm femoral patch angioplasties inoculated locally with *S aureus* for 30 minutes and then irrigated with either 100 cc saline or kanamycin/bacitracin solution. At reharvest 7 days later, there was 100% positive clinical infection and arterial disruption, and 100% were culture-positive. An extended model then delayed harvest to 6 weeks, at which point all grafts were said to be incorporated and culture-negative.[37] Digiglia suggested a prolonged antibiotic activity for this surprising finding, a curious notion that does not explain the initial 100% positive cultures at 7 days, as well as being at best tenuous in its logic. In addition, other studies note culture positivity in grafts that appear clinically noninfected. A more reasonable explanation for the study findings would be that at least for dogs presented with a small synthetic patch angioplasty, complete graft incorporation and subsequent bacterial eradication are possible. Canine models testing complete grafts do not show this phenomenon, nor is it possible to extrapolate the finding to humans. It does raise the possibility that a simple synthetic patch angioplasty that became infected in the human might heal in similar fashion. There is little concrete clinical evidence for this, however, I would note the reported ease of obtaining wound healing with local therapy of both femoral- and carotid-infected femoral patch angioplasties as suggestive evidence that this is so.

The same study was subsequently reported by Baker (1972), who did not reach either the same results or conclusions. Baker used a similar canine model with a 5-mm Dacron graft implanted in the infrarenal aorta and then locally inoculated with 1.5×10^6 *S aureus*. At reharvest 3 to 5 days later, eight saline-soaked grafts showed 100% infection with four dogs dying; nine cephaloridine-soaked grafts demonstrated one clinical infection only, but a 75% rate of positive graft cultures. Even when systemic cephaloridine was added for three days, the grafts remained culture-positive in 16% of cases (2/12). Baker specifically refuted the conclusion from Digiglia that somehow antibiotics could remain effective for days, or that the grafts were remaining uninfected.[38]

The differences between the two studies, however, may be of real clinical importance. Baker studied aortic graft segments while Digiglia studied patch angioplasties. The rate of intimal coverage and fibrous incorporation for each of these is different. Perhaps, the models indicate a real difference in healing capacity and therefore infection resistance that has relevance to the clinical situation.

Ultimately, these three models for topical antibiotic prophylaxis do not show any clear cut data to support advocacy of that regimen in the human situation of synthetic graft implantation in a clean field. They do demonstrate that in situ grafting of a fresh synthetic graft into a grossly contaminated field cannot be done safely, even if specific antibiotics are irrigated into the operative field, since 20% to 80% of such grafts will remain culture-positive. It should be clearly recognized that the euphemism *culture-positive graft* may be translated as infected graft, with all the long-term problems attendant to it.

There are equally conflicting clinical

studies, mostly from the general surgery literature, about the efficacy of topical antibiotics in otherwise clean wounds. A representative study is that of Scherr (1973), who demonstrated sterilization of wounds contaminated with any of 19 various bacterial strains after exposure to 1 minute of polymycin-B, bacitracin, or neomycin sulfate solutions. All three solutions were 100% effective versus *S aureus*; neomycin was 100% but bacitracin only 95% versus *S epidermidis.*; and both were 100% effective versus *E. coli.*[39] The model is not truly one of a wound incidentally contaminated during exposure and dissection. However, it does suggest that frequent wound irrigations with topical antibiotic solutions may aid in decreasing if not eliminating wound contamination, provided the irrigation follows wound exposure to bacteria at some (undetermined) close interval.

Indeed, there are little data in the literature on topical antibiotics from which to make extrapolative conclusions: how many vascular wounds are actually culture positive; what is the usual concentration of organisms; are they simply spread over the wound surface or has tissue penetration been obtained in these few short hours; and does the local environment contribute, e.g., local, protein, fibrin, blood, or even the graft itself positively or negatively to the ability of whatever bacteria are present to develop a frank wound or graft infection, or of topical antibiotics to eradicate them before the process begins. We have more questions than data to provide answers.

Pharmacology of Antibiotics

A brief review of the basic pharmacologic principles involved in antibiotic usage is particularly relevant to the question of whether currently accepted regimens could even be expected, much less actually prove, to be beneficial. Several related questions need to be addressed. What is the purpose or purposes of the regimen? How may antibiotics best be delivered? What are the limitations of that expected efficacy? What bacteria are effectively or expectantly prophylaxed?[15]

The purpose of antibiotics generically is multifold:

1. To prevent subcutaneous wound infections that may later involve the deeper seated graft by extension.
2. To protect against contamination or seeding of the graft matrix by local skin, tissue, or fluids at time of implantation.
3. To protect against secondary matrix contamination by potentially contaminated fluids (lymph, blood, seroma fluid).
4. To protect against both early (1 week) and long-term contamination of the graft during bacteremias or septicemias.

It is implicit to this broadened concept of antibiotic purpose that we look at the complete problem holistically (prevention of a graft infection) and not focus too narrowly on the concept of selecting a specific prophylactic intravenous antibiotic regimen. The possible methods of securing antibiotic prophylaxis versus GIF would then be as follows, each with its specific usefulness.

1. Intravenous perioperative prophylaxis: This would be defined best as a two or three dose regimen given in the immediate perioperative period (to be defined precisely below).

2. Intravenous perioperative therapeutic: defined as a round-the- clock multidose/multiday, culture- or situation-directed course of antibiotics instituted for specific clinical indications (to be defined below).

3. Topical prophylaxis: defined as local wound irrigations with an antibiotic solution during or at the completion of the surgery.

4. Graft-antibiotic impregnation: chemical or physical bonding of then slowly re-

leased or eluted antibiotic/antiseptic compounds from a graft matrix.

5. Bacteremic prophylaxis: institution of single dose prophylaxis against graft seeding by late bacteremias arising from dental or visceral instrumentation, if indeed these are of any importance (see below).

The methods of prophylaxis, the expected pathogens of graft infection, particularly those most expected at different sites or for different clinical situations should all be considered.[40] Our review of the literature to 1983 noted the relative incidences of bacteria, which have changed little except for an increase in *S epidermidis*. Acute postoperative or 30-day infections tend to be predominantly *S aureus* for both aortic and peripheral infections. Gram-negative species are less common as primary agents, but are common secondary contaminants once the wound has been treated in open fashion for some time. Gram-negative species are also and quite self evidently associated with GEF and GEE due to the effects of visceral contamination. Thus, the relative incidence of Gram-negative infection increases with increasing time of onset.[41]

S epidermidis has been demonstrated in the past decade to be a significant cause of GIF, particularly those with delayed onset or recognition. Usually the infection presents as delayed limb thrombosis or pseudoaneurysm. *S epidermidis* as an etiologic agent was actually described by a number of early series on GIF, but its virulence was not well recognized until the work of Bandyk's group. Schmitt (1984) described 10 aortic graft infections, 8 of which were due to *S epidermidis*. The group described the pathogenetic slime producer SP-12 and noted that its identification was difficult without accurate retrieval and handling. Seeger (1983) noted that 5 of 10 inguinal wound infections were due to *S epidermidis*; Yeager (1985) noted in a review of the Portland series that half were due to *S epidermidis*; my own recent (1993) 8-year experience with 22 aortic graft infections showed

18 of the 22 to be due to *S epidermidis*, with 9 presenting as limb thrombosis and 5 as pseudoaneurysms.[42–45]

Sources of Bacteria

The exact etiology or source of the *S epidermidis* that is now recognized with increasing frequency is uncertain. It would be easy to ascribe it to local skin contamination of the graft at the inguinal incision. Yet, that readily offered postulate does not explain why the inguinal incision but not the abdominal portion is so often affected; nor why one seldom sees *S epidermidis* infections either of the proximal end of either axillofemoral or iliacofemoral grafts, or of the distal end of femoropopliteal grafts.

Lymphatic Effluent One disconcerting possibility has been raised by a number of authors who implicate indolent contamination of the implanted graft by either local lymph node effluent or by the arterial wall itself. Initial attention to this problem was drawn by the Arizona group in three successive studies that all demonstrated a high incidence of positive *S epidermidis* cultures at arterial sites.[46–48]

We have also looked at the potential for both arterial and the lymphatic node contribution. In 1985, 45 patients undergoing groin dissection for elective clean revascularization had cultures taken at incisional opening and incisional closing, and of a representative bit of transected lymph node and artery at the arteriotomy site. All patients were on cephalosporin prophylaxis. Twenty-five percent of the arterial and 30% of the lymph node cultures were positive, 95% of which grew *S epidermidis*. No opening culture was positive. Twenty percent of closing cultures were positive but there was no defined correlation between tissue and closing cultures to suggest cross contamination.[49,50]

Gayless performed a similar study of routine culture on the periaortic lymph nodes obtained during aortic dissection for aortic surgery, and found negative cultures routinely. No GIFs occurred in the series.[51]

There is not, as yet, a consensus as to the clinical relevance of these studies, with many feeling that the positive arterial or lymph node cultures are either spurious or at least not important. However, there has to be a source of S epidermidis at the groin incision where it is most often detected; there has to be a reason why it is not seen at other incisions of seemingly equal vulnerability to incidental skin contamination. The fact that S epidermidis sets up indolent infections with small numbers of actual organisms suggests that the original source is small and/or that antibiotic prophylaxis is at least partially effective in its suppression. The question of the relevance of these positive cultures is more than moot; elimination of S epidermidis as an ever increasingly common pathogen of delayed onset GIF must start with an understanding of how it gets there, must address appropriate antibiotic penetration and susceptibility factors, and may well end with surgeons being advised to handle lymph nodes and/or arteriotomies differently than they do now.

In examining the pathogens that must be considered when selecting a prophylactic regimen, consideration must be given to S aureus for the first week and S epidermidis, which may be a contaminant for the first week or may also be a more long-term risk until lymph effluent ceases and/or graft incorporation occurs.

Pedal Infection In addition, there is the consideration of whether or not there can be contamination of the graft by bacteria in the lymphatic effluent that may bathe the graft postoperatively if lymphatics are transected. Clinical evidence for this has been little better than anecdotal. Most of the evidence rests on the canine study reported by Malone's group (as above).[46–48]

Hoffert noted in his series of 10 graft infections, all presenting at the groin from local or peripheral (e.g., nonaortic) procedures, that 75% had the same bacteria cultures from the groin infection as had been cultured previously from the distal pedal infection.[52]

We looked at the problem prospectively in 1985, comparing the incidence of positive inguinal lymph nodes cultures in 30 elective clean cases as opposed to 15 done in the face of active distal gangrene or infection. Twenty-seven percent of the clean cases grew S epidermidis as did 12% of the infected, but an additional 12% of the latter also grew additional bacteria. Two patients subsequently developed a groin presentation of GIF with the same bacteria that was cultured from the foot and from the lymph node.[49–50]

However, other authors describing their series of GIFs have minimized the importance of concomitant pedal infection. Thus, there is some laboratory and some clinical evidence for the phenomenon of graft contamination by bacteria carried in the lymphatic drainage from an infected distal site. However, it is only uncommonly cited as a suspected or proven cause of an actual clinical case of GIF.

Bacteremias Bacteria may thus be a significant problem in the acute postoperative period, arriving in the graft by local skin, lymph, arterial wall, or ascending from distal infection.[52] What about bacteremic infection?

As noted previously, the major thrust to this scenario comes from the lab, where bacteremic challenges with S aureus have been the standard canine model for producing GIF. Clinical evidence is, however, decidedly lacking. Review of the literature from 1954 to 1992 reveals, at most, only 10 cases in which documented bacteremias could be reasonably expected to have produced the GIF; this out of over 1200 cases.(See Section X) Certainly this is not a dominant cause of clinical GIF! It is, of course, theoretically possible that the clinical situation sometimes mimics the canine model, and that some GIFs are occurring due to unrecognized bacteremias and are mistakenly assumed to be due to other causes.

There are some authors who suggest that secondary infection of EABs post-GIF resection may represent bacteremic GIFs, particularly since many occur as midshaft or otherwise localized infections and not at inguinal or axillary at incision. However, I would suggest that it remains more likely that these were due to local contamination, despite all efforts to place the EAB in a clean field, rather than being due to presumed bacteremias during the staged secondary infected graft resection when the EAB was already in place. There has not been a documented decrease in such EAB infections when sequential and staged operations are compared. Of course, bacteremias occurring simultaneously or several days post-EAB are probably of similar potential virulence. The point is indeterminate at present.

Pharmacokinetics

There are a number of theoretical considerations that bear review when determining the optimal antibiotic for intravenous usage.[53] Basically, to be effective, an antibiotic must:

1. attain and maintain sufficient serum and relevant tissue levels (whether or not this is the MIC or therapeutic ratio is discussed below).
2. have an appropriate spectrum against suspected or real pathogens.
3. attain high levels in particularly sensitive tissues of relevance to graft infection (arterial wall, fibrin clot, subcutaneous tissue).
4. Have a prolonged half-life (or be redosed, as discussed below).
5. have limited or controllable side effects.

Serum half-lives are available for all antibiotics, one summary of which is summarized in Table 4. An appropriate half-life for most vascular surgery would be at least 3 hours so that levels above the necessary MICs are maintained for the duration of the operation.

The Minimum Inhibitory Concentration (MIC) is defined as the lowest tissue level necessary for inhibition of bacterial growth and is routinely used in infectious disease situations as a definition of bacterial efficacy. Some authors, notably Lalka,[54] suggest that maintenance of serum or tissue levels above the geometric mean of the MICs for the expected pathogens of GIF is reasonably a therapeutic goal. Others, including myself, use the same concept as is used in most infectious disease treatment and suggest that the therapeutic ratio is a safer ratio to maintain—the ratio of obtained antibiotic concentration to the minimum concentration for bactericidal activity. Successful or positive ratios are usually arbitrarily set as being a ratio in excess of 10 to 1. One might term this the standard prophylactic therapeutic ratio (PTR), recognizing that there is no firm consensus on either the ratio itself nor of the necessity to obtain that ratio to obtain prophylaxis.[1,2]

This point is more than moot or an exercise in semantics. Simple MIC levels against common GIF pathogens are easily obtained by most antibiotics: review of Table 4 shows that many currently used drugs, however, do not obtain PTRs versus *S epidermidis*. It is my published contention that this is, in part, responsible for the increased recognition of *S epidermidis* as an agent of GIF, despite fairly routine use of prophylactic antibiotics at all centers.[53]

Dose duration curves (DDC) are another useful concept. The DDC describes the length of time that a given antibiotic will maintain the MIC or the PTR. Dose duration curves are implicitly a function of the serum half-life and therefore relate, in part, to the amount, duration, and tightness of serum protein binding.

There are different DDCs for different tissues, although few antibiotics come with this information fully worked out and described. The DDC can further be modified by the amount of the initial dose and by additional or redosing with time. In general, an adequate antibiotic for prophylaxis

Table 4
Pharmacologic Attributes of Commonly Used Antibiotics

		MIC-90 (μg/mL)			Peak serum	Half-life
Antibiotic	Dose	S. aureus	S. epidermidis	E. coli	μg/mL	(hours)
Penicillin G	24×10^6 qd	12.5	25	>100	200	0.5
Ampicillin	1g IV	12.5	3.1	>100	40	1
Nafcillin	500mg IV	0.8	3.1	>100	11	0.5
Methicillin	1g IV	3.1	12.5	>100	60	1.0
Mezlocillin	3g IV	2.0	8	>100	310	1.0
Piperacillin	4g IV	3.1	8	>100	244	—
Erythromycin	500g IV	0.39	25	>100	10	1.4
Clindamycin	600mg IV	0.2	25	>100	10	2.5
Tetracycline	500mg IV	0.1	>100	>100	8	8.5
Vancomycin	500mg IV	0.78	3.12	>100	35	6.0
First-Generation Cephalosporin						
Cephalothin	2g IV	0.78	1.56	25	90	0.8
Cefazolin	1g IV	1.56	12.5	12.5	188	1.9
Second-Generation Cephalosporin						
Cefamandole	2g IV	1.0	12.5	16	165	0.7
Cefoxitin	1g IV	4.0	50	8	117	0.8
Cefonicid	1g IV	6.3	10	0.8	150	4.4
Ceforanide	1g IV	4	8	2	135	3.0
Third-Generation Cephalosporin						
Cefotaxime	2g IV	2	8	0.25	85	1.0
Moxalactam	2g IV	16	32	0.25	150	2.2
Cefoperazone	2g IV	4	8	16	200	2.1
Ceftizoxime	1g IV	8	25	6.2	100	
Imipenem-cilastatin	1g IV	0.5	0.5	0.25	73	1.0
Gentamicin	1.5mg/kg IV	0.4	0.8	3.5	6	2.3
Tobramycin	1.5mg/kg IV	0.4	0.8	3.5	6	2.0

would have a DDC that translated into prolonged serum half-life, and presumed or proven prolonged tissue half-life.

Penetration into special tissues would also be of theoretical import, since control of bacteria in lymph, the arterial wall, or the fibrin clot surrounding an implanted graft or the thrombus on its matrix would all involve different DDCs. Penetration into fibrin clot and thrombus may be a function of protein binding. A theoretically ideal antibiotic would maintain high lymph, tissue, and arterial wall levels. Selective leukocyte sequestering is a further refined antibiotic

quality, one currently ascribed to rifampicin only.

A number of authors have specifically addressed the pharmacokinetics of antibiotics during vascular surgery. Fradet (1986) studied the distribution of cephalosporin given as a 25 mg/kg dose in a canine aortic replacement model and correlated tissue levels with the MICs for the three most common pathogens. They used a PTR of 10 at an arbitrary 3-hour interval. Levels were measured in the aortic wall, serum, subcutaneous tissue (SQ), and muscle. Moxalactam and cefazolin both maintained PTRs in all four tissues for all three pathogens, and both achieved significantly ($P < .05$) higher levels than cefoxitin or moxalactam. All four antibiotics obtained satisfactory levels in all tissues versus *Enterococcus*. However, both moxalactam and cefoxitin failed to attain adequate levels in the blood, aorta, SQ, and muscle for *S aureus* and *S epidermidis*.[55]

Mutch (1982) studied a clinical model in 24 patients on three-dose perioperative antibiotics who were undergoing aortic surgery. Serum levels were measured at aortic cross-clamp, the aortic wall at anastomosis, and the subcutaneous tissues at the time of closure. They also used a PTR of 10. One gram of cefazolin obtained 9.3 ± 5.5 mg/mL at the aorta, 15.7 ± 4.13 in the cross-clamp aortic blood, and 3.1 ± 1.3 in the closing subcutaneous tissues; 600 mg of clindamycin obtained $1.1 \pm .55$ aorta, $13.8 \pm .39$ blood, and $0.66 \pm .38$ tissue; and cefoxitin 2 grams obtained 9.5 ± 3.08 aorta, 32.6 ± 4.17 aorta, and 2.2 ± 2.5 at tissue. Minimum inhibitory concentrations for the studied pathogens were 0.2 to 1.2 for *S aureus*, except cefoxitin which required 4.8 µg/kg.[56]

Thus, cefazolin obtained therapeutic ratios for all three pathogens at all three tissues. Clindamycin was therapeutic against *S aureus* and *S epidermidis* but not *E coli*. Cefoxitin did not maintain PTRs against any of the three pathogens at the time of closure, although sufficient levels were maintained in the serum and aortic wall. These samples, however, were obtained earlier in the case.

Robbs (1984) looked at the distribution of 1-gram intravenous cefuroximine given to 10 patients at induction of anesthesia for aortic surgery and then at subsequent operative intervals. The serum levels were 66.8 ± 19 mg/mL at 1 hour, 71.3 ± 27.3 at 2 hours, 60.4 ± 27.8 at 3 hours, and 54.5 ± 24.0 at 4 hours. Aortic wall levels taken at aortotomy averaged 7.3 ± 3.2 mg/mL; subcutaneous levels at opening averaged 2.1 ± 1.8 and at closure 2.0 ± 1.9; and peripheral tissue levels were 7.4 ± 4.2 at 2 to 3 hours and 6.4 ± 2.3 at 4 hours. The half-life for cefuroximine was 60 minutes, prompting the authors to recommend redosing. Even with this frequent redosing, subcutaneous levels were sufficient for 90% of *S aureus* (although not for methicillin-resistant *S aureus*) and were adequate for most Gram-negative cultures. All tissue levels were one tenth that of serum, indicating poor tissue penetration. Although the authors state that the tissue levels were adequate, they barely meet the PTR for *S aureus* and *S epidermidis* and therefore cannot be regarded as completely safe levels.[57]

Almgren (1986) studied the kinetics of dicloxacillin given as a 2-gram infusion at 3 time intervals; the induction of anesthesia, 3 hours preoperatively, or 6 hours preoperatively. He studied tissue levels, serum levels, and aortic wall biopsies at two time intervals. The study showed concentrations of dicloxacillin to be > 100 mg/kg in the serum and > 20 mg/kg in the aorta shortly postinfusion, and that the elution curves were parallel, with levels falling below 5 mg/kg in the serum at 7 hours, and below 5 mg/kg in the aorta at 4 hours. They concluded that the most efficacious use of the antibiotic would indicate infusion at induction of anesthesia. Redosing was not discussed.[58]

Lalka (1989) studied the biologic distribution of cefamandole and cefazolin in 47 patients undergoing elective primary prosthetic aortic or infrainguinal reconstruction. Specimens were taken of serum, subcutaneous fat, and three surgically dissected portions of artery divided into local thrombus, atheroma, and arterial wall. Each specimen was analyzed for bacterial cultures, MIC, and absolute drug level.

Serum half-lives were 1.43 ± 0.36 hours for cefamandole and 2.22 ± 0.4 hours for cefazolin; measured serum levels were therefore correspondingly higher for cefazolin for the first 2 hours of surgery ($P < .025$). Tissue samples at all sampling times demonstrated higher levels of cefazolin than cefamandole ($P < .005$). However, positive arterial wall cultures were still obtained in 41% of patients and 20% of arterial specimens, with 69% growing *S epidermidis* subspecies.[54]

Lalka's study looked specifically at cefamandole because of its in vitro increased activity versus *S epidermidis*; however, the study raised questions about the actual in vivo bioactivity, since cefazolin maintained better serum and tissue levels. Tissue half-lives per se could not be calculated, but at all time intervals of sampling there was a higher absolute concentration of cefazolin than cefamandole for arterial wall and atheroma, although not for arterial thrombus. If the tissue to serum ratios were analyzed for all tissue types, there was no statistical difference between the two drugs.

Although the paper reads initially as showing cefazolin to be a better drug, close reading would indicate that both drugs maintained adequate ratios, and that the decreased serum levels but increased thrombus levels of cefamandole were an expected result of cefamandole's high protein binding. Furthermore, the calculated arterial penetration of cefamandole was 32% versus 16% for cefazolin. It would seem that the paper shows differential pharmacokinetics between the two drugs in terms of absolute distribution, but that both drugs maintained reasonable levels above the geometric median MIC for the major GIF pathogens.

Gugiliemo (1989), speaking for the San Francisco group, studied eight patients for aortic surgery for the potential differential pharmacokinetics of a 1-gm intravenous cefamandole dose given in the preoperative steady state 1 to 3 days prior to surgery as compared to a dose given intraoperatively. They noted an increase in serum half-life from 67 ± 19 minutes to 93 ± 23 minutes intraoperatively. The volume for distribution also increased from 16.8 ± 5.3 liters to 25.2 ± 11.9 liters, a change they attributed to a major change in extravascular distribution, since total body clearance remained unchanged at 192 ± 90 mL/minute. Absolute plasma concentrations were low at the time of graft placement (mean 223 ± 62 minutes postantibiotic administration), with mean peak plasma levels of 144.1 ± 53.4 mg/mL falling to 0.6 to 27 mg/mL at time of graft placement. The MIC for *S aureus* was calculated at 1 to 2 µg/mL. The obvious conclusion of the study was that the pharmacokinetics of cefamandole (and therefore presumably other antibiotics) was altered by the operative state, and that a single preoperative dose did not allow adequate levels at graft placement 2 to 3 hours into the case. Their recommendation was to redose antibiotics just prior to graft placement.[59]

Recommendations

Prophylactic antibiotic usage should be carefully thought out and individualized for each patient in each situation; the appropriate use of such agents should be as well conceived as are decisions for therapeutic antibiotics. Utilization should proceed logically from what is known and understood about:

the potential sources of infection
the pathogens that may be expected
the potential for secondary graft contamination and bacteremias
the pharmacology of the antibiotic used, particularly its dose response curve, tissue penetration, and bacterial spectrum
any effects the graft itself may have (e.g., differential infectability).
the length of time that cross-contamination of the graft by local or bacteremic phenomenon may be expected to occur

Prophylactic antibiotics should not be used on a routine basis in the same way for all patients. They should be given selectively and individually to address the clinical situation presented by that patient. Considerations in this decision-making process should include:

the potential for positive arterial wall cultures

the potential for aneurysmal wall cultures
the presence of distal pedal infection
the presence of other or nosocomial infection
the requirement for long-term invasive monitoring lines
whether or not the planned procedure is likely to involve an inguinal incision
whether dissection at the groin is a redo situation
consideration of the patient's immunologic status

In addition, it is our strong belief that *S epidermidis* graft infections have been noted with increasing frequency in this past decade. Although their now predominant place as an etiologic infective agent may be, in part, a factor of increased recognition of their commonly occult presentations, it is still clear that recognized or not, current antibiotic regimens do not afford adequate prophylaxis versus *S epidermidis* infections. As discussed elsewhere, there are multiple factors involved in the insidious pathogenicity of *S epidermidis*. The one that can cur-

rently be addressed is whether or not there is an adequate dosing regimen to maintain an adequate MIC level versus this organism. As pointed out in Table 4, the therapeutic ratios of many drugs are barely if at all adequate. Strong consideration should be given to better dosing mechanisms and antibiotic selection to minimize *S epidermidis* infections.

Finally, consideration must also be given to the choice of an antibiotic regimen for such distinct points of concern as:

whether it is specific for the organism cultured from distal or remote infective sites
whether high-fibrin clot penetration is important for early protection of Dacron grafts, which show increased bacterial adherence/affinity at this juncture as a direct function of that same fibrin binding
whether leukocyte sequestration is of theoretical benefit to the specific situation, e.g., placing a new graft in a potentially contaminated field.

Table 5
Specific Drug Recommendation

First Choice Routine Cases

		Rationale
A. FP, FD, EAB	Oxacillin or Nafcillin	1. *S aureus* most common pathogen 2. Limited morbidity of GIF if occurs
B. FP, FD, AR, or EAB with pedal sepsis	Specific drug for culture of septic site	
C. AR, AAA, IF, ThF	Rifampicin or Cefazolin	Need *S epidermidis* coverage
D. D. EAB: AXF, CF, subclavin/carotid, AXA	Oxacillin Nafcillin Cefazolin Cefamandole	*S aureus* most common pathogen
E. CEA	None	Incidence GIF too infrequent to warrant prophylaxis

---

FP = femoropopliteal bypass; FD = femorodistal bypass; EAB = extra-anatomic bypass; AR = aortic reconstruction; AAA = abdominal aortic aneurysmorrhaphy; IF = iliacofemoral; THF = thoracofemoral; AXF = axillofemoral; CF = cross-femoral; AXA = axilloaxillary; CEA = carotid endarterectomy; GIF = graft infection.

whether the regimen may be extended by simple redosing, or will require a cognitive gearshift to a therapeutic regimen

whether redosing intraoperatively should be done at the expected half-life time interval, and/or whether it should be specifically added prior to subcutaneous wound closure, since most studies indicate inadequate tissue levels at closure

whether silver- or antibiotic-impregnated grafts will provide an additional measure of local prophylaxis over a more extended time frame.

Our broad recommendations attempt to take into account the various permutations of clinical presentation, and are summarized in Table 5.

References

In this chapter, the references are listed by section, which Dr. Bunt considers the most useful presentation of these references.

General Measures

1. Bunt TJ. Synthetic vascular graft infections I: Graft infections. *Surgery*. 1983;93:6:233–246.
2. Bunt TJ. Synthetic vascular graft infections II: graft enteric erosions and graft enteric fistulae. *Surgery*. 1983;94:1:1–9.
3. Bunt TJ. Personal experience with 55 vascular graft infections. *J Cardiovasc Surg*. 1993.
4. Bunt TJ, Haynes JL. Synthetic vascular graft infections: the continuing headache. *Am Surg*. 1984;50:43.
5. Bunt TJ. Thoughts on evolving a protocol for selection of extra-anatomic bypass vs. aortic reconstruction. *Arch Surg*. 1986;121:10: 1166–1172.
6. Read R in discussion of Ernst C, et al. Incidence and significance of intraoperative bacterial cultures during abdominal aortic aneurysmectomy. *Ann Surg*. 1977;185:6:626–629.
7. Edwards MJ, Richardson JD, Klamer TW. Management of aortic prosthetic infections. *Am J Surg*. 1988;155:2:327–331.
8. Cruse PJE, Foord R. A five year prospective study of 23,649 surgical wounds. *Arch Surg*. 1973;107:2:206–210.
9. Ad Hoc Committee of the Committee on Trauma. Division of Medical Sciences, National Academy of Sciences. National Research Council: The influence of ultraviolet of the operating room and other various factors. *Ann Surg*.1964;(suppl):100:2.
10. Birkenstock WE. Surgical sepsis. *S African Med J*.1973;47:436.
11. Edwards LD. The epidemiology of 2,056 remote site infections and 1966 surgical wound infections occurring in 1865 patients. *Ann Surg*. 1976;184:6:758.
12. Hammarsten J, Holm J, Schersten T, et al. Infections in vascular surgery. *J Cardiovasc Surg*. 1977;18:543–545.

Long-Term Prophylaxis

1. Paquin O. Bacteremia following the removal of diseased teeth. *J Am Dent Assoc* 1941;28:6: 879–881.
2. Lindemann RA, Henson JL. The dental management of patients with vascular grafts placed in the treatment of arterial occlusive disease. *J Am Dent Assoc*. 1982;104:5:625–627.
3. Lefrock JL, Ellis CA, Turchik JB, et al. Transient bacteremia associated with sigmoidoscopy. *N Eng J Med*. 1973; 8:30:467–468.

Differential Infectability

1. Sugerman B. In vitro adherence of bacteria to prosthetic vascular grafts. *Infection*. 1982; 10:9.
2. Goeau-Brissoniere O, Pechere JC, Guidoin R, et al. Experimental colonization of vascular grafts with *Staphylococcus aureus*. *Can J Surg*. 1983;26:6:540–545.
3. Bennion RS, Williams RA, Wilson SE. Comparison of infectibility of vascular prosthetic materials by quantitation of median infective dose. *Surgery*. 1984;95:1:22–25.
4. Rosenman JE, Pearce WH, Kempczinski W. Bacterial adherence to vascular grafts after in vitro bacteremia. *J Surg Res*. 1985:38:648–655.
5. Schmitt DD, Bandyk DF, Pequet AJ, et al. Bacteria adherence to vascular prostheses: a determinant of graft infectivity. *J Vasc Surg*. 1986;3:5:732–740.
6. Bergamini TM, Bandyk DF, Govostis D, et al. Infection of vascular prostheses caused by bacterial biofilms. *J Vasc Surg*. 1988;7:1: 21–30.
7. Bricker DL, Beall AC Jr, DeBakey ME. The differential responses to infection of autogenous vein vs. dacron arterial prosthesis. *Chest*. 1970;58:6:566–570.
8. Shah P, Katsuki I, Clauss RH, et al. Expanded PTFE graft in contaminated wounds: experi-

mental and clinical study. *J Trauma.* 1983;23: 12:1030–1034.

9. Akhondzadeh L, Wilson SE, Williams RA, et al. Infection of materials used in vascular access surgery: an evaluation of dacron, bovine heterograft, teflon, and human umbilical vein grafts. *Dialysis Transplant.* 1980;9:7: 697–700.

10. Stone KS, Walshaw R, Sugiyama GT, et al. PTFE vs. autologous vein grafts for vascular reconstruction in contaminated wounds. *Am J Surg.* 1984;147:5:692–696.

Preventive Measures

11. Busuttil RW, Rees W, Baker JD, et al. Pathogenesis of aortoduodenal fistula: experimental and clinical correlates. *Surgery.* 1979;85:1: 1–8.

12. Hertzer NR. A rotated aneurysm cuff for separation of aortic graft and duodenum. *Surg Gynecol Obstet.* 1985.

13. Deweese MS, Fry WJ. Small bowel erosion following aortic resection. *JAMA.* 1962:179: 882–886.

14. Robiscek F, Dougherty HK, Mullen DC, et al. Is there a place for wall reinforcement in modern aortic surgery? *Arch Surg.* 1972;105: 6:824–829.

15. Miller DR. Prevention of aortoduodenal fistula by duodenal reflection. *Am J Surg.* 1979; 138:8:332–333.

16. Sauvage LR. *Grafts for the 80s: New Knowledge in Vascular Biology: Advances in Prosthetic Technology.* Seattle: Providence Medical Center Press; 1980;29.

17. Fry WJ, Lindenauer SM. Infection complicating the use of plastic arterial implants. *Arch Surg.* 1967;94:5:600–609.

18. Slidenberg B, Gitlitz GF, Hurwitt ES. Management of infected arterial prostheses. *Surg Gynecol Obstet.* 1965;3:585–586.

19. Buchbinder D, Leather R, Shah D, et al. Pathologic interactions between prosthetic aortic grafts and the gastrointestinal tract. *Am J Surg.* 1980;140:8:192–195.

20. Ray A, Hayes DF. Closure of an aortic stump: a new method. *Am J Surg.* 1983;145:3: 403–404.

21. Cogbill TH. Secure aortic stump closure with autogenous vein pledgets. *Surgery.* 1984;96: 5:940–942.

22. Bacourt F, Goeau-Brissoniere O, Koskas F. Aortic stump closure: a new technique. *Ann V Surg.* 1986;1:271–272.

23. Goldsmith HS, de los Santos R, Vanamee P, et al. Experimental protection of vascular prosthesis by omentum. *Arch Surg.* 1968;97: 6:872–878.

24. Bunt TJ, Doerhoff CR, Haynes JL. Retrocolic omental pedicle flap for routine plication of abdominal aortic grafts. *Surg Gynecol Obstet.* 1984;158:6:591–592.

25. Moulton S, Adams M, Johansen KH. Aortoenteric fistulae: a 7-year urban experience. *Am J Surg.* 1986;151:5:607–610.

Antibiotic Prophylaxis

26. Szylagyi ED, Smith RG, Elliott SP, et al. Infection in arterial reconstruction with synthetic grafts. *Ann Surg.* 1972;176:321.

27. Jamieson GG, Deweese JA, Rob CG. Infected arterial grafts. *Ann Surg.* 1975;181:6:850–852.

28. Goldstone J, Moore WS. Infection in vascular prostheses: clinical manifestations and surgical management. *Am J Surg.* 1974:128: 225–233.

29. Lord JW, Rossi G, Daliana M. Intraoperative antibiotic wound lavage: an attempt to eliminate postoperative infection in arterial and clean general surgical procedures. *Ann Surg.* 1977;185:6:634–641.

30. Pitt HA, Postier RG, Macgowan WA, et al. Prophylactic antibiotics in vascular surgery: topical, systemic, or both? *Ann Surg.* 1980; 192:3:356–364.

31. Kaiser AB, Clayson KR, Mulherin JL, et al. Antibiotic prophylaxis in vascular surgery. *Ann Surg.* 1978;188:3:283–288.

32. Salzmann G. Perioperative infection prophylaxis in vascular surgery: a randomized prospective study. *J Thorac Cardiovasc Surg.* 1983; 31:239–242.

33. Hasselgren P, Ivarsson L, Rigberg B, et al. Effects of prophylactic antibiotics in vascular surgery. *Ann Surg.*1984;200:1:86–92.

34. Edwards WH, Kaiser AB, Kernodle DS, et al. Lefuroxime vs. cefazolin as prophylaxis in vascular surgery. *J Vasc Surg.* 1992;15:1: 35–42.

35. Lord JW. Intraoperative antibiotic wound irrigation. *Surg Gynecol Obstet.* 1983;157:4: 357–359.

36. Richardson RL, Pate JW, Wolf RY, et al. The outcome of antibiotic-soaked arterial grafts in guinea pig wounds contaminated with *E. coli* or *S aureus. J Thorac Cardiovasc Surg.* 1970; 59:635.

37. Digiglia JW, Leonard GL, Ochsner JL. Local irrigation with an antibiotic solution in the prevention of infection in vascular prostheses. *Surgery.* 1970;67:5:836–840.

38. Baker WH, Cram AE, O'Connor JE. An evaluation of combined routes of antibiotic administration in vascular reconstruction surgery. *J Thorac Cardiovasc Surg.* 1972;64:2: 301–303.

39. Scherr DD, Dodd TA. Brief exposure of bacteria to topical antibiotics. *Surg Gynecol Obstet.* 1973;137:7:87–90.
40. Bunt TJ. Prophylactic antibiotics in vascular surgery. *Compl Surg.* 1991;10:1:46–50.
41. Bunt TJ. Synthetic vascular graft infections part I: selected readings in general surgery 1987.
42. Bandyk DF, Berni GA, Thiele BL, et al. Aortofemoarl graft infections due to *Staphylococcus epidermidis. Arch Surg.* 1984;119:102–108.
43. Seeger JM, Wheeler JR, Gregory RT, et al. Autogenous graft replacement of infected prosthetic grafts at the femoral position. *Surgery.* 1983;93:1:39–43.
44. Yeager RA, Moneta GL, Taylor AM. Improving survival and limb salvage in patients with aortic graft infection. *Am J Surg.* 1990; 159:5:466–470.
45. Bunt TJ. A personal experience with 55 vascular graft infections. *J Cardiovasc Surg.* 1993.
46. Durham JR, Malone JM, Bernhard VM, et al. The impact of multiple operations on the importance of arterial wall cultures. *J Vasc Surg.* 1987;5:160–169.
47. Macbeth GA, Rubin JR, McIntyre KE. The relevance of arterial wall microbiology to the treatment of prosthetic graft infections: graft infection vs. arterial infection. *J Vasc Surg.* 1984;1:6:750–756.
48. Malone JM, Lalka SG, McIntyre KE, et al. The necessity for long-term antibiotic therapy with positive arterial wall cultures. *J Vasc Surg.* 1988;8:262–267.
49. Bunt TJ. Sources of synthetic vascular graft infection during lower extremity revascularization. *Am Surg.* 1986;52:9:472–474.
50. Bunt TJ, Mohr JD. Incidence of positive lymph node cultures at time of peripheral arterial revascularization. *Am Surg.* 1984;50: 10:522–524.
51. Gayless WM In discussion of Bacourt F, Goeau-Brissoniere O, Koskas F. Aortic stump closure: a new technique. *Ann V Surg.* 1986;1:271–272.
52. Hoffert PW, Gensler S, Haimovici H. Infection complicating arterial grafts. *Arch Surg.* 1965;90:3:427–434.
53. Bunt TJ. Antibiotics in vascular surgery. *Compl Surg.* 1991;10:1:46–50.
54. Lalka SG, Malone JM, Fisher DF, et al. Efficacy of prophylactic antibiotics in vascular surgery: an arterial wall microbiologic and pharmacokinetic perspective. *J Vasc Surg.* 1989;10:5:501–510.
55. Fradet G, Brister S, Richards GK. Antibiotic prophylaxis in vascular surgery: pharmacokinetic study of four commonly used cephalosporins. *J Vasc Surg.* 1986;3:535–539.
56. Mutch D, Richard G, Brown RA, et al. Bioactive antibiotic levels in the human aorta. *Surgery.* 1982;92:6:1068–1071.
57. Robbs JV, Kharsany A. Serum and tissue concentrations of intravenous cefotaxime during aortic surgery. *Br J Antimicrob Ther.* 1984;14(suppl B):113–116.
58. Almgren B, Cars O, Eriksson I, et al. Pharmacokinetics of dicloxacillin in serum and aortic all during aneurysmal surgery. *Acta Chir Scand.* 1986;152:19–21.
59. Gugliemo BJ, Hohn DC, Koo PJ, et al. Antibiotic prophylaxis in surgical procedures: a critical analysis of the literature. *Arch Surg.* 1983;118:2:943–953.

Chapter 6.1

Overview of Antibiotic-Impregnated Grafts

T.J. Bunt

Introduction

A number of authors independently arrived at the theoretical construct of bonding antibiotics directly to the graft matrix to prevent bacterial adherence and secondary infection. The basic methods have involved either direct chemical bonding of the antibiotic to the graft itself via an intermediate structure, either a catalytic agent (benzalkonium to polytetrafluoroethylene [PTFE]) or a matrix impregnation (collagen, albumin, keratin to Dacron), or by increasing the levels of antibiotics in the naturally occurring clot matrix that lines the luminal surface.

Initial enthusiasm was stunted by the report from Kempczinski in 1962 that both cephalosporin and penicillins added to the preclot blood for Dacron grafts was rapidly eluted out and retained no significant activity. Kempczinski noted that the addition of cephalothin to the preclot blood for Dacron grafts was eluted out by a saline wash within 45 seconds.[1] A similar model with implantation of the grafts in the canine carotid resulted in elution within 2 minutes. subsequent authors have noted that this may have been largely a function of the low protein binding of the cephalothin used, with little residual antibiotic in the matrix thrombus. However, a series of researchers from 1974 to 1990 then reported successful methods of obtaining longer antibiotic retention.

Literature Review

Clark et al. (1974) demonstrated an incidental decrease in graft infectability while looking at a model for combined thromboresistance and infection resistance. They extended the concept of bacteriostasis in burn wounds by silver nitrate to vascular procedures by first demonstrating that, although aqueous silver nitrate itself added no resistance to surgical sutures, a silver-allantoin complex did confer *Staphylococcus aureus* bacterial reduction of 90% to 99%. The preliminary studies were then extended to a canine implant model. Twelve-mm woven Dacron grafts were treated with SAH (silver-allantoin-heparin) complex, dried, sterilized, and then tested ex vivo versus solutions of 2×10^3 *S aureus*, 3.4×10^3 *Escherichia coli*, 5.2×10^3 *Proteus mirabilis*, and 1×10^5

Pseudomonas. All treated grafts inhibited plate-culture growth. Silver-allantoin-heparin-treated 12-mm Dacron prostheses were then implanted in the superior vena cava of dogs; 6 weeks later, patency of the graft was confirmed by venography and 5×10^4 *S aureus* bacteremia was produced without antibiotic coverage. Harvest of the segments was then performed 1 week later, and the grafts again tested for bacterial inhibition; all five control dogs showed *S aureus* overgrowth, while the SAH-treated grafts showed nearly complete bacterial inhibition.[2]

Clark noted that the study indicated continued silver release from the SAH complex with resultant inhibition from the graft at 7 weeks. He was, however, nonplussed by the phenomenon, because he did not see how the silver ion could be effective in the local milieu, since he thought that it should be bound quickly by rapid protein and tissue chloride binding. However, he felt that the bacterial resistance conferred might be useful in the early postoperative time frame.

Unfortunately, the study did not look at the actual incidence of graft infection (GIF), but only at whether or not there were confirmed zones of inhibition or bacterial plates at the 7-week period. No mention is made of the clinical findings at explantation. It may be that the dose of *S aureus* used for the bacteremia was 1) too small at 5×10^4 organisms/cc; and/or 2) delayed to near total pseudointimal formation such that no grafts became infected.

Clark's seminal work was not duplicated until 10 years later, but by then the concept had developed numerous permutations. Rutledge et al. (1982) wrote the first of several papers for the North Carolina group, demonstrating that rifampicin could be passively bonded to Dacron. They chose rifampicin as a semisynthetic nonmethyl piperazine with a broad spectrum activity via inhibition of DNA-dependent ribonucleic acid polymerase activity. The group used implants of 3-mm PTFE in canine carotids with a local inoculation of 1×10^3 *S aureus.*

At graft explant 5 days later, control dogs showed 7/7 infections; 7/12 animals pretreated with a single dose of cefazolin 50 mg/kg were infected $P < .05$) as opposed to only 2/12 of dogs pretreated with rifampicin 50 mg/kg ($P < .05$).[3]

Powell (1983) followed up that paper, looking at passive antibiotic bonding via addition of the antibiotic to Dacron graft preclot solutions. Eight-mm Dacron grafts were immersed briefly in a 60 mg/mL solution and then triply preclotted with a 1:10 solution of antibiotic and blood. A ring of the material was removed to test for plate inhibition of *S aureus;* the remainder was implanted using the canine infrarenal aorta model. A second ring was then researched for sensitivity studies after 15 minutes of flow reestablishment, at 60 minutes, and at a reexploration at 24 hours. In an additional two dogs, supplementary intravenous rifampicin was also given as 500 mg doses every 12 hours. Similar studies were done for cefazolin, cefamandole, cefotaxime, oxacillin, tobramycin, gentamycin, tetracycline, and clindamycin. There was no residual activity demonstrated by graft-ring plate inhibition for any of the antibiotics except rifampicin. A mean dialysis curve for rifampicin was constructed, showing 94% activity at 60 minutes and 91% at 24 hours. The addition of parenteral rifampicin did not materially increase the zone of inhibition.[4]

In a follow-up study McDougal (1986) reported a longer canine implant study. Fifteen dogs underwent infrarenal aortic replacement with 8-mm knitted Dacron grafts; five were controls, five had 237 mg cefazolin and five had 60 mg rifampicin added to the preclot blood. At wound closure, a 1×10^7 *S aureus* bacteremia was induced. At 3 weeks, grafts were explanted and a ring of each graft analyzed for residual antibiotic activity. Three of five control grafts were clinically infected as were all cefazolin-treated grafts. In contrast, none of the rifampicin-treated grafts were clinically infected or culture-positive ($P < .05$). Interestingly, there was no residual antibiotic activity noted in any of the grafts.[5]

Bennion (1984) noted, in a paper primarily reviewing the differential infectability of grafts as measured by graded bacterial inocula, that an otherwise undescribed silver-complexed human umbilical vein (HUV) graft showed tenfold resistance to *S aureus* bacteremic infection over standard HUV grafts. However, the graft was reliably infected at 1×10^3 organisms, which was inferior to Dacron grafts.[6]

Webb (1986) presented supporting studies with oxacillin bonded to PTFE with benzalkonium; an in vitro immersion model was used for 1 hour at 1 mg/mL oxacillin; disc inhibition was supplemented by scanning electron microscopy (SEM) for detection of bacterial adhesiveness. This interesting adjunct supplied the surprising finding that although there was bacterial inhibition by the antibiotic solution, there was still significant bacterial adhesion noted on SEM.[7]

Some researchers explored other avenues in this field of antibiotic bonding. A series of papers came from the Columbia group. White (1984) first looked at passive bonding by adding the highly protein-bound antibiotics nafcillin, cefamandole, and cefazolin to preclot blood. Knitted Dacron grafts were analyzed in vitro after saline centrifugal wash. Increasing doses of antibiotic were used to calculate a transfer curve (from blood to graft). An average of 84% nafcillin, 67% cefazolin, and 56% of cefamandole were transferred. Concentrations higher than 50 mg/mL cefazolin and 10 mg/mL cefamandole had no further effect on *S aureus* plate inhibition. In addition, nafcillin at > 2 mg/mL and cefazolin at > 10 mg/mL had significant and undesired anticoagulant effects. Washout curves showed significant antibacterial activity at 6 hours that persisted at 96 hours.

A second protocol used silver pefloxacin, a silver nalidixic acid analogue with intense antistaphylococcal activity. These grafts maintained activity out beyond 18 days of in vitro washing and at day 6 had an inhibitory zone 67% of normal. Two-cm canine infrarenal aortic replacements with nafcillin or pefloxacin Dacron grafts were then performed, with 1×10^7 *S aureus* bacteremia 30 minutes later. At 3 weeks explantation, 0/14 nafcillin and 1/6 silver pefloxacin grafts showed clinical or culture-positive infection, versus 9/11 controls.[8]

It should be pointed out that the dialysis studies quoted in this study were of saline washes over days; these may not necessarily represent the same effect as might be seen with serum exposure. However, the small canine series did indicate the ability of those grafts to repel an immediate postoperative bacteremia of a sensitive bacteria. Since one can expect high matrix antibiotic levels at this early juncture, the model may not be clinically relevant and only represents the effect of a large dose of topical or local antibiotic at the time of the early bacteremia.

Modak reported for the group again in 1987, using PTFE bonded with tridodecylmethylammonium (TDMAC) and either norfloxacin or pefloxacin. Bonding was simply accomplished by soaking the PTFE graft in a 5% ethanol solution of TDMAC for 1 hour, followed by air drying and then a 5-minute soak at room temperature in a 1:25 acetic acid-chloroform or 4:1 ethanol-chloroform solution. Silver salts were then added by a second 5 minute room temperature soak in a 25-mmol silver nitrate, zinc nitrate, or cerium nitrate solution of the ethanoic metal salt, followed by a dark drying and resoaking in the antibiotic.

Grafts were studied by direct bonding (defined as organic solvent binding of antibiotics) versus TDMAC-coated bonding. The results showed comparative efficacy in bonding antibiotics with either procedure with 4 to 5-μmol norfloxacin and oxacillin being bonded. Adding silver to the process increased bonding to 7 to 8 μmol per 2 cm of graft. Zinc was also tried, with slightly better results. All grafts demonstrated strong in vitro *S aureus* inhibition. Saline irrigations decreased the amount of bound antibiotic, but sufficient antibiotic was retained for bacterial inhibition. A blood perfusion model was then tested and metal-antibiotic-bonded grafts showed strong activity up to 7 days.

The authors noted that direct bonding with solvents was looked at because it did not involve coating the graft with a compound cationic anchor such as TDMAC, and that silver was added for its antibacterial activity, but required intermediary fixation with the antibiotic because silver salts were not soluble in organic solvents. The rationale for the silver-antibiotic complex was that these more stable compounds could retain antibacterial activity for longer periods of time. They noted that these hypotheses were all borne out by the in vitro studies. Furthermore, toxicity for the silver salts would be unexpected, since the 10-cm grafts contained a total of 10 mg of silver, whereas 500 gm of silver sulfadiazine is routinely administered daily in burn patients, and the calculated ID_{50} for silver in humans is between 1 and 10 gm, depending on the silver salt. Of course, one could argue that there would be a potentially higher total exposure to silver if, for example, a totally coated 20 × 10-cm aortofemoral graft were used, and that the silver exposure might then increase toward perhaps 50% to 60% of the toxic level.[9]

Benvinisty in 1988 updated the experience with an in vivo model. Seven-mm PTFE grafts were treated with silver-oxacillin and silver-amikacin. A canine infrarenal aortic replacement model was used. In vivo efficacy was tested by local inoculations of 0.1 cc of 10^8/cc S aureus, with graft explantation at 10 minutes and 1 week. Seventy-four percent of oxacillin silver and 47% of amikacin-silver complex was retained at 10 minutes. This fell to 19.5% silver oxacillin at 1 week (the amikacin graft was not further tested). At 1 week, no graft appeared clinically infected; quantitative bacterial counts were reduced from a control of 1.3×10^6 to 1.72×10^2 for oxacillin ($P < .05$) and 2×10^2 for amikacin ($P < .06$).[10]

Although the authors noted the ability of the oxacillin-silver graft to retain strong antibacterial activity at 1 week, their implant study is curious for the fact that frank and complete sterilization of the grafts did not occur (residual 10^2 organisms) despite local antibiotic activity. Correlating this with the absence of clinical infection suggests that the grafts might well demonstrate persistent infection and perhaps recrudescence to clinical infection if a longer time interval had been used.

Sobinsky (1986) entered one paper for the Illinois group, studying the bonding of cefoxitin to PTFE via a glycosaminoglycan-keratin luminal coating. Glycosaminoglycan-keratin is a bilayered material that can be bonded to a PTFE graft and cefoxitin then bonded to the keratin. Glycosaminoglycan-keratin itself has no antibacterial activity. It is biodegradable so that there is no permanent graft impregnation. Bonding at various doses of antibiotic was then plotted versus inhibition zones to show an experimental increase in antibiotic activity. Forty-four 2.5-cm PTFE grafts were then placed in dogs with subsequent inoculation bacteremias of 1×10^8 S aureus performed at wound closure. Grafts were then harvested at intervals from 1 to 28 days. Ten out of 10 control grafts showed culture-positive infection versus 1/ 10 study grafts ($P < .0001$). Antibiotic activity was shown to wash out gradually over 1 week, with no activity at 10 and 14 days. This occurred in stepwise fashion on regression analysis ($r = 0.9654$).[11]

Avramovic et al. (1991) presented a paper from Milwaukee on their experience with passive impregnation of an albumin-sealed Dacron graft. They implanted 2-cm grafts in the carotids of sheep, half of which had 600 mg of rifampicin added to the saline storage solution. The wounds were inoculated with 1×10^8 S aureus at closure. At graft explantation 3 weeks later, 9/9 control grafts were infected versus 1 of 9 rifampicin grafts; there were three positive-tissue cultures where graft cultures were negative (P

< .002). There was no residual antibacterial activity noted on plate inhibition analysis.[12]

Ney (1990) has looked at the possibility of incorporating antibiotics into a fibrin glue that could be instilled as a temporary barrier around vascular grafts or anastomoses. Cryoprecipitate was mixed with bovine thrombin, aminocaproic acid, and 5 mg/cc tobramycin. In vitro kinetics of the mixture were determined to decrease from an initial greater than 8,000 to greater than only 2 μg/cc at 4 days. The standard canine infrarenal aortic replacement model was then used, with 1-cm segments of PTFE that had been bathed in a solution of 6×10^8 E coli and 3×10^8 S aureus. The dogs received intravenous cefonicid for 2 weeks. Four of four control dogs had graft infections within 4 days; four of four dogs with a fibrin-glue-sealed graft also died of graft infection within 4 days; four of four antibiotic fibrin-glue-sealed graft dogs, however, survived without clinical signs of infection at day 17 (P < .0025). However, three of four graft cultures still showed weak S aureus with one also positive for E coli. Serum tobramycin levels were negligible by 12 hours; local levels were not assayed.[13] Again, although clinical graft infection at the short 3-week follow-up was aborted, occult graft infection persisted, and had the experiment been carried out longer, a more recrudescent clinical infection might have been observed.

This interesting initial study also raises the question of whether the in vitro tobramycin elution curve was changed by the implantation and exposure to tissue fluids and catabolism. Furthermore, the persistent positive cultures, despite evidence of local healing, would indicate occult GIF and the possibility of later redevelopment of clinical graft infection. Indeed, the model is peculiar in that the infection is being produced in the graft matrix and walled off from the surrounding tissues, whereas the converse anatomic situation is usually the concern, e.g., a clean graft in a potentially contaminated field. Still, it offers yet another concept in producing local concentrations of antibiotics at the site of graft implantation.

Shenk (1991) reported the evaluation of a tobramycin adhesive in both the prevention and treatment of vascular graft infections using and expanded PTFE. They produced their grafts by mixing tobramycin powder with N-butyl-2-cyanoacrylate. In a prophylaxis model, grafts were immersed in E coli and S aureus. The treatment group was significant in comparison to the control group (P < 0.0002). The 10 surviving infected dogs served as an established graft infection protocol. These dogs were randomized into two groups, a control group and a treatment group in which the grafts were treated with the tobramycin adhesive. Again, the experimental group was superior to the control (P < 0.005).[14] There is no additional comment about the effect of the adhesive on perigraft tissues, but one wonders about the difficulty of subsequently excising a graft so clinically treated.

Haverich (1992) described the efficacy of perioperative antibiotic prophylaxis with a gentamycin derivative and fibrin sealant as an antibiotic carrier in Dacron prostheses. These studies were conducted in vitro and in vivo, and in the latter, grafts were directly contaminated with S aureus. After 1 week, the grafts and their corresponding implantation sites were excised for measurement of the antibiotic content. The antibiotic-fibrin compound bound far more antibiotic than the control (P < 0.0005).[15] However, in the in vivo studies of infection resistance, all the Dacron prostheses without pretreatment and those with the fibrin sealant alone were infected, while five of 10 antibiotic-fibrin grafts remained sterile. Recently, Phaneuf et al. demonstrated that Dacron grafts could be altered with textile-dyeing technology to bond ciprofloxacin. Though preliminary, these studies add another interesting technology to an ever burgeoning number of strategies to develop an infection-resistant vascular graft.[16]

The most comprehensive and long-term studies of antibiotic graft bonding have been performed by Greco's group in New Jersey and Moore's group at UCLA.

References

1. Kempczinski RF. Discussion following Moore et al: Development of an infection-resistant vascular prosthesis. *Arch Surg.* 1981;116:407.
2. Clark RE, Margraf HW. Antibacterial vascular grafts with improved thromboresistance. *Arch Surg.* 1974;109:2:159–162.
3. Rutledge R, Baker VV, Sherertz R, et al. Rifampin and cefazolin as prophylactic agents. *Arch Surg.* 1982;117:3:1164–1166.
4. Powell TW, Burnham SJ, Johnson G. A passive system using rifampin to create an infection-resistant vascular prosthesis. *Surgery.* 1983;94:5:765–769.
5. McDougal EG, Burnham SJ, Johnson G. Rifampin protection versus experimental graft sepsis. *J Vasc Surg.* 1986;4:1:5–7.
6. Bennion RS, Williams RA, Wilson SE. Comparison of infectability of vascular prosthestic materials by quantitation of median infective dose. *Surgery.* 1984;95:1:22–25.
7. Webb LX, Myers RT, Cordell R, et al. Inhibition of bacterial adhesion by antibacterial surface pretreatment of vascular prostheses. *J Vasc Surg.* 1984;4:1:16–21.
8. White JV, Benvenisty AJ, Reemstz K, et al. Simple methods for direct antibiotic protection of synthetic vascular grafts. *J Vasc Surg.* 1984;1:2:372–380.
9. Modak SM, Sampath L, Fox CL, et al. A new method for the direct incorporation of antibiotic in prosthetic vascular grafts. *Surg Gynecol Obstet.* 1987;164:2:143–147.
10. Benvenisty AI, Tannenbaum G, Ahlborn TN, et al. Control of prosthetic bacterial infection: evaluation of an easily incorporated, tightly bound, silver antibiotic PTFE graft. *J Surg Res.* 1988;44:1–7.
11. Sobinsky KR, Flanigan DP. Antibiotic binding to PTFE via glucosaminoglycon-keratin luminal coating. *Surgery.* 1986;100:4:629–634.
12. Avramovic J, Fletcher JP. Prevention of prosthetic vascular graft infection by rifampicin impregnation of a protein-sealed dacron graft in combination with parenteral cephalosporin. *J Cardiovasc Surg.* 1992;33:70–73.
13. Ney AL, Kelly PH, Tsukayama DT, Bubrick MP. Fibrin glue antibiotic suspension in the prevention of prosthetic graft infection. *J Trauma.* 1990;30:1000–1006.
14. Shenk JS, Ney AL, Tsukayama DT, Olson ME, Bubrick MP. Tobramycin adhesive in preventing and treating PTFE vascular graft infections. *J Surg Res.* 1989;47:487–492.
15. Haverich A, Hirt S, Karck M, Siclari F, Wahlig H. Prevention of graft infection by bonding of gentamycin to dacron protheses. *J Vasc Surg.* 1992;15:187–193.
16. Phaneuf MD, Ozaki CK, Bide MJ, et al. Application of the quinolone antibiotic ciprofloxacin to Dacron utilizing textile dyeing technology. *J Biomed Mater Res.* 1993;27:233–237.

Chapter 6.2

Therapeutic Strategies Based on Antibiotic Bonding

R.S. Greco

R.A. Harvey

Infections have been a dominant theme in surgical practice since before the birth of Christ. Early surgeons had little understanding of the mechanisms of infections and even less ability to alter the course of microbial growth. However, the development of antibiotics in the mid-twentieth century for the first time promised to alter the struggle between bacterial and surgical wounds in favor of healing rather than suppuration. Soon after this development came the evolution of surgical implants and prostheses which altered the equation once again. Indeed, the last few decades have seen an ever-expanding array of vascular grafts, prosthetic heart valves, neurosurgical devices, orthopedic prostheses, breast implants, hernia repair devices, genitourinary prostheses, ocular implants, and an ever increasing inventory of tubes, pumps, and catheters playing a role in virtually every disease process affecting the human organism.

Infection in these devices is the most catastrophic complication associated with their use and has produced a unique type of infection quite unlike its predecessors. In particular, vascular prosthetic infections are notably intransigent clinical dilemmas associated with excessive morbidity and mortality. The goal of this chapter is to characterize the pathobiology of vascular prosthetic infections and to review the current and future role of methodologies of antibiotic bonding in the prevention and treatment of vascular prosthetic infections.

The Pathobiology of Vascular Prosthetic Infections

The pathogenesis of vascular prosthetic infections remains enigmatic. The host, the foreign body, and contaminating bacteria conspire in some way to potentiate the development of a group of infections that show two distinct features. First, the infections are unresponsive to the administration of systemic antibiotics and are frequently caused by bacteria, such as *Staphylococcus epidermidis*. They are not pathogenic in the absence of a foreign body. Second,

From Bunt, TJ: *Vascular Graft Infections.* Armonk: Futura Publishing Co., Inc.; © 1994.

vascular grafts are foreign bodies which provoke an inflammatory response that is certainly a factor in their healing, but is also responsible for their propensity to become infected and thrombosed as well. The classic paper of Elek and Cohen published 35 years ago set the stage for this concept by demonstrating the effect of silk sutures on staphylococcal abscess formation in human volunteers.[1]

In general, tissue injury in the absence of a foreign body can be coped with by host defenses even when large numbers of bacteria are involved. The foreign body, however, subverts these defenses and facilitates the development of infections; the mechanism of this synergism is largely unknown.

The interaction between the host and the foreign body even in the absence of bacteria is complex. Earlier work demonstrated that the foreign body caused phagocytic activation and oxidative burst. Neutrophils contain a wide variety of armaments designed to kill bacteria but are capable as well of destroying any living tissue or cell. These enzymes are expelled from the cell when the leukocyte is exposed to the foreign body and play a role in the potentiation of infection. The burst of oxidative metabolism produces another group of highly reactive intermediates capable of local tissue injury. Complement activation may also be a primary mechanism by which foreign bodies provoke inflammation.[2] Recent evidence that Dacron and expanded polytetrafluoroethylene (ePTFE) are associated with increased binding of antibodies against the B_2 integrins, the intracellular adhesion molecule ICAM-1, and the leukocyte adhesion molecule ELAM-1 gives further credibility to the inflammatory potential of vascular grafts.[3–5]

Clinical evidence has pointed to a number of pathogens that are commonly associated with vascular prosthetic infections. The most common of these are *Staphylococcus aureus, S epidermidis, Escherichia coli,* and *Pseudomonas aeruginosa.* Of great interest is the recent demonstration by Hook and his associates that *S aureus* contains specific receptors for matrix proteins, such as fibronectin, fibrinogen, and collagen which have been demonstrated to quickly occupy the surface of an implanted prosthesis.[6] Thus, while there are a number of clues about the pathogenesis of these infections, extensive work in cellular and molecular biology will be required before the mystery is resolved.

Despite our incomplete knowledge of the mechanisms of vascular prosthetic infection, the pragmatic issue of treatment universally focuses on the use on antimicrobial agents to eliminate bacteria at the surgical site. This has led to the routine use of systemic antibiotic prophylaxis; one prospective randomized trial supports the use of this form of prevention.[7] Though there have been anecdotal clinical reports of vascular prosthetic infections caused by bacteremia and experimental evidence that bacteremia in a freshly implanted graft can cause a graft to become infected, a great majority of observers support the contention that infection occurs because of a local contamination in the perioperative period. This conclusion appears to be supported by clinical data indicating a variation in the incidence of infection according to the anatomic site of graft implantation.

When a vascular prosthetic infection occurs, treatment is more controversial and the outcome is dire. There have been increasing advocates of a more conservative approach, including antibiotic irrigation and systemic antibiotic therapy.[8] Nevertheless, despite the universal use of prophylactic systemic antibiotics, a number of investigators have sought alternatives to this approach for practical and theoretical reasons. For example, despite the use of systemic antibiotics, vascular prosthetic infections continue to occur and exact an outrageous toll, including a reported 50% mortality rate and limb loss in one half of the survivors. In addition, while experimental models use large numbers of bacteria to cause perioperative contamination, virtually all investigators agree that clinical infections occur because of contamination of the prosthesis by very small numbers of bacteria in the perioperative period. It seems likely that such contamination is greatest on the surface or in the interstices of the prosthesis. It is not at all clear whether parenteral antibiotics are capable of eliminating bacteria in this location. This, together with the likelihood that such bacteria may be protected by adsorbed plasma proteins or the constituents of the graft itself, has led to attempts to create a graft containing large doses of antibiotics which, hopefully, would completely eliminate any bacteria contaminating the prosthesis.

Antibiotic Bonding

During the 1960s, Gott and his associates developed the concept of noncovalently bonding heparin to implantable surfaces.[9] Heparin bonding has therefore gained a modest following as an adjunct in the prevention of implant-related thrombosis. In 1969, Krajicek and his associates at the Prague Medical School reported an infection-resistant synthetic vascular graft in which antibiotics were impregnated using collagen.[10] In 1974, Clark et al. reported studies of a graft with antibacterial activity, although the aim of the experiment was thromboresistance.[11] Later, McDivitt studied the incorporation of tetracycline into Dacron grafts by heat and pressure and demonstrated a decrease in *E coli* sepsis in a canine model.[12]

In 1979, we first reported *Studies of a Graphite Benzalkonium Oxacillin Surface*.[13] In these studies, we examined the efficacy of the biochemical bonding of an antibiotic to a prosthetic surface and the ability of such a surface to eliminate an infection caused by local contamination with *S aureus*. This research was predicated on our observation that the penicillins are negatively charged as is heparin and, therefore, might be used in conjunction with a positively charged quaternary ammonium compound, benzal-

konium chloride. Indeed, these surfaces were superior in infection prevention than surfaces exposed to this antibiotic alone in vitro and in vivo. In 1980, we reported at the Surgical Forum of the American College of Surgeons on the *Prevention of Graft Infection by Antibiotic Bonding*.[14] In these studies, control grafts were commercially available expanded polytetrafluoroethylene. Bonded grafts were prepared by soaking the grafts in 50% aqueous benzalkonium chloride and 10 mg of oxacillin. Both groups of grafts were locally contaminated with 1×10^7 *S aureus* after implantation in the canine aorta. Grafts were harvested 6 weeks after implantation; there was a statistically significant reduction in infection ($P < 0.03$) by antibiotic bonding.

In 1981, we further characterized the process of antibiotic bonding using benzalkonium chloride as the bonding agent. In both an in vitro bioassay and in a subcutaneous pouch in the rat, the grafts bonded to oxacillin demonstrated superior antibacterial activity when compared to either control grafts or grafts simply soaked in the antibiotic. These studies were noteworthy because they also characterized the biochemical interactions in the process by using radiolabeled antibiotics. This showed that the interaction was at least in part ionic and that the process could be manipulated by both altering the antibiotic as well as the surfactant-treated grafts. At the time, this seemed most interesting in the case of antibiotics which had double-negative charge, such as carbenicillin and ticarcillin. These studies indicated that appropriately charged antibiotics could be bound to vascular prostheses by means of a surfactant with complementary charge. The process using ePTFE as the substrate without the need for graphite, which had been used in the first group of studies, suggested a method of prophylaxis with potential clinical implications.[15]

Later in the same year, we further evaluated the interactions between cationic surfactants and anionic antibiotics. In these studies, antibiotics were bound to ePTFE using a group of surfactants. The interaction between ^{14}C-penicillin and ^{3}H-benzalkonium was studied to demonstrate the length of binding, as well as the differential specificity of bonding among different drugs. The dissociation constant of penicillin was also investigated.(Fig. 1) These studies were important because they began the development of an understanding of the interaction between the bound ligands, characterized the concentration of drugs in the bioassay, and compared this to the binding measured by liquid scintillation counting. These data demonstrated a difference between the concentration of the loosely bound antibiotic measured in the bioassay and the total amount of bound antibiotic measured by radiolabeling techniques. This heterogeneity of binding was deemed possible by the sensitivity of the microbiologic assay to the weakly bound antibiotic. The linear Scatchard plots of penicillin binding indicated that the bulk of the antibiotic was bound at sites with similar dissociation constants. That led us to believe that the binding of antibiotics to ePTFE surfaces might play a pivotal role in the prevention of vascular prosthetic infections.[16]

In the next series of experiments, grafts soaked or bonded to ^{14}C-penicillin were placed in subcutaneous pockets in rats and harvested at various time intervals.[17] This allowed us to characterize both the concentration of ^{14}C-penicillin present in the grafts over time in vivo, albeit not in the vascular tree, and also to characterize local tissue concentrations over time. These studies indicated that the elution of antibiotic was biphasic, presumably caused by the initial elution of the antibiotic from the surfactant and the later dissociation of both antibiotic and surfactant from the graft. In addition, local tissue concentrations were consistent with this type of dissociation from the graft. In 1982, we published an expanded version of the Surgical Forum presentation of the previous year in which oxacillin was bonded to PTFE grafts using the cationic surfactant benzalkonium chloride. Control ePTFE grafts and bonded grafts were prepared both at room temperature and at 90°C, placed in the infrarenal aorta of dogs and challenged by local contamination with S aureus. These studies demonstrated the markedly superior performance of both groups of bonded grafts in terms of a positive culture for the S aureus of both the graft and the site, as well as histologic evaluation, patency, and survival. This study indicated the likelihood that an antibiotic-bonded graft would be both an effective method of

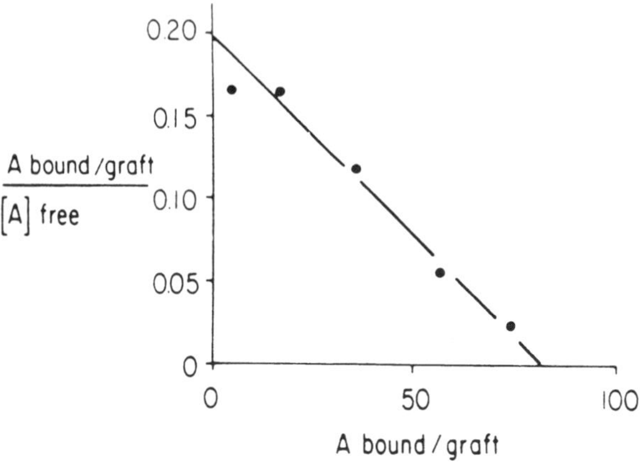

Figure 1. Scatchard plot of the binding of ^{14}C-penicillin to benzalkonium-treated grafts.

prophylaxis as well as a potential treatment for established vascular prosthetic infections.[18]

Further studies were performed using the oxacillin benzalkonium graft in which the implantation in the canine aorta was followed by harvesting 6 and 12 weeks after implantation to evaluate light, scanning, and transmission electron microscopy with regard to healing. In these studies, no histologic differences could be demonstrated between control and antibiotic-bonded grafts. Significant antibacterial activity was demonstrated at the time of graft implantation. However, none remained 6 and 12 weeks later.[19] Finally, a new method for binding benzalkonium chloride and oxacillin was developed in which much larger concentrations of antibiotics were achieved. These grafts were then implanted in the canine aorta and harvested 6 weeks later. Again, whether the bonding was performed at 100°C or with ethanol at room temperature as a solvent, the antibiotic-bonded grafts performed in a superior manner to controls and to grafts simply soaked in the antibiotic when cultures of the graft and site were evaluated. They were superior also in terms of patency and survival.[20]

In 1982, our work on antibiotic bonding took a more quantitative direction using the cationic surfactant tridodecylmethylammonium chloride (TDMAC) and a group of anionic antibiotics. In these studies, the binding of surfactants was performed using radiolabeled TDMAC, as well as C-14-labeled penicillin and a group of surfactants of varying hydrophobicity. In addition, in these studies, the ability to simultaneously bind penicillin and heparin was evaluated. The most important result of this study was that TDMAC bound substantially more ^{14}C-penicillin than did benzalkonium chloride at various concentrations of ^{14}C-penicillin in graft preparation (Fig. 2). In addition, the TDMAC-treated surfaces were able to bind both heparin and penicillin to the same surface. These studies set the stage for a detailed evaluation of TDMAC as a more effi-

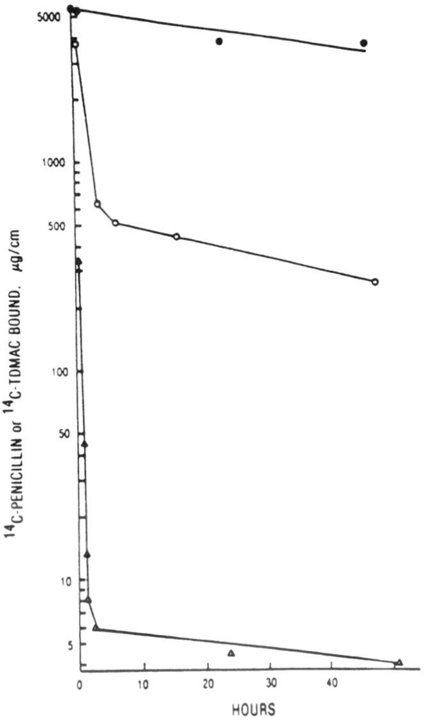

Figure 2. Retention of penicillin or TDMAC on PTFE incubated in plasma. Each point represents the average of three grafts incubated in plasma for the times indicated. Open circles, PTFE bound with unlabeled TDMAC and ^{14}C-penicillin; closed circles, PTFE bound with ^{14}C-TDMAC and unlabeled penicillin; triangles, PTFE bound with unlabeled benzalkonium and ^{14}C-penicillin. TDMAC = tridodecylmethylammonium choloride; PTFE = polytetrafluoroethylene.

cient method for producing an antibiotic-bonded ePTFE graft and supported the contention that a quaternary ammonium compound with three rather than one hydrophobic side chains would further stabilize surfactant binding. Another interesting aspect of these studies was that implantation of TDMAC-treated grafts in animals given parenteral antibiotics indicated that it would be possible to recharge the surface after implantation.[21]

In 1984, we described the bonding of cefoxitin to an ePTFE surface using TDMAC. Bactericidal concentrations of this cephalosporin were achieved with very low concentrations of the antibiotic. Elution of cefoxitin was almost identical to that achieved with penicillin and, once again, it was possible to absorb the antibiotic to the TDMAC-pretreated ePTFE after implantation when the antibiotic was administered locally or intravenously. These studies expanded our prior observations to the cephalosporin family of antibiotics and enhanced the types of antibiotics that might be usable with such a system.[22]

In 1984, we expanded our studies further by evaluating antibiotic bonding using TDMAC and Dacron vascular grafts. Our prior work had all been with ePTFE. In these studies, Dacron grafts adsorbed the radiolabeled surfactant TDMAC and were able to bind therapeutic amounts of both penicillin and cefazolin. Interestingly, these studies showed that the binding of the surfactant and both antibiotics and the retention of bound antibiotics were virtually identical to that achieved with ePTFE. In addition, local tissue concentrations of both drugs after implantation in a rat muscle pouch was very similar to what had previously been described with ePTFE. Finally, the ability to bind intravenously administered penicillin or cefazolin was similar to that which had been described previously with penicillin alone and ePTFE. These studies set the stage for the development of an antibiotic-bonded vascular graft with clinical application for the prevention of vascular prosthetic infections.[23]

A number of practical and clinical issues remained before antibiotic bonding could be brought to the bedside. In 1984, we reported on the stability of antibiotics bound to ePTFE with cationic surfactants. This study evaluated the effect of prolonged storage and sterilization on the noncovalent bonding of penicillin to ePTFE. Tridodecylmethylammonium choloride was unaffected by prolonged storage or sterilization and its ability to bind penicillin remained constant for as long as 3 months. Steam and ethylene oxide sterilization markedly diminished any bacterial activity of bound an-

tibiotic. However, the antibacterial properties of TDMAC-bound penicillin remained constant for up to 12 weeks when grafts were stored at either 4°C or at room temperature. From these studies we concluded that the bonding process appeared to increase the stability of the antibiotic and suggested a method of manufacturing that would facilitate clinical use of these grafts (Fig. 3). That system would involve the manufacturer applying the surfactant to the surface during the manufacturing process and the surgeon adding antibiotic of choice from among all of the penicillins and cephalosporins in the operating room at the time of graft implantation.[24]

By this time, our group received the

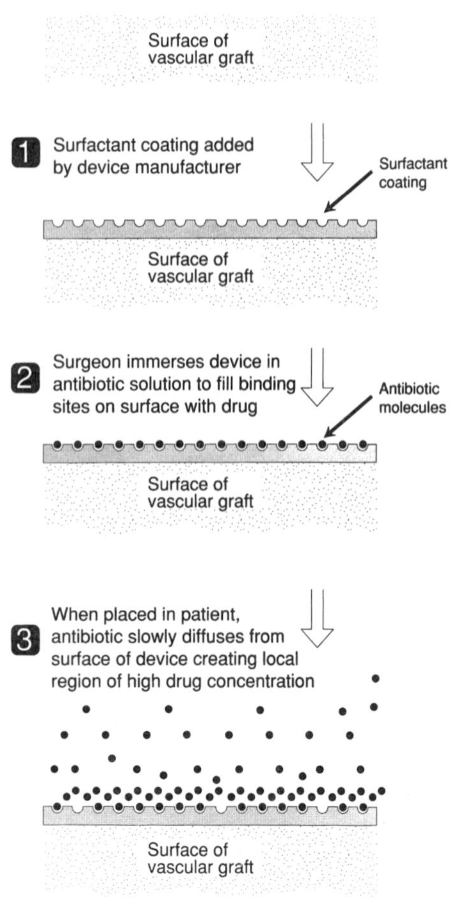

Figure 3.

first of three United States patents that would ultimately be issued involving the process of antibiotic bonding to a number of different types of prostheses. It seemed to us that two major studies had to be concluded during the same time frame so that research and development agreements might begin with the manufacturers of implantable devices. The first of these would test the hypothesis that an antibiotic-bonded vascular graft might not only prevent vascular prosthetic infections as in our prior work, but be able to treat established vascular prosthetic infection with in situ replacement. This study, presented at the annual meeting of the Surgical Infection Society, was, in our minds, the most important and complex of the studies we had done in vivo involving antibiotic bonding. The infected graft protocol consisted of implanting ePTFE grafts in the infrarenal aorta and infecting 40 control grafts with 1×10^7 S aureus. Three weeks later, all animals were reexplored and grafts excised with gross signs of infection observed. Culture and sensitivity of the excised graft, the adjacent aorta, and the surrounding tissue were performed. At this operation, the excised graft was replaced in situ. In addition, a local antibiotic irrigation of penicillin was performed but no systemic antibiotics were given. Animals with negative cultures after the reimplantation operation were then discarded and this left nine animals in each of three groups—control, animals that received a benzalkonium penicillin-bonded graft, and animals that received a TDMAC penicillin-bonded graft. Animals were explored at 3 weeks and grafts reexcised after making notations about the presence of gross infection or thrombosis. Both groups of antibiotic-bonded grafts behaved in a markedly superior manner to the control group and the results of positive cultures or total cultures per animal were significantly different from control in both the benzalkonium group and the TDMAC-bonded group. Control animals had a high thrombosis rate secondary to infection. All the

benzalkonium-bonded grafts were patent and a smaller number of the TDMAC-bonded grafts were also patent. The latter instance was the only time that the TDMAC-bonded grafts had a higher thrombosis rate in all of the studies we performed (and in all of the later research and development studies that were performed which were unpublished but shared with the Food and Drug Administration.) The thrombosis rate in the TDMAC-bonded grafts in these studies remains enigmatic to us.

Another extremely important aspect of these studies was that all of the animals received ^{14}C-labeled penicillin. This enabled us to characterize the amount of antibiotic originally bonded to the grafts and the amount remaining at the time of explant. Both the benzalkonium- and the TDMAC-bonded grafts contained over 4 mg of penicillin per centimeter of graft at the time of implantation, which resulted in a mean implantable dose of over 17 mg for each of the 4-cm grafts. Compared to this, untreated PTFE adsorbed only 1.03 μg of penicillin per centimeter or 4.12 μg per 4-cm graft. Despite the fact that the TDMAC grafts contained as much as 122 μg per centimeter of penicillin at explantation 3 weeks later compared to only 0.76 μg per centimeter in the benzalkonium-bonded group, both groups performed well in preventing infection. This was an extremely important observation because it indicated to us that the efficacy of antibiotic bonding is predicated not on the time that the antibiotic is present but on the huge dose present at the time of implantation. This supports our hypothesis that vascular prosthetic infection occurs because of perioperative contamination and that the complete killing of all bacteria would be associated with an elimination of infection in both the prophylaxis and the treatment models.

Finally, another interesting aspect of these studies was that we attempted to characterize whether or not surfactant-treated ePTFE could adsorb antibiotics given parenterally in an animal model, the rat, in which TDMAC-treated grafts were implanted. The animals were then given 14C-labeled penicillin at various intervals. These studies indicated that the TDMAC-bonded grafts, indeed, adsorbed greater concentrations of antibiotic than the control. Most importantly, in control grafts, there was only a small, less than bactericidal, dose of antibiotic in the graft for as much as 96 hours after graft implantation (Fig. 4). This may be why vascular prosthetic infections occur despite the use of systemic antibiotic prophylaxis.[25]

The last major in vivo study of antibiotic bonding was published in 1988. The study differed from our prior work in three major ways. First, we used Dacron in the vascular system. Second, a cephalosporin was the bound antibiotic in a model of infection in the canine aorta. Third, we compared antibiotic bonding to parenterally administered antibiotic whereas in the past we had always compared bound drug to the same concentration of antibiotic given by local irrigation. In these studies, antibiotic bonding performed in a far superior manner in all categories, especially cultures of the suture lines.[26]

We also evaluated the median infective dose of bonded cephalosporin in a rat subcutaneous pouch. The evaluation of median infective dose indicated a marked shift to the right in favor of antibiotic bonding which increased the infection resistance of Dacron-bonded to TDMAC 500-fold when compared to control and fivefold when compared to simply soaking the grafts in the same antibiotic. It appeared from these observations that surfactant-mediated antibiotic bonding was a valid method of pre-

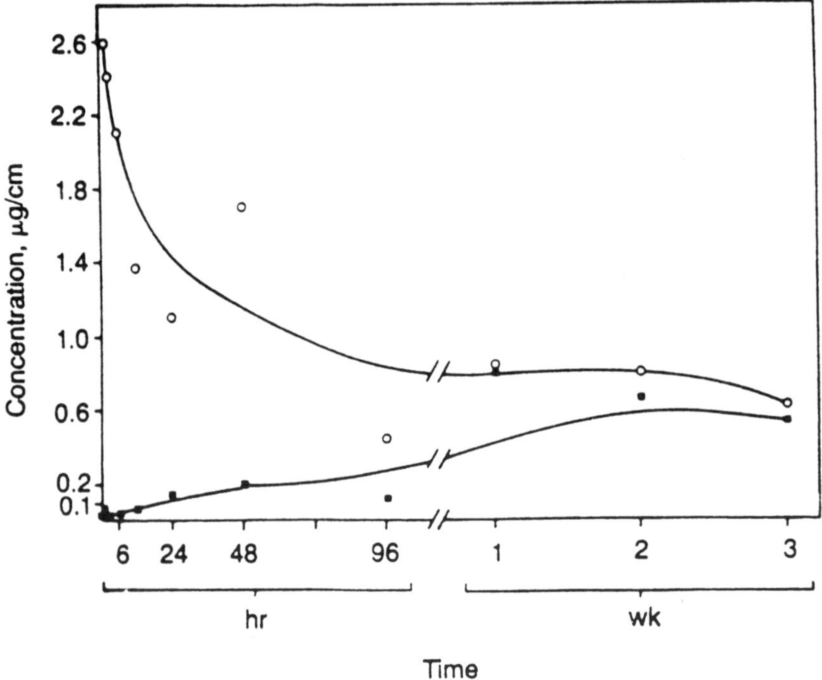

Figure 4. Concentration of penicillin-G labeled with radioactive carbon in control (closed squares and tridodecylmethylammonium chloride (TDMAC)-treated polytef (open circles) versus time of intravenous penicillin-G administration. Concentration in TDMAC-treated polytef is significant compared with control grafts for 4 days ($P < .001$).

venting vascular prosthetic infections using a Dacron graft and built on our prior work showing the similar preventive role with ePTFE, and the in situ treatment of infected vascular grafts. At this time, a multicenter clinical trial sponsored by Bard Cardiosurgery was planned.

It should be noted here that beginning in 1983, we started a corollary series of studies characterizing the effect of antibiotic bonding on catheter-related sepsis. The studies indicated that antibiotic bonding prevented locally induced catheter sepsis in animal models. This methodology could be extended to animal models of hyperalimentation by both in vitro studies of the elution of bound ligands to silicone elastomer and polyethylene, and in an in vivo bioassay using polyethylene tubing inserted into the jugular vein.[27-29] Later studies in animal models and in a prospective randomized clinical trial in chronic peritoneal dialysis catheters demonstrated efficacy, although this did not persist over an extended period of time.[30] Perhaps the most noteworthy of antibiotic-bonded catheter clinical trials was recently published in *Journal of the American Medical Association* by Kamal et al.[31] This double-blind, prospective, randomized trial of intra-arterial and intravenous catheters in humans indicated a significant advantage in infection resistance of antibiotic-bonded catheters and is the first study of its kind which may lead to general use of these devices in humans.

To summarize our more recent work in this arena, we have turned our attention to the binding of antithrombogenic and thrombolytic agents to vascular grafts using surfactants.[32] This technique has been used with both tissue plasminogen activator and the prostacyclin analogue, Iloprost. Studies of the interactions indicate that it is possible to bind both drugs with TDMAC and that such surfaces are highly resistant to thrombosis. Of interest is that the combination of tPA and the antibiotics appears to increase infection resistance.[33] Recently, we have demonstrated an increased patency of a small vessel prosthesis bonded to tPA and Iloprost simultaneously.[34]

Other Strategies-Antibiotic Bonding using Different Techniques

The first alternative method to surfactant-mediated antibiotic bonding was described by Moore et al.[35] Dacron grafts bonded to amikacin with collagen and challenged by bacteremia were found to be statistically and significantly superior to control in terms of infection prevention. The precise methodology of the collagen binding was incompletely described, however, and this made corroboration by other investigators difficult. Almost a decade later, the same group of investigators described the efficacy and duration of antibiotic bonding with a collagen release system and three different antibiotics, the most promising of which was rifampicin rather than amikacin.[36] A year later, the same investigators described the prevention of graft infection by the use of a Dacron graft bonded with rifampicin and collagen in the canine aorta. The results indicated that rifampicin bonded to Dacron with collagen protected the graft from bacteremic infection for 7 days after implantation.[37] More recently, the same group described the efficacy of antibiotic bonding with collagen and rifampicin in the treatment of established prosthetic infection with in situ replacement.[38] Of concern in the collagen binding systems is the recent observations of Hook et al. that *S aureus* contains specific binding domains for collagen. The fact that a significant number of such grafts continue to become infected might reflect the influence of collagen in this system. Furthermore, the collagen release system appears, at the present time, to be applicable to Dacron only.

An alternative method for antibiotic bonding was described by Benvenisty's group at Columbia. Beginning in 1984, they described a method in which nafcillin, cefazolin, and cefamandole were bound to the graft in the preclotting of Dacron. In addition, they were the first to describe the complexing of antibiotics with silver as a method of antibiotic bonding. Later, this same group described the silver antibiotic complex in a series of experiments using ePTFE, but in a nonvascular model. Though the biphasic release was similar to that achieved with TDMAC and other surfactants, ultimate application to an intravascular model was not included with this study.[39,40] Finally, in 1988, the same group described the use of silver oxacillin or ciprofloxacin in a canine abdominal aortic model. They were able to demonstrate the retention of antibacterial activity for the time of implantation.[41] Finally, Bandyk and Town used a silver ciprofloxacin-bonded graft of ePTFE and found that it reduced the incidence of perioperative infections with *S epidermidis*. They concluded that bonding with silver ciprofloxacin with and without TDMAC was equivalent. It is not possible to explain the use of TDMAC in these studies since ciprofloxacin is not negatively charged. Nevertheless, this group of experiments expanded interest in metals as a potential method for antibiotic bonding.[42]

Three separate recent studies have described different methods of antibiotic bonding. Ney et al. in 1990 described the use of a fibrin glue antibiotic suspension used with ePTFE grafts.[43] The cryoprecipitate was a mixture of bovine thrombin, aminocaproic acid, and tobramycin. Initial antibiotic activity was high, although only half of that reported previously with TDMAC. When grafts were placed in the infrarenal aorta and challenged with *E coli* and *S aureus*, the grafts treated with the fibrin glue antibiotic suspension performed in a much superior manner to controls.

Another group has described a different sealant. This graft was produced by Vascutek of Inchinnnan, Scotland and is sealed with gelatin dissolved at 65°C and impregnated under pressure throughout the interstices of a double-velour warp-knitted pros-

thesis. The evolution of this graft was to avoid the preclotting technique needed with the classic knitted Dacron prosthesis. This problem has been the subject of great debate in the vascular surgical literature and manufacturers have sought alternatives before, including collagen and albumin.[50] These seemingly unrelated phenomena reported on in a little known abstract presented at the 16th Annual Meeting of the Society for Biomaterials in 1990. Ashton and his associates compared the Gelsoft®, (Vascutek Limited, Inchinnan Scotland) grafts and grafts sealed with collagen, albumin, and a different gelatin which were then soaked in a 1 mg/mL solution of rifampicin. Their studies indicated that the antibacterial activity of rifampicin bound in this manner lasted for as long as 4 days and that alteration with pH indicated that the bonding was ionic in nature.[51] Their work was followed by a study by Lachapelle et al. in which the in vivo drug retention and antibacterial activity of the gelatin rifampicin grafts was studied in a swine model. These studies indicated that rifampicin retention was significant for 3 days in the vascular system, that the mean drug concentration was highly bactericidal, and that there was inhibitory activity against both *S aureus* and *S epidermidis* using this technique.[52]

The use of the Gelsoft® Dacron graft has become particularly interesting to the Europeans. In 1992, Goeau-Brissonniere and colleagues reported on the efficacy of rifampicin bonding in a canine model of thoracoabdominal aortic bypass. The rifampicin-bonded grafts withstood bacteremic challenge by the parenteral route.[53] They concluded that soaking the gelatin-sealed Dacron graft in rifampicin was efficacious and reported their plan to develop a prospective randomized trial in Europe involving as many as 3000 patients. The details of this bold plan have yet to be published, but it is anticipated that patient accrual will begin by the time this book is published. Thus, it appears that the gelatin rifampicin graft may become the first clinically used antibiotic-bonded graft to be prospectively studied in a clinical trial of prophylaxis. Clearly, it also indicates the greater ease of developing such protocols in Europe rather than in the United States.

In Situ Graft Replacement in Humans

As noted in a number of methodologies described experimentally, there are two potential roles for antibiotic bonding. The first of these is in the prevention of vascular prosthetic infection and the second is in the in situ replacement of an infected graft. In the recent past, a number of exciting and perhaps adventuresome studies have been reported in the use of antibiotic bonding in humans.

Strachan has reported the use of rifampicin gelatin-bonded grafts in four patients at high risk of developing subsequent infections.[54] The investigators point to the benefits of the gelatin coating which: eliminates the need for preclotting, reduces blood loss to a minimum, does not allow elution of antibiotics because of its low porosity, and allows for a simple procedure requiring nothing more than the gelatin-sealed graft produced by the manufacturer and simple soaking in rifampicin in the operating room. More recently, Torsello et al. have described the use of the rifampicin-bonded graft in five patients using in situ replacement after the development of vascular prosthetic infections. With at least 6 months of follow-up, all grafts are patent without evidence of infection by a computerized tomographic scan. They agree with Strachan that infected vascular prostheses can be safely replaced in situ by the gelatin-rifampicin-bonded Dacron graft.[55]

On the other hand, it is important to point out that other investigators have reported the successful in situ replacement of vascular prostheses using systemic antibiotics, graft excision, and local debridement *without* antibiotic bonding.[56,57]

Conclusions

Vascular prosthetic infections are notably intransigent clinical dilemmas associated with excessive morbidity and mortality. Despite the use of prophylactic systemic antibiotics (which are quite costly), these infections continue to occur and to exact an excessive toll in both morbidity and mortality. It is quite clear from all the investigations in this field that the host, the foreign body, and the bacteria synergize to create a milieu in which these unique infections occur. The prevailing hypothesis is that small numbers of bacteria implanted in the perioperative period colonize the foreign body and are protected in some way from host defenses and systemically administered antibiotics. This has led to the concept that an antibiotic capable of killing these bacteria, which is bonded to the surface and interstices of the biomaterial, would remove all living bacteria and thereby eliminate infections. The number of techniques described indicates that none are perfect but serves to clarify how important a clinical dilemma these infections represent and give a general indication for the direction of future research.

Obviously, one direction is the development of vascular conduits based on autogenous tissue; however, the development of such materials is a daunting task which requires them not only to be infection resistant and thrombosis resistant but to demonstrate all of the mechanical properties of current prosthetic materials.

The second option is the modification of prosthetic materials to improve their biologic performance. All of this has occurred at a time when the era of bionic man remains in its infancy. The next few decades should see the development of a wide array of prosthetic devices, many of which will be designed to replace organs as well as blood vessels. The development of such biomaterials will require a careful characterization of the cellular and molecular effects on the host and may, thereby, lead to the evolution of truly biocompatible devices.

At the present time, antibiotic bonding has yet to fulfill its promise. The surfactant-mediated technology we described more than a decade ago remains feasible and appears to be efficacious in both the prophylaxis and treatment modes. Clinical trials have been suspended both as a result of the decisions by manufacturers to further upgrade the mechanical performance of their grafts, and because of the regulatory climate in the United States at the present time. The Europeans, less beleaguered by regulation, appear to be the most likely to develop a prospective randomized trial in the near term.

At this time, it is tempting to recount an interesting irony in the evolution of research in this compelling area. One of the first antibiotic-bonded vascular grafts, which actually was the instigator of our research, was conceived as an attempt to physically incorporate tetracycline into grafts under pressure in 1977. Tetracycline was used because of its yellow color, which provided a means to crudely measure the amount of bound antibiotic. The most recently described antibiotic-bonded graft, notably the gelatin-rifampicin graft, results in an orange color to the vascular prosthesis soaked in rifampicin. Thus, after almost 15 years of investigation, the shade of the bonded graft has been changed ever so slightly.

The goal remains the same however—the eradication of a relatively rare complication in vascular surgery with devastating implications for the patients thus affected.

References

1. Elek SD, Cohen PE. The virulence of *Staphylococcus pyogenes* for man: a study of the problems of wound infection. *Br J Exp Pathol.* 1957;38:573.
2. Dougherty SH, Simmons RL. Current problems in surgery. 1992;19:268–318.
3. Margiotta MS, Robertson FM, Greco RS. Selective induction of intercellular adhesion molecule (ICAM-1) expression by human endothelial cells following adherence to vascular grafts using an in vitro model. *Surg Forum.* 1990;41:339–341.
4. Margiotta M, Benton L, Bijur G, Robertson F, Greco RS. The role of adhesion molecules in neutrophil binding to endothelial cells adherent to vascular grafts. *Surg Gynecol Obstet.* (Submitted).
5. Benton LD, Purohit UM, Khan M, Greco RS. The biologic role of B2 integrins in the host response to ePTFE. (Submitted).
6. Froman G, Switakski LM, Speziale P, Hook M. Isolation and characterization of a fibronectin receptor from *Staphylococcus aureus. J Biol Chem.* 1987;262(14):6564–6571.
7. Kaiser AB et al. Antibiotic prophylaxis in vascular surgery. *Ann Surg.* 1979;188:283–289.
8. Ehrenfeld WK, Wiebur BC, Olcott CN, Stoney RJ, Wylie EJ. Autogenous tissue reconstruction in the management of infected prosthetic grafts. *Surgery.* 1979;85:82–92.
9. Whiffen JD, Gott VL. In vivo absorption of heparin by graphite-benzalkonium intravascular surfaces. *Surg Gynecol Obstet.* 1965;121:287.
10. Krajicek M, Dvorak J, Chvapil M. Infection-resistant synthetic vascular substitutes. *J Cardiovasc Surg.* 1969;10:453–457.
11. Clarke RE, Margraf HW. Antibacterial vascular grafts with improved thromboresistance. *Arch Surg.* 1974;109:159–162.
12. McDivitt NB. Development of an infection-resistant vascular prosthesis. *Arch Surg.* 1981. Commentary. 116:1403–1467.
13. Jagpal R, Greco RS. Studies of a graphite-benzalkonium-oxacillin surface. *Am Surg.* 1979;45:774–779.
14. Greco RS, Harvey RA, Henry R, Prahlad A. Prevention of graft infection by antibiotic bonding. *Surg Forum.* 1980;31:29–30.
15. Harvey RA, Greco RS. The non-covalent bonding of antibiotics to a polytetrafluoroethylene graft. *Ann Surg.* 1981;194:642–647.
16. Henry R, Harvey RA, Greco RS. Antibiotic bonding to vascular prostheses. *J Thorac Cardiov Surg.* 1981;82:272–277.
17. Prahlad A, Harvey RA, Greco RS. Diffusion of antibiotics from a polytetrafluoroethylene (PTFE) surface. *Amer Surg.* 1981;194:642–647.
18. Greco RS, Harvey RA. The role of antibiotic bonding in the prevention of vascular prosthetic infections. *Ann Surg.* 1982;95:168–171.
19. Greco RS, Tesoriero JV, Smilow PC, Harvey RA. Light and electron microscopic studies

of an antibiotic bonded vascular graft. *J Cardiov Surg.* 1984;25:489–497.

20. Greco RS, Harvey RA, Smilow PC, Tesoriero JV. Prevention of vascular prosthetic infection by a benzalkonium-oxacillin bonded polytetrafluoroethylene graft. *Surg Gynecol Obstet.* 1982;155:28–32.

21. Harvey RA, Alcid DV, Greco RS. Antibiotic bonding to polytetrafluoroethylene with tridodecylmethylammonium chloride. *Surgery.* 1982;92(3):504–512.

22. Harvey RS, Tesoriero JV, Greco RS. The noncovalent bonding of penicillin and cefazolin to Dacron. *Amer J Surg.* 1984;147:205–209.

23. Greco RS, Harvey RA. The biochemical bonding of cefoxitin to a polytetrafluoroethylene graft. *J Surg Res.* 1984;36:237–243.

24. Donetz AP, Harvey RA, Greco RS. The stability of antibiotics bound to polytetrafluoroethylene with cationic surfactants. *J Clin Microbiol.* 1984;19:1–3.

25. Greco RS, Trooskin SZ, Donetz AP, Harvey RA. The application of antibiotic bonding to the treatment of established vascular prosthetic infection. *Arch Surg.* 1985;120(1):71–75.

26. Shue WB, Worosilo SC, Donetz AP, Trooskin SZ, Harvey RA, Greco RS. Prevention of vascular prosthetic infection with an antibiotic bonded Dacron graft. *J Vasc Surg.* 1988;8(5):600–605.

27. Trooskin SZ, Harvey RA, Greco RS. Prevention of catheter sepsis by antibiotic bonding. *Surg Forum.* 1983;34:132–133.

28. Trooskin SZ, Donetz AP, Harvey RA, Greco RS. Prevention of catheter sepsis by antibiotic bonding. *Surgery.* 1985;97(5):547–551.

29. Rodriguez JL, Trooskin SZ, Greco RS, Herbstman RA, Doillon C, Donetz AP, et al. Reduced bacterial adherence to surfactant coated catheters. *Curr Surg.* 1986;43(5):423–425.

30. Trooskin SZ, Harvey RA, Donetz AP, Baxter J, Greco RS: Infection resistant continuous peritoneal dialysis catheters. *Nephron.* 1987;46:263–267.

31. Kamal GD, Pfaller MA, Rempe LE, Jebson PJR. Reduced intravascular catheter infection by antibiotic bonding. *JAMA* 1991;265(18):2364–2368.

32. Harvey RA, Kim HC, Pincus J, Trooskin SZ, Wilcox JN, Greco RS. Binding of tissue plasminogen activator to vascular grafts. *Thromb Haemostasis* 1989;61(1):131–136.

33. Greco RS, Harvey RA. Utilizing vascular prostheses for drug delivery. *J Vasc Surg.* 1991;13(5):753–755.

34. Greco RS, Kim HC, Donetz AP. Harvey RA. Patency of a small vessel prosthesis bonded

to tissue plasminogen activator and iloprost. Submitted.

35. Moore WS, Chvapil M, Seiffert G, Keown K. Development of an infection-resistant vascular prosthesis. *Arch Surg.* 1981;116:1403–1407.

36. Chervu A, Moore WS, Chvapil M, Henderson T: Efficacy and duration of antistaphylococcal activity comparing three antibiotics bonded to Dacron vascular grafts with a collagen release system. *J Vasc Surg.* 1991;13:897–901.

37. Chervu A, Moore WS, Gelabert HA, Colburn MD, Chvapil M. Prevention of graft infection by use of prostheses bonded with rifampin/collagen release system. *J Vasc Surg.* 1991;14:521–525.

38. Colburn MD, Moore WS, Chvapil M, Gelabert HA, Quinones-Baldrich WJ. Use of an antibiotic-bonded graft for in-situ reconstruction following prosthetic graft infections. *J Vasc Surg.* (In press).

39. White JV, Benvenistry AI, Reemtsma K, Voorhees AB, Fox CL, Modak S, Nowygrod R. Simple methods for direct antibiotic protection of synthetic vascular grafts. *J Vasc Surg.* 1984;1:372–380.

40. Modak SM, Sampath L, Fox CL, Benvenisty A, Nowygrod R, Reemstmau K. A new method for the direct incorporation of antibiotic in prosthetic vascular grafts. *Surg Gynecol Obstet.* 1987;164:143–147.

41. Benvenisty AI, Tannenbaum G, Ahlborn TN, Fox CL, Modak S, Sampath L, et al. Control of prosthetic bacterial infection: evaluation of an easily incorporated, tightly bound, silver antibiotic PTFE graft. *J Surg Res.* 1988;44:1–7.

42. Kinney EV, Bandyk DF, Seabrook GA, Kelly HM, Towne JB. Antibiotic-bonded PTFE vascular grafts: the effect of silver antibiotic on bioactivity following implantation. *J Surg Res.* 1991;50:430–435.

43. Ney AL, Kelly PH, Tsukayama DT, Bubrick MP. Fibrin glue-antibiotic suspension in the prevention of prosthetic graft infection. *J Trauma* 1990;30:1000–10006.

44. Shenk JS, Ney AL, Tsukayama DT, Olson ME, Bubrick MP. Tobramycin-adhesive in preventing and treating PTFE vascular graft infections. *J Surg Res.* 1989;47:487–492.

45. Sobinsky KR, Flanigan DP. Antibiotic binding to polytetrafluoroethylene via glucosaminoglycan-keratin luminal coating. *Surgery.* 1986;100(4):629–634.

46. Haverich A, Hirt S, Karck M, Siclari F, Wahlig H. Prevention of graft infection by bonding of gentamycin to Dacron prostheses. *J Vasc Surg.* 1992;15:187–193.

47. Phaneuf MD, Ozaki CK, Bide MJ, Quist WC, Alessi JM, Tannenbaum GA, et al. Application of the quinolone antibiotic ciprofloxacin to Dacron utilizing textile dyeing technology. *J Biomed Mater Res.* 1993;27:233–237.

48. Powell TW, Burnham SJ, Johnson G. A passive system using rifampin to create an infection-resistant vascular prosthesis. *Surgery.* 1983;94(5):765–769.

49. McDougal EG, Burham SJ, Johnson G. Rifampin protection against experimental graft sepsis. *J Vas Surg.* 1986;4:5–7.

50. Jonas RA, Ziemer G, Schoen FJ, Britton L, Castaneda AR. A new sealant for knitted Dacron prostheses: minimally cross-linked gelatin. *J Vasc Surg.* 1988;7:414–419.

51. Ashton TR, Cunningham JB, Paton D, Maini R. Antibiotic loading of vascular grafts. *Transactions of the Society for Biomaterials 235;* 1990.

52. Lachapelle K, Graham AM, Symes JF. A simple technique of antibiotic impregnation using a gelatin sealed Dacron graft: in vivo drug retention and antibacterial activity. *J Vasc Surg.* (In press).

53. Goeau-Brissonniere O, Leport C, Bacourt F, Lebrault C, Comte R, Pechere JC. Prevention of vascular graft infection by rifampin bonding to a gelatin-sealed Dacron graft. *Ann Vasc Surg.* 1991;5:408–412.

54. Strachan CJL, Newsom SWB, Ashton TR. The clinical use of an antibiotic-bonded graft. *Eur J Vasc Surg.* 1991;5:627–632.

55. Torsello G, Sandmann W, Gehrt A, Jungblut RM. In situ replacement of infected vascular prostheses with rifampin-bonded vascular grafts: early results. *J Vasc Surg.* 1993; 17(4)768–773.

56. Bandyk DF, Bergamini TM, Kinney EV, Seabrook GR, Towne JB. In situ replacement of vascular prostheses infected by bacterial biofilms. *J Vasc Surg.* 1991;13:575–583.

57. J. Andrew Robinson, Johansen K. Aortic sepsis: is there a role for in situ graft reconstruction? *J Vasc Surg.* 1991;13:677–684.

Chapter 6.3

Development of an Antibiotic-Protected Vascular Prosthesis Using a Collagen-Bonded Release System

W.S. Moore

H.A. Gelabert

M.D. Colburn

Introduction

The concept of incorporating an antibiotic into a vascular prosthesis has long been proposed for both the prevention of graft contamination and the treatment of established graft infections. The ideal infection-resistant prosthesis should contain several qualities. First, the antimicrobial agent must be effective against the organisms that are most commonly encountered in vascular graft infections. Second, the bonding agent must be nontoxic and have no adverse effect on either graft healing or thrombogenicity. Third, the binding process should be easily accomplished and not compromise the mechanical characteristics of the graft. Lastly, the completed prosthesis must provide a prolonged duration of local antibiotic activity that is sufficient to protect the graft during the early healing process.

Research into the development of an in-fection-resistant vascular graft has been conducted by several investigators. These efforts have ranged from passive coating of grafts with antimicrobial agents, to covalently bonding the antibiotics using a variety of bonding materials (Table 1). Unfortunately, differences in antibiotic doses, tested organisms, and methods of evaluation make comparison of these bonding techniques difficult. In our laboratory, we have been interested in the development of an antibiotic-protected Dacron graft using a collagen-bonded release system. The purpose of this chapter is to highlight the important steps in the development of this new vascular prosthesis and to review the experimental data supporting its use.

Clinical Problem

The incidence of prosthetic graft infec-tion has remained stable and no recent sig-

Table 1
Reported Methods of Bonding Antibiotics to Prosthetic Vascular Grafts

Author	Year	Graft	Antibiotic	Bonding Agent	Bond Type
Clark et al.[40]	1974	Dacron	Silver	Allantoin	Ionic
Moore et al.[33] Retention	1981	Dacron	Amikacin	Collagen	
Prahlad et al.[24]	1981	PTFE	Penicillin G	Benzalkonium Chloride	Ionic
Henry et al.[25]	1981	PTFE	Oxacillin	Benzalkonium Chloride	Ionic
Greco et al.[26]	1982	PTFE	Oxacillin	Benzalkonium Chloride	Ionic
Harvey et al.[28]	1982	PTFE	Penicillin G	TDMAC	Ionic
Greco et al.[27]	1984	PTFE	Cefoxitin	TDMAC	Ionic
Sobinsky et al.[31]	1986	PTFE	Cefoxitin	GK	?
Benvenisty et al.[21]	1986	PTFE	Amikacin Oxacillin	AgNO$_3$	Ionic
Modak et al.[22]	1987	Dacron PTFE	Norfloxacin Oxacillin	TDMAC AgNO$_3$	Ionic
Shue et al.[29]	1988	Dacron	Oxacillin	TDMAC	Ionic
Shenk et al.[30]	1989	PTFE	Tobramycin	NBCA	Topical
Ney et al.[32]	1990	PTFE	Tobramycin	Fibrin	Topical
Kinney et al.[23]	1991	PTFE	Ciprofloxacin	TDMAC AgNO$_3$	Ionic
Chervu et al.[34] Retention	1991	Dacron	Rifampin	Collagen	

PTFE = Polytetrafluoroethylene; TDMAC = Tridodecylmethylammonium chloride; GK = Glucosaminoglycan-keratin; AgNO$_3$ = Silver nitrate; NBCA = N-butyl-2-cyanoacrylate.

nificant advance in the prevention of this devastating problem has occurred. The true incidence is difficult to quantify. This is due to the absence of any prospective randomized studies documenting this complication. With the combination of optimal surgical technique and appropriate prophylactic antibiotics, the incidence has persistently been reported in several retrospective series to be between 1% to 5%.[1-4] Clinically, these infections may present any time following implantation. In two reports, over half of the observed graft infections occurred within 1 month of operation.[1,4] However, we and others have noted the manifestation of this complication following an interval of up to 10 years.

Once a graft infection does occur, the clinical outcome remains dismal. Overall, the mortality rate in patients with a prosthetic graft infection is 30% to 40%, and up to 30% will require a subsequent amputa-tion.[2,3,5] In one report, 82% of patients treated for an aortic graft infection were dead at 5 years.[6] Furthermore, those patients who do survive the initial removal of the infected prosthesis continue to suffer from a relatively high morbidity related to their remote extra-anatomic bypasses. The primary graft patency rate of these reconstructions is 43% at 3 years in those grafts whose primary indication was an infected graft. This can be improved to 65% after secondary procedures.[7] Subsequent limb loss associated with a failed axillobifemoral graft is as high as 34%.[7] Furthermore, the recurrence of infection in an extra-anatomic bypass graft is significant at about 20%.[7]

Thus, research directed toward devising methods of both preventing contamination of prosthetic grafts, as well as treating established graft infections, is of great importance. An effective antibiotic-protected graft should be capable of reducing the incidence of graft contamination in the perioperative period. Furthermore, these prostheses may also be successful in reducing the chance of secondary infections following either in situ or remote reconstructions and thereby eliminating the numerous problems associated with an extra-anatomic bypass.

Experimental Design of an Antibiotic-Protected Prosthesis

The two main routes by which prosthetic grafts are believed to become infected following implantation are direct contamination and bacteremic seeding. Therefore, it follows that the clinical success of an antibiotic-protected prosthesis will largely be determined by its ability to resist infection by these mechanisms. Direct contamination is thought to occur intraoperatively either from intestinal translocation or breaks in sterile surgical technique. Theoretically, bacteremic contamination could occur at any time following implantation; however, in experimental models it has been difficult to document infectability of a healed vascular prosthesis. In one study by Malone and Moore, Dacron aortic grafts were placed in dogs and challenged with a 30-minute infusion of 1×10^7 *Staphylococcus aureus* organisms administered at sequential time intervals.[8] Three weeks following the bacteremic challenge, each group of dogs was returned to the operating room where the grafts were removed under sterile conditions. The grafts were cultured and the status of neointimal development inspected. The incidence of positive graft cultures was 100% in all grafts challenged at healing intervals of up to 2 weeks. At 1 month after implantation, the infection rate was 93%; at 3 months 57%; 4 months 75%; 5 months 38%; 6 months 15%; and at 1 year the rate was only 30%. When the data were correlated with the appearance of the pseudointima, it was most remarkable that none of the 26 grafts

with a complete lining developed a graft infection, whereas 54 of the 57 grafts (95%) with either incomplete or ulcerated pseudointimal lining became infected. Thus, it would appear that, like direct contamination, infection of a prosthetic graft by bacteremic seeding is also more likely to occur in the early perioperative period. Confusingly, the onset of clinical graft sepsis rarely occurs in the perioperative period. Goldstone and Moore reported a mean duration from operation until the onset of symptoms of 15 months.[2] This delayed onset of clinical graft infection has also been noted by other researchers.[9] Furthermore, at the time of presentation, a likely source of bacteria is rarely found. Thus, although clinically there is a long latent period before the onset of graft sepsis, it is likely that the origin of most cases of graft infection is related to contamination, which occurs at the time of graft implantation. The prosthesis is colonized early before an intimal lining is formed, but the infection remains indolent. Later, clinical graft sepsis occurs when the immune balance has been compromised.

Thus, protecting a prosthesis in the perioperative period and allowing adequate healing to occur, should reduce the incidence of subsequent graft infection. Because the experimental data suggest that complete healing of a vascular prosthesis takes several weeks, it is critical that any antibiotic-protected graft retain its antimicrobial activity for at least a similar duration. The antibiotic must therefore be delivered by a slow release system. The important components of this system are the graft itself, the bonding method, and the antibiotic agent incorporated into the prosthesis.

Selection of the Graft Material

The first reported use of synthetic vascular prostheses in humans was made in 1954.[10] Since that time, a large number of synthetic materials have been tested. Currently, several different prosthetic graft materials are available and they all differ in their biologic characteristics. The two most commonly used materials are Teflon and the synthetic textiles. Polytetrafluoroethylene (PTFE) is the most popular Teflon graft. Of the available textile grafts, Dacron has become the most widely used material due to its ease of handling and relative biocompatibility. When contrasting the various virtues of any vascular prosthesis, traditionally compared characteristics include; thrombogenicity, healing properties, and the incidence rate of secondary infection.

Several factors contribute to the overall surface thrombogenicity of a vascular graft. These include biomechanical, electrostatic, as well as hemodynamic and healing properties. To date, most data related to the thrombogenicity of a specific vascular prosthesis have been implied from the results of platelet activation and clotting factor generation studies. Using these techniques, several studies have suggested that PTFE grafts accumulate a relatively fewer number of platelets following implantation. In one study by Callow et al. indium 111 labeled platelets were infused into baboons 1 hour after the implantation of either a Dacron or a PTFE graft.[11] Following the measurement of platelet deposition by gamma imaging, it was determined that Dacron grafts accumulated greater numbers of platelets than did those made from PTFE. In a related study, Ito et al. found similar levels of platelet reactivity on Dacron prosthetic surfaces by measuring thromboxane B_2 levels along the length of the implanted grafts.[12] Ito's results also suggested that platelet activation along implanted Dacron grafts lasts as long as 1 year following their implantation. Despite this experimental data, clinical studies in humans have failed to demonstrate any difference in platelet activation among different types of graft materials.[13] Furthermore, no data linking an increase in platelet deposition or activation to the subsequent incidence of graft failure are currently available.

Ideal healing of a vascular prosthesis is a delicate balance between solid incorporation and hyperplastic fibrous growth. Some interaction between the prosthetic material and the host's immune responses is a desirable graft characteristic. This reaction is critical to the ingrowth of both neovasculature and fibrous connective tissue into the interstices of the graft. Pseudointimal healing on the luminal surface of the graft is dependent on this process, as is the incorporation of the outside of the graft to the surrounding host tissue. On the other hand, too much graft-host interaction can lead to a hyperplastic inflammatory tissue reaction and eventual graft failure due to luminal obstruction. This latter process has been termed anastomotic intimal hyperplasia because it is invariably clinically relevant only at the graft-native vessel suture line. A graft anastomosis is a highly complex region and several factors contributing to the development of intimal hyperplasia have been recognized. These include; hemodynamic parameters, compliance mismatch, platelet activation, inflammatory cell pathways, as well as the liberation of countless locally active growth and humoral factors. Cantelmo et al. compared the development of anastomotic intimal hyperplasia in carotid interposition grafts composed of either Dacron or PTFE.[14] In this study, both materials stimulated the development of intimal hyperplasia and there was no significant qualitative or quantitative difference between the two.

The final property of prosthetic materials that is frequently compared is susceptibility to infection. Once an organism comes in contact with the prosthetic graft, several steps must occur in order for colonization and subsequent graft infection to develop. First, there must be adhesion of the organism to the prosthesis. Next, there must be sufficient structural and nutritional support for microcolony formation to occur. Lastly, the infecting organisms must stimulate the activation of host defenses including the development of inflammation and the infiltration of leukocytes. Thus, it is clear that the prosthetic graft and the colonizing organism act synergistically to activate the host defense mechanisms which eventually lead to the development of a clinically significant graft infection. In an in vitro study, Sugarman has demonstrated that there is no significant difference in the adherence of *Staphylococcus* to either Dacron or PTFE prostheses.[15] Experimentally, many studies comparing graft infectability of Dacron versus PTFE have been reported in the literature. In one study by Weiss et al., no difference in the infectability of these grafts was noted in a canine perioperative bacteremic model.[16] In contrast, Moore et al. reported a significant difference in the susceptibility of healed prosthetic grafts to infection following a bacteremic challenge.[17] In this study, three different Dacron grafts were compared to two types of PTFE prostheses. The grafts were implanted into the aortas of mongrel dogs and subsequently challenged with an intravenous infusion of *S aureus* at both 3- and 6-month intervals. In the 6-month series, all three types of Dacron grafts had a lower infection rate than both PTFE grafts. Furthermore, this observed difference was associated with a more complete neointimal healing of the Dacron prostheses.

In summary, neither the Dacron nor PTFE vascular prostheses seem to demonstrate any important clinical advantage with regards to thrombogenicity. The Dacron grafts however, while not increasing the risk of intimal hyperplasia, do appear to heal with a greater degree of tissue incorporation which may reduce their susceptibility to infection. Other important properties of a vascular prosthesis being considered for antibiotic impregnation include the ability to incorporate a bonding agent, as well as ease of technical handling following drug incorporation. These requirements are also satisfied by the Dacron grafts. For these reasons, we have chosen the Dacron textile graft for our investigations into the development of a antibiotic-impregnated vascular prostheses.

Selection of a Bonding Agent

The purpose of a bonding agent is twofold. First, one of the major drawbacks of the Dacron prosthesis has been its porosity. The textile in synthetic Dacron contains large interstices that leak after implantation into the vascular system. As a result, these grafts have generally been preclotted with the patient's own blood to seal the gaps in the textile fiber and prevent large amounts of blood loss during surgery. Prior application of a bonding agent to the prosthetic surface essentially eliminates this leaking and greatly facilitates implantation of the graft. Second, the bonding agent serves as a method of temporarily attaching the antibiotic to the graft surface.

Currently, four biocompatible substances are used to seal commercially manufactured synthetic vascular grafts: bovine collagen, bovine gelatin, human albumin, and silicone. Silicone is used primarily on (PTFE) to coat dialysis catheters. Type 1 bovine collagen is a structural protein found in bone, tendons, and fascia, and is the sealant used in the Hemashield® graft produced by Meadox Medicals, Inc., (Oakland, NJ). Heating of collagen denatures the structural protein and produces a soluble derivative called gelatin. Gelatin is used as the sealant in both the Gelsoft® and Uni-Graft® prostheses. Both collagen and gelatin provide a flexible coating that effectively seals the textile graft without compromising its handling characteristics. Collagen-based preparations have been criticized, however, for their potential immunogenicity and thrombogenicity. In one randomized study, the Hemashield® graft was found to produce an antigenic response in four of 11 patients, although no patient had an adverse clinical reaction.[18] Also, collagen is known to be a potential platelet activator and has been shown to cause platelet adhesion and aggregation.[19,20] However, no increase in thrombogenicity associated with the use of a collagenated prosthesis has been demonstrated clinically. In addition, the increased reactivity surrounding these grafts may enhance their healing characteristics. Nonetheless, these concerns have led to the investigation into the use of albumin as an alternative graft sealant. Dacron grafts coated with human albumin have been produced but are currently available for investigational use only.

Experimentally, several substances have been used as bonding agents for the purpose of attaching antibiotics to vascular prostheses. These include heavy metals such as silver nitrate,[21-23] the surfactants tridodecylmethylammonium chloride (TDMAC) and benzalkonium chloride,[22-29] chemical glues such as N-butyl-2-cyanoacrylate,[30] as well as biologic proteins.[31-34] Direct bonding of an antibiotic with a heavy metal such as silver nitrate has been shown to produce a stable impregnated graft.[22] However, concerns have been raised regarding the potential of in vivo toxicity of these bonding agents. The surfactant-bonding agents are also effective and have been studied extensively. These compounds are positively charged substances that can easily be absorbed onto a prosthetic surface. The coated graft then serves as a cationic anchor for the binding of any negatively charged antibiotic. A theoretical concern regarding this system is the potential thrombogenic effect of the implanted graft. Once the ionically bound antibiotic elutes away from the graft, the positively charged coating remains and may serve to activate circulating clotting mechanisms. Finally, like heavy metals, chemical glues are highly toxic compounds and further research is needed before their use in humans can be considered safe. Therefore, we have focused on the use of biologic proteins as a method of impregnating vascular grafts with antimicrobial agents.

The use of collagen as a bonding agent in an antibiotic delivery system was first reported by Krajicek et al. in 1969.[35] Since that time our laboratory has accumulated considerable experience with this technique. Currently, our protocol involves preparing a solution of type 1 collagen that is layered onto a knitted double-velour Dacron graft and then minimally cross-linked with formalin vapor. The grafts are then aerated and dried prior to implantation. When impregnating the prosthesis with antibiotics, the antimicrobial agent is mixed into the collagen slurry prior to its application onto the graft.

Among our first experiments using this new prosthesis was a study designed to determine whether or not there was any adverse effect of collagen impregnation with respect to healing.[36] Forty-five dogs had their infrarenal abdominal aortas resected. Thirty had vascular continuity restored by the implantation of 6-cm collagen-impregnated double-velour grafts placed in a double end-to-end fashion. Fifteen had their vascular continuity restored using 6-cm double-velour Dacron grafts without collagen impregnation. The dogs were then allowed to return to normal kennel activity. At 3, 6, and 9 months following implantation, 10 dogs with experimental grafts and five dogs with control grafts were selected for harvest. The experimental and control grafts were compared with regard to gross appearance and retroperitoneal response to healing, as well as the microscopic healing response with sections taken at the proximal, middle, and distal portion of the grafts. Observers were blinded with regard to the evaluation of the experimental versus control prostheses. A grading system was established with respect to neointimal healing, fibroblastic infiltration, and perigraft capsular thickness and bonding. Using this evaluation, there was absolutely no difference between the healing response of the collagen-impregnated graft when compared to control prostheses.

Selection of an Antibiotic Agent

When choosing an antimicrobial agent for incorporation into a vascular prosthesis, several properties are important to consider. First, the drug selected must be sensitive to the known spectrum of organisms that are commonly encountered in vascular graft infections. These include *S aureus*, *Staphylococcus epidermidis*, *Streptococcus* species, as well as Gram-negative bacteria including *Escherichia coli*, *Pseudomonas aeruginosa*, and others.[2,3,5] Second, the agent should be easily incorporated by the bonding compound and not lose any appreciable antimicrobial activity during this process. Third, the relationship between the antibiotic's chemical affinity for the bonding agents and its aqueous solubility in the surrounding tissue must be favorable. This is important so that the incorporated drug elutes from the graft slowly, providing a prolonged duration of local antimicrobial activity. Fourth, the selected agent should have a low antigenic potential and minimal associated toxicity. Lastly, the antibiotic must be stable and not altered by commonly used graft sterilization techniques including gas treatments and γ-radiation.

As mentioned, many different antibiotics have been incorporated into vascular grafts using a variety of bonding agents and resulting in varying success. Many of these investigations are summarized in Table 1. In our laboratory, we have tested the efficacy of combining several antibiotics with a Dacron graft using a collagen-bonded release system. In this system, the antibiotic is first mixed with the collagen solution and then layered onto an otherwise untreated prosthesis. After minimally cross-linking the collagen-antibiotic coating with formalin vapor, the antibiotic becomes trapped within the interstices of the collagen protein fibers and is nearly completely retained even following aqueous soaking. After implantation of the treated graft into the host circulation, the biodegradable collagen is gradually degraded by host-enzymatic systems which thus slowly release the antibiotic into the surrounding tissues. Theoretically, this process provides high tissue levels of antibiotic activity for a prolonged interval.

To test the hypothesis that collagen-antibiotic release system would indeed provide prolonged antimicrobial activity, and to compare several possible antibiotics that were considered for incorporation into our antibiotic-impregnated prosthesis, an in vitro elution system was developed. Two-hundred and fifty milliliters of 5% albumin was placed in a flask. Graft samples, 6 mm in diameter were dropped into the flask and placed on continued agitation. The fluid in the flask was totally removed and replaced every 24 hours. Two graft disk samples were removed from the flask each day and placed on a blood agar plate infected with *S aureus*. The zones of inhibition found on each plate were measured and recorded daily. Samples were studied until no bacteriostatic effect was noted. Using this system, two sets of experiments were carried out.

The first experiment used amikacin as the antibiotic and adjusted the cross-linking of the collagen release system in three different ways: 1) three coats of collagen, uncross-linked; 2) three coats of 1.5% collagen cross-linked with hexamethyline diisocyanate; and 3) three coats of collagen cross-linked with formaldehyde. Control grafts consisted of the three processes without amikacin. The results demonstrated that the control grafts showed no bacteriostatic activity at time zero. The experimental grafts each maintained a zone of inhibition averaging approximately 5 sq cm, but for 2 days only. This experiment was repeated using a lightly formalin cross-linked collagen graft to bond the amikacin. The average maximal initial zone of inhibition was 5.75 sq cm, but again all activity was totally gone after 48 hours. Because it appeared that the soluble nature of amikacin accelerated its removal from the prosthesis in this model, we decided to change our antibiotic to rifampicin, which is known to be a water insoluble agent.

In the next experiment, amikacin, chloramphenicol, and rifampicin were bonded to double-velour Dacron grafts with minimally cross-linked type 1 collagen.[34] A fourth experiment in which a graft without collagen was preclotted with blood mixed with rifampicin was also tested. Each graft was tested at daily intervals in our bioassay for antistaphylococcal activity after continuous elution in the in vitro agitation system. The results demonstrated that the collagen-bonded graft impregnated with rifampicin was superior to either amikacin or chloramphenicol and had an overall duration of activity of 22 days. In addition, rifampicin alone without collagen, although not as effective as the collagen-bonded rifampicin graft, was superior to both amikacin and chloramphenicol when mixed with blood and used to preclot the grafts. This finding confirms the results reported by Powell et al., in which grafts demonstrated prolonged antimicrobial activity after being preclotted with blood containing rifampicin.[37] The superiority of rifampicin in models incorporating an antibiotic onto a vascular prosthesis is likely related to its relatively low solubility in aqueous solutions.

To summarize, using a series of in vitro experiments, it appears that a Dacron graft treated with the combination of rifampicin antibiotic and minimally cross-linked collagen provides the longest duration of antimicrobial activity.

In Vivo Results Using a Collagen-Rifampicin-Impregnated Graft

Having determined the most effective combination of bonding material and antibiotic agent in vitro, the next step in the development of the antibiotic-impregnated graft was to establish its efficacy in vivo.

The first experiment was designed to test the resistance of the rifampicin-impregnated collagen graft to a bacteremic challenge as a function of time following implantation.[38] Our model used the rifampicin-protected graft in a previously established canine graft sepsis model. Fifty

6-mm Dacron grafts, impregnated with either collagen (control) or collagen plus rifampicin (experimental), were implanted end-to-end into the infrarenal aorta. The retroperitoneum and abdominal wall were closed in layers and the animals allowed to recover. The dogs were then divided into four groups; each with an experimental and control arm. At 2, 7, 10, or 12 days after graft implantation, sequential groups were challenged with 1.2×10^8 organisms of *S aureus* intravenously. Three weeks after this hematogenous seeding, the grafts were harvested under sterile conditions. Control and experimental grafts were compared by evaluating patency and culture-proven infection as a function of implantation time prior to the bacteremic challenge. Three dogs died after bacterial infusion and were excluded from further analysis. The results of this study showed that collagen-coated grafts could be infected up to 7 days after implantation (Table 2). After 7 days, it appeared that healing of the collagen graft surface interfered with delayed bacterial seeding. The experimental rifampicin-impregnated graft could not be infected when challenged up to several days after implant. At 10 days and 12 days, one graft and two grafts, respectively, had positive cultures in the experimental group. Therefore, this study indicated that a vascular prostheses, protected with rifampicin in a collagen-release system could maintain prolonged resistance to infection in a challenging bacteremic model.

Having demonstrated that the rifampicin-impregnated collagen graft was effective in resisting infection when challenged intravenously, a second experiment was designed to test whether this ability extended to a bacterial challenge by direct contamination.[39] Again, we used our previously established canine graft model with some modification. For this study, experimental antibiotic-protected grafts were implanted in situ into a previously infected aortic bed. Eighty-three adult mongrel dogs underwent implantation of a 3-cm untreated Dacron graft into the infrarenal aorta. This ini-

Table 2
Results of the Experiment Investigating the Resistance of Collagen-Rifampin-Impregnated Grafts
to a Bactermic Challenge as a Function of Time Following Implantation

	2 days Patency	Infected	7 days Patency	Infected	10 days Patency	Infected	12 days Patency	Infected
Control	6/6	4/6	6/6	5/6	6/6	2/6	4/5	1/5
Experimental	6/6	0/6	6/6	0/6	6/6	1/6	6/6	2/6
	N.S.	$P = .030$	N.S.	$P = .008$	N.S.	N.S.	N.S.	N.S.

tial graft was deliberately infected at the time of operation with 10^2 organisms of *S aureus* by direct inoculation. One week later, the dogs were reexplored, the retroperitoneum debrided, and the animals randomized to undergo an end-to-end in situ graft replacement with either one of two types of prosthetic grafts; group 1 (collagen n = 36) received control collagen-impregnated knitted Dacron grafts, and group II (rifampicin n = 47) received experimental collagen-rifampicin bonded Dacron grafts. Each group of animals was then subdivided to receive one of our treatment protocols: 1) no antibiotic therapy (no abx); 2) cephalosporin peritoneal irrigation solution (cefazolin 500 mg/1000 cc) during surgery and two doses of cephalosporin (cefazolin 500 mg I.M., B.I.D.) (1 week), and 3) perioperative plus 2 weeks of cephalosporin (cefazolin 500 mg I.M., B.I.D.) (2 weeks). All grafts were removed under sterile conditions, 4 weeks after implantation. There were no anastomotic disruptions and all

grafts were patent at the time of removal. Cultures were obtained from the grafts and perigraft tissues separately. Analysis included determination of the culture positivity of tissue and graft samples combined (T&G Cx), as well as of the graft segments alone (Graft Cx) irrespective of the results of the surrounding tissue cultures. Results were expressed as the percentage of animals which were culture-positive at sacrifice. In all four treatment groups, the reduction of positive graft cultures (Graft C) following in situ replacement of a previously infected aortic prosthesis with a collagen-rifampicin bonded graft, was statistically significant (Table 3). When overall infection rates (T & G Cx) were evaluated, this reduction was statistically significant only in the subset of animals treated with 2 weeks of supplemental antibiotics. In conclusion, it appears that the collagen-rifampicin bonded graft reduces the incidence of graft colonization following in situ replacement of an infected graft. However, a course of supplemental

Table 3
Results of the Experiment Investigating the Ability of Collagen-Rifampin-Impregnated Grafts to
Resist Infection Following In Situ Replacement of a Previously Infected Prosthesis

	No Abx			Periop			1 Wk			2 Wks		
	n	T&G Cx	Graft Cx	n	T&G Cx	Graft Cx	n	T&G Cx	Graft Cx	n	T&G Cx	Graft Cx
Collagen	5	100	100	16	87.5	87.5	5	100	100	10	80	80
Rifampin	16	62.5	50	16	62.5	50	5	60	20	10	20	20
p Value		N.S.	< 0.05		N.S.	< 0.05		N.S.	< 0.05		< 0.02	< 0.02

T&G Cx = tissue and graft combined.

antibiotics is required to sterilize the surrounding perigraft tissues.

In summary, the available experimental evidence clearly suggests that a Dacron vascular prosthesis impregnated with rifampicin using a collagen release system is effective in resisting contamination in a canine model. Also, results following an in situ reconstruction using this graft have been encouraging. Whether these laboratory data will translate into any clinical benefit must await the completion of properly performed randomized controlled clinical trials.

Future Directions

One potential weakness in the design of the collagen-rifampicin impregnated prosthesis is the failure of the graft to retain any significant antimicrobial activity after 3 weeks. This property suggests that, although protected in the immediate perioperative period, these grafts remain susceptible to late bacteremic challenges. Thus, one logical future modification of any antibiotic-protected prosthesis would be the ability to prolong the duration of antimicrobial activity. Possible ways to achieve this goal include: 1) alteration of the properties of the bonding agent; and 2) development of methods to reload the graft with antibiotics.

Currently, the use of type 1 collagen as a bonding agent has several advantages. These include its nontoxicity, ease of handling following impregnation, as well as its biodegradability which allows for the steady release of the antimicrobial agent following implantation. Unfortunately, this degradation is complete within 1 month after which no antimicrobial activity remains in the graft. Therefore, if a more stable collagenlike polymer could be developed, which was capable of delivering high doses of antibiotics for a much longer duration of time, this would represent a major advance in this area of research.

The ability to reload the graft with sub-sequent doses of an antimicrobial agent is an intriguing idea. Theoretically, this would also allow for prolonged protection of the graft. One possibility is the union of the sciences of immunology and antimicrobial therapy. Conceptually, this would require the development of an antigen-specific prosthetic graft coating material. This coating material should be separate from the bonding agent and stable from all biodegradation. Next, a monoclonal antibody-bound antibiotic could be given any time following graft implantation. This could be used clinically, either to extend prophylactic prosthetic protection or as therapy for an already established graft infection. Furthermore, if the infecting organism is known, the type of antibiotic bound to the monoclonal antibody could be changed accordingly. This would allow for the administration of high doses of organism-specific antibiotic therapy to be delivered directly to the infected graft. Unfortunately, the development of such a system is in its earliest stages only. However, as we enter the 21st century, the possibilities of this line of research represents an exciting new area of investigation.

References

1. Szilagyi DE, Smith RF, Elliott JP, Vrandecic MP. Infection in arterial reconstruction with synthetic grafts. *Ann Surg.* 1972;176:321–323.
2. Goldstone J, Moore WS. Infection in vascular prostheses: clinical manifestations and surgical management. *Am J Surg.* 1974;128: 225–233.
3. Bunt TJ. Synthetic vascular graft infections I: graft infections. *Surgery.* 1983;93:6:733–746.
4. Lorentzen JE, Nielsen OM, Arendrup H. Vascular graft infection: an analysis of sixty-two graft infections in 2411 consecutively implanted synthetic vascular grafts. *Surgery.* 1985;98:81–86.
5. Liekweg WG, Greenfield LJ. Vascular prosthetic infections: collected experience and results of treatment. *Surgery.* 1977;81:3: 335–342.
6. O'Harra PJ, Hertzer NR, Beven EG, Krajewski LP. Surgical management of infected ab-

dominal aortic grafts: review of a 25 year experience. *J Vasc Surg.* 1986;3:725–731.

7. Quinones-Baldrich WJ, Hernandez JJ, Moore WS. Long-term results following surgical management of aortic graft infection. *Arch Surg.* 1991;126:507–511.

8. Malone JM, Moore WS, Campagna G, Bean B. Bacteremic infectability of vascular grafts: the influence of pseudointimal integrity and duration of graft infections. *Surgery.* 1975;78:211–216.

9. Fry WJ, Lindenauer SM. Infection complicating the use of plastic arterial implants. *Arch Surg.* 1967;94:600–609.

10. Blakemore AH, Voorhees AB. The use of tubes constructed from vinyon "N" cloth in bridging arterial defects: experimental and clinical. *Ann Surg.* 1954;140:324–334.

11. Callow AD, Connolly R, O'Donnell TF, et al. Platelet-arterial synthetic graft interaction and its modification. *Arch Surg.* 1982;117:1447–1455.

12. Ito RK, Rosenblatt MS, Contreras MA, Brophy CM, LoGerfo FW. Monitoring platelet interactions with prosthetic graft implants in a canine model. *ASAIO Transactions.* 1990;36:M175–M178.

13. Wakefield TW, Shulkin BL, Fellows EP, Petry NA, Spaulding SA, Stanley JC. Platelet reactivity in human aortic grafts: a prospective, randomized midterm study of platelet adherence and release products in Dacron and polytetrafluoroethylene conduits. *J Vasc Surg.* 1989;9:234–243.

14. Cantelmo NL, Quist WC, LoGerfo FW. Quantitative analysis of anastomotic intimal hyperplasia in paired Dacron and PTFE grafts. *J Cardiovasc Surg.* 1989;30:910–915.

15. Sugarman B. In vitro adherence of bacterial to prosthetic vascular grafts. *Infection.* 1982;10:2–12.

16. Weiss JP, Lorenzo FV, Campbell CD, Myerowitz RL, Webster MW. The behavior of infected arterial prostheses of expanded polytetrafluoroethylene (Gore-Tex). *J Thor Cardiovasc Surg.* 1977;73:4:630–636.

17. Moore WS, Malone JM, Keown K. Prosthetic arterial graft material: influence on neointimal healing and bacteremic infectibility. *Arch Surg.* 1980;115:1379–1383.

18. Norgren L, Holtas S, Parsson G, Ribbe E, Saxne T, Thorne J. Immune response to collagen impregnated Dacron double velour grafts for aortic and aortofemoral reconstructions. *Eur J Vasc Surg.* 1990;4:379–384.

19. Baumgartner HR. Morphometric quantitation of adherence of platelets to an artificial surface and components of connective tissue. In: Didisheim P, ed. *Platelets, Thrombosis and Inhibitors.* Stuttgart: Schattauer Verlag; 1973;38–49.

20. Mason RG, Read MS. Some effects of a microcrystalline collagen preparation of blood. *Haemostasis.* 1974;3:31–45.

21. Benvenisty A, Tannenbaum G, Ahlborn TN, et al. Control of prosthetic bacterial infection: evaluation of an easily incorporated, tightly bound, silver antibiotic PTFE graft. *J Surg Res.* 1986;44:1–7.

22. Modak SM, Sampath L, Fox CL, Benvenisty A, Nowygrod R, Reemstmau K. A new method for the direct incorporation of antibiotic in prosthetic vascular grafts. *Surg Gynecol Obstet.* 1987;164:143–147.

23. Kinney EV, Bandyk DF, Seabrook GA, Kelly HM, Town JB. Antibiotic-bonded PTFE vascular grafts: the effect of silver antibiotic on bioactivity following implantation. *J Surg Res.* 1991;50:430–435.

24. Prahlad A, Harvey RA, Greco RS. Diffusion of antibiotics from a polytetrafluoroethylene-benzalkonium surface. *Am Surg.* 1981;47:515–518.

25. Henry R, Harvey RA, Greco RS. Antibiotic bonding to vascular prostheses. *J Thorac Cardiovasc Surg.* 1981;82:272–277.

26. Greco RS, Harvey RA, Smilow PC, Tesoriero JV. Prevention of vascular prosthetic infection by a benzalkonium-oxacillin bonded polytetrafluoroethylene graft. *Surg Gynecol Obstet* 1982;155:28–32.

27. Greco RS, Harvey RA. The biochemical bonding of cefoxitin to a microporous polytetrafluoroethylene surface. *J Surg Res.* 1984;36:237–243.

28. Harvey RA, Alcid DV, Greco RS. Antibiotic bonding to polytetrafluoroethylene with tridodecylmethylammonium chloride. *Surgery.* 1982;92:3:504–512.

29. Shue WB, Worosilo SC, Donetz AP, Trooskin SZ, Harvey RA, Greco RS. Prevention of vascular prosthetic infection with an antibiotic-bonded Dacron graft. *J Vasc Surg.* 1988;8:600–605:

30. Shenk JS, Ney AL, Tsukayama DT, Olson ME, Bubrick MP. Tobramycin-adhesive in preventing and treating PTFE vascular graft infections. *J Surg Res.* 1989;47:4387–4492.

31. Sobinsky KR, Flanigan DP. Antibiotic binding to polytetrafluoroethylene via glucosaminoglycan-keratin luminal coating. *Surgery.* 1986;100:4:629–634.

32. Ney AL, Kelly PH, Tsukayama DT, Bubrick MP. Fibrin glue-antibiotic suspension in the prevention of prosthetic graft infection. *J Trauma.* 1990;30:8:1000–1006.

33. Moore WS, Chvapil M. Sieffert G, Keown K. Development of an infection resistant vascular prosthesis. *Arch Surg.* 1981;116: 1403–1407.

34. Chervu A, Moore WS, Chvapil M, Henderson T. Efficacy and duration of antistaphylococcal activity comparing three antibiotics bonded to Dacron vascular grafts with a collagen release system. *J Vasc Surg.* 1991;13: 897–901.

35. Krajicek M, Dvorak J, Chvapil M. Infection-resistant synthetic vascular substitutes. *J Cardiovasc Surg.* 1969;10:454.

36. Quinones-Baldrich WJ, Moore WS, Ziomek S, Chvapil M. Development of a "leak-proof" knitted Dacron vascular prosthesis. *J Vasc Surg.* 1986;3:6:895–903.

37. Powell TW, Burnham SJ, Johnson G. A passive system using rifampin to create an infection-resistant vascular prosthesis. *Surgery.* 1983;94:5:765–769.

38. Chervu A, Moore WS, Gelabert HA, Colburn MD, Chvapil M. Prevention of graft infection by use of prostheses bonded with a rifampin/collagen release system. *J Vasc Surg.* 1991;14:4:521–525.

39. Colburn MD, Moore WS, Gelabert HA, Chvapil M, Quinones-Baldrich WJ. Use of an antibiotic-bonded graft for in situ reconstruction following prosthetic graft infections. *J Vasc Surg.* 1992;16:651–660.

Diagnosis

Most complications are the result of omission rather than commission. Failure to completely examine, failure to consider a complete differential diagnosis, failure to check out an abnormal test or vital signs—these all lead to failure of surgical care.

Chapter 7

Diagnosis of Vascular Graft Infections

P.F. Lawrence
R.J. Pitsch
S.W. Merrell

Introduction

Optimal treatment of vascular graft infections is predicated on the timely diagnosis of the process. Successful diagnosis depends upon a high index of clinical suspicion and aggressive workup of the problem when graft infection is suspected. The diagnosis may be fairly obvious in the case of a superficially located graft, especially in the early postoperative period, since wound complications often herald the presence of (or secondarily cause) graft infection. On the other hand, vascular graft infections that involve prosthetic material deep within the abdomen or chest pose a much more difficult diagnostic challenge. The presenting signs and symptoms tend to be vague and nonspecific. The clinical picture is often rather unimpressive, reflecting the indolent nature of many late infections that may exist in virtual symbiosis with the patient and present many months to years after graft implantation.[1-6]

In this chapter, a comprehensive review of the various modalities available for the diagnosis of vascular graft infections is presented. These include basic clinical laboratory testing, general radiologic studies, tomographic imaging, and nuclear medicine scans. The adjunctive role of gastrointestinal endoscopy, the vascular laboratory, and operative graft exploration will also be discussed. Finally, we present a practical strategy for the evaluation of possible graft infections in various clinical scenarios.

Blood Tests

Serologic tests in patients with suspected prosthetic graft infections are nonspecific and often unreliable. White blood cell counts ranged from 1400 to 13,100 in 15 afebrile patients with graft infection, reported by Bandyk.[7] The erythrocyte sedimentation rate and C reactive protein are often elevated but are also nonspecific.[8] Neither routine peripheral blood cultures nor arterial blood cultures obtained distal to the graft have proven reliable for detection of prosthetic graft infections (PGI).[9,10] Thus documentation of suspected PGIs in patients with vague, nonspecific complaints usually requires a more extensive workup involving the nuclear medicine and noninvasive imaging departments of radiology.

Direct Culture and Graft Exploration

The role of exploration and direct culture of graft material is still important in the patient with a vague symptomatic presentation if clinical suspicion remains high. Direct exploration of the graft may identify signs of infection such as purulent fluid or exudate surrounding the graft, a perigraft capsule, or lack of graft incorporation.[11] These findings will confirm the diagnosis of graft infection, even when less invasive tests have been negative (Fig. 1). Lack of graft incorporation is the sine qua non confirming graft infection. Routine cultures of perigraft fluid should be obtained. If the graft is excised, part of the graft should be sent for ultrasonification. The yield of positive graft cultures after ultrasonification is significantly higher compared to routine cultures because ultrasonification disrupts the surface biofilm.[7] Generally, direct exploration is performed in cases where suspicion of PGI remains high despite a negative noninvasive workup. If PGI has been confirmed by previous studies, exploration of the noninfected graft area may be performed to confirm noninvolvement of a graft segment as part of a staged bypass and partial excision procedure.

General Radiology

Plain Radiographs, Sinograms, and Enteral Contrast Studies

Plain radiographs are rarely helpful in the evaluation of vascular graft infections. On the other hand, they may be obtained early in the course of evaluating a patient with nonspecific abdominal complaints who is later found to have a graft infection. In most cases, films are normal or show a paralytic ileus, which may be a response to retroperitoneal infection. The identification of intragraft air is pathognomonic for a graft infection, but this is a rare finding.[12]

Some authors feel that contrast sinography should be done routinely when draining sinuses are present in the vicinity of a vascular graft (Fig. 2). Sinus tract communication with the vascular graft or with adjacent bowel is presumptive evidence of infection.[9,10,13–16] If the entire graft is outlined by contrast material, one may reliably conclude that there is paninfection of the graft.

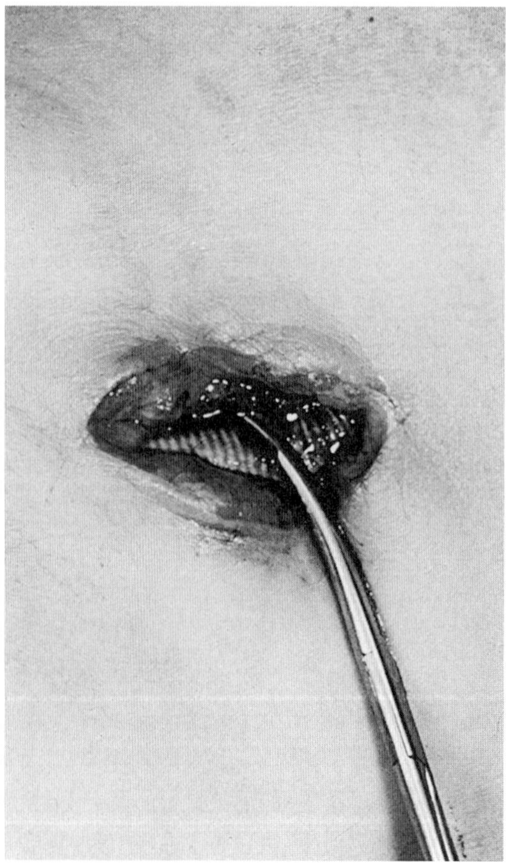

Figure 1. Direct exploration identifies an unincorporated graft.

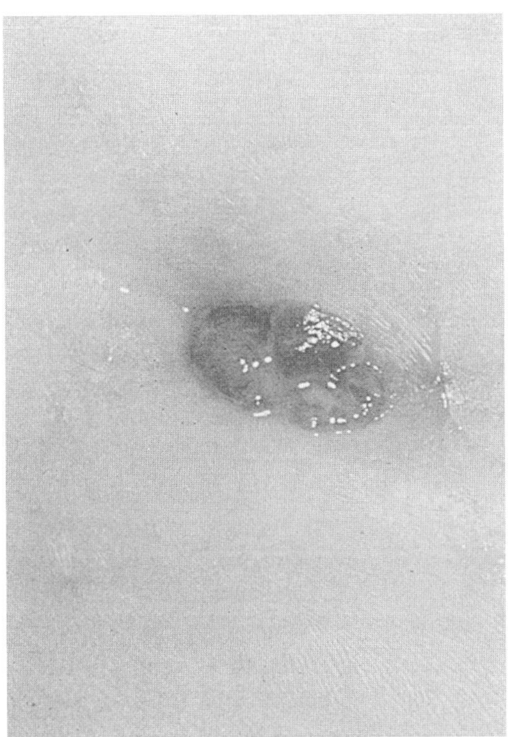

Figure 2. Draining groin sinus overlying a femoral anastomosis of an aortobifemoral graft.

However, the accuracy of determining the extent of infection is not known when only a portion of the graft is visualized, since the experience with sinograms has been anecdotal (Fig. 3). Sinogram procedures may induce bleeding, bacteremia, or an extension of local bacterial contamination. Due to these potential complications and the lack of proven diagnostic accuracy, we do not recommend contrast sinography in the routine workup of vascular graft infections.

Enteral contrast studies are obtained occasionally to work up cases of gastrointestinal bleeding. However, as Reilly and associates showed in a previous study,[17] gastrointestinal bleeding is more often a result of the stress response to a graft infection rather than related to a graft-enteric erosion or graft-enteric fistula. Further, enteral contrast studies rarely show direct evidence of a graft-enteric fistula or graft-enteric ero-

sion. Finally, the standard evaluation of patients who present with gastrointestinal bleeding has shifted to reliance upon endoscopy rather than contrast studies. The presence of barium within the gastrointestinal tract may interfere with the interpretation of subsequent computed tomography scans or arteriography. Due to all of these considerations, enteral contrast studies are rarely indicated in the workup of vascular graft infections.

Ultrasonography

There have been several reports which have documented the usefulness of ultrasound in the evaluation of vascular grafts.[9,13,18–20] Duplex scanning has improved the ability to diagnose graft patency and adjacent pathology, such as perigraft fluid collections and pseudoaneurysms.[21,22]

The benefits of ultrasound include the lack of radiation exposure and the portability of equipment, which allows bedside evaluation of patients.[20,22] Although ultrasound equipment is available in most hospitals, the major disadvantage of ultrasound is the variability in the quality of the study due to variable technical skills. Abdominal ultrasound images are often technically inadequate in the early postoperative period due to excessive bowel gas, limiting their usefulness for evaluation of aortic grafts.[20,23] Due to all of these considerations, ultrasonography has been largely supplanted by other imaging techniques, such as computed tomography (CT) or magnetic resonance imaging (MRI), both of which provide better anatomic detail and specificity for diagnosis of graft infections. In current practice, ultrasound studies are mainly used to evaluate grafts in superficial locations and perigraft masses or suspected graft occlusion. The finding of an anastomotic pseudoaneurysm, particularly if there is a fluid collection around the graft or pseudoaneurysm, is the most typical finding associated with graft infection.[20,24]

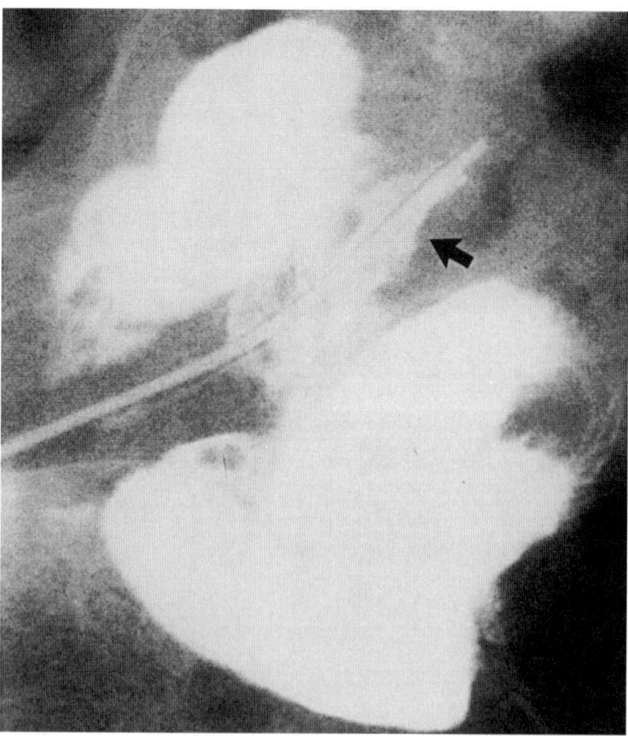

Figure 3. A sinogram demonstrates a catheter passed through a groin sinus and up alongside the femoral limb of an aortobifemoral graft. Contrast is seen along side the graft limb (arrow), and passes via an enteric fistula into several loops of adjacent small bowel.

Computed Tomography

Computed tomography has been widely used for patients with suspected graft infections, especially for retroperitoneal grafts.[9,13,23,25–32] The characteristic appearance of a graft infection with computed tomography includes abnormal collections of fluid or air around the graft, as originally described by Haaga, et al.[25] However, in the early postoperative period, these characteristics may be present in the absence of infection.[25,33,34] Air around the graft is common in the first week after implantation, but the presence of air beyond that time implies the presence of infection with a gas-forming organism or communication with the lumen of an adjacent hollow viscus (Fig. 4).[33,34] Perigraft fluid collection is also frequently seen in the early postoperative period, but gradually diminishes over time. In one series, 5% of patients without graft infection had persistent fluid collections around their abdominal aortic grafts at a mean of 102 days postoperatively.[34] Fluid collections were even more common in the femoral position at that late interval (Fig. 5). However, the lack of perigraft fluid or air is very useful for the exclusion of graft infection.[29] If a fluid collection is demonstrated in close proximity to a graft, serial examinations that show progressive resolution of the process are evidence against infection. Finally, early postoperative diagnosis with CT scanning may be enhanced by performing a needle aspiration of perigraft fluid collections, with Gram stain and culture of the specimen (Fig. 6).[31,35]

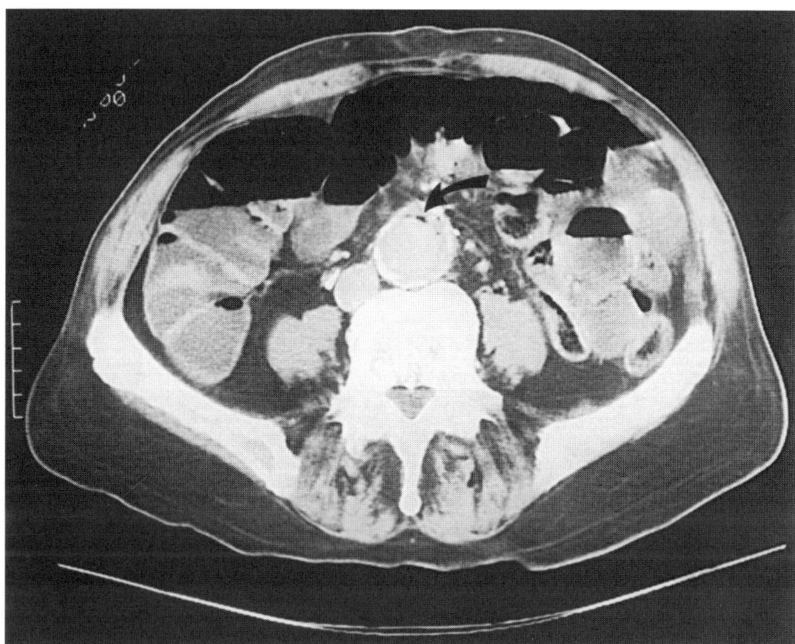

Figure 4. Computed tomography scan reveals air (arrow) around the proximal aspect of an infected aortic graft.

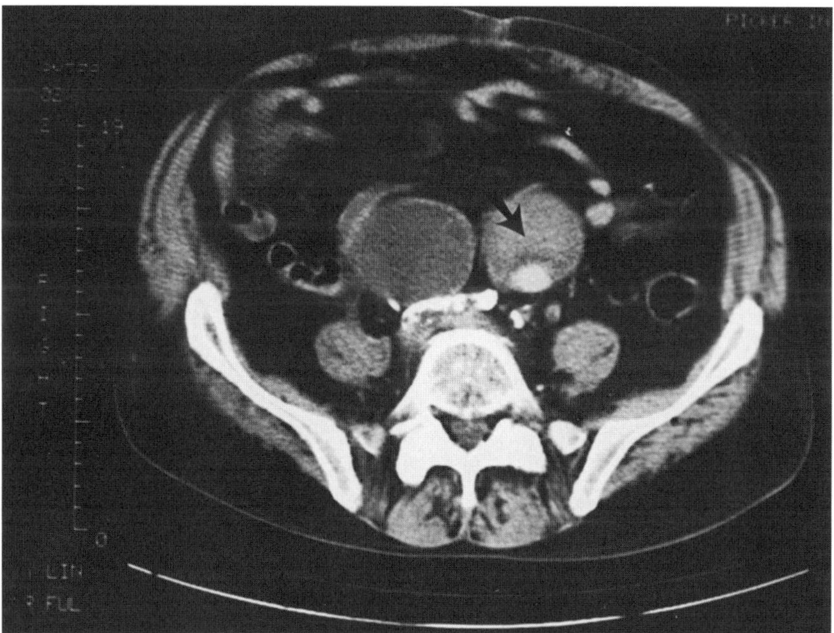

Figure 5. Computed tomography scan demonstrates perigraft fluid around the femoral limbs of an aortobifemoral graft. Note pseudoaneurysm in left limb suggested by the enhancement with I.V. contrast (arrow).

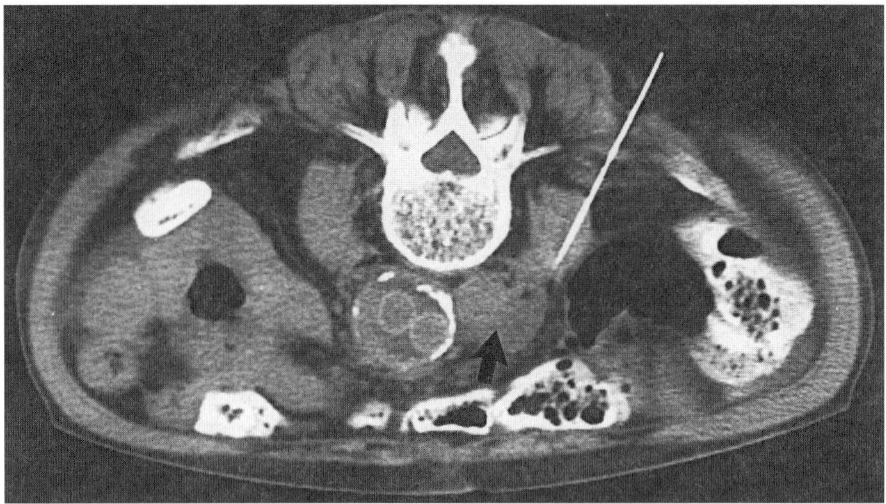

Figure 6. Computed tomography guided-needle aspiration of a perigraft fluid collection (arrow), provides fluid for Gram stain and culture in a prone patient.

Computed tomography is clearly most useful in the diagnosis of late vascular graft infections. In addition to the classic findings associated with graft infection, CT scanning may also demonstrate graft occlusion, pseudoaneurysm, or intra-abdominal processes which may provide an alternative explanation for the patient's septic presentation. Computed tomography is now widely available in most community hospitals, and is preferred by some researchers as the best single test for evaluation of graft infection.[36]

Magnetic Resonance Imaging

The first study using MRI for the diagnosis of vascular graft infections was published in 1985 by Justich et al.[37] The major diagnostic criteria for infection are similar to those used in CT exams: inflammation of adjacent soft tissues or the presence of perigraft fluid collections. Studies of noninfected vascular grafts in the postoperative period have yielded results similar to CT studies: perivascular fluid collections are present in 90% to 100% of cases early on,[38,39] but this finding resolved in 77% by 8 to 12

weeks and 100% of cases by 24 weeks. The appearance of a collar of low-signal intensity in T_1-, and T_2-weighted images around the graft is believed to correlate with graft incorporation, essentially excluding the presence of graft infection. The accuracy of MRI for detection of graft infection has been as high as 94% in published series. When compared to CT scanning in small numbers of patients, the sensitivity of MRI has been superior, which probably relates to improved resolution of tissue-fluid interfaces.[23,40–42]

The major advantage of MRI is the ability to reconstruct images in multiple planes to accurately delineate the extent of infection.[37] A black *flow-void* represents flowing blood on the MR image, so administration of intravenous contrast is not required for the performance of MRI scans.[37] One disadvantage of MRI scanning is the lack of differentiation between air and calcium in the native vessel wall.[41] This finding is one of the most useful and specific criteria for infection in computed tomography scans.[25]

Data suggest that MRI is an excellent method for the diagnosis of graft infections, but the published experience with MRI is much more limited than CT in this setting. Guided-needle aspirations of perigraft fluid are cumbersome with MRI, the scans take more time, generally are more expensive, and are not as widely available as CT. For all of these reasons, CT is the study of choice for the evaluation of abdominal vascular grafts in most institutions.

Angiography

Angiographic findings that have been associated with graft infection include anastomotic false aneurysms and graft occlusion, but these findings are nonspecific and insensitive for establishing the diagnosis. In rare cases where other studies are normal and the clinical suspicion for graft infection is strong, demonstration of a pseudoaneurysm by angiography may provide enough evidence to justify surgical exploration.[13,14,16,43,44]

Angiography is most useful in planning surgical therapy and should be obtained in all cases when the patient is stable and the diagnosis of infection is already established.[9,14,23,45,46] It is important to document the status of proximal and distal vessels, since initial revascularization followed by staged removal of infected grafts is often the best surgical strategy for managing these patients.[9,43,46]

Gastrointestinal Endoscopy

Gastrointestinal bleeding is fairly common in patients following aortic surgery, occurring in up to 21% of patients.[47] Graft-enteric fistulae (GEF) are much less common, comprising only 1% of those patients with gastrointestinal blood loss. Furthermore, as many as 39% of patients with graft-enteric fistula or graft-enteric erosion (GEE) present with no clinical history of significant gastrointestinal bleeding. These figures notwithstanding, the vast majority of graft-enteric fistulae or erosions occur in the dis-

tal duodenum, and are accessible to direct visualization by endoscopy.[15–17]

Due to the extremely high mortality related to late diagnosis of a graft-enteric fistula, expeditious endoscopic evaluation should be undertaken in any patient with an aortic vascular prosthesis who presents with gastrointestinal bleeding. The examination should include a concerted effort to evaluate the distal duodenum. The presence of a graft-enteric fistula may be indicated by ulcerations or adherent thrombus on the posterior aspect of the distal duodenum, active hemorrhage, a pulsatile posterior mass, or direct visualization of graft material within the lumen.[16,48] Endoscopy may induce severe hemorrhage from graft-enteric fistulae. For this reason, the procedure should be performed with cross-matched blood available and a surgeon on standby when there is clinical suspicion for a graft-related fistula. Some authors advocate performance of the endoscopic procedure in the operating room. In addition, when adherent thrombus is identified in the typical location (posterior aspect, fourth portion of the duodenum), no attempt should be made to remove it in order to visualize the underlying pathology.[49,50]

Alternative sources of hemorrhage, such as gastritis or peptic ulceration, must be excluded simultaneously. Reilly, et al. showed that such findings are frequently present in patients who have infected vascular grafts without fistula or erosion formation.[17] This association presumably reflects the stress response to the graft infection.

Nuclear Medicine Studies

Indium 111 Labeled Leukocyte Scans

Indium 111 labeled leukocyte scans require less than a 50 cc specimen of the patient's blood. The white blood cells are separated, labeled with indium 111 and reinjected into the patient prior to scanning. Because indium 111 binds to all cell types indiscriminately, it is necessary to separate leukocytes from the remainder of the whole blood prior to labeling. Mixed cell preparations are obtained by gravity sedimentation of blood, and contain leukocytes, erythrocytes, and platelets. Centrifugation is then performed to reduce the number of platelets contaminating the leukocytes and to reduce the amount of plasma in the buffy coat, because plasma transferrin has a high affinity for indium 111. The indium 111 is mixed with oxine, a lipophilic ligand which chelates indium 111. The leukocytes are then incubated with indium 111 oxine. During incubation, Indium 111 oxine enters the leukocytes where indium 111 bonds intracellularly. Oxine and excess indium 111 oxine is then washed out of the labeled leukocyte preparation. The indium 111 labeled leukocytes are then reinjected intravenously into the patient. Serial scans can be performed starting as early as 30 minutes after injection, and then at 4 hours; however, many institutions do not image for 24 hours.[51–54]

In 1977 Thakur described a technique for indium labeled leukocyte scanning. Subsequently, Stevick and Fawlett reported detection of an aortoarterial graft infection in 1981 and Serota documented that radiolabeled leukocyte scans were both sensitive and specific in identifying PGI in animals.[55–57] Lawrence reported on 31 scans in 21 patients with possible prosthetic graft infections in 1985 (Figs. 7,8). These studies were 86% sensitive and 100% specific.[58] Similar results were found by Williamson reporting 100% sensitivity, and 88% specificity. Williamson also correlated 11 out of 21 cases with CT scans. The sensitivity of CT scans was 75% and the specificity 100% in the same patients, using the presence of perigraft fluid, gas, or soft tissue mass as the CT criterion.[59]

Indium labeled leukocyte scans are the

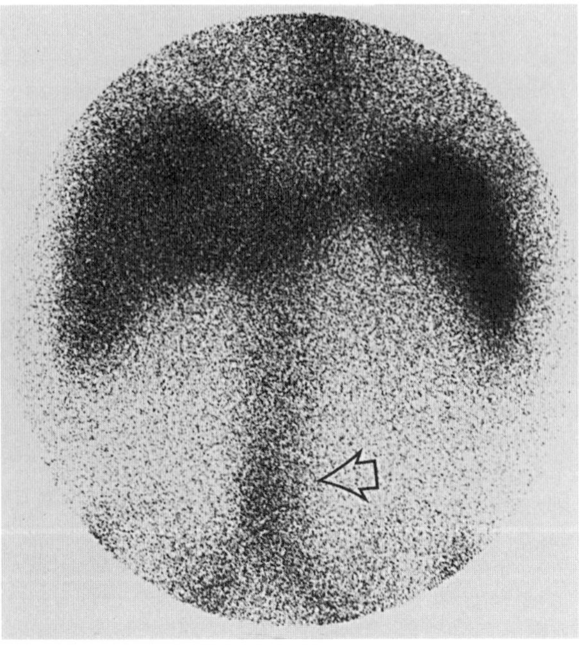

Figure 7. Indium 111 WBC scan demonstrates normal uptake in the liver, spleen, and bone. Area of abnormal focal uptake identifies an infected proximal anastamosis of an aortic graft (arrow).

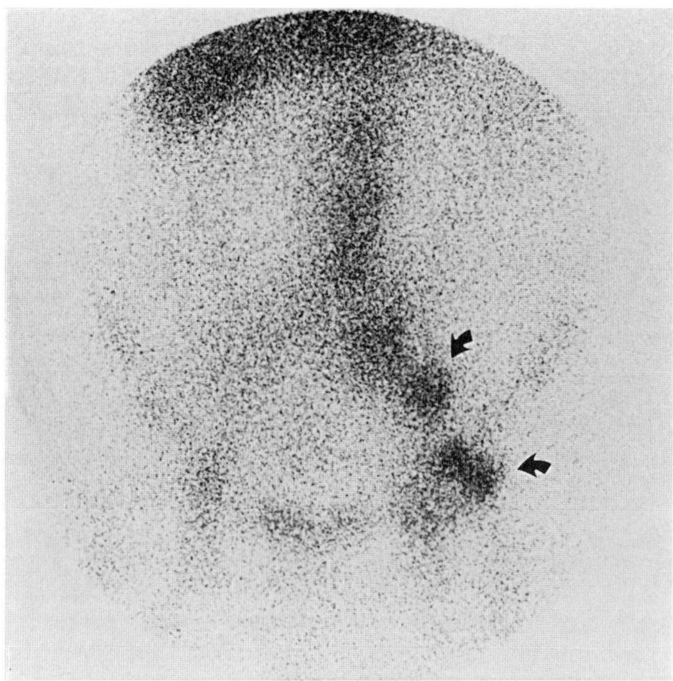

Figure 8. Indium 111 WBC scan demonstrates an intense focal area of uptake in the left limb (arrows), and a mild area of uptake in the right limb of an aortobifemoral graft. Exploration revealed lack of incorporation and purulent fluid associated with the left graft limb.

most commonly used nuclear medicine study for graft infection in clinical medicine as it is practiced currently. Advantages of indium labeled leukocyte scans include preservation of labeled PMN function, ability to detect infection 4 to 24 hours after injection of labeled cells, minimal nonspecific bowel uptake, higher target to background ratio than Gallium 67 scans, greater specificity for abscesses than Gallium 67, and widespread experience.[60]

False-positive scans can occur for many reasons. Platelets and RBCs are found in the white cell pellets after centrifugation and, like leukocytes, erythrocytes and platelets bind indium. After reinjection of the labeled cells, platelets may accumulate on the inner surface of the graft, causing a false-positive scan. In animal studies Dries reported 100% specificity, detecting no false positives in early scans.[61] However, Sedwitz reported a clinical series of 30 patients studied before and after discharge from the hospital following prosthetic vascular graft placement. False-positive early scans occurred in 53% of patients prior to discharge. Abnormal indium 111 white blood cell (WBC) scans were more common after graft placement in the groin region but were unusual after placement of grafts confined to the abdomen. Sedwitz concluded that the indium 111 labeled WBC scan has low specificity in the early postoperative period, although the technique of leukocyte preparation may have caused contamination with a large number of platelets.[62]

Other authors have proposed the use of purified leukocyte preparations to minimize platelet contamination and improve specificity. Using discontinuous density gradient centrifugation, Becker lowered the red cell contamination by a thousandfold and the platelet contamination by tenfold. With a more purified granulocyte preparation, the blood pool is still visible at 20 minutes but not on 4-hour and 24-hour scans. Theoretically, purified granulocytes should improve specificity; using pure granulocyte preparations, any vascular uptake is pathologic.[51] Reilly reported no false positives in early postoperative scanning on nine control patients using purified WBC preparations. The only false positive occurred in a patient with an inflammatory aneurysm.[63] This contrasts with a 53% positive early scan rate in the Sedwitz series.[62] Discontinuous density gradient centrifugation decreases inadvertent labeling of platelets and appears to improve the reliability of indium 111 scans in the early postoperative period; however, at this time it usually is not clinically available.

False positives may also be caused by hematomas, accessory spleens, bowel, bladder, lung in cystic fibrosis, pseudoaneurysms, inflammatory aneurysms, primary and secondary neoplasms, lymphoceles, and graft thrombosis.[64,65]

False-negative scans with indium 111 labeled WBC scans are rare. The sensitivity of indium 111 labeled WBC scans has been questioned in patients on antibiotics. Reviewing 23 scans performed on patients receiving antibiotic therapy for a mean duration of 22 days, Chung reported no false-negative scans in patients on antibiotics. Overall sensitivity was 100% and specificity 85%. Neither sensitivity nor specificity was adversely affected by antibiotics.[66]

Indium labeled WBC scans are also useful for identifying the extent of infection and to localize other nongraft sites of infection. Graft infections may appear either as localized uptake, full length, or multifocal uptake on scans.[67] Detection of localized graft infections may help in planning treatment. Extravascular sites of infection may also be detected during scanning. Williamson reported finding pseudomembranous

colitis, a suprapubic catheter wound infection, a subphrenic abscess, and an amputation site infection.[59] Normal wound healing does not interfere with scan results.

Technetium 99m Hexametazine Labeled Leukocyte Scans

Technetium is a metallic element, number 43, that does not exit in nature. Technetium 99 is the metastable form which emits γ-radiation and has a 6-hour half-life. Technetium 99m is widely used as a label in nuclear medicine. It is obtained as pertechnetate (TcO_4) which is dissolved in saline solution prior to being labeled with the compound of choice.[54]

Technetium 99m labeled leukocyte scans start with a sample of the patient's blood. Sedimentation and centrifugation of the venous blood will separate white blood cells from red blood cells and platelets. Technetium 99m hexametazine is then added to the leukocytes. After a 10-minute period of incubation the technetium 99m hexametazine labeled leukocytes are reinjected intravenously. Scans are usually obtained at 30 minutes, 4 hours, and 24 hours.[8,68–70]

The technetium 99m hexametazine labeled leukocyte scans have been recommended by some authors as an alternative to indium 111 labeled leukocyte scans. Vorne reported on 51 scans performed on eight control patients and 19 patients with suspected graft infections in 1989. The studies were 100% sensitive and 96% specific for the diagnosis of prosthetic graft infection.[8] Subsequently, two more series have been reported adding 54 more patients. The results have been similar to Vorne's results. Both authors reported 100% sensitivity; specificity ranged from 89% to 94.4%.[68,69] Each of the three series reported one false positive. One patient was studied 3 days postoperatively and had a positive scan, but there was no evidence of infection in subsequent clinical follow-up.[8] Another patient with a groin hematoma had a false-positive scan.[68] The third patient with a false-positive study had an anastomotic aneurysm.[69] False-negative scans did not occur in these series.

The reliability of technetium 99m leukocyte scans in the early postoperative period has been a concern of some authors. In 1991, Insall reported on 20 consecutive patients undergoing aortic bypass graft surgery who underwent routine 99m technetium labeled leukocyte scanning at 2 to 5 days and 7 to 10 days after surgery. Early postoperative scans had an overall 82.5% specificity at 2 to 5 days and 95% specificity at 10 days after surgery. At 20 days postoperatively all scans were negative, resulting in 100% specificity. Based on this study it appears that the specificity of technetium 99m labeled WBC scans is not significantly reduced 7 to 10 days after surgery.[71] This is in contrast to indium labeled WBC scans; Sedwitz reported only 47% of patients had true negative initial postoperative scans and the specificity for acute wound problems was only 50%.[62] However, the low specificity reported by Sedwitz using indium 111 scans in the early postoperative period may have been associated with platelet contamination causing false positives. Thus technetium 99m labeled leukocyte scans have few false positives in the early postoperative period and are reliable studies.

Fiorani compared technetium 99m leukocyte scans to CT scans in a series of 37 patients with suspected aortic graft infection. The sensitivity of 99m technetium WBC scans was 100% versus 78.9% for CT scans. The specificity of technetium 99m WBC scans was 94.4% versus 100% for CT scans. This suggests that technetium 99m WBC studies are more sensitive than CT scans, because technetium 99m WBC scans are able to detect graft infections before there are obvious anastomotic changes that could be detected by CT scan.[69]

There are several advantages of technetium 99m labeled WBC scans over gallium 67 and indium 111 scans. These advantages include better image quality, lower radiation dose, comparable cost, ready availability of materials, better reliability in the early postoperative studies, diagnostic information available after a few hours, and better sensitivity than gallium 67 scans. Other benefits that technetium 99m labeled WBC scans share with other nuclear medicine scans include: detection of other infected sites, localized and diffuse graft uptake is detectable, and false negatives rarely occur.[72]

Disadvantages of 99m technetium labeled leukocyte scans include: 20% have activity in the small bowel and proximal colon by 3 to 6 hours, the colon is usually visualized at 18 to 24 hours, and similar to indium 111 WBC scans, technetium 99m WBC scans are labor-intensive and require skilled technicians for the WBC-labeling process.[8,68,73]

Indium 111 Labeled Immunoglobulin G Scans

A technique for indium 111 labeling of polyclonal immunoglobulin G (IgG) was reported by Fischman in 1988. Both animal and human clinical studies have shown that radiolabeled, polyclonal IgG accumulates at the site of infection.[39,74,75]

Antibody fragment studies in animals indicate that the binding of antibody to inflammatory cells probably occurs on the Fc portion of IgG. The Fc portion of IgG is involved in nonspecific binding, whereas the Fab portion binds to specifically recognized sites only. This indicates that localization of graft infections by indium 111 labeled IgG is probably associated with nonspecific binding of IgG to inflammatory cells.[39,74]

Indium 111 labeled IgG is easily prepared. Nonspecific human polyclonal immunoglobulin can be purchased commercially and stored on the shelf (Sandoglobulin, Sandoz, Inc. East Hanover, NJ). After conjugating the antibody with diethylenetriamine pentaacetic acid (DTPA) it can be stored and then labeled with indium 111 chloride prior to use. After the antibody is labeled with indium 111, it is injected intravenously. Diagnostic images are available in 24 hours.[74,76]

LaMuraglia reported a series of 25 patients with possible graft infection; 11 graft infections were subsequently documented. The studies were 91% sensitive and 100% specific. One false-negative study was associated with an aortoduodenal fistula. An indium 111 labeled WBC scan and a CT scan were also negative in this patient. There were no false positives. Thus indium 111 labeled IgG scans are both sensitive and specific for PGI.[77]

Advantages of IgG labeled scans are: scans are able to delineate the site and extent of graft infection, they appear reliable in the early postoperative period, and because less indium 111 accumulates in the spleen with IgG labeled scans than with leukocyte-labeled scans, more indium can be used in IgG scans. Other advantages include: long shelf life of the reagent, ease of preparation, increased safety, no exposure to blood products, no inadvertent platelet labeling, and minimal accumulation of radioactive material in normal bowel.

Disadvantages of IgG labeled scans include: lack of localization of IgG in early images (5 to 30 minutes) and accumulation in areas of inflamed bowel, phlebitis (indium 111 labeled leukocyte scans also share this characteristic), tumors, and sites of endothelial injury. Diagnostically useful images are not obtained until 24 hours after injection. Immunoglobulin G may localize at sites of experimental atherosclerosis and areas of endothelial injury. Also, high blood pool activity up to 72 hours after injection may occur which could conceal subtle abnormalities in vascular graft locations (Fig. 9).[75,77,78]

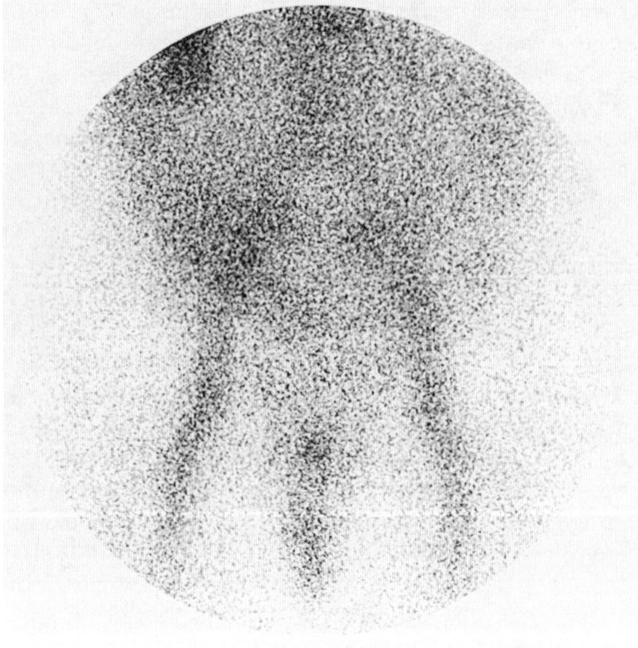

Figure 9. Normal Indium 111 IgG scan of an aortobifemoral graft with diffuse blood pool activity which could overshadow small focal areas of graft uptake.

Iodine 123 Labeled Immunoglobulin Scans

Graft infections can also be detected by iodine 123 labeled antigranulocyte antibody. The antibody is a murine monoclonal antibody against the glycoprotein NCA 95 on mature human granulocytes. In 1991, Cordes reported on 27 patients who were suspected of having PGI. The studies had a 94% sensitivity at 4 and 24 hours and an 83% specificity at 4 hours and a 70% specificity at 24 hours. This compared to a CT scan sensitivity of 67% in the same study. One false-negative scan in an axillofemoral bypass was also negative on CT; however a follow-up iodine 123 scan and CT were positive. False-positive results were seen in early postoperative patients and were associated with noninfected hematomas or wound healing. Advantages include image quality and safety, and diagnostic scans at 4 hours after injection.[79,80] The major disadvantage is the limited general availability of this reagent for most hospitals.

Gallium 67 Scintigraphy

Gallium is a group III B metal. Gallium 67 citrate is injected intravenously. It is not labeled with leukocytes or immunoglobulin and therefore does not require preparation of the patient's blood. Gallium 67 binds to plasma transferrin and is excreted by the kidneys and colon. The mechanism of gallium uptake is associated with cellular inflammation; however, the precise mechanism is unclear. After intravenous injection, initial scans may be obtained at 6 and 24 hours, although imaging at 48 or 72 hours is often desirable. Areas of normal activity include the liver, spleen, bone marrow, nasopharynx, lacrimal glands, and lactating breasts.[54]

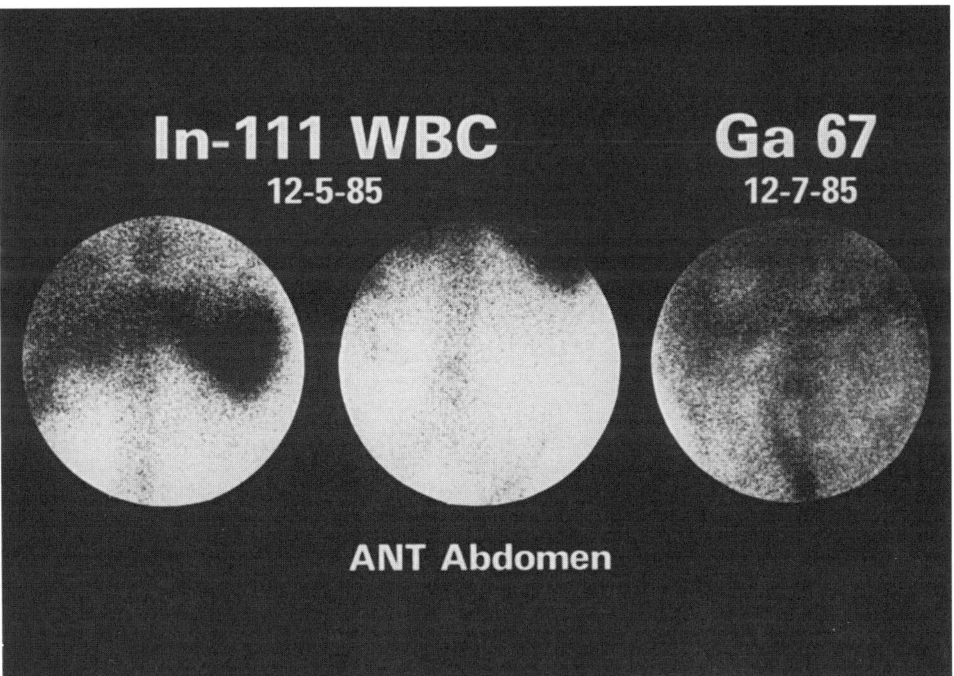

Figure 10. Gallium 67 scan compared to an Indium 111 WBC scan demonstrates the difficulty encountered with bowel uptake of gallium 67 which can significantly diminish image quality for abdominal graft positions. (Courtesy of Kathryn A. Morton, M.D.)

An initial experience with gallium 67 scintigraphy was reported by Causey in 1980.[81] Five patients with suspected PGI involving aortic grafts were evaluated and found to have abnormal uptake of gallium 67 around their grafts. All five had true positive scans. Subsequently other authors have published reports with sensitivities ranging from 78% to 100%, and specificities of 94% to 100%.[82,83]

Johnson et al. compared gallium 67 scans to CT scans in a series of 16 patients. Gallium 67 scans were significantly more specific than CT scans (94% versus 72%). The difference in sensitivity was not statistically significant.[83]

Advantages of gallium scans include wide experience with the tracer, less expensive than other scans, absence of special preparation prior to scanning, and visualization of infection by 24 hours (Fig. 10).[82,83] Characteristics that are considered problems by some authors include hepatic and splenic uptake, and excretion of radionuclide into the colon, bladder, and surgical incision. Fortunately, the site of inflammation or infection is not usually adjacent to the liver or spleen; therefore the site of interest, (the aorta and iliac vessels), usually can be visualized. Most patients can tolerate a cathartic bowel preparation prior to scanning which may diminish tracer in the intestine. Lastly, radionuclide uptake at the incision is not usually visible after the first week.[81] While most centers prefer indium 111 WBC scans over gallium 67 scans, some centers still use the gallium 67 scan.[83]

Limitations of Clinical Prosthetic Graft Infection Research

The prosthetic graft infection that presents with open wound, exposed graft, or a draining sinus is more obviously a PGI than an aortic graft confined to the abdomen in a patient who has vague complaints. Unfor-

Table 1
Diagnostic Modalities

Scan	Sensitivity	Specificity	Advantage	Disadvantage
CT	(65.3)	(84.1)	available late PGI needle aspiration	I.V. contrast radiation exposure
MRI	(75.0)	(100.0)	no x-rays saggital views	air vs Ca^{++} unable to aspirate
^{111}In WBC	70–100% (97.0)	83–100% (85.6)	experience minimal bowel uptake False negatives rare	rare false positives
^{99m}Tc WBC	89–100%	82–100%	image quality lower radiation dose False neg rare	few clinical trials bowel uptake labor intensive
^{111}In IgG	91% (90)	100% (100)	lower radiation dose no exposure to blood no plt labeling	few trials blood pool activity no early images
^{123}I IgG	94%	83% @ 4h 70% @ 24h	image quality early scans no exposure to blood	few clinical trials
Gallium	78–100% (90.5)	94–100% (95.2)	no exposure to blood	background activity

* numbers in parenthesis from meta-analysis[84] PGI = perigraft infection; CT = computer tomography; MRI = magnetic imaging; WBC = white blood cell; IgG = immunoglobulin.

tunately most authors lump both types of patients together when reporting on the sensitivity and specificity of the various diagnostic modalities. It is not clear what the sensitivity or specificity is of most studies in the patient who presents with vague symptoms only and no signs of infection. While graft infections are a relatively rare occurrence overall, diagnosis of the silently smoldering graft infection is extremely difficult. Many late graft infections are associated with *Staphylococcus epidermidis,* which causes infections that are indolent and associated with less inflammation. Routine culture techniques result in significantly fewer positive cultures. Many graft specimens are culture-positive only after ultrasonification which disrupts the graft's surface biofilm, freeing the bacteria.[7,51] Many authors have not correlated the culture results with the results of diagnostic scans.

As a result, the sensitivity and specificity of the various diagnostic modalities (Table 1) are unknown in a patient with vague, nonspecific complaints, and an intra-abdominal aortic graft, which is later found to be infected with *S epidermidis.* Until more studies correlate the microorganism and the diagnostic scan's sensitivity and specificity, the best test for diagnosis of PGI caused by specific bacteria will not be known.[84]

Current Approach to Patients with Suspected Prosthetic Graft Infection

Patients with prosthetic graft infections may present in many ways, some subtle and others obvious. They may present with vague, nonspecific symptoms and signs which only indirectly suggest a graft infection, or they may present with a local soft tissue infection in an area near the graft but with no direct evidence of graft infection. For example, prosthetic grafts which are entirely intra-abdominal rarely present with purulent drainage (10.4%) compared to aor-

tofemoral (43.6%), ileofemoral (42.8%), or femoropopliteal (74.5%) grafts.[85] Initially a radionuclide scan is usually obtained. Most centers use indium 111 labeled leukocyte scans. If this is positive no further tests are necessary. However, if the initial test fails to confirm a graft infection, a CT scan is usually obtained next, looking for air, soft tissue swelling, or perigraft fluid. Aspiration of perigraft fluid may be helpful in some cases.[35] If all tests are negative and clinical suspicion is low, the patient can be observed and testing may be repeated at a later time. However, if all tests are negative and clinical suspicion is high, then exploration of the graft may be indicated. At the time of operation, signs of infection associated with grafts include purulent fluid or exudate surrounding the graft, a perigraft capsule, or a lack of tissue incorporation of the graft[11](Fig. 11).

Secondly, patients may present with a definite graft infection, such as a purulent femoral wound with exposed graft. As mentioned above, purulent drainage is rare in patients with grafts confined to the abdomen and more common in patients with femoral anastomoses. This scenario does not require confirmation of PGI; however, imaging studies are useful to determine the extent of graft involvement and to rule out multiple sites of involvement. When only a limited area of radionuclide uptake occurs, it may be possible to excise the infected portion of the graft and salvage the uninfected portion (Fig. 12).

Occasionally patients who have an aortic graft and present with nonspecific complaints do have evidence of gastrointestinal bleeding. The unstable patient with an aortic graft and a hemorrhagic bleed should go straight to the operating room for a diagnostic laparotomy and treatment. These patients may have a graft-enteric fistula (GEF). However, a stable patient with an aortic graft and evidence of a gastrointestinal bleed should be evaluated urgently. An esophagogastroduodenoscopy using a colonoscope should be performed to visualize the fourth portion of the duodenum where a

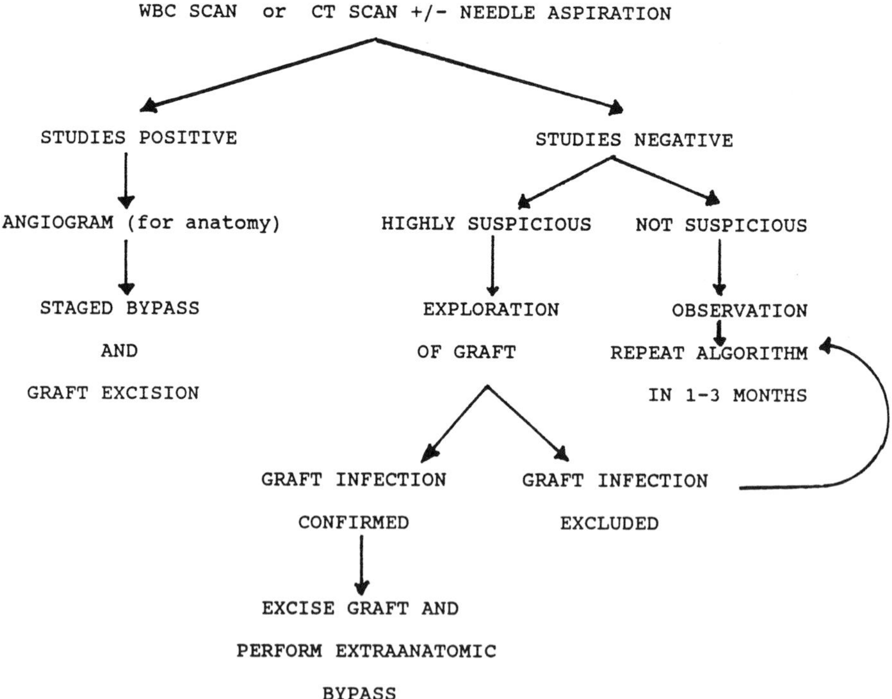

Figure 11. Suspected graft infection.

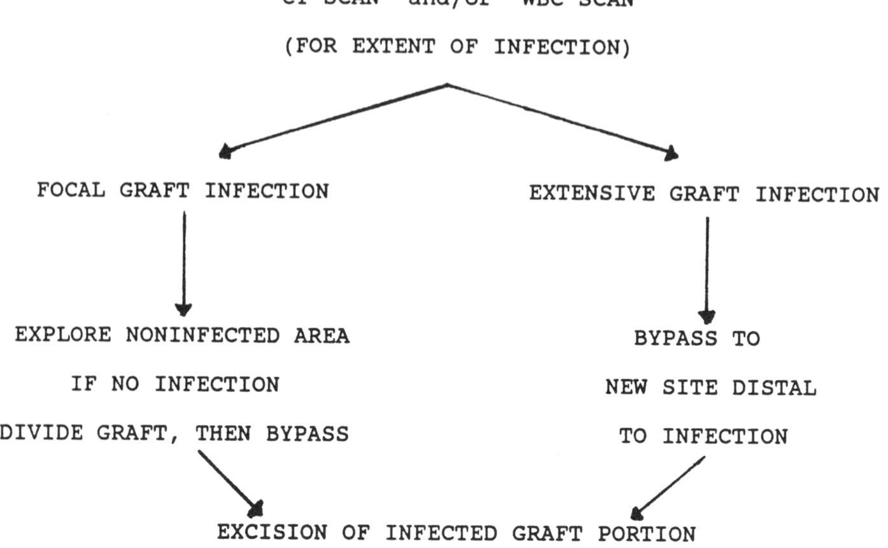

Figure 12. Established graft infection (purulent drainage or exposed graft).

GEF may be identified. If a GEF is highly suspected, endoscopy should be performed in an operating room, in the event massive hemorrhage ensues. If endoscopy is negative, angiography or a RBC scan may be able to locate the source of bleeding. If all of the above tests are negative yet the suspicion of PGI remains, proceed with a WBC scan, CT scan, or lastly, surgical exploration.[17,78]

Aknowledgment: The authors are grateful to Alyssa Hickman for her assistance with manuscript preparation, and to Katherine A. Morton, MD for comments related to nuclear medicine evaluation of patients and critical review of the manuscript and photographs.

References

1. Bunt TJ, Haynes JL. Synthetic vascular graft infection: the continuing headache. *Am Surg.* 1984;50:43–48.
2. Lorentzen JE, Nielsen OM, Arendrup H, et al. Vascular graft infection: an analysis of sixty-two graft infections in 2411 consecutively implanted synthetic vascular grafts. *Surgery.* 1985;98:81–86.
3. Jamieson GG, DeWeese JA, Rob CG. Infected arterial grafts. *Ann Surg.* 1975;181:850–852.
4. Edwards WH Jr, Martin RS III, Jenkins JM, et al. Primary graft infections. *J Vasc Surg.* 1987;6:235–239.
5. Szilagyi DE, Smith RF, Elliott JP, et al. Infection in arterial reconstruction with synthetic grafts. *Ann Surg.* 1972;176:321–333.
6. Plecha FR, Plecha FM. Femorofemoral bypass grafts: ten-year experience. *J Vasc Surg.* 1984;1:555–561.
7. Bandyk DF, Berganmini TM, Kinney EV, et al. In situ replacement of vascular prostheses infected by bacterial biofilms. *J Vasc Surg.* 1991;13:575–583.
8. Vorne M, Laitinen J, Lehtonen J, et al. 99mTc-leukocyte scintigraphy in prosthetic vascular graft infections. *Nucl Med.* 1989;28:95–99.
9. Golan JF. Vascular graft infection. *Infect Dis Clin North Am.* 1989;3:247–258.
10. Bunt TJ. Synthetic vascular graft infections. I. Graft infections. *Surgery.* 1983;93:733–746.
11. Seabrook GR, Schmitt DD, Bandyk DF, et al. Anastomotic aneurysms after vascular reconstruction: problems of incidence, etiology, and treatment. *Surgery.* 1975;78:800–816.
12. Campbell C, Robertson DAR. Gas in an infected vascular prosthesis: an unusual finding on plain radiographs. *Clin Radiol.* 1990;41:60–62.
13. Yeager RA, McConnell DB, Sasaki TM, et al. Aortic and peripheral prosthetic graft infection: differential management and causes of mortality. *Am J Surg.* 1985;150:36–43.
14. Freischlag JA, Moore WS. Infection in prosthetic vascular grafts. In: Rutherford RB, ed. *Vascular Surgery, 3rd ed.* Philadelphia: WB Saunders; 1989:510–521.
15. Reilly LM, Altman H, Lusby RJ, et al. Late results following surgical management of vascular graft infection. *J Vasc Surg.* 1984;1:36–44.
16. Bunt TJ. Synthetic vascular graft infections, II: graft-enteric erosions and graft-enteric fistulas. *Surgery.* 1983;94:1–9.
17. Reilly LM, Ehrenfeld WK, Goldstone J, et al. Gastrointestinal tract involvement by prosthetic graft infection: the significance of gastrointestinal hemorrhage. *Ann Surg.* 1985;202:342–348.
18. Wolson AH, Kaupp HA, McDonald K. Ultrasound of arterial graft surgery complications. *AJR.* 1979;133:869–875.
19. Gooding GAW, Herzog KA, Hedgcock MW, et al. B-mode ultrasonography of prosthetic vascular grafts. *Radiology.* 1978;127:763–766.
20. Gooding GAW, Effeney DJ, Goldstone J. The aortofemoral graft: detection and identification of healing complications by ultrasonography. *Surgery.* 1981;89:94–101.
21. Lewis BD, James EM, Welch TJ. Current applications of duplex and color doppler ultrasound imaging: carotid and peripheral vascular system. *Mayo Clin Proc.* 1989;64:1147–1157.
22. Polak JF, Donaldson MC, Whittemore AD, et al. Pulsative masses surrounding vascular prostheses: real-time US color flow imaging. *Radiology.* 1989;170:363–366.
23. Goldstone J. Infected prosthetic arterial grafts. In: Haimovici H, ed. *Vascular Surgery, 3rd ed.* Norwalk: Appleton-Lange; 1989:564–574.
24. Yashar JJ, Baxter JC, Burnard RJ, et al. Ultrasonic investigation of infected vascular prostheses. *Int Surg.* 1979;64:51–53.
25. Haaga JR, Baldwin GN, Reich NE, et al. CT detection of infected synthetic grafts: preliminary report of a new sign. *AJR.* 1978;131:317–320.
26. Mark AS, McCarthy SM, Moss AA, et al. Detection of abdominal aortic graft infection: comparison of CT and In-labeled white blood cell scans. *AJR.* 1985;144:315–318.
27. Hilton S, Megibow AJ, Naidich DP, et al. Computed tomography of the postoperative

abdominal aorta. *Radiology.* 1982;145: 403–407.

28. Vogelzang RL, Limpert JD, Yao JST. Detection of prosthetic vascular complications: comparison of CT and angiography. *AJR .* 1987;148:819–823.

29. Freimanis IE, Kozak B, Taylor LM Jr, et al. Failure of CT scanning to diagnose aortic graft infection. *J Vasc Surg.* 1987;6:531–532.

30. Tobin KD. Aortobifemoral perigraft abscess: treatment by percutaneous catheter drainage. *J Vasc Surg.* 1988;8:339–343.

31. Cunat JS, Haaga JR, Rhodes R, et al. Periaortic fluid aspiration for recognition of infected graft: preliminary report. *AJR.* 1982;139: 251–253.

32. Wittenberg J. Computed tomography of the body: second of two parts. *N Engl J Med.* 1983;309:1224–1229.

33. 0'Hara PJ, Borkowski GP, Hertzer NR, et al. Natural history of periprosthetic air on computerized axial tomographic examination of the abdomen following abdominal aortic aneurysm repair. *J Vasc Surg.* 1984;1:429–433.

34. Qvarfordt PG, Reilly LM, Mark AS, et al. Computerized tomographic assessment of graft incorporation after aortic reconstruction. *Am J Surg.* 1985;150:227–231.

35. Rabinovici R, Fields S, Berlatzky Y, et al. CT guided pepriaortic fluid aspiration diagnosing aortic graft infection. *J Cardiovasc Surg.* 1988;29:318–319.

36. Calligaro KD, Veith FJ. Diagnosis and management of infected prosthetic aortic grafts. *Surgery.* 1991;110:805–813.

37. Justich E, Amparo EG, Hricak H, et al. Infected aortoiliofemoral grafts: magnetic resonance imaging. *Radiology.* 1985;154:133–136.

38. Auffermann W, Olofsson PA, Rabahie GN, et al. Incorporation versus infection of retroperitoneal aortic grafts: MR imaging features. *Radiology.* 1989;172:359–362.

39. Fischman AJ, Rubin RH, Khaw BA, et al. Detection of acute inflammation with 111-In-labeled nonspecific polyclonal igg. *Sem Nucl Med.* 1988;18:335–344.

40. Auffermann W, Olofsson P, Stoney R, et al. MR imaging of complications of aortic surgery. *J Comput Assist Tomogr.* 1987;11: 982–989.

41. Olofsson PA, Auffermann W, Higgins CB, et al. Diagnosis of prosthetic aortic graft infection by magnetic resonance imaging. *J Vasc Surg.* 1988;8:99–105.

42. Spartera C, Morettini G, Petrassi C, et al. Role of magnetic resonance imaging in the evaluation of aortic graft healing, perigraft fluid collection, and graft infection. *Eur J Vasc Surg.* 1990;4:69–73.

43. Bernhard VM. Aortoenteric fistulas. In: Rutherford RB, ed. *Vascular Surgery, 3rd ed.* Philadelphia; Saunders; 1989:528– 535.

44. Flye MW, Thompson WM. Aortic graft-enteric and paraprosthetic-enteric fistulas. *Am J Surg.* 1983;146:183–187.

45. O'Hara PJ, Hertzer NR, Beven EG, et al. Surgical management of infected abdominal aortic grafts: review of a 25-year experience. *J Vasc Surg.* 1986;3:725–731.

46. Reilly LM, Stoney RJ, Goldstone J, et al. Improved management of aortic graft infection: the influence of operation sequence and staging. *J Vasc Surg.* 1987;5:421–431.

47. Pabst TS III, Bernhard VM, McIntyre KE, et al. Gastrointestinal bleeding after aortic surgery: the role of laparotomy to rule out aortoenteric fistula. *J Vasc Surg.* 1988;8:280–285.

48. Brand EJ, Sivak MV, Sullivan BH Jr. Aortoduodenal fistula: endoscopic diagnosis. *Dig Dis Sci.* 1979;24:940–944.

49. Yeager RA, Sasaki TM, McConnell DB, et al. Clinical spectrum of patients with infrarenal aortic grafts and gastrointestinal bleeding. *Am J Surg.* 1987;153:459–461.

50. Mir-Madjlessi SH, Sullivan BH Jr, Farmer RG, et al. Endoscopic diagnosis of aortoduodenal fistula. *Gastrointest Endosc.* 1973;19: 187–188.

51. Becker W, Dusel W, Berger P, et al. The 111-In-granulocyte scan in prosthetic vascular graft infections: imaging technique and results. *Eur J Nucl Med.* 1987;13:225–229.

52. Berridge DC, Frier M, Perkins AC, et al. A comparison between visual and quantitative analysis in a prospective evaluation of labeled 111-In leucocyte imaging in vascular infection. *Nucl Med Comm.* 1989;10:487–495.

53. Datz FL. Hematologic imaging. In: Osborn, ed. *Nuclear Medicine.* Chicago: Year Book Medical Pub; 1988:272–280.

54. Alazraki NP, Mishkin FS. Inflammatory and infectious processes. In: Alazraki NP, ed. *Fundamentals of Nuclear Medicine.* New York: The Society of Nuclear Medicine; 1984: 115–119.

55. Thakur ML, Coleman RE, Welch MJ. Indium-111-labeled leukocytes for the localization of abscesses: preparation, analysis, tissue distribution, and comparison with gallium-67 citrate in dogs. *J Lab Clin Med.* 1977; 89:217–228.

56. Stevick CA, Fawcett HD. Aortoiliac-graft infection: detection by leukocyte scan. *Arch Surg.* 1981;116:939–942.

57. Serota AI, Williams RA, Rose JG, et al. Uptake of radiolabeled leukocytes in prosthetic graft infection. *Surgery.* 1981;90:35–40.

58. Lawrence PF, Dries DJ, Alazraki NP, et al. Indium 111-labeled leukocyte scanning for detection of prosthetic vascular graft infection. *J Vasc Surg.* 1985;2:165–173.

59. Williamson MR, Boyd CM, Read RC, et al. 111 In-labeled leukocytes in the detection of prosthetic vascular graftinfections. *AJR.* 1986;147:173–176.

60. McKeown PP, Miller DC, Jamieson SW, et al. Diagnosis of arterial prosthetic graft infection by indium-111 oxine white blood cell scans. *Circulation.* 1982;(suppl 1)66:130–134.

61. Dries DJ, Alazraki NP, Lawrence PF, et al. Detection of acute synthetic vascular graft infection with 111-In-labeled leukocyte scanning: an animal study. *AJR.* 1985;145:1053–1056.

62. Sedwitz MM, Davies RJ, Pretorius HT, et al. Indium 111-labeled white blood cell scans after vascular prosthetic reconstruction. *J Vasc Surg.* 1987;6:476–481.

63. Reilly DT, Grigg MJ, Cunningham EJ, et al. Vascular graft infection: the role of indium scanning. *Eur J Vasc Surg.* 1989;3:393–397.

64. Chung CJ, Wilson AA, Melton JW, et al. Uptake of In-111 labeled leukocytes by lymphocele: a cause of false-positive vascular graft infection. *Clin Nucl Med.* 1992;17:368–370.

65. Forstrom LA, Dewanjee MK, Chowdhury BS, et al. Indium-111 labeled purified granulocytes in the diagnosis of synthetic vascular graft infection. *Clin Nucl Med.* 1988;13:859–862.

66. Chung CJ, Hicklin OA, Payan JM, et al. Indium-111-labeled leukocyte scan in detection of synthetic vascular graft infection: the effect of antibiotic treatment. *J Nucl Med.* 1991;32:13–15.

67. Berridge DC, Earnshaw JJ, Frier M, et al. 111-In-labelled leucocyte imaging in vascular graft infection. *Br J Surg.* 1989;76:41–44.

68. Insall RL, Jones NAG, Chamberlain J, et al. New isotopic technique for detecting prosthetic arterial graft infection: 99mTc-hexametazime-labeled leucocyte imaging. *Br J Surg.* 1990;77:1295–1298.

69. Fiorani P, Speziale F, Rizzo L, et al. Early detection of low-grade aortic graft infection. *J Vasc Surg.* 1993;17:87–96.

70. Danpure HJ, Osman S, Carroll MK. In vitro studies to develop a clinical protocol for radiolabelling mixed leukocytes with ^{99m}Tc-HMPAO. *Nucl Med Commun.* 1987;8:280.

71. Insall RL, Keavey PM, Hawkins T, et al. The specificity of technetium-labelled-leucocyte imaging of aortic grafts in the early postoperative period. *Eur J Vasc Surg.* 1991;5:571–576.

72. Vorne M, Laitinen R, Lantto T, et al. Chronic prosthetic vascular graft infection visualized with technetium-99m-hexamethylpropyleneamine oxime-labeled leukocytes. *J Nucl Med.* 1991;32:1425–1427.

73. Mortelmans L, Verlooy H, Nevelsteen A, et al. Clinical usefulness of Tc-99m HMPAO labeled white blood cell imaging in prosthetic vascular graft infections. *Clin Nucl Med.* 1992;17:11–13.

74. Fischman AJ, Wilkinson R, Khaw BA, et al. Imaging of localized bacterial infections with radiolabeled non-specific antibody fragments. *J Nucl Med.* 1988;29:887.

75. Fischman AJ, Rubin RH, Khaw BA, et al. Radionuclide imaging of experimental atherosclerosis with nonspecific polyclonal immunoglobulin G. *J Nucl Med.* 1989;30:1095–1100.

76. Rubin RH, Fischman AJ, Callahan RJ, et al. 111-In-labeled nonspecific immunoglobulin scanning in the detection of focal infection. *N Engl J Med.* 1989;321:935–940.

77. LaMuraglia GM, Fischman AJ, Strauss HW, et al. Utility of the indium 111-labeled human immunoglobulin-G scan for the detection of focal vascular graft infection. *J Vasc Surg.* 1989;10:20–28.

78. Merrell SW, Lawrence PF. Diagnosis of graft infection: anatomic and functional imaging techniques. *Semin Vasc Surg.* 1990;3:89–100.

79. Cordes M, Hepp W, Langer R, et al. Vascular graft infection: detection by 123I-labeled antigranulocyte antibody (anti-NCA95) scintigraphy. *Nucl Med.* 1991;30:173–177.

80. Cordes M. Diagnostic evaluation of radioimmunoscintigraphy (ris) with use of iodine 123-labeled antibodies against human granulocytes (123I-anti-NCA95) for the detection of prosthetic vascular graft infection. *J Vasc Surg.* 1991;14:703–705.

81. Causey D, Fajman WA, Perdue GD, et al. 67 Ga scintigraphy in postoperative synthetic graft infections. *AJR.* 1980;134:1041–1045.

82. Thivolle P, Varenne L, Heyden Y, et al. Gallium-67 citrate whole body scanning for the localization of infected vascular synthetic grafts. *Clin Nucl Med.* 1985;10:330–332.

83. Johnson KK, Russ PD, Bair JH, et al. Diagnosis of synthetic vascular graft infection: comparison of CT and gallium scans. *AJR.* 1990;154:405–409.

84. Lawrence PF, Merrell SW. Diagnosis of vascular graft infections: a meta-analysis. Presented at the 44th meeting of the Society for Vascular Surgery, June 4–6, 1990; Los Angeles, Ca.

85. Liekweg WG, Greenfield LJ. Vascular prosthetic infections: collected experience and results of treatment. *Surgery.* 1977;81:335–42.

SECTION V

Treatment Options for Graft Infections

Intellectual dishonesty is exemplified by the disclaimer that the patient was a poor risk for the procedure. It is the surgeon's judgment and skill that overcomes the perceived risk or avoids the risk for the patient in the first place. Having taken the risk for the patient, it is the surgeon's responsibility to fulfill the contract.

Chapter 8

Treatment Options for Graft Infections

T.J. Bunt

Introduction

The choice of therapy for a graft infection should follow as logically as possible from an understanding of the underlying pathophysiology, seeking to expeditiously correct the life and limb threat without further compromising the patient with injudicious (either overly or inadequately aggressive) treatment. Thoughtful review of the problem beforehand is indicated and should encompass the principles that are presented in this book.

In 1983 I suggested that graft infection management entailed more than a simple indication as to whether it was aortic or at the groin—that recognition of all of the vagaries and variables of the individual situation is necessary to direct appropriate treatment selection.[1] Thus, the graft infection (GIF) should be further classified as to:

a. type of graft: Dacron, Teflon, knitted, woven, autologous
b. site of graft: aortic reconstruction (AR), iliacofemoral (IF), axillofemoral (AxF), cross-femoral (CF), femoropopliteal (FP), etc.
c. site of infection: groin, midshaft, aortic shaft
d. complication: anastomotic involvement, graft-enteric fistula (GEF), pseudoaneurysm, etc.
e. bacterium(a): particularly as to whether it is Gram positive or negative.

Choice of therapy would then logically draw on these facts of the situation and application of the facts to the patient involved, including :

a. age
b. compromising medical conditions, particularly quality of life and expected extent of survival
c. psychosocial, particularly cognitive ability and ambulatory capability
d. presence of clinical sepsis
e. level and severity of underlying occlusive disease

The choice of therapy cannot logically be a de rigueur or rote application of one modality to all situations or even to one site and type of infection. All of the individualizing variables must be placed and weighted in the equation. This principle can be applied as critically and appropriately to published series extolling a specific method of management, as it can to the management of an individual situation.

This section will attempt to provide fairly definitive options for treatment:

first, by listing and vigorously critiquing all the extant literature to show what has been tried, with what success, and with what distinct and important errors, (recognized or not by the authors).

second, by a series of selected monographs in certain therapy options, each presented by an expert in that field and.

lastly, by a summary with our carefully considered recommendations based on analysis of all that has been detailed and tempered by what is clearly the largest single author experience in the field (80 cases).

Literature Review

Critical surveys of well-observed and carefully followed angioplastic operations are sorely needed. I am afraid that in the past too much stress has been placed on the reporting of brilliant early results, the observation of which often seemed to have stopped in the recovery room or at the discharge office.

D. Emerick Szylagyi (1962)[2]

The first aortic aneurysmorrhaphy was reported by Dubost in 1952, the first aortic reconstruction by Oudot in 1951, the first femoropopliteal graft by Kunlin in 1948, and the first axillofemoral graft by Blaisdell and Hall in 1962. The advent of these innovative approaches to vascular disease by synthetic-autologous reconstruction was soon followed by recognition of the potential for major infectious complications, with Claytor and then Brock reporting the first aortic graft infections in 1956.[3–8]

Blaisdell (1961) reported the first successful thoracofemoral bypass grafting for recurrent aortic GIF.[9] The case is instructive on its own merits. A 66-year-old man presented 2 months after urgent aortic aneu-

rysmorrhaphy and aortoiliac grafting with the postoperative course marred by persistent low-grade fever. He was discharged only to present with acute aortic disruption. An in situ replacement was performed despite positive *Escherichia coli* cultures of the field. He presented with repeat rupture 1 month later. The aortic stump was oversewn with catgut and a thoracofemoral graft was placed for severe limb ischemia. The patient died of sepsis 1 month later with a patent graft and an intact aortic stump but with continued retroperitoneal sepsis.

The first series of graft infections was reported by Javid (1962). He noted the development of late complications in 13% (18/240) of abdominal aortic aneurysmorrhaphy (AAA) versus only 3.5% (12/420) of aortic reconstructions (AR). There were in the series 6 GEFs and 5 GIFs, 4 of which presented as infected pseudoaneurysms (PA). The GIFs and PAs occurred predominantly in the AR series. Javid also first noted (although he did not ascribe importance to) *Staphylococcus epidermidis* as a significant factor in the late presentation of PAs, with 4 of 8 groin PAs culturing out *S epidermidis*, 1 of these with systemic *S epidermidis* sepsis. The management of these cases was highly individualized, since there were no antecedent guidelines for the authors to follow. Local repair of the *S epidermidis*-infected PAs led to 2 recurrences and 2 thromboses. Local treatment of 2 groin GIFs led to ascending infection in both and subsequent mortality from proximal anastomotic hemorrhage. Three other groin GIF presentations were managed by limb resection and extra-anatomic bypass (EAB) reconstruction, all successfully.[10]

Javid's analysis of these varied results suggested some of the earliest management postulates. He believed that the graft represented a foreign body that potentiated the infection and noted that attempts at local treatment only left the patient vulnerable to ascending infection with catastrophic secondary hemorrhage. His paper also first noted the potential for *S epidermidis* graft infections, although it did not recognize the now commonly accepted secondary problem of delayed graft thrombosis and pseudoaneurysm formation.

Carter and Whelan (1963) presented a vigorous advocacy of local therapy that would be quoted by many authors in the following decades. Unfortunately, the results when closely analyzed do not really support their belief in the superiority of local treatment. They presented seven cases, six of which were GIFs and all presenting at the groin. All were Dacron grafts—four AR and two FP. The bacteria were *Micrococcus*, *Streptococcus*, and *S aureus*, with secondary *Aerobacter* and *Proteus mirabilis* in two cases. Carter used local therapy in all and claimed good results.[11] However, one patient died (16% mortality) and four grafts thrombosed at intervals of 1 to 8 months, with one amputation. In reality therefore only one of six patients was alive with a patent graft at 1 year. These are hardly the stellar results with which to advocate therapy! Despite the inadequacy of the real results, every subsequent author on the local therapy of graft has used Carter as a primary reference. That in itself is a cogent condemnation of our medical literature insofar as the accuracy of its literature review is concerned!

Hoffert, writing for Haimovici's group (1965), described 12 cases of GIF, all presenting at the groin or peripherally, and involving 8 FP and 4 femoral reconstructions. The affected grafts were Nylon in 5, Dacron in 5, and homograft in 2. He noted a 6% rate of GIF in 201 grafts placed over a 7-year period. Bacteria were *S aureus* in 7, *E coli* in 5, *P mirabilis* in 4, *Pseudomonas* in 3, *S epidermidis* in 2, and 1 each *Enterococcus* and *Streptococcus*. Nine of the 12 cases had involved revascularization in the face of an infected pedal lesion, 7 ipsilateral, and 2 contralateral. He noted the same bacteria on cultures of subsequent GIFs. Six of the 12 had wound problems at initial surgery. Hoffert treated 10 of these cases with total graft excision, 1 with partial, and 1 with local therapy only.

The mortality rate for these peripheral graft problems was 25% (3/12) and the amputation rate 75% (9/12), in large part because he made no attempt at reconstruction for most of these peripheral infections. He did perform an in situ reversed saphenous vein (RASV) reconstruction in one patient, which also became infected with secondary hemorrhage, and an in situ synthetic replacement of an infected FP led to ascending infection of a more proximal aortic aneurysm with fatal proximal disruption.[12]

Hoffert's study initiated the study of the epidemiology of GIF, with his notations that postoperative wound hematomas occurring in the face of distal pedal sepsis were a prominent factor in the development of GIF. His paper also first noted the prohibitive amputation rate and high mortality associated with peripheral graft infection if reconstruction was not carried out.

Fry and Lindenauer (1967) presented the Michigan experience, noting 12 GIFs over 13 years and 890 cases for a 1.34% incidence. The mean presentation was 8 months postoperatively. No prophylactic antibiotics were used in the primary cases, although they had initiated routine prophylactic antibiotic usage at the time of publication. Presenting symptoms were well described and included graft thrombosis, sinus formation, postoperative groin abscess, pseudoaneurysm, and anastomotic bleeding. They recommended complete graft resection and extra-anatomic reconstruction. They also noted that infection ascended up three thrombosed graft limbs to involve the aortic shaft, but did not do so in two patent limbs. They also noted a seemingly long-term survivor of no treatment of an AR-GIF who then at 3 1/2 years died of multiple embolic infarcts and sepsis. The mortality for this early series was 75%; of the survivors, one was a bilateral amputee, and one had severe claudication, leaving only one symptom-free survivor.[13] The paper thus indicated not only a high operative mortality, but an even more prohibitive long-term morbidity to be associated with aortic GIF.

Fry's paper was instrumental in establishing the concept of GIF as a highly morbid complication of aortic surgery, and perhaps also in establishing a fatalistic attitude toward its management that persisted over the next 15 years. Despite the high mortality, the paper did establish the basic tenets of GIF management, particularly total graft excision and extra-anatomic reconstruction. The concept of infection ascending along thrombosed versus patent grafts has never been fully validated, but has been repeatedly echoed by subsequent authors. Many subsequent series have noted ascending infection in patent grafts as well.

Najafi (1968) updated the experience in Javid's group to 12 GIFs, describing 5 AR GIFs presenting at the groin (duplicate of Javid's paper?) and adding 4 FPs, 1 IF, 1 thoracic AR, and a carotid Dacron reconstruction. The four FPs were midshaft problems and responded to local therapy without complications. Two of the 5 ARs were treated with graft excision and EAB and did well. One graft infection ascended during local therapy and the patient died of aortic disruption and one presented as a PA due to *S epidermidis* and underwent in situ reconstruction with recurrence requiring excision. The thoracic GIF fatally ruptured before therapy. The IF was a failure on local therapy and required EAB; the carotid healed on local therapy.[14] Their conclusions from this expanded experience were that local therapy was successful in peripheral GIFs if there was no bleeding or signs of systemic sepsis, and if the process was well localized. These tenets were established for the management of GIFs with local therapy. However, since in their initial experience, local infection frequently ascended with fatal results, they recommended a more complete graft excision with EAB.

Cohn (1968) presented 11 patients with graft complications managed in a private practice setting; 3 of these were GIFs 2 of whom died from PA rupture prior to surgical intervention. The third had uneventful graft excision without revascularization.

Diethrich (1970) similarly presented three patients with groin presentations of GIF. All three underwent successful graft resection and EAB uneventfully.[15]

Conn (1970) presented a series of 12 patients at Mississippi in which he emphasized the prevalence and virulence of Gram-negative GIFs. The GIFs were of AR in 7, FP in 4, and carotid in 1. This represented a 5% incidence of GIF at their institution (22/435). The bacteria were Gram negative in 68% and these resulted in an 83% mortality. The bacteria were *P mirabilis*, Pseudomonas, S aureus, and *Klebsiella* in 5, *E coli* and *Aerobacter* in 4, *Serratia* and *E coli* in 3, and an assortment of *S epidermidis*, *Streptococcus*, and *Enterococcus*. For AR cases, 4 underwent graft excision with only 2 mortalities and amputation; 5 had local therapy with only 2 fatal failures; and 2 underwent excision and EAB with 1 mortality and amputation. For FP infections, 4 were treated locally with 3 mortalities and 1 amputation, and 4 underwent graft excision with 3 amputations.[16]

Such uniformly poor results do not lend themselves to advocacy of any one treatment modality. The series certainly underscored a worse prognosis for Gram-negative infections, which tended to result in sepsis and/or anastomotic disruptions. It also underscored the futility of attempts at local therapy with Gram-negative infections; 8 attempts led to 5 mortalities and 3 amputations. As an incidental footnote, the paper also noted the first case of secondary infection of an axillofemoral EAB placed for reconstruction.

Szylagyi (1972) surveyed the extensive experience at Henry Ford Hospital, noting a 1.9% incidence of GIF in 3347 cases, which varied from 0.7% for AR and AAA to 3.0% for FP cases. No perioperative antibiotics were used in the primary revascularizations. Szylagyi also defined three levels of groin wound infections, with a III being actual involvement of the graft. Sixty-five percent of the GIFs presented as 30-day postoperative problems, and the remainder presented at intervals from 13 to 60 months. There was only one case of proven hematogenous GIF which arose from an abscess of the hand; all others occurred as local wound problems or after visceral erosion-perforation. The predominant bacteria were therefore *S aureus* or *S epidermidis* at the groin and *E coli* for aortic shaft infections, and constituted *S aureus* in 13, *E coli* in 9, *S epidermidis* in 6, *P mirabilis* in 3, *Pseudomonas* in 1, and 5 miscellaneous.

Szylagyi detailed the varied treatment results in this group. For 20 AR GIFs, 2 were treated locally, 1 with in situ reconstruction. Both of these cases were successfully treated. Ten underwent partial graft excision with 1 mortality and 4 amputations, 5 underwent excision without revascularization, with 3 mortalities and 1 amputation, and 3 underwent excision with EAB, all with fatal outcomes. For 10 FP GIFs, 8 were resected without revascularization with no mortality but 4 amputations, 1 was treated locally and did well, and 1 excision with EAB resulted in both amputation and mortality. Szylagyi summarized the experience by noting that he had good success with partial graft excision and revascularization but strangely had uniformly fatal outcomes with a more complete graft excision and EAB.[17]

Szylagyi vigorously opined against the use of prophylactic antibiotics for vascular surgery, noting that the incidence of GIF in his extensive experience was equal to or less than any other series, and suggesting that routine prophylactic antibiotic use would lead to complications, emergence of resistant organisms as agents of presumably more virulent GIFs, and suppression of otherwise signal symptoms of occult GIF.

Bouhotsous (1974) presented a study of GIFs occurring in two hospitals and 532 patients over a 15-year period. Complications occurred in 2 of 790 intra-abdominal anastomoses, 2 of 365 suprainguinal anastomoses approached via the groin, and 10 of 201 inguinal anastomoses ($P < .001$). Five of the 12 groin infections were preceded by wound

hematomas and 2 of 35 GIFs occurred in patients with foot infections. The paper goes on to describe the management. Eight patients underwent graft excision only, with 1 mortality and 2 amputations; a single attempt at EAB resulted in death. Four patients were supposedly treated with antibiotics alone; however, documentation of the diagnosis of GIF is poor. For that matter, one can easily question if most of the series even had GIFs, since there is little definitive evidence presented and most cases were treated presumptively.[18]

Goldstone (1974) presented the Arizona experience, totaling 27 cases over a 14-year period. Prophylactic antibiotics had not been used from 1959 to 1965, but were routinely used from 1966 to 1973; topical antibiotics were, however, routinely used. The GIF rate fell nonsignificantly from 4.1% (9/222) to 1.5% (5/344) with the institution of intravenous antibiotics. The study also looked at etiologies: 5 patients had groin wound hematomas, 2 had distal pedal sepsis, and 2 had potential concomitant peritoneal contamination, 1 with incidental appendectomy and 1 with postoperative peritonitis. Two additional patients had a urinary tract infection and ureteral injury, respectively. The series also noted a tendency to see *S aureus* in early, and *S epidermidis* in late inguinal infections. Overall, there were 11 *S aureus*, 7 *S epidermidis*, and 7 Gram-negative infections. Presentation was by groin abscess or sinus in 14, PA in 13, graft thrombosis in 8, anastomotic hemorrhage in 7, sepsis in 5, and distal emboli in 2. The average time of presentation was 15 months (range 1 to 87). Forty-six percent (12/22) involved a redo case and 77% of GIFs initiated at the groin.[19]

Goldstone's experience with local therapy was uniformly unsuccessful, with failure in all 11 tries and 1 immediate mortality; of these failures 2 underwent partial excision, both with fatal results, and 8 total excisions with 2 further mortalities. Thus, they saw 5 mortalities in 11 tries at local therapy. Six partial excisions resulted in 2 mortalities (as above) and 1 amputation. Their preferred treatment modality was total graft excision. Fourteen cases handled without revascularization were done, with 3 deaths and 5 amputations, while 6 done with concomitant EAB all did well. Their overall mortality was therefore 37% with 37% amputation, but the best results were seen with total graft excision and EAB. However, the paper emphasized their feeling that revascularization could be delayed or even avoided in many patients after aortic limb or full aortic graft excision, and they felt that revascularization should be done only when clinically indicated by profound ischemia following graft excision. This point is interesting because it is not truly borne out by their results. As they state in the paper, the mortality was 75% for combined therapy versus 21% for graft excision only, but their best results were no mortality in six patients who underwent total excision and immediate EAB.

Spanos (1975) presented 7 cases from Minnesota, 2 of which were GIFs. Both presented shortly after surgery, one with an abscess and the second with an infected PA. Both underwent graft resection and EAB successfully. They made the further point that only 2 of the 4 long-term survivors of the series of 7 were actually symptom free.[20]

Jamieson (1975) reported the Rochester experience with 15 GIFs. He noted a 7.3% incidence of GIF in 664 revascularizations and reported that while antibiotics were not always used, that in cases in which they definitely were used, the rate of GIF decreased to 2.2% (11/510). Graft infections occurred in 3.2% (10/315) cases involving a groin incision but only 0.9% (3/325) (NSS) of cases not involving the groin. Groin wound complications were also implicated; there were 4 in 22 cases with wound problems versus 6 in 293 cases without wound problems (P < .01). The incidence was higher after ruptured (4/53) versus elective (5/314) aneurysmorrhaphy but not significantly. Bacteria were *S aureus* in 7, *E. coli* in 6, *Klebsiella* in 2, and 1 each of *Streptococcus*

and *Pseudomonas*. All of these findings echoed those of previous institutional surveys. Treatment varied over this 18-year period. Four patients receiving no specific treatment had fatal results. Three underwent graft excision only, with 1 mortality, 1 amputation, and 1 persistent GIF. Five underwent graft resection and EAB with 2 mortalities.[21] The report added little to the known protocols of decisions for management, but underscored the problems of the inguinal incision in urgent and/or redo situations as an etiologic agent in development of GIF.

Becker (1976) presented 14 cases of which 9 were GIFs. Infected grafts were Teflon in 6, Dacron in 5, and unknown in 3. Presenting symptoms were abscess in 8 and PA in the remainder; presentation was acute in 4 cases and from 3 to 7 months postoperatively in 4. Bacteria were *S aureus, S epidermidis,* and *E. coli* in 4 each; *Enterococcus* and *P mirabilis* in 2 each, and *Klebsiella* and *Candida* in 1 each. His paper noted poor results with attempts at local therapy and suggested that it was appropriate only if intra-abdominal infection was ruled out; however, he did not specify how that determination should be made. A further unsupported conclusion was that the pseudointima did not harbor infection and the suggestion that exposed graft sections were the problem (note: laboratory evidence now would not support this conclusion, See Section II). Three patients in the series had undergone prior cholecystectomy or gastrostomy, but no visceral procedure was involved in the other 11 cases. Treatment was by local therapy in 9 with 4 failures, 3 mortalities, and 2 amputations, and only 1 survivor with both limbs intact. Four patients underwent graft excision and EAB after failure of local therapy, with 2 additional mortalities and 2 amputations. The overall results in their small series were poor, but emphasized the morbidity and mortality after failure of attempts at local therapy.[22]

Crawford (1977) presented a large series of aortic graft complications in 1287 patients undergoing AR or AAA over 20 years; there was an overall 6.4% incidence of late complications with a 12% mortality and 6% amputation rate. I would be remiss at this point in the literature review if I did not quietly emphasize these statistics regarding the true morbidity of aortic surgery and suggest that more vascular surgeons should remember these figures when they so blithely recommend (on grounds of improved patency rates) that aortic surgery should always be considered the first approach to revascularization in obstructive disease.

Seven of Crawford's cases were GIFs, all in Dacron grafts. All occurred after reoperation and were delayed presentations at the groin. Concomitant visceral surgery had been done routinely during the series, including cholecystectomy, colostomy, a gastric procedure, and appendectomy, yet there was no GIF associated with those visceral procedures. Therapy involved local therapy in 1 with amputation and mortality, graft excision only in 4 with 2 mortalities and 2 amputations, and 6 were treated with graft excision and EAB with only 1 amputation and 1 mortality.[23] Despite the actual good experience with this last modality, the authors recommended that aortic GIFs presenting as groin problems be suppressed with antibiotics for as long as possible until secondary complications forced graft excision. This recommendation was based on anecdotal experience with a single patient (a federal judge) who went 16 years with a draining groin sinus and a patent graft. Their stated indications for more aggressive therapy included uncontrolled infection, graft thrombosis, or hemorrhage. If an EAB were to be done, they performed the EAB first and total graft resection second to avoid prolonged limb ischemia. The paper thus underscores the reality of long-term complications following with aortic surgery, and suggested for the first time that axillofemoral grafting precede graft resection to minimize operative trauma via increased limb ischemic times.

Christenson (1977) presented a series from Sweden of 14 patients seen over 15 years. Graft infections occurred in 2% (4/180) of abdominal anastomoses and 19% (10/54) of groin anastomoses ($P < .001$); 6 of the 10 groin infections were preceded by wound hematomas. The bacteria were *S aureus* in 12, *Enterococcus* in 3, and *Streptococcus* or *E. coli* in 1 each. Treatment was not specified as to aortic or peripheral site, but stated that excision and EAB was successful in 5. Local therapy was successful in 3, but this included thrombosis of the graft with limb salvage by collaterals. Overall there were 4 deaths (28%) and 4 amputations (35%). The authors noted that antibiotics alone failed in two patients who then underwent EAB.[24]

The results are confusingly presented but consistent with the few centers then reporting. The discussion, however, was important for emphasizing the surgeon's role at the primary revascularizations and outlined various principles of wound management, avoidance of concomitant nosocomial infections, and short preoperative hospitalizations.

Liekweg (1978) presented the first collective review of GIFs, and added 12 aortic and 11 peripheral GIFs from the Virginia experience. The incidence of GIF was 2.6% (22/859). Presenting symptoms were a sinus in 12, PA in 3, hemorrhage in 3, sepsis in 2, and thrombosis in 1. Overall mortality and amputation rates were 46% (3/11) and 50% for aortic GIFs, and 27% (3/11) and 63% for peripheral cases. For aortic cases, 5 were treated locally with no deaths and 2 amputations, 3 had graft excision, all with fatal results, and 3 underwent graft excision with EAB, all with fatal results. For peripheral cases, 9 attempts at local therapy resulted in 2 deaths and 5 amputations, while 2 patients who underwent excisions with EAB recovered uneventfully.[25]

This paper was one of the first to use the poetic license of combining aortic and peripheral results in an effort to show an overall lower mortality; however, the results of either category taken individually were equivalently as poor as other series of that time frame. Taken at face value, their results would suggest that peripheral GIFs were best handled with EAB, and that no conclusion could be made for aortic GIFs, since they had uniform fatality with any aggressive treatment and little better results with local therapy, where only two patients of five did well. Despite this paper being a frequently cited source for management protocols (as a review paper), the truth is that the results are too poor to lend themselves to a recommendation of any sort.

Scobie (1978) presented 11 patients culled from 407 aortic grafts done in Ottawa over 10 years for a 2.7% incidence; 6 of these were GEF or graft-enteric erosion (GEE). All patients had been on a protocol of 8 days perioperative prophylactic antibiotics and careful perioperative care. Routine intestinal bag cultures were performed in 144 patients and positive in 14, none of which correlated with GIFs. Graft infection-graft-enteric erosion occurred in 5.5% of 73 ruptured aneurysms, 2.8% of 181 elective aneurysms, and 1.3% of aortic reconstructions; 5 were Dacron and 6 Teflon. Bacteria were Gram negative in 7 and positive in 5; 7 *E coli*, 4 *S aureus*, 3 *Klebsiella*, 2 each *Pseudomonas*, *Proteus mirabilis*, *Enterobacter*, and 1 each *Streptococcus* and *Bacteroides*. A potential source of nosocomial infection was noted in 2 of the 11 patients; 1 from wound infection of prior herniorrhaphy and 1 from genitourinary surgery performed 24 months following grafting. Presentation was by PA in 4, thrombosis in 3, and septic emboli in 3. Treatment was uniformly unsuccessful with aortic shaft involvement, with six of seven patients dying. For aortic GIF patients, 1 died at laparotomy for excision; 2 were unilateral onlay aortofemoral grafts and were successfully excised without reconstruction; 2 had partial resection and EAB, 1 of whom died.[26]

Scobie's emphasis was properly placed on preventive measures, since operative results were uniformly poor with an overall 65% mortality (7/11) for the combined procedures. He carefully outlined all of the perioperative measures to reduce nosocomial infection and intraoperative measures to reduce GEF, most of which are covered in detail in Section II.

Yashar (1978) reviewed the institutional experience at Rhode Island in 590 patients over 11 years. The incidence of GIF was 9% in 230 RASV peripheral reconstructions and 2.5% in 590 prosthetic reconstructions. This varied from 1.3% (4/300) aneurysm cases, 2.4% (5/210) for aortobifemoral bypass (ABFB), 4.6% (3/65) for FP, to 20% (3/15) for AxF cases. In this last category, 5 AxFs were done for other GIFs and 2 of these 5 resulted in a secondary AxF GIF. Two GIFs were shown to be of hematogenous origin; one following abdominal wound infection and dehiscence, the other from pedal sepsis. In addition, one aortic GIF was secondary to ureteral injury with leakage. Thirty-three percent of the GIFs followed groin wound hematomas at initial operation. Bacteria were *S aureus* and *Pseudomonas* in 6 cases each. Presentation was acute in 8 and delayed in 7. Treatment of 5 aortic GIFs was by total excision and EAB, with 2 mortalities and 1 amputation. One additional aortic case was treated locally without problem. Six peripheral GIFs were treated without specific description of that treatment, with no deaths but 2 amputations.[27]

A paper by Yashar et al. suggested that trials of local therapy be limited to 6 weeks. If patients are unsuccessfully treated up to that point, they should undergo graft excision and EAB. Local therapy should not be considered if anastomoses were involved, if the GIF was of early onset, and if the graft was thrombosed. All of these represented reasonable speculations on their part, if not per se supported by the limited data of their clinical experience, and have become basic tenets of a preliminary trial of local therapy.

Casali (1980) presented the Arkansas experience with 20 cases, representing a GIF rate of 3.1% for 652 total reconstructions.

The paper described 14 AR GIFs, 3 FPs, and 3 assorted cases. The bacteria were *S aureus* in 14, *E coli* or *Pseudomonas* in 5 apiece, *Enterococcus* in 4, and 1 each for *Serratia*, *Salmonella*, and *Bacteroides*. The overall mortality was 64% for AR and 33% for FP. They recommended a trial of local therapy first, followed by partial graft excision and EAB. In 9 graft excisions alone, they had 6 mortalities and 3 amputations, and with 5 excisions and EAB, they had 3 mortalities. All three attempts at total graft excision in this series resulted in fatalities. Basically, the universal high mortality in this series precludes any meaningful conclusions as to appropriate therapy.[28]

Courmier (1980) presented a confusing mixture of cases which appear to be 2 GEFs, 10 infected aortoiliacofemoral thromboendarterectomies and 17 GIFs, 12 primary and 5 reinfections. The incidence of GIF was 0.76% at that institution (8/1057). Four cases in the series were culture proven to be due to bacteremias, 1 perioperatively and 3 at later periods of graft implantation with GIF then becoming evident 3 to 4 months subsequently. The management for an iliac-ofemoral-infected thromboendarterectomy was obturator or cross-femoral grafts with exclusion of the infected segment. For GIFs, 7 underwent excision only with 4 amputations and 1 death, and 17 underwent excision and EAB with 4 septic deaths. Courmier also noted routine usage of omental plications in 49 patients with poor duodenal tissue, inadequate retroperitoneal tissue for closure, or postmycotic aneurysm resection, and stated that all healed uneventfully.[29]

In the early 1980s a rash of articles appeared describing successful treatment of inguinal presentation GIFs by local antiseptic or antibiotic irrigations, indicating a resurgence of interest in this seemingly less rigorous approach to GIF management.

Popovsky (1980) presented 3 cases of GIF at the groin, after 2 AxF and 1 femoral reconstruction. All were treated locally with continuous antibiotic irrigation and debridement and all healed and stayed free of

problems for 3-years follow-up. Kwaan and Connolly (1981) presented a similar small series of locally treated patients, describing successful management of inguinal presentation of GIF in 10 patients using continuous povidone-iodine irrigations followed by wound closure. The grafts were AR in 5, AxF in 3, and CF in 2, all Dacron grafts. Bacteria were *S aureus* in 6 and *Pseudomonas* in 4. There was one late graft thrombosis. Knight (1983) presented a single case of an aortic shaft GIF with *Fusobacterium necrophorum* treated with povidone-iodine irrigation for 18 days. Follow-up CAT scan at 2 years showed no residual infection. The novel therapy was chosen because the patient was 88 years old and developed the GIF as a complication of colonic ischemia following ruptured aortic aneurysmorrhaphy.[30–32]

Ghosn (1983) reported on 13 ABFB GIFs presenting at the groin, representing a 2% incidence in 605 grafts performed over a 10-year period. All grafts were Dacron. Four presented early and 9 later than 1 year. Bacteria were *S aureus* in 10, and 1 each *P mirabilis*, *Bacteroides*, and *E coli*. All were treated with local debridements and irrigations, with 3 mortalities, and 3 amputations. In addition there were 2 late thromboses, 2 late PAs, and 1 persistent GIF (sinus).[33] The authors presented these data as enthusiastic support for local therapy, comparing their results equivalent to the current mortality rates with formal resection. I would submit that there were realistically only two long-term successes in 13 tries, which hardly supports their advocacy of local treatment.

Lorentzen in 1984 published the national experience of Denmark with local treatment, presenting 62 GIFs representing a 2.6% incidence in 2411 synthetic graft placements over 4 years. Fifty-three percent of cases presented within 30 days of reconstruction; the incidence of aortic GIF was the same for primary AR and AAA. All cases involved an inguinal incision at primary surgery. The highest incidence was 5.9% for ABFB/AAA, while AR-ABFB had a 3%, and FP a 3.5% incidence. The type of graft was also studied and involved knitted Dacron in 2.1%, woven Dacron in 2.3%, PTFE (mostly peripheral grafts) in 4.8%, and velour Dacron in 3%. Thirty-six percent of patients had pedal sepsis (ulcer or gangrene) at original operation but the culture of their GIF correlated with pedal culture only in four. Twenty percent had a urinary tract infection or pneumonia at first operation. Forty-eight percent suffered inguinal wound complications and 11% represented reoperations. Bacteria were *S aureus* in 47%, *S epidermidis* 27%, *Enterococcus* 15%, *E coli* 11%, *Bacteroides* 8%, *Klebsiella* 6.5%, *P mirabilis* 3.2%, *Pseudomonas* 1.6%, and other in 6.5%.

The authors attempted to apply the principles of orthopedic prosthesis infection management to GIFs. Eighty-five procedures were done in 62 patients. For aortic GIF, local therapy in 31 patients failed in 13; partial graft excision was then attempted in 26 and failed in 5. Five total graft excisions were successful. Tables, which summarize the last treatment the patient underwent and give the mortality and morbidity results, are somewhat confusingly presented in the paper . Local care in 18 resulted in 9 deaths and 2 amputations. Partial excision without revascularization in 3 resulted in 1 death and 2 amputations; partial excision with revascularization in 18 resulted in 2 deaths, 3 amputations, and 2 persistent GIFs. Total excision without revascularization in 3 patients resulted in amputation in all 3 while total excision and EAB in 2 was successful in both.

For FP GIFs, there were 2 failures in 7 attempts at local therapy and failure in 4 of 6 partial graft excisions. All 11 patients undergoing total graft excision did well. Listed in terms of the last procedure performed, there were 2 amputations and 1 death for 5 treated locally, 1 death and 1 amputation for 2 undergoing partial graft resection without revascularization, 1 death and 6 amputations for total graft excision without revascularization, and no problems

in the 2 treated by total graft excision and EAB.[34]

The authors use this extensive and well-tabulated experience with 62 patients to advocate a graduated plan of local therapy followed by partial graft excision, with total resection reserved as a last resort. I do not feel that their data support that claim. The group with the most success was the total graft excision-EAB group. Conversely, they had a 33% failure rate for aortic GIF treated locally and when this was the only treatment modality there was a 50% mortality! For FP GIFs, only total graft excision was uniformly successful in eliminating infection, and if revascularization was not simultaneously offered, the amputation rate was 85%! Their data would support partial graft resection with revascularization for single limb aortic GIF cases. A 20% failure rate with 10% mortality and 15% amputation is certainly reasonable.

The major conclusions of the authors regarding etiology are, however, well documented and certainly bear reemphasis. They stressed the role of expert, gentle, careful vascular surgical technique in avoiding the initial problem which might lead to subsequent GIF. Seventy-five percent of their series had postoperative complications and half had problems with the inguinal incision. No differential resistance for the types of synthetic graft used could be discerned in this report. The authors drew the appropriate parallel with orthopedic surgical methods of managing total hip or knee prosthetic replacements and noted that their sister service had managed to historically decrease the incidence of catastrophic infection in their specialty by strict protocols of perioperative antisepsis and surgical technique.

Almgren (1985) presented a varied series of 43 patients treated preferentially with local therapy. The series included 12 autologous grafts as well as 31 synthetic and/or composite grafts, so that evaluation of its conclusions must be colored by that inclusion. The incidence of AR GIF was

2.8% (22/780) and of FP GIF 2.1% (21/910). Bacteria were *S aureus* in 16 AR and 9 FP, and *E coli* in 8 AR and 6 FP. Local treatment of 9 aortic GIFs was successful in all 9; graft excision alone in 5 led to 1 mortality and 2 amputations; graft excision with EAB in 6 led to 2 mortalities and 1 amputation. For FP GIFs, local therapy was successful in 6 of 9 attempts of which 7 were autologous. Three grafts thrombosed within 3 months. Ten patients underwent graft excision only with 6 amputations, all of whom had patent but infected grafts initially. Follow-up was stated to be 5 to 130 months with a mean of 50 months, but was not specifically further classified as to the type of graft.[35]

The authors use these data to advocate local therapy for both aortic and peripheral GIFs. The data for aortic grafts are certainly supportive of that conclusion, although one would have liked to see the specific data on how the nine aortic GIFs did, how thoroughly they were reevaluated, and over what time frame. The conclusion for peripheral GIF is logical and valid only for autologous grafts and cannot be applied to the management of synthetic grafts.

The next phase of the literature saw a series of papers reporting on moderate sized series of GIFs seen at major university centers and for the most part handled by formal graft resection. A steady trend toward decreasing operative mortalities was also with the most aggressive surgical approaches. The first of these was for the San Francisco group by Ehrenfeld in 1979, with that data updated by Reilly in 1984 and then again in 1988. A similar UCLA experience was reported by Martin-Paredo in 1983 and updated by Quinnones-Baldrich in 1990. Yeager presented the Oregon experience in 1984 and updated it in 1990. (One can ask the obvious question as to why there were so many GIFs centered on the West Coast during that decade?) My own experience with 20 patients was dismally reported in 1983 and then updated to a much more sanguine report with 55 new patients in 1992.

Ehrenfeld (1979) presented a series of 24 GIFs (16 aortic, 4 peripheral, and 4 miscellaneous) who were all managed by total graft excision and some variety of immediate revascularization. The operative mortality was said to be 13% and amputation rate 9%. Actually, the mortality for aortic GIF was 20% (3/15) and amputation rate 14% (2/15). Typical of the presentations from this group over the next decade, the abstract heralded a lower mortality than was actually documented in the paper. Reconstruction involved composite synthetic/autologous grafts in 5, venous grafts in 3, arterial graft in 1, and endarterectomized superficial femoral artery aortoiliac conduits in 4. This latter technique was used for in situ reconstruction and was said by the authors to hold up both acutely in the face of infection and long-term in terms of continued patency. However, no supporting data were given.[36]

Endarterectomized superficial femoral artery (SFA) presents an interesting conceptual problem as to long-term patency since it effectively represents a technical model for thrombosis. The graft is a collagen tube further compromised by total ex vivo operative handling to induce the maximum conditions for intense fibrointimal hyperplasia. One would therefore expect a high thrombosis rate at 18 months to 3 years. In addition, the natural history of the homograft collagen tube in an infected field was aneurysmal formation and/or disruption. It is not unlikely that the SFA tube would display a similar predilection. None of the several USF articles on GIF have delineated the 3- and 5-year patency or secondary graft failure rates of these SFA reconstructions, which are certainly necessary in order to know precisely how viable this reconstruction fares as compared to synthetic revascularizations.

The other conceptual problems to SFA use are technical. Less than one third of all GIF/GEF patients will have an available thrombosed SFA to use. In addition, the modality demands graft excision combined with revascularization, which makes for maximum operating times and operative stress (both to patient and surgical team). All of these would seem to lessen the appeal of the SFA graft.

Reilly (1984) gave an expanded follow-up on the USF series, which now totaled 92 GIFs over 17 years. (All statistics listed here are corrected for 12 GEEs and 33 GEFs also in the series, but covered later in that section.) The mean presentation of 51 aortic GIFs was 25 months, with 20% (10/51) presenting as graft thrombosis and 9% (8/51) as PA. The authors stressed that final diagnosis of a suspected GIF required formal exploration in 15% (9/59), with CAT scans, sinograms, and angiography being variably used or useful. All patients underwent total graft excision and EAB; 15 by prosthetic EAB and 39 by autologous in situ techniques. The overall mortality for these was stated to be 16% (8/51) with a 26% (13/51) amputation rate (the actual stated figure was 14% (8/59) and 25% (13/59) but are corrected to reflect 51 actual GIFs). However, the paper notes that an additional 12% died of "secondary infection and/or aortic stump sepsis," so that the real mortality for this series is closer to 28%! Long-term survival and quality of life was said to be normal in all cured patients.

Partial graft excision was attempted initially in 23 patients. One third died of sepsis or aortic stump sepsis, one third required total graft excision which was done without further mortality after the delay, and one third did well with that treatment alone. Secondary infection occurred in 3 of 15 EABs. They also noted differential mortality for the type of reconstruction, varying from 14% (8/56) treated by autologous reconstruction versus 41% (12/29) treated by prosthetic reconstruction (this includes cases of GEE/GEF). Aside from the under-reporting of the true mortality rate in their series, this extensive experience underscored the failure rate of partial graft excision and detailed a successful experience with total graft excision, particularly if autologous reconstruction could be obtained.[37]

Reilly again updated the experience in 1987,[38] specifically addressing the concept of staged versus sequential EAB grafting. There were 43 GEFs and 58 GIFs studied, resulting from 71 ABFBs, 26 AIBs, and 4 tube grafts. Mortality was again minimized in the abstract to 19% for GEF and 14% for GIF; however, 12 additional graft-related deaths occurred within 6 months, so that the actual mortalities were 37% and 21%, respectively.[39] Reilly defined four types of operative treatment:

> *traditional*: total graft excision and immediate secondary EAB
> *synchronous*: total graft excision and immediate in situ autologous reconstruction
> *staged*: initial EAB, followed at a median 5-day interval by graft resection
> *sequential*: initial EAB, followed immediately by graft resection

Other institutions presented small series during this decade, detailing good results. Fulenwider (1983) noted within a series of aortic redo cases that the Emory group had managed 11 patients with GIFs with total excision and EAB without mortality. Four of four attempts at partial graft resection were unsuccessful. They also specifically noted that three patients had undergone tertiary formal AR at a minimum 2-year interval, all without problem. Seeger (1983) presented 11 patients with groin infections, 10 after ABFB and 1 after AxF. Bacteriae were *S aureus* in 4, negative cultures (? *S epidermidis*) in 5, and 1 each *Enterobacter, Streptococcus,* and *Pseudomonas.* Fistulograms were positive in one of four, and gallium scans in one of three patients. Four patients were tried on local therapy, all with failure. Total graft resection and autologous reconstruction was performed with one mortality and one amputation. There were, however, six late failures with the saphenous vein reconstructions, usually due to vein graft stenosis that could be salvaged by secondary procedure.[40]

Trout (1984) summarized the literature

to that point to support his contention that staged bypass prior to formal aortic graft removal would result in lowered mortality rates. He stated that mortality fell from 75% (10/14) if resection preceded revascularization for GIF to 26% (6/23) if revascularization came first. Similar reduction was seen with GEF/GEE, where it fell from 53% (40/75) to 17% (5/29). He also presented 8 new cases from George Washington, of which 3 were aortic GIFs and 1 was peripheral. Two aortic GIFs were treated with sequential EAB followed at 72 hours by graft resection, with both patients dying from aortic stump sepsis. The third underwent single limb excision and EAB successfully.[41]

Edwards (1988) presented the Louisville experience with 18 patients over 6 years (three of whom had GEFs). Computerized tomography scan was positive in 3 of 4, and sinograms in 6 of 6. Three patients had undergone visceral procedures at initial surgery; 1 pyloroplasty, 1 cholecystectomy, and 1 gastrostomy. In three patients a definite hematogenous seeding could be delineated. All had *S aureus* GIFs after *S aureus* culture-positive septic venous thrombophlebitis. Local therapy was unsuccessful in 7 of 9 patients, which led to 7 partial graft excisions with 1 mortality and 2 aortoduodenal fistulae, and only 4 successes. Eight total graft excisions were done with 1 mortality only.[42]

Martin-Paredo (1983) presented the initial UCLA experience with 15 patients. The incidence of GIF was 2.6% (15/671)–sinograms were positive in 5 of 15. Bacteria were Gram negative in 50% and Gram positive in 25%. One patient underwent excision only; the remainder of the patients had total excision and EAB. Mortality was 39% (7/16) and amputation rate 28% (5/16). Those data were updated by Quinones-Baldrich (1990) to describe 45 patients. Thirty-seven involved Dacron, 3 PTFE, and 5 unknown material grafts. Mean interval to presentation was 40.3 months. Symptoms were abscess in 40%, PA in 20%, and GEF in 16%. Bacteria were *S aureus* in 21% and *Pseudomonas* in 21%. Nine patients underwent graft excision only with 4 mortalities; 36 underwent total graft resection and EAB with a 16% (6/36) mortality; overall mortality for the series of GIFs and GEFs was therefore 24% (11/45) with an amputation rate of 33% (15/45). Some cases were done as 1-stage procedures and some in staged fashion. There was no difference in the rate of secondary GIF; 5/33 for 1 stage and 1 of 3 2-stage procedures. Eighty-two percent of the series mortality occurred when there was total graft infection. Long-term survival of patients in the series was 55% at 3 years and 49% at 5 years.[43,44]

Yeager (1985) presented the initial Oregon experience noting 25 cases (10 AR, 11 FP) over 10 years. Eight involved GEE or GEF, leaving 6 aortic and 11 FP GIFs for analysis. All grafts were Dacron. Presentation was at a median 260 weeks for aortic versus 35 weeks for peripheral grafts ($P <$ .05). Nine of 11 aortic GIFs presented with groin abscesses. Computer tomography scans were positive in 5 of 5, sinograms in 2 of 3, and indium scans in 1 of 2. Partial resection was attempted in 5 and was unsuccessful in all. Total graft excision with EAB was performed in six with 50% mortality. Peripheral GIFs were treated by excision alone in 6, with 3 mortalities and 2 amputations, and by excision with EAB in 5, with 1 mortality and amputation. Autogenous reconstruction was performed in 5 AR and 5 FP GIFs and all did well.

That experience was updated by Yeager (1990) with 23 GIFs being presented among 38 total cases. Computer tomography scan proved useful in 12 of 16 cases, with 10 showing definite signs and 2 more showing inflammatory changes without fluid. Indium scans were positive in 5 of 6, and sinograms in 2 of 2. Bacteria were *S epidermidis* in 12, *S aureus* in 5, *Streptococcus* in 5, *E coli* in 2, and 1 each for *Enterococcus*, *Bacteroides*, *Klebsiella*, and *Candida*. In the combined series of 23 GIFs and 15 GEFs, total excision with EAB was performed in 38 with 26% mortality (10/38) and 5-year survival of 52%; the mortality was 22% for 23 aortic GIFs. Twenty-two percent of EABs become secondarily infected, with high amputation rates; the cumulative 5-year survival was, however, 76%.[45,46]

Three successive series were then published that gave considerable impetus to the concept that local management of graft infections could be carried out safely. All three gave 80% to 90% cure rates in a mixed series of aortic, peripheral, and unusual site graft infections.

The first of these was Mixter (1989), who presented 8 aortic grafts among 21 patients. Seventeen of these were groin wound infections (20 wounds). The overall rate of successful wound healing was 92%, with one failure and one death; the mortality occurred in the aortic cohort. Follow-up averaged 30 months (4 to 102 months) with 11 of the 20 survivors being followed less than 3 years. The authors used mafenide for their dressing changes, stating that wounds were more rapidly sterilized, and advocated wound closure within 7 days to prevent secondary Gram-negative or fungal wound colonization. They also clearly delineated between an early wound infection with the graft bathed in purulence and the early wound infection that exposes but only contaminates the graft by contiguous soft tissue inflammation. They felt that bacterial penetration into the graft matrix mitigated against successful local control and specifically noted that "grafts with transmural infection, anastomotic breakdown (pseudoaneurysm), gastrointestinal fistulae, or limb occlusions" were not considered for local therapy and that these grafts required excision.[47]

The second series was presented in a series of related papers by Calligaro et al. (1990 to 1992). Calligaro (1990) summarized the 20-year experience at Montefiore with local treatment of GIFs presenting at the groin. In this and two related articles from 1991 to 1992, Calligaro outlined the generic principles for local therapy that include both contraindications to its use and specifics of management.

Calligaro (1990) reported on 28 patients with groin presentations of GIF, including two Dacron aortic and 31 peripheral PTFE grafts. He recommended incomplete excision of thrombosed grafts, leaving a rim of graft on the donor vessel, and local therapy if there was no systemic sepsis or anastomotic hemorrhage. The follow-up on these cases averaged 3 years (1 to 10) and resulted in an 11% (3/28) hospital mortality and 13% (4/30) amputation rate. Failure of the local treatment occurred in 13%. An additional three patients had late disruption at 8 months, 2 years, and 4 years after treatment.[48]

Looking at these figures in detail, there were 10 patients with graft preservation, with 1 septic death and 1 failure; and 16 cases with occluded grafts, 8 of which were revascularized after excision. Of 28 total patients, 3 died; 1 of sepsis, 1 of anastomotic hemorrhage, and the third of a myocardial infarction. Then there were four immediate and three late failures for a failure rate (death/failure) of 36% (10/28). There were no data given as to the long-term PA or thrombosis rate that might have indicated further failures.

This widely publicized study involved only two aortic grafts and is therefore a study of graft preservations at the groin of peripheral grafts. An 11% mortality and 13% amputation rate are acceptable but certainly not the best reported results in this situation. The salient point of graft preservation is credible, but I would point out that EAB reconstruction and graft excision is certainly a more cost-effective way of dealing with this problem. Conversely, local therapy of an aortic graft leaves the patient at a distinct risk for potentially fatal complications of ascending infection. Finally, the long-term follow-up notes recurrent infection only and does not mention unexplained (? septic-anastomotic) deaths, nor does it indicate the rates of subsequent PA or thrombosis, both of which would be expected long-term complications of an occultly infected graft.

Perler[49] presented the Johns Hopkins experince with local rotational flap therapy for 22 wounds in 19 patients, of which 9 were aortofemoral grafts. Local therapy with antibiotics and wound debridements were performed for up to 30 days prior to definitive wound closure with rotational muscle flaps. The operative mortality was 5.3%, and failures during hospitalization noted in an additional 17.6%. For aortic patients there was one mortality and one failure with ascending infection that led to mortality at excision and EAB. Follow-up for the entire series was for a mean 30 months. There was one graft thrombosis and four deaths within 6 months that were not further characterized. Perler noted success with all 12 infections in the series that presented acutely, but only 3 of 5 which presented chronically. They furthermore did not have difficulty with Gram-negative infections.

Ricotta (1991) presented a series culled from several surgeons at different sites and included 24 GIFs over 15 years. The mean interval to presentation was 34 months; presentation was groin sepsis in 11, PA in 9, and graft thrombosis in 6. Computer tomography scan was positive in 16 of 17 cases. Three of 12 partial resections recurred and required total excision, with 1 interval mortality. Partial excision with or without revascularization was performed in 12 patients with 4 mortalities and 1 amputation, so that nearly half of that cohort failed treatment. Total excision without revascularization was done in 2, with 1 mortality and 1 amputation, and total with EAB was done in 18 with 17% mortality and 13% amputation rates. Life-table analysis of survival for this last treatment group was 71% at 6 years.[50]

We presented our initial experience with 20 graft infections in 1983; 14 of these were aortic, including 1 each of GEE and GEF. Within that series was the first *Salmonella* primary GIF[51]; most of the series were Gram-negative infections. Operations were combined and averaged more than 10 hours. The mortality for the aortic GIFs was 80%.[52]

In 1983, we began a prospective protocol of management that included routine staged operations (revascularization first followed by graft excision 4 to 5 days later) and routine ventricular function monitoring as well as nitroglycerine-induced volume loading. In 1993 we published our results with a 9% (2/22) mortality for aortic GIFs and no mortality in 33 peripheral graft infections.[53] Although 18 of the 22 were *S epidermidis* chronic GIFs presenting with PA or limb thrombosis, we saw no mortality or amputation in the 18 patients handled with total graft excision and EAB. There were no subsequent episodes of ASS or GEF, and the short-term (1 year) EAB patency was 92% (17/18) and secondary patency 100%. These results need to be kept in mind when evaluating studies advocating in situ or local therapy of *S epidermidis* infections. Such series usually compare mortality and morbidity results to the collective review statistics on GIF or to recent studies that include more virulent organisms.[52,53]

Bandyk (1991) presented a carefully outlined plan for highly selective use of in situ replacement of synthetic grafts with highly successful early results in 15 patients. All had *S epidermidis* infections, 14 of these being of aortofemoral grafts; all were chronic presentations at an average 70 ± 16 months postinitial revascularization. Seven presented with pseudoaneurysm, 6 with graft purulence, and 4 with sinus tracts. All were treated by complete local graft excision as well as debridement of the infected tissue bed, followed by an in situ PTFE prosthesis. There were no deaths, graft infection recurrences, or thromboses at an average 21 month (5 to 50 months) follow-up. There were 4 late deaths said to be unrelated to infection; 2 of these showed no signs of infection at autopsy at 5 and 24 months. Follow-up duplex scans were performed and demonstrated three persistent perigraft fluid collections, and one patient had a late thrombosis (3 years) responding to thrombectomy. The authors limited their patients to those with limited groin presentation of *S epidermidis*, and specifically recommended that the technique not be attempted if it was an early or acute GIF (< 4 months), with sepsis with bacteria other than *S epidermidis*, current anastomotic hemorrhage, or proximal problems such as GEF or GEE.[54]

This study was based on a wealth of careful supporting studies from the laboratory, which are presented elsewhere (Section II). The most recent studies by Bandyk's group have used antibiotic-impregnated PTFE grafts in a canine model of in situ intra-abdominal aortic graft treatment. It is of great interest in that model that nearly half of the nonimpregnated grafts showed persistent biofilm infection despite clinical healing. This was reduced significantly, but not eliminated by the silver pefloxacin-impregnated graft. Bandyk presents these data elsewhere, but I would strongly caution against an in situ replacement of a nonimpregnated graft at this time, since the laboratory clearly shows persistence of infection (e.g., inadequate treatment) in 30% to 50%.

Finally, rereading the data presented above would show that 14 aortic graft infections treated with in situ management resulted in no deaths but technically in three (20%), all of whom had perigraft fluid demonstrable at the aortic prosthesis just proximal to the in situ graft. That to me is an ominous sign of potential future aortic GIF and GEF/ASS, which must be considered in the evaluation of the success of this technique. It certainly would indicate extreme caution in attempting in situ replacement with any other bacteria than *S epidermidis*. One would not want to incur proximal aortic prosthetic infection as a failure of the method with some more virulent bacteria.[51]

Staged versus Sequential Operations

Although the potential advantages of staged resection-revascularization had been theorized by Crawford (1979), the first series detailing the potential benefits of this approach was by Reilly (1987), as above. Other series have also suggested the benefits of staged procedures.[23,39,53,55]

Turnipseed (1983) studied 12 GIFs and 8 GEFs seen over a 4-year period, all treated by total graft excision and EAB. Forty-five percent of these had encountered early postoperative complications at first surgery. Nine presented as PA, 7 as graft thrombosis, and 2 as a kinked graft. Bacteria were *S aureus* in 10, *E coli* in 4, *Pseudomonas* in 4, and *Klebsiella* or *Bacteroides* in 1 each. Two attempts at partial excision failed and came to total resection. Seven patients underwent combined resection and EAB with 4 mortalities and 1 amputation, whereas 13 undergoing resection followed by revascularization delayed from 8 hours to 3 months, had 4 mortalities and 2 amputations. Average anesthesia time decreased from 7.5 to 5.5 hours and average transfusions from 5 to 3 units.[55]

Turnipseed asserted that collateral flow at the groins should be maintained by patch angioplasty rather than vessel ligation, and that an on-table ankle-arm index of 0.3 at the conclusion of the graft resection demonstrated sufficient collateral limb flow to indicate delayed revascularization. One can argue that the results in the two groups are not really comparable, since delayed reconstructions were done in those patients with sufficient flow to warrant it and conversely that patients further compromised by the acute ischemia were forced into the prolonged operative stress and would therefore have predictably suffered a higher mortality. The series does, however, support the concept of staged procedures.

Reilly's paper on sequential versus staged versus combined procedures presented an extensive analysis of various parameters of metabolic and physiologic stress which were interpreted in the text to show an advantage to staged resections for reduced operative time, crystalloid infusion, and transfusion requirements. In addition, there was a significant ($P < .05$ to $P < .01$) reduction in operative-perioperative acidosis for any procedure involving initial EAB placement.

Operative mortality tended to be lower with staged procedures 26% (5/19) and sequential 24% (9/38) as opposed to traditional 43% (3/7) or synchronous 35% (7/20). However, this trend did not reach significance. Amputation rates were significantly ($P < .05$) decreased for sequential (11%) and nonsignificantly($P = 0.17$) for staged (16%) as compared to synchronous (25%), traditional (57%), or excision without revascularization (47%). They further looked at new GIFs of the implanted EAB reporting an overall 20% incidence, falling from 43% with traditional to 16% staged and 18% sequential.

Reilly interpreted these results to show that preliminary EAB would reduce total physiologic stress to the patient by providing flow to the limbs and thus preventing the advent of perioperative acidosis. They stated that staged procedures offered less metabolic stress than sequential. Although I agree in principle, I fail to see that the data generated within the paper actually prove their point. In fact, the comparison made is not valid because the parameters for the first of the two staged operations only are compared to the combined parameters of both operations for sequential and traditional methods. If one adds the two operations of staged procedures together, there is actually more operative time and crystalloid used than in the combined operations. Such sleight of hand use of the statistics is inappropriate.

The third point to Reilly's article is that secondary EAB GIF occurs quite frequently (20% of cases) and may be a factor in considering synchronous operations. Furthermore, this group saw no differences in the incidence of secondary GIF for staged or sequential. At face value, the latter statement makes little sense. One would expect a very low GIF rate for what is essentially a clean elective EAB, unless secondary bacteremias are the cause of the secondary GIFs, an unproven point. Yet the paper could not correlate septicemias with the development of GIF-EAB.

I would suggest that the 20% rate seen is excessive, and that other factors are responsible. However, the theoretical risk of what is essentially a *nosocomial* secondary GIF due to the presence of the remote primary GIF source might suggest that a prudent course is to provide staged procedures only when: a) there is no concomitant sepsis, and b) a suitable time interval for wound healing of the EAB can be secured before graft resection is required (7 to 10 days?).

In the discussion of this paper when it was presented, I noted that we had specifically addressed the effect of the prolonged operative times necessary to do a combined (sequential, synchronous, or traditional) procedure by looking at ventricular function. At the time we were involved in an intensive perioperative monitoring protocol, and were able to perform aortic surgery on 60 patients of all degrees of cardiac decompensation, without seeing the expected decreases in cardiac function at aortic cross-clamping and declamping. We looked at the time courses of ventricular function in several patients undergoing traditional versus staged procedures and were able to show that there was a steady decline in ventricular function in patients undergoing prolonged procedures (> 7 hours), whereas that function could be preserved if the operations were staged and each was less than 6 hours.[56,57]

My personal experience is in favor of staged operations and was presented in 1993. I have personally managed 33 aortic graft infections. The first 11 were performed as staged operations, usually lasting 10 to 12 hours, and with an 80% mortality. In 1983, I began a prospective protocol for management that included routine staging and have performed resection-EAB in 22 patients with 9% (2/22) mortality. Other factors figured in this low mortality rate, but staging was undoubtedly a major factor.[53]

Thus, on theoretical grounds (decreased operative stress, limited limb ischemia), clinical experience, and some small laboratory corroboration, we would advocate routine staged procedures.

The major remaining problem with EAB is the question of patency. There are now a number of reports detailing 75% to 80% 5-year patencies of axillofemoral grafts, indicating better patency rates associated with an increased familiarity with this operation. However, we would take the position that interval redo retroperitoneal AR or thoracofemoral grafting be strongly considered for those patients who return with axilofemoral thromboses, particularly if they are younger and/or in good health.

Discussion

The complete review of all graft infection papers published to date and presented in the preceding pages should provoke some conclusions on the reviewer's part (Table 1).

First, few published series involved sufficient numbers of any one variety of infection to actually make valid conclusions about the management of specific clinical situations. Only 9 had 10 or more patients for review, and only 4 had more than 50. Seven of these involved a mix of aortic and peripheral GIFs with GEFs. It is clear that the results of management of each of these are as different as their clinical presentations and their pathophysiologic etiologies. In contrast, the extended series from UCLA, USF, and Denmark *do* represent an adequate experience at one institution, and also are useful for the fact that treatment protocols had some coherency and therefore comparative results could be analyzed. Similarly, my own published experience with 55 patients treated by one surgeon offers a reasonable control on the variables of multiple surgeons, multiple institutions.

Secondly, much of the poor image of GIF stems from this proliferation of papers detailing small experiences with GIF with multiple surgeons each handling few individual cases, almost on a random basis. Most major problems such as GIF require a distinct learning curve before mortality rates can be expected to decrease. Collected reviews such as my own (1983), or Liekweg (1977) and Calligaro (1991)[1,58] therefore tend

---

Table 1
Historical Perspective on the Development of Management Principles for Graft Infection

Javid	(1962)	The graft is a foreign body that potentiates infection and must be removed; in situ repairs therefore fail.
Hoffert	(1965)	Excessive amputation rates are seen after graft excision if revascularization is not done.
Fry Lindenauer	(1967)	Control of aortic infections requires total graft excision; partial excisions result in ascending infection.
Najafi	(1968)	Local therapy can be successful if there was now bleeding or systemic sepsis, and process is well localized.
Conn	(1970)	Gram-negative infections are more virulent than Gram positive.
Crawford	(1977)	Total graft excision should be done in stages to minimize ischemic time.
Yashar	(1978)	Attempts at local therapy should be limited to 6 weeks and failure at that time interval indicates graft excision.
Ehrenfeld	(1979)	Autologous reconstruction fares better than synthetic reconstruction in the infected field and can therefore be used to avoid extra-anatomic routes of reconstruction.

to collate the melange of poor results and provide what I believe is a decidedly distorted image of the problem. They also incidentally present an average that some author use (probably an invalid assumption) as a comparison for their own treatment protocols in an effort to show *improved* results. This has been particularly true for papers extolling the virtues of local therapy for the treatment of aortic graft infections at the groin.

I would candidly suggest that the real mortality of GIF management has markedly changed over the years, and that equivalently good mortalities may be obtained with a variety of either aggressive or less aggressive measures.

Whatever management modality is chosen, the current mortality for aortic GIF rate should be less than 20% and probably should more closely approach 10%; with amputation rates at 10% to 15%; and for peripheral infections should approach zero mortality and amputation rates. The long-term survival and subsequent lifestyle of survivors of GIF management should also be better than commonly held factors would suggest; 70% to 80% of these patients should do well.

However, as has been shown in related studies on the long-term morbidity of redo surgery, a fairly high percentage can be expected to need further revision. If the EAB reconstruction were AxF, then 25% to 30% will require subsequent thrombectomy to maintain patency. There will certainly be increasing utilization of delayed secondary aortic, ventral aortic, or thoracofemoral reconstruction to provide better long-term patencies in a sizable number of these patients.

A third summary point to this literature review is that most authors indulged themselves in a fair amount of speculation as to appropriate management despite the fact that they either had inadequate cases to support their speculation, or (as pointed out in the review) their actual results were inconsistent with their conclusions. This is one field in vascular surgery in which reams

of opinions have been voiced, but few hard data conclusions have been reasonably reached! The major purpose of this book, and the reason each paper has been so thoroughly critiqued, is to present the reader with a more balanced fact sheet on which to draw his own conclusions.

Treatment

The treatment of (synthetic) vascular graft infections has evolved over 40 years of clinical experience, with only a moderate amount of directly supportive evidence from the laboratory. A thoughtful surgeon should synthesize the myriad bits of evidence from all of these authors into a rational management plan.

First, it should be stated that there is no one single answer to the problem—that one method of management cannot and should not be routinely applied to all clinical situations. Rather, treatment must be highly individualized to include an appreciation of:

the age and medical condition as risk factors and likelihood long-term survival

the presence or absence of systemic sepsis

psychosocial factors including the likelihood of ambulation and cognitive abilities

the bacteria involved, particularly as to the presence of Gram-negative species

the site and presumed extent of infection

the type of graft involved

the site of graft (aortofemoral, iliacofemoral, etc).

the extent of revascularization that will be required

All of this is then to be modified by what is probably the most important factor in the decision—the institutional capability for support services coupled with the surgeon's experience with these difficult cases and willingness to commit a major portion of patient care time for what will probably be a week to month time frame.

Vascular graft infections represent the most difficult long-term complication of our revascularizations, with high mortality and morbidity rates. Vascular surgeons therefore have a real responsibility to be more keenly aware of their potential. Too often revascularization is urged on a patient for what, on reflection, are only moderately debilitating symptoms, and in my experience, too often without full reiteration of the potential disasters that such a revascularization might entail. This condemnatory critique applies as well to endovascular and nongraft-related vascular procedures in terms of the more usual acute complications of death or thrombosis resulting in worse symptoms or even limb loss. Claudication is a relatively benign situation. It is not in itself a cause of death except for those unfortunate few patients who then collectively comprise our operative mortality-morbidity statistics.

There is much that is understood regarding GIFs-GEFs, much that remains controversial, and much that needs more definitive study. Treatment modalities have been dominated by the concept of the synthetic graft as foreign body that potentiates the infection, which then leads logically to the concept of graft extirpation as a mainstay of treatment. Yet, there are active proponents of both local and in situ replacement therapy, neither of which conform to that maxim.

The basic principles of management have long been (Table 2):

1. excision of the graft as a foreign body
2. wide and complete debridement of devitalized and/or infected tissue to provide a clean wound for healing
3. maintain or reestablish flow to the distal bed
4. prolonged and specific antibiotic treatment to prevent and/or control systemic sepsis and locally invasive cellulitis

Table 2
Principles of Management for Graft Infection

1. Excision of the graft as a foreign body potentiating the infection
2. Wide and complete debridement of devitalized, infected tissue to provide a clean wound in which healing may occur
3. Maintain or establish vascular flow to the distal bed
4. Institute intensive and prolonged antibiotic coverage to reduce sepsis and prevent secondary graft infection

However, the actual application of these principles has been a number of extrapolations and interpretations.

1. Excision of the graft can be interpreted as total graft excision, excision totally or in part with in situ reconstruction, or as partial (one limb) excision with or without revascularization in situ or EAB.

2. Wide debridement to some is excision of the graft and its adherent debris, to other surgeons, excision of the fibrous sheath, or to some nibbling away the proximal aortic stump of obvious debris, while to others it requires resection of a sizable aortic segment back to normal nonfibrotic tissue.

3. Reestablishment of flow, while clearly accepted, has been felt by some to be best performed first (staged / sequential), by others to be after graft resection, and by a few authors to be avoided entirely unless obvious limb ischemia dictates it.

4. Long-term antibiotics although empirically obvious, are rarely used.

Furthermore, extra-anatomic reconstruction is being totally revamped, from the initial argument between an in situ autologous reconstruction versus axillofemoral, to now a resurgence of in situ allograft versus EAB, and even consideration of *newer* (forgetting Blaisdell in 1961) EABs such as thoracofemoral or retroperitoneal reconstructions.

It is of some interest to watch the evolution of the closely related issue of axillofemoral-iliacofemoral EAB versus AR as a primary operation. Ten years ago those of us who were advocates of EAB to reduce the perceived morbidity and mortality of AR, were routinely castigated for that advocacy; patency rates were so important, and the complications of aortic surgery were minimized. Now we have major groups on both coasts extolling EAB as a viable, long-term alternative to AR. This increased familiarity with primary EAB must effectively affect the efficacy of this reconstruction for GIF, and one can expect to see routine 70% to 80% 5-year patencies rather than some of the 30% to 50% rates currently being published for AxF post-GIF treatment.

We must not forget that the real common denominator to a successful result is the surgeon, demonstrated by the depth of understanding of the principles and wisdom in applying surgical judgment to each case (Table 3).

Specifically important are the details of the surgeon's:

Table 3
10 Principles for Aortic Graft Infection Management

---

1. Total graft excision is the best management protocol.
2. Staged procedure preferred to sequential procedure, and either to simultaneous.
3. Extra-anatomic clean plane reconstruction preferred to in situ reconstruction.
4. Intense hemodynamic monitoring is indicated for all aortic infections.
5. In-hospital total parenteral nutrition.
6. Single-layer closure aortic stump acceptable if normal aortic tissue is present.
7. Routine omental pedicle to aortic stump and aortic shaft bed.
8. Aortic cultures done routinely to direct long-term care.
9. Long-term antibiotics for positive aortic stump cultures.
10. Tertiary thoracofemoral reconstruction at 2 years.

---

technique: whether fast or slow—translated as increased tissue contamination and wound infection rates with increased operative times; sloppy or meticulous—translated as the frequency of wound hematomas, seromas, lymphococeles, all associated with GIF; or having too large a graft tunnel, with poor incorporation leading to perigraft fluid, or the attention paid to wound closure.

knowledge: in the choice of antibiotics, in the choice of reconstructive surgery to fix the clinical problem, in the choice of graft type.

carefulness: taking the time to perform careful dissections, taking the time to prevent GEF by various maneuvers, careful selection of graft size, careful attention to the hood of onlay grafts and to kinking or anterior angulation, check of mesenteric flow and/or inferior mesenteric artery reimplantation to avoid colonic ischemia.

malleability: to be able to change technique when faced with unusual anatomy (caval abnormalities, for example), pathology (inflammatory or mycotic aneurysm), or situations (hostile abdomen, dense adhesions, prior peritonitis).

All this preamble aside, the choice of therapy must be examined, first sequentially by each available method, and then, in summary, both of the results of such therapy and with our own critical footnotes.

Treatment Options

Some initial points need to be made in comparing the success rates of various therapies, which may skew the results of the summary statistics at the end of this section.

Graft exposure versus graft infection: a wound infection that causes wound breakdown and subsequent exposure of the anterior aspect of a deeper seated graft does not present the same clinical picture as a graft or graft limb that is freely submerged in pus and totally unincorporated. It is difficult to statistically address this issue, but conceptually the exposed graft is likely to be easier to handle and probably will respond to local therapy. Conversely, proximal extension of pus along the nonincorporated graft is a more likely possibility. Of course, the basic concept of persistent occult GIF due to matrix adherence by bacteria would remain a theoretical concept.

Whether or not the graft is thrombosed is a major factor in the decision for revascularization, since tolerance of the thrombosed graft without distal ischemia obviously mitigates the need for revascularization. This is not always clear in an author's tabulation of results and skews the morbidity rates accordingly. Conversely, many of the cases included in the excision only category did not undergo what was obviously a necessary revascularization, leading to amputation and sometimes death. Clearly excision alone is best and perhaps only indicated for management of a chronically thrombosed graft without distal ischemia.

Whether systemic sepsis is present: clearly systemic sepsis as a presenting clinical feature is associated with increased mortality, both from associated multiorgan and system failure and from the tendency toward uncontrolled or unrelieved postoperative sepsis leading to death.

Gram-positive versus Gram-negative infections, as opposed to merely being contaminants of the graft such as a positive culture from the graft at a GEE. Specific Gram-negative organisms (*Salmonella, Pseudomonas, Serratia, Proteus*) are recognized by most authors to carry prohibitive morbidity rates if complete graft excision and specific antibiotic control is not initiated and monitored. Pseudoaneurysms, anastomotic hemorrhages, and aortic stump sepsis are all common problems. Clearly these Gram-negative infections skew the results of authors if not clearly differentiated and managed appropriately.

S epidermidis versus *S aureus* or other Gram-positive organisms clearly affects both the clinical presentation (occult rather than acute presentation) and probably the result of therapy. Low mortality rates are associated with even total graft excision and EAB due to the absence of systemic sepsis and dense local inflammation complicating dissections.

Excision

Excision of the graft without revascularization clearly follows all the principles of GIF management, except revascularization. It therefore follows that excision alone is indicated for chronically (or sometimes acutely) thrombosed grafts in which there is no evidence of clinical ischemia due to preservation of collateral flow.

One must be careful to reassess distal flow on the operating table and in the first 6 to 12 hours because there may be compromise of that collateral circulation either due to operative dissection, to stenosis of the vessel by patch angioplasty or simple closure of the artery at time of excision, or due to unforeseen thrombosis/embolus into the collateral bed, usually associated with intraoperative hypotension. The safety of excisional therapy alone can not be assumed simply because the graft is already thrombosed.

The overall results of excisional therapy are not sanguine—33% (24/73) mortality and amputation rates in 73 tries. However, these are skewed by cases in which excision of patent grafts without revascularization led to problems.

Partial Graft Excision

Partial graft excision theoretically applies all of the principles of graft infection management, with the caveat that removal of the synthetic foreign body was indeed sufficiently accomplished by the removal of the one presumably infected segment. Revascularization is usually accomplished via an EAB approach, with obturator or crossfemoral approaches predominating.

Partial graft excision most usually applies to cases in which one limb of an aorto-femoral graft was resected for infection presumed to be limited to one groin. Documentation of this presumption has been based on CAT/leukocyte scans demonstrating no contralateral limb or aortic shaft problem and the notation of graft incorporation at time of initial approach. However, there is still room for error by failure to identify occult infection, a principle and problem clearly outlined in all the laboratory studies.

It may also be possible that some cases represent true reinfection of the graft stump via bacteremias or from ascending lymphatic draining the more distal infection where they find a convenient culture medium in the fresh retroperitoneal incision (hematoma), or by ascent along the non-obliterated residual fibrous tunnel.

The basic theoretical and indeed practical problem with this approach is the certainty that indeed foreign body removal has been attained. This is heightened by the disturbing realization that recurrent, persistent infection will of necessity involve the aortic shaft and thereby raise the specter of fatality from ASS. Indeed, this clinical scenario has been played out repeatedly. As a result, the literature is not very sanguine about the feasibility of the approach, with a 44% (47/106) failure rate. Although there is only a 19% (7/106) mortality and 20% (20/106) amputation, it is because most of these failures have then gone on to total excision usually with EAB and fatalities are reported in those categories (incidentally skewing the mortality for EAB as a class, since it includes patients requiring multiple operations). Failures have been reported in 2 of 2 by Turnipseed, 4 of 4 by Fulenwider, 5 of 5 by Yeager, 4 of 6 by Bunt, 4 of 8 by Edwards, and 3 of 12 by Ricotta. Reilly's series detailed attempts in 23 patients, one third of whom died with persistent infection and/or ASS, one third of whom required total excision-EAB, and only one third of whom actually did well with that therapy alone. Lorentzen similarly described 10 failures in

21 tries, with 2 mortalities and 6 amputations.[37,40,42,46,50,53,54]

Basically, we no longer advocate partial excisional therapy as optimal—the rate of failure is too high, and the risks of that failure are also too high. Conversely, the steadily improving results with formal graft excision and EAB warrant its preferential use.

We recognize that 30% to 40% of patients will do well with what is undeniably a smaller procedure, but do not believe the risk of recurrent, continuing infection warrants that approach in anything but a clearly limited chronic inguinal presentation of a *S epidermidis* GIF, or a medically compromised patient unlikely to survive the additional surgery.

Local

Local therapy essentially ignores the first principle of GIF management in that graft excision is not performed in lieu of a purported sterilization of the graft matrix to allow local healing. When practiced appropriately, the other tenets (especially wound debridement) are adequately met. We must emphasize, however, that local therapy is not a simple wound dressing protocol, which by itself is doomed to failure. The full tenets of management are clearly outlined by Calligaro and Perler, and entail frequent and complete debridement, systemic antibiotics, and early wound closure.

Dr. Perler's well-researched article delineates the theoretical advantages of rotational muscle flaps in creating a more advantageous milieu for graft sterilization and wound healing by increased vascularity, tissue oxygen tension, and probable cellular immunologic improvement. The actual data for the situation of a graft foreign body infection are limited to the three models cited—all are acute *S aureus* inoculations of a freshly implanted graft that is overlaid with a muscle flap. However, this is not the same anatomic or histologic situation that is presented by a previously implanted graft becoming infected and then having secondary flap coverage. In the real world, there is scarring, a diffuse hypoxic environment, and quite potentially a more thorough matrix bacterial permeation than that achieved by the laboratory model of local inoculation. Furthermore, the clinical graft is not restricted to the local field, but rather has a proximal limb(s) extending out of the field (and the muscle flap) where persistent or recurrent infection may be a problem.

Furthermore, the actual results of the studies are disturbing for the fact that there was no sterilization of the grafts even in the laboratory model. Cruz, for example, noted a 60% persistent infection rate at a 1×10^5 inoculum, certainly within the realm of the bacterial levels seen in clinical wounds.[49,58]

The few clinical studies of muscle flaps rely heavily on clinical healing percentages and a low perioperative mortality rate. Perler appropriately emphasized the major economic costs of such treatment. In his own series, the absolute failure rate was reported as 17% (3/18) but is actually 50% (9/18) when one includes four early deaths (we all have to include such deaths in our statistics, even if they were not per se due to treatment; most deaths are due to MI or cardiovascular accident, not sepsis or ASS!) and the one reported failure with thrombosis and recurrent infection. Thus, the technique failed in half of attempted cases and at a real mortality of 40% (5/18). Calligaro's failure rate was 36% (10/28) mirroring the same problems.

Furthermore, the long-term follow-up of these reported studies focuses on recurrent infection only that is clinically recognized; however, long-term complications that may be ascribed to persistent occult infection include late thrombosis and pseudoaneurysm formation as well as clinical infection. These data are either not provided or not recognized by the authors and included in their statistics.

A healed wound does not per se indicate cure of the infection. The laboratory indicates that bacteria may be demonstrated in the matrix and on the luminal surface of grafts that appear clinically healed. Their natural history, whether they may cause subsequent clinical problems, and over what time frame is unknown. This may be of little clinical import for peripheral grafts where such complications will be predominantly limb threatening, but for aortic grafts, the possibility of later ascending infection is a risk that needs quantification.

Summary of the literature does not offer a very sanguine support either (Table 4). Local therapy has been attempted 139 times with 58 (42%) failures for groin presentations of proximal grafts; the mortality 17% (23/134) and amputation 13% (18/134) have been respectable. It must be clearly stated that local therapy has been shown to be an effective and safe management protocol for angioaccess or other upper extremity grafts, and for peripheral (FP, FT, CF) grafts presenting at the inguinal and/or distal incisions (see Section X). This is the major finding of studies such as Calligaro's, but too often the generic destination of successful local therapy for GIFs is taken to indicate widespread success with that modality for aortic or other inflow cases when in actuality the major area of success with that modality has been with peripheral grafts.

Failure of local therapy was reported by Becker in 8 of 9 cases, 11 of 11 by Goldstone, 11 of 11 by Crawford, 6 of 8 by Conn, 4 of 4 by Seeger, and 8 of 9 by Edwards.[15,18,22,23,42] Conversely, Kwaan and Connolly reported success in 10 of 10, Almgren 9 of 9, Lorentzen 18 of 31, and Calligaro 5 of 5; Ghosn reported 10 of 13 successful tries, but had two PAs on follow-up suggesting late failure in an additional 2. Lorentzen had 9 failures in 18 tries, with 9 mortalities and 2 amputations.[31–35,49] One may well ask why the wide range of successful and completely unsuccessful attempts at local therapy?

Furthermore, there has to be differentiation between the exposed versus the infected graft. A wound infection that exposes a small surface of the graft appears to be

Table 4
Summary of Literature for the Results of Aortic Graft Infection Management

Type Treatment	No. of Patients	Mortality	Amputation	Recurrent GIF
None	8	7	—	1
Local	139	23 (17%)	18 (13%)	58 (42%)
In situ	1	—	—	—
Partial	106	20 (19%)	9 (8%)	47 (44%)
Excise	73	24 (33%)	24 (33%)	—
EAB	238	59 (25%)	32 (13%)	—
Total	565			

EAB = total graft excision and extra-anatomic bypass; GIF = graft infection.

handled very effectively by local therapy, whereas ascension along the limb or its perigraft sheath seems to occur more frequently and rapidly if the graft is immersed in pus and nonincorporated.

Our feeling is that although local therapy with or without adjunctive vascular pedicle therapy is clearly a reasonable and safe way to approach peripheral GIFs, that the theoretical as well as actual clinical experience with the modality simply does not support its use in aortic infections. As was true for partial graft excision, the stakes are too high and the safety and efficacy of total excision with EAB too well proven to advocate its routine use.

However, when the psychosocial situation or medically compromised condition of the patient mitigates against a formidable operation as posed by EAB, then local therapy under the constraints and principles outlined by Calligaro seem a reasonable judgment call.

In Situ In situ regrafting in the contaminated bed of the GIF violates two principles of GIF management; first, that there is foreign body retention, and second, that adequate debridement of contaminated tissue has been provided.

Prior to 1990, only one documented attempt at GIF treatment with in situ replacement had been made successfully. Johansen's and Bandyk limited experiences will be presented. Bandyk's experience is lim-

ited to specific groin presentations of *S epidermidis* GIFs, and Johansen's centers on low-pathogenicity organisms at the aortic bed and really does not focus on the treatment of GIF per se. Their experiences are preliminary.

The technique holds most appeal if the reimplanted graft is fortified by antibiotic impregnation. In this scenario, the laboratory holds strong promise that the graft might heal successfully.

Our reservation with this technique at the moment is the same as for local and partial therapy—recurrence of infection is likely to be with life-threatening ASS or GEF, which seems a steep price to pay when EAB works so well. Certainly the onus is on the surgeon to closely follow-up with CAT and leukocyte scans to make an early diagnosis of recurrent GIF if it occurs. Furthermore, with the known virulence of Gram-negative infections we would not support an in situ treatment for a Gram-negative infection.

Extra-anatomic Bypass

Clearly the major principles of GIF management are met by total graft excision and revascularization by EAB through clean anatomic planes.

Extra-anatomic bypass has become the dominant method of treatment. Of 530 cases (excluding the 104 cases of GIF, GEF, GEE in mixed series), more than half (238 cases) were managed by this protocol, with 25% (59/238) mortality and 13% (32/238) amputation rates. The mortality rate for EAB has steadily decreased and in series from 1985 onwards approaches 15%. Furthermore, total summary mortality is skewed by series in which local or partial therapy preceded EAB so that multiple operations were being performed.

The standard operation is graft excision with axillofemoral bypass, with the anatomic exigencies of which incisions are contaminated, and what potential recipient outflow vessels remain patent and usable.

The major question is whether the EAB should be performed as a staged or sequential operation. Staged operations are based on the concepts that total operative stress is decreased by dividing the operations with time for interval recovery, and that preliminary limb revascularization obviates the major additional stress of prolonged limb ischemia with resultant lactate acidosis, thromboxane production, and hyperkalemia—all major cardiac depressants and arrhythmic agents when suddenly flooded into the systemic circulation by delayed reperfusion.

The downside to staged revascularization is the potential for interval thrombosis of the EAB when there are parallel competing flows (only anecdotally reported, however), and the purported risk of bacteremic infection of the EAB from septicemias induced at secondary graft resection. Although the incidence of secondary EAB GIF has been reported at 7% to 15%, it is hardly clear that this results from bacteremia rather than being simply a problem of maintaining any sterile field in these circumstances.

Proponents of sequential revascularization note the prolonged total operative times and the potential for prolonged limb ischemia, but point out that both are better tolerated in today's climate of improved hemodynamic monitoring. They further point out that use of autologous in situ techniques requires this approach, and that partial graft

excision may be elected with lesser EAB reconstruction if clinical parameters so indicate.

As discussed earlier, we strongly advocate sequential EAB and graft excision and indeed advocate this as the standard therapy for GIF (Table 5).

Treatment Recommendations

In a field as complex as this and one that has received such a plethora of literature attention over 30 years, it is unlikely that a firm consensus will ever be reached as to all encompassing tenets of management. Perhaps that is as it should be, that there be room for individual judgment and thought. To my mind, this is one of the major differences between general and vascular surgery—the latitude of therapy options and the need for real conceptual visualizing to bring the best therapy to each patient.

Therapy must begin with a complete assessment of the clinical variables as previously noted.

1. The infection: the types of bacteria, the site of infection, the extent of spread, involvement of an anastomosis or viscus, signs of sepsis, acute versus chronic, sinus tract or abscess, aortic versus peripheral, patent versus thrombosed.
2. The patient: old or young, medically compromised and to what degree, ambulatory or other psychosocial issues.
3. The institution: capability of the ICU (TPN, monitoring) and of the operating room, as well as real consideration of the financial cost involved in potential 30- to 60-day hospitalizations.

Philosophically, graft infections should be strictly the province of the certified and experienced vascular surgeon, and preferably at an institution equally experienced and capable with such major problems.

Table 5
Recommendations for the Treatment of Graft Infections

Graft type	Patient type	Recommendation
I. Aortoiliac Aortic tube Aortofemoral shaft	Younger, healthier Gram positive	1. Sequential total excision and a) in situ autologous b) in situ allograft c) retroperitoneal aorta
	Older, sicker Gram negative	1. Staged EAB 2. Total excision 3. Long-term antibiotics
II. Aortofemoral Iliacofemoral Groin presentation	Younger, healthier Gram positive	1. Attempt partial resection
	Younger, healthier Gram negative Anastomotic bleeding Systemic sepsis	1. Total graft excision with sequential EAB 2. Delayed tertiary thoracofemoral
	Older, sicker Gram positive	1. Trial local therapy 2. Partial resection with sequential EAB
	Older, sicker Gram negative	1. Staged EAB 2. Total graft excision
III. Aortofemoral onlay Patent aortoiliac		1. Excise graft autologous patch aortotomy 2. Cross-over graft if unilateral occlusion
IV. Axillofemoral Cross-femoral with shaft presentation	Younger, healthier Gram negative	1. Local excision 2. EAB reconstruction
	Older, sicker Gram positive	1. Trial local therapy
V. Axillofemoral Cross-femoral Groin presentation Patch angioplasty		1. Trial local therapy 2. Muscle flap
VI. Femoropopliteal Femorodistal with shaft presentation	Gram positive	1. Trial local therapy 2. Marsupialization 3. Muscle flap
	Gram negative	1. Total graft excision 2. Autologous EAB
VII. Femoropopliteal, Femorodistal with anastomosis involved	Gram positive	1. Graft excision 2. EAB autologous
	Gram negative	1. Graft excision 2. EAB autologous 3. Muscle flap to arteriotomy

EAB = extra-anatomic bypass.

These are tier II cases. The only study I am aware of that looked specifically at the ability of general surgeons without vascular training to handle these cases was my own in 1990.

In that study, all lower extremity revascularization cases were done over a 4-year period prior to and after the establishment of a defined vascular surgery service run by certified vascular surgeons. Caseloads were divided into tier I as cases done by general surgeons with some vascular experience and included aortic reconstruction or aneurysmorrhaphy, femoropopliteal bypasses, extra-anatomic bypass, trauma, and thromboembolectomy, and tier II, cases usually seen in tertiary care centers and done by more experienced vascular surgeons, included visceral revascularization, redo cases,graft infections, etc.

In tier I there were 49 cases (30 inflow, 19 outflow) with 14% (7/49) mortality, 32% (21/67) limb thrombosis or embolus, and 10% (5/49) graft infections; 80% (39/49) of operations were done for claudication; 20% (10/49) were done for inappropriate indications ($P < .005$). In tier II there were 110 cases (47 inflow, 63 outflow); the increase was predominantly due to increased use of EAB and complex infrapopliteal reconstruction. Seventy percent (77/110) of cases were done for limb salvage. There was a 3% (4/110) mortality ($P < .025$), 11% (13/137) limb thrombosis or embolus ($P < .005$), and no graft infections ($P < .001$). Thus lower extremity revascularization was offered to more patients at lower morbidity and mortality rates with more complex procedures.[55]

Decision for management should not be based on tradition or one's training, but on analysis of all the available facts (as for example, presented in this book). I cannot overemphasize that the results in this difficult field come with thought as well as direct experience.

That prologue aside, our general recommendations and our rationale are presented in Table 5.

References

1. Bunt TJ. Synthetic vascular graft infections I: graft infections. *Surgery.* 1983;93:6:733–746.
2. Szylagyi DE. In discussion: Javid H, Julian OC, Dye WS, et al. Complications of abdominal aortic grafts. *Arch Surg.* 1962;85:142–161.
3. Dubost C, Allary M, Oeconomos N. Concerning the treatment of aneurysm of the aorta: ablation of the aneurysm-reestablishment of continuity by graft of the preserved human aorta. *Arch Surg.* 1952;64:405.
4. Oudot J, Beaconsfield P. Thrombosis of aortic bifurcation treated with resection and homograft replacement: report of five cases. *Arch Surg.* 1953;66:3:365–370.
5. Kunlin J. The treatment of arterial ischemia by the long venous graft memoirs. *Academic de Chirurgie.* 1948;74:567.
6. Blaisdell FW, Hall AD. Axillofemoral artery bypass for lower extremity ischemia. *Surgery.* 1963;54:563.
7. Claytor H, Birch L, Caldwell ES, et al. Suture line rupture of a nylon aortic bifurcation graft into the small bowel. *Arch Surg.* 1956;73:947–949.
8. Brock RC. Aortic homografting: a report of six successful cases. *Guy's Hosp Rep* 1953;102:204–208.
9. Blaisdell FW, Demattei GA, Guader PJ. Extraperitoneal thoracic aorta to femoral bypass graft as replacement for an infected aortic bifurcation prosthesis. *Am J Surg.* 1961;102:583–586.
10. Javid H, Julian OC, Dye WS, et al. Complications of abdominal aortic grafts. *Arch Surg.* 1962;85:142–161.
11. Carter SC, Cohen A, Whelan TJ. Clinical experience with management of the infected Dacron graft. *Ann Surg.* 1963;158:2:249–255.
12. Hoffert PW, Genster S, Haimovici H. Infection complicating arterial grafts. *Arch Surg.* 1965;90:427–432.
13. Fry WJ, Lindenauer SM. Infection complicating the use of plastic arterial implants. *Arch Surg.* 1967;94:600–606.
14. Najafi H, Javid H, Dye WS, et al. Management of infected arterial implants. *Surgery.* 1969;65:539–550.
15. Cohn R, Angell WW. Late complications from plastic replacement of aortic abdominal aneurysms. *Arch Surg.* 1968;97:5:696–698.
16. Conn JH, Hardy JD, Chavez CM, et al. Infected arterial grafts: experience in 22 cases with emphasis on unusual bacteria and techniques. *Ann Surg.* 1970;171:5:704–710.
17. Szylagyi DE, Smith RF, Elliott JP, et al. Infec-

tion in arterial reconstruction with synthetic grafts. *Ann Surg.* 1972;176:321.

18. Bouhoutsos J, Chavatzas D, Martin P, et al. Infected synthetic arterial grafts. *Br J Surg.* 1974;61:108–111.

19. Goldstone J, Moore WS. Infection in vascular prostheses: clinical manifestations and surgical management. *Am J Surg.* 1974;128:225–233.

20. Spanos P, Gilsdorf RB, Sako Y, et al. The management of infected abdominal aortic grafts and graft enteric fistulae. *Ann Surg.* 1976;183:4:397–402.

21. Jamieson CG, Deweese JA, Rob CG. Infected arterial grafts. *Ann Surg.* 1975;181:6:850–852.

22. Becker RM, Blundell PE. Infected aortic bifurcation grafts: experience with fourteen patients. *Surgery.* 1976;80:5:544–550.

23. Crawford ES, Manning LG, Kelly TF. Re-do surgery after operations for aneurysm and occlusion of the abdominal aorta. *Surgery.* 1977;81:1:41–52.

24. Christenson J, Eklof B. Synthetic arterial grafts II: infection complications. *Scand J Thorac Cardiovasc Surg.* 1977;11:43–50.

25. Liekweg WG, Greenfield LJ. Vascular prosthetic infections: collected experience and results of treatment. *Surgery.* 1977;81:3:335–342.

26. Scobie TK, Elder RH, McPhail N. Infected abdominal aortic grafts. *Can J Surg.* 1978;21:6:527–531.

27. Yashar JJ, Weyman AK, Burnard RJ, et al. Survival and limb salvage in patients with infected arterial prostheses. *Am J Surg.* 1978;135:4:499–504.

28. Casali RE, Tucker ET, Thompson BV, et al. Infected prosthetic grafts. *Arch Surg.* 1980;115:577.

29. Courmier JM, Ward AS, Lagneau P. Infection complicating aortoiliac surgery. *J Cardiovasc Surg.* 1980;21:303–314.

30. Popovsky J, Singer S. Infected prosthetic grafts. *Arch Surg.* 1980;115:2:203–207.

31. Kwaan JHM, Connolly JE. Successful management of prosthetic graft infection with continuous povidone-iodine irrigation. *Arch Surg.* 1981;116:716–720.

32. Knight CD, Farwell MB, Hollier LH. Treatment of aortic graft infection with povidone-iodine irrigation. *Mayo Clin Proc.* 1983;58:472–475.

33. Ghosn PB, Rabbat AG, Trudel J. Why remove an infected graft? *Can J Surg.* 1983;26:4:330–332.

34. Lorentzen JE, Nielsen OM, Arendrup H, et al. Vascular graft infection: an analysis of sixty-two graft infections in 2411 consecutively implanted synthetic vascular grafts. *Surgery.* 1985;98:1:81–87.

35. Almgren B, Eriksson I. Local antibiotic irrigation in the treatment of arterial graft infections. *Acta Chir Scand.* 1981;147:33–36.

36. Ehrenfeld WK, Wiebur BG, Olcott CN, et al. Autogenous tissue reconstruction in the management of infected prosthetic grafts. *Surgery.* 1979;85:1:82–91.

37. Reilly LM, Altman H, Lusby RJ, et al. Late results following surgical management of vascular graft infection. *J Vasc Surg.* 1984;1:1:36–41.

38. Reilly LM, Stoney RJ, Goldstone J. Improved management of aortic graft infection: the influence of operation sequence and staging. *J Vasc Surg.* 1987;5:3:421–429.

39. Bunt TJ: In discussion of #38;

40. Fulenwider JT, Smith RB III, Johnson RW. Reoperative abdominal arterial surgery: a ten year experience. *Surgery.* 1983;93:1:20–30.

41. Trout HH, Kozloff L, Giordana JM. Priority of revascularization in patients with graft enteric fistulas, infected arteries, or infected arterial prostheses. *Ann Surg.* 1984;199:6:669–680.

42. Edwards MJ, Richardson JD, Klamer TW. Management of aortic prosthetic infections. *Am J Surg.* 1986;155:2:327–331.

43. Martin-Paredo V, Busuttil RW, Dixon SM. Fate of aortic graft removal. *Am J Surg.* 1983;146:2:194–197.

44. Quinones-Baldrich WJ, Hernandez JJ, Moore WS. Long-term results following surgical management of aortic graft infection. *Arch Surg.* 1991;126:4:507–510.

45. Yeager RA, McConnell DB, Sasaki TM, et al. Aortic and peripheral prosthetic graft infection: differential management and causes of mortality. *Am J Surg.* 1985;150:1:36–43.

46. Yeager RA, Moneta GL, Taylor LM, et al. Improving survival and limb salvage in patients with aortic graft infection. *Am J Surg.* 1990;159:5:466–469.

47. Mixter RC, Turnipseed WD, Smith DJ Jr, et al. Rotational muscle flaps: a new technique for covering infected vasclar grafts. *J Vasc Surg.* 1989;9:472–478.

48. Calligaro KD, Veith FJ, Gupta SK, et al. A modified method for management of prosthetic graft infections involving an anastomosis to the common femoral artery. *J Vasc Surg.* 1990;11:4:485–491.

49. Perler BA, Vanderkolk CA, Dufresne CA, et al. Can infected prosthetic grafts be salvaged with rotational muscle flaps? *Surgery.* 1991;110:30–34.

50. Ricotta JJ, Faggioli GL, Stella A, et al. Total excision and extra-anatomic bypass for aortic graft infection. *Am J Surg.* 1991;162:2:145–149.
51. Wooldridge WD, Doerhoff CA, Bunt TJ. Primary *Salmonella* aortic graft infection: 1st reported case. *Am Surg.* 1983;49:679–681.
52. Bunt TJ, Haynes JL. Synthetic vascular graft infections: the continuing headache. *Am Surg.* 1984;50:43.
53. Bunt TJ. A personal experience with 55 vascular graft infections. *J Cardiovasc Surg.* 1993;1:5:489–493.
54. Bandyk DF, Bergamini TM, Kinney EV, et al. In situ replacement of vascular prostheses infected by bacterial biofilms. *J Vasc Surg.* 1991;13:575–583.
55. Turnipseed WD, Berkoff HA, Detmer DE, et al. Arterial graft infection: delayed versus immediate vascular reconstruction. *Arch Surg.* 1983;118:4:410–414.
56. Bunt TJ. Commentary: Reilly LM, Stoney RJ, Goldstone J. Improved management of aortic graft infection: the influence of operation sequence and staging. *J Vasc Surg.* 1987;5:3:421–429.
57. Bunt TJ, Manczuk M, Varley K. Nitroglycerine-induced volume loading. *Surgery.* 1988;5:549–559.
58. Cruz NI, Canario QM. Muscle flaps in the management of vascular grafts in contaminated wounds: an experimental study in dogs. *Plast Reconstr Surg.* 1988;82:480–483.

Bibliography

These miscellaneous articles are not cited but were used in determination of review data.

Bunt TJ, Malone JM. The impact of vascular certification on lower extremity revascularization at one institution. *Am Surg.* 1992;58:463–469.

Diethrich EB, Noon GP, Liddicoat JE, et al. Treatment of infected aortofemoral arterial prosthesis. *Surgery.* 1970;68:6:1044–1052.

Grafe WR, Watson RC, Dineen P. Infections of vascular anastomoses. *Vasc Surg.* 1971;5:204.

Moran KT, Jewell ER. Local antiseptic treatment of infected prosthetic vascular grafts in the groin. *Br J Surg.* 1988;75:10:1037–1038.

Quick CRG, Vascallo DJ, Colin JF, et al. Conservative treatment of major aortic graft infection. *Eur J Vasc Surg.* 1990;4:63–67.

Smith RF, Szylagyi DE. Healing complications with plastic arterial implants. *Arch Surg.* 1961;82:1:34–44.

Van de Water JM, Goal PG. Management of patients with infected arterial prostheses. *Am Surg.* 1965;31:651.

Vellar IDA, Doycle JC. Axillofemoral bypass in the management of infected aortic bifurcation dacron graft. *Aus NZ J Surg.* 1970;40:1:58–60.

Willwerth BM, Waldhausen JA. Infection of arterial prostheses. *Surg Gynecol Obstet.* 1974;139:3:446–452.

Chapter 9

Antibiotic Therapy Alone for Graft Infection

T.W. Wakefield

Introduction

It has been suggested that prosthetic vascular graft infections may be treated conservatively without graft excision in certain situations. For example, the use of continuous povidine-iodine irrigation[1] and continuous antibiotic irrigation in areas of an infection localized to the groin have been advocated.[2] If infection is limited to the bed of a graft without suture line involvement and the graft is patent without evidence of septic embolization, local debridement with or without topical antibiotics has also been recommended[3,4] in addition to the use of muscle flap transposition.[5,6] However, in all of these reports, systemic antibiotics have been used in an adjunctive fashion only with further surgical therapy being the primary modality.

Rifampicin and Clindamycin

In order to determine the efficacy of treating established vascular graft infections with rifampicin and clindamycin, antibiotics that are preferentially concentrated in leukocytes, a study was performed in a canine model.[7] Infrarenal aortic grafts, 6 mm × 6 cm made of knitted Dacron double-velour construction, were implanted and infected with 10^8 colony-forming units (CFU) of coagulase-positive *Staphylococcus aureus* organisms injected intravenously immediately after graft placement. Antibiotic therapy was instituted at 3 months postimplantation.

Three groups of animals were studied: 1) untreated controls (n = 3); 2) animals treated with intravenous cephazolin 15 mg/kg per 8 hours for 28 days; 3) animals treated with combined therapy consisting of intravenous rifampicin 13 mg/kg per 24 hours and intravenous clindamycin 13 mg/kg per 8 hours for 28 days (n = 7). The grafts were removed for quantitative bacteriologic studies after the 28-day course of therapy.

Two group 1 control grafts remained patent with 6.4×10^6 and 8.1×10^3 CFU *S aureus* per gram of graft. The third control graft was thrombosed. Two group 2 animals demonstrated 1.6×10^7 and 2.3×10^5 CFU *S aureus* organisms per gram of graft, respectively, while the remaining five group 2 grafts were free of organisms. All group 3

From Bunt, TJ: *Vascular Graft Infections.* Armonk: Futura Publishing Co., Inc.; © 1994.

grafts were sterile, a statistically significant difference from group 1 grafts. This study demonstrated that in this experimental canine model, established prosthetic vascular graft infections could be successfully treated by intensive administration of antibiotics preferentially concentrated in leukocytes.

Although the ability of leukocytes to preferentially concentrate antibiotics may be responsible for the results reported above, other explanations are possible for the improved results with the use of this antibiotic combination. For example, the MIC for rifampicin against *S aureus* is well below the drug levels that were achieved in this investigation. Likewise, the MIC for *S aureus* inhibition by clindamycin was also well below the levels achieved. Thus, improved drug pharmacokinetics may be responsible for the observed effect of graft sterilization. On the other hand, not all group 2 grafts were sterile despite the excellent levels of cefazolin achieved (well above its MIC for *S aureus*), suggesting an effect over and above a pure pharmacokinetic effect.

Certain drugs, including lipid-soluble antibiotics, appear to be concentrated in leukocytes. Such is the case with clindamycin in which fivefold to fiftyfold increases over serum levels are noted, and with rifampicin in which twofold to fivefold increases over serum levels exits.[8] In this regard, phagocytosis due to *S aureus* caused a marked uptake of clindamycin by human polymorphonuclear leukocytes (PMNs) in an energy-dependent membrane transport system.[8] Clindamycin will also inhibit *S aureus* proliferation in bacteria that survive ingestion by human PMNs over a 24- to 48-hour period. Clindamycin not only inhibits and reduces the number of viable organisms, but also prevents the death of PMNs due to late bacterial growth.[8] Both clindamycin and rifampicin are effective at killing intracellular *S aureus* in vitro,[9] considered to be due to direct antimicrobial activity within the PMNs.

Other neutrophil functions have been evaluated in patients receiving clindamycin. In patients, it has been found that intracellular killing of clindamycin-resistant strains of *S aureus* is possible with no evidence of altered neutrophil chemotaxis, phagocytosis, or chemoluminescence.[10] Clindamycin has also been shown to be effective, even at subinhibitory concentrations, at decreasing or preventing the production of glycocalyx formation by *S aureus.*

Rifampicin appears to be an ideal antibiotic for vascular graft infections based on its excellent activity against *S aureus*, methicillin-resistant staphylococci, and multiresistant slime-forming coagulase-negative staphylococci species from peripheral vascular patients.[11,12] Rifampicin has been impregnated in or bonded to vascular grafts in the hope of preventing contamination at the time of graft insertion with promising results.[11–16] A theoretical problem in the treatment of prosthetic vascular graft infections is the inability to achieve a sufficient antibiotic concentration on the fabric surface to sterilize the graft. Use of antibiotics that concentrate in leukocytes might offer a solution to this problem, because white blood cells preferentially attach to infected grafts and in so doing, might provide an effective carrier system for the antibiotics. The usual leukocyte attraction to infected prosthetic grafts has been clearly documented by the accumulation of indium 111 oxine labeled white blood cells on these grafts.[17]

Although one may conclude from our experimental data that an established vascular graft infection of 3 months duration may be eradicated in a majority of cases by means of antibiotics such as rifampicin and clindamycin (antibiotics that may be given orally in addition to intravenously), the applicability of such results to the clinical area remains in question for at least four reasons.

First, it is not known if the graft sterilization produced will persist over time. Second, the experimental study that we performed related to pure *S aureus* infection only, while other organisms have been found to be more prominent than *S aureus* in prosthetic vascular graft infection today. In fact, *Staphylococcus epidermidis* is the most frequent pathogen found at the present time. Third, the experimental model presented best mimics infection when the pathogenesis involves hematogenous seeding of organisms onto the implanted graft. Infections complicating graft placement in which direct contamination occurs intraoperatively, may not be expected to behave in a similar manner. The whole question of hematogenous seeding as the primary etiology in vascular graft infections must be questioned in view of the fact that most authors today recommend placement of extra-anatomic bypasses prior to graft removal for prosthetic vascular graft infections[18] and find no higher incidence of infection of these extra-anatomic bypasses than if they are placed after the infected graft is removed first, despite the bacterial *shower* that must occur during graft removal. Finally, the number of animals in this experimental study is small; statistical analysis of the data must therefore be cautiously interpreted. Furthermore, one cannot directly extrapolate from an animal study to the clinical condition.

Literature Review

The use of antibiotics alone in the treatment of prosthetic vascular graft infections has been reported in 13 cases with success noted in 5 of these instances. Bouhoutsos et al.[19] reported infections in 3 grafts in the aortoiliac location (2 and 3 weeks after insertion) and 1 graft infection in the femoropopliteal location (1 week postoperatively) all successfully treated with antibiotics. In one of these cases, antibiotic usage was accompanied by drainage of an abscess in the left iliac fossa. Crawford et al.[20] reported on the treatment of 11 patients with aortic graft infection of whom 1 patient was treated with antibiotics only without graft removal; this patient expired.

Knight et al.[21] presented the case of an 88-year-old woman with an aortic graft infection 2 months following repair of a rup-

tured abdominal aortic aneurysm. A woven Dacron graft had been placed. Postoperatively, the patient had developed ischemic colitis limited to the mucosa. After conservative treatment, the patient was discharged. Eight weeks later, the patient developed a fecal fistula from a presumed sigmoid stricture and a large retroperitoneal abscess was found on exploration surrounding the aortic graft. The abscess was drained. The entire graft including both anastomoses was found to be bathed by pus. Cultures grew *Fusobacterium necrophorum.* Drains were placed, the graft irrigated with 2500 mL/day of 0.5% povidine-iodine solution for 18 consecutive days, and systemic antibiotics consisting of penicillin, tobramycin, and clindamycin used for 11 days. The patient recovered, was instructed to take Cephradine® 500 mg B.I.D. indefinitely, and was well 2 months later.

Christenson and Eklof[22] reported two cases of aortic graft infection treated with antibiotics only in which failure resulted in the need for reconstructive vascular surgery. In the first case, a 57-year-old male had undergone resection of a ruptured abdominal aortic aneurysm and placement of a right aortoiliac, left aortofemoral bypass. Postoperatively, he developed disseminated intravascular coagulation but recovered rapidly. Approximately 2 months later, he presented with a fistula in the left groin connecting to the aortic graft with *S aureus* recovered. Local irrigation of the fistula with antibiotics and systemic chloramphenicol, cloxacillin, and cephalosporin failed to eradicate the infection and the patient was forced to undergo extra-anatomic bypass and removal of the infected left limb of the graft. In the second case, a patient with mycotic aortoiliofemoral aneurysms underwent right axillopopliteal bypass with a femorofemoral crossover and left femoropopliteal bypass, all with velour Dacron. Postoperatively, a right groin infection with *E. coli* and *Pseudomonas aeruginosa* was treated with gentamycin, ampicillin and benzyl penicillin. Within the next 6 months, the reconstruction thrombosed twice with *S aureus* recovered from the graft. The infected portion of the graft was subsequently removed and the patient recovered. The patient died approximately 11 months later with an intact extra-anatomic reconstruction.

Jamieson and colleagues[23] reported on a series of 15 infected grafts out of 664 patients between 1955 and 1973 who had undergone arterial reconstructive surgery. Four patients were treated with antibiotics only. In these cases, all died of septicemia 15, 21, 22 days, and 12 months after their respective operations. Finally, Fry and Lindenauer[24] reported one case of the use of systemic antibiotics for 3 1/2 years in a patient with an infected Teflon aortofemoral bypass that eventually resulted in the patient's death. In this case, *E. coli* and *S aureus* appeared to be the organisms involved.

We have likewise had the opportunity to treat two patients with infected prosthetic vascular graft infection with antibiotics only. The first patient presented with a large infected fluid collection around both limbs of an aortofemoral bypass that had been placed 14 years previously. The patient was treated with aspiration and 2 weeks of I.V. vancomycin and gentamycin. His cultures were initially all negative suggesting coagulase-negative *Staphylococcus.* After initial I.V. treatment, the fluid accumulations had resolved. He was then treated with a full 6-month course of P.O. clindamycin and Bactrim.™ Unfortunately, a 6-month repeat computer tomography (CT) scan revealed reaccumulation of fluid around the right limb of the graft. Two months later, he had reaccumulated fluid around both graft limbs despite continued P.O. antibiotics and required extra-anatomic bypass and removal of the aortofemoral bypass. His cultures were positive for coagulase-negative *Staphylococcus* and α-hemolytic *Streptococcus.*

The second patient had developed an infected left femoral expanded polytetrafluoroethylene (ePTFE) patch after repair of a pseudoaneurysm resulting from the use of cannulas for the institution of extracorporeal membrane oxygenation (EMCO). This patient, a 29-year-old male, had required ECMO for severe pancreatitis. He was treated with I.V. antibiotics for 2 months, but required removal of the ePTFE patch and replacement with a saphenous interposition graft followed by a rectus muscle flap due to systemic sepsis and evidence of septic embolization to the left foot. His cultures grew out *Pseudomonas* and *S aureus.* He subsequently was treated with a 6-month course of I.V. vancomycin and is now 18 months status post-ePTFE excision, doing well with no evidence of infection.

Both patients had failed aggressive antibiotic therapy only and required more traditional excisional therapy combined with antibiotics and blood flow restoration through either an extra-anatomic route with prosthetic material or through clean-contaminated tissue planes with autogenous tissue.

Summary

In summary, the use of antibiotics alone in the treatment of prosthetic vascular graft infection is clearly controversial, has met with limited success only, and must be used with extreme caution. The use of antibiotics alone, especially those concentrated in leukocytes, may be indicated and effective for the occasional case in which suspicion of infection exists, as in a femoral pseudoaneurysm excision with a negative intraoperative Gram stain only to eventually grow a few colonies of staphylococci from the resected graft tissue postoperatively. However, even the use of antibiotics only in this situation requires diligent follow-up, both clinically and with appropriate imaging studies.

The use of antibiotics combined with local therapy may have a more definitive role to play in the management of certain high-risk patients. The use of continuous povidine-iodine irrigation,[1,21] continuous antibiotic irrigation,[2] local debridement with or without topical antibiotics,[3,4] and muscle flap transposition[5,6] has been recommended. Likewise, two recent reports have advocated appropriate percutaneous drainage associated with systemic antibiotic therapy. Tobin[25] reported on a 64-year-old male with a complex fluid collection around the right limb of an aortofemoral bypass graft which had been placed 1 month previously. This collection grew methicillin-resistant *S aureus* and was successfully treated with percutaneous drainage and systemic vancomycin that was switched eventually to nafcillin therapy. The drain was removed after 41 days and a follow-up CT scan 7 months later revealed no abscess recurrence. The patient is presently on lifelong oral dicloxacillin. Matley et al.[26] operated on a patient with a leaking thoracoabdominal aortic aneurysm and inserted a woven Dacron graft. Postoperatively, a number of infectious complications occurred including a *Klebsiella* urinary tract infection. Forty days postoperatively (and 1 week after discharge), the patient developed a large abscess around the graft. Percutaneous aspiration with a large 12-French stump drainage catheter revealed *Klebsiella* species and 1000 mL of purulence was drained. The catheter remained in place for 22 days and each day, purulence drained. One gram of cefotaxime was introduced daily. The catheter was reinserted on postaspiration day 26 and remained for another week. Additionally, the patient was treated with I.V. amikacin and cefotaxime. Five months after the initial aspiration, small quantities of pus containing *Klebsiella* continued to drain from the catheter site. Two years after drainage, the patient is asymptomatic, CT scan is negative, as are gallium 67 and indium 111 leukocyte scans. The patient remains on oral cotrimoxazole daily.

The use of systemic intravenous antibiotics combined with local topical therapy or aspiration plus topical therapy would seem to offer an alternate for high-risk situations in which more aggressive excisional ther-apy places the patient at increased operative risk, such as those patients with severe cardiopulmonary disease. Patients with grafts in place in the thoracoabdominal location where excision is not possible would also be candidates for such local plus systemic therapy. Additionally, the advisability of such an approach may also be dependent on the type of graft material involved in the infectious process. Bacteria penetrate the interstices of Dacron prostheses more deeply than ePTFE grafts[27]; ePTFE grafts have been used to successfully replace infected, distal anastomotic sites of Dacron aortofemoral bypass grafts with no recurrence of infection at a mean follow-up of 14 months.[28] It has been recommended recently that Dacron infrainguinal anastomotic infections must be treated by immediate excision while graft preservation is the treatment of choice for Gram-positive anastomotic infections of patent ePTFE or vein grafts.[29] Finally, areas where such a regimen would be contraindicated include cases in which infection involves vascular prosthetic graft anastomoses placed in locations that are not readily accessible such as the intra-abdominal retroperitoneal location and infections involving virulent Gram-negative organisms, especially strains of *Pseudomonas*. Gram-negative organisms appear to be more virulent than Gram-positive organisms in prosthetic vascular graft infections.[30,31] In these instances, despite isolated case reports to the contrary, more traditional excisional therapy must remain the treatment of choice.

References

1. Kwaan JH, Connolly JE. Successful management of prosthetic graft infection with continuous povidine-iodine irrigation. *Arch Surg.* 1981;116:716–720.
2. Popovsky J, Singer S. Infected prosthetic grafts: local therapy with graft preservation. *Arch Surg.* 1980;115:203–205.
3. Almgren B, Eriksson I. Local antibiotic irrigation in the treatment of arterial graft infections. *Acta Chir Scand.* 1981;147:33–36.

4. Almgren B, Eriksson I. Local treatment of infected arterial grafts. *Acta Chir Scand Suppl.* 1985;529:92–94.

5. Cherry KJ Jr, Roland CF, Pairolero PC, et al. Infected femorodistal bypass: is graft removal mandatory? *J Vasc Surg.* 1992;15:295–305.

6. Dacey LJ, Miett TO, Huntsman WT, Colen LB, Schned AR, McDaniel MD. Efficacy of muscle flaps in the treatment of prosthetic vascular graft infections. *J Surg Res.* 1988;44:566–572

7. Wakefield TW, Schaberg DR, Pierson CL, et al. Treatment of established prosthetic vascular graft infection by antibiotics preferentially concentrated in leukocytes. *J Vasc Surg.* 1987;102:8–14.

8. Hand WL, King-Thompson NL, Steinberg TH. Interactions of antibiotics and phagocytes. *J Antimicrob Chemother.* 1983;12:(suppl C):1–11.

9. Jacobs RF, Wilson CB. Intracellular penetration and antimicrobial activity of antibiotics. *J Antimicrob Chemother.* 1983;12:(suppl C):13–20.

10. Faden H, Hong JJ, Orga PL. In-vivo effects of Clindamycin on neutrophil function. *J Antimicrob Chemother.* 1985;16:649–657.

11. Chervu A, Moore WS, Gelabert HA, Colburn MD, Chvapil M. Prevention of graft infection by use of prostheses bonded with a rifampin/collagen release system. *J Vasc Surg.* 1991;14:521–525.

12. Strachan CL, Newsom SB, Ashton TR. The clinical use of an antibiotic-bonded graft. *Eur J Vasc Surg.* 1991;5:627–632.

13. McDougal EG, Burnham SJ, Johnson G Jr. Rifampin protection against experimental graft sepsis. *J Vasc Surg.* 1986;4:5–7.

14. Goeau-Brissonniere O, Leport C, Bacourt F, Lebrault C, Comte R, Pechere JC. Prevention of vascular graft infection by rifampin bonding to a gelatin-sealed Dacron graft. *Ann Vasc Surg.* 1991;5:408–412.

15. Avramovic J, Fletcher JP. Prevention of prosthetic vascular graft infection by rifampin impregnation of a protein-sealed Dacron graft in combination with parenteral cephalosporin. *J Cardiovasc Surg.* 1992;33:70–74.

16. Avramovic JR, Fletcher JP. Rifampin impregnation of a protein-sealed Dacron graft: an infection-resistant prosthetic vascular graft. *Aust NZ J Surg.* 1991;61:436–440.

17. Wakefield TW, Whitehouse WM Jr, Sawnson DP, et al. Late discriniation of infected synthetic arterial grafts using indium-111-labeled leukocyte scans. *Surg Forum.* 1983;34:452–454.

18. Reilly LM, Stoney RJ, Goldstone J, Ehrenfeld WK. Improved management of aortic graft infection: the influence of operation sequence and staging. *J Vasc Surg.* 1987;5:421–431.

19. Bouhoutsos J, Chavatzas D, Martin P, Morris T. Infected synthetic arterial grafts. *Br J Surg.* 1974;61:108–111.

20. Crawford ES, Manning LG, Kelly TF. Redo surgery after operations for aneurysm and occlusion of the abdominal aorta. *Surg.* 1977;81:41–52.

21. Knight CD, Farnell MB, Hollier LH. Treatment of aortic graft infection with povidine-iodine irrigation. *Mayo Clin Proc.* 1983;58:472–475.

22. Christenson J, Eklof B. Synthetic arterial grafts II: infection complications. *Scand J Thorac Cardiovasc Surg.* 1977;11:43–50.

23. Jamieson GG, DeWeese JA, Rob CG. Infected arterial grafts. *Ann Surg.* 1975;181:850–852.

24. Fry WJ, Lindenauer SM. Infection complicating the use of plastic arterial implants. *Arch Surg.* 1967;94:600–609.

25. Tobin KD. Aortobifemoral perigraft abscess: treatment by percutaneous catheter drainage. *J Vasc Surg.* 1988;8:339–343.

26. Matley PJ, Beningfield SJ, Lourens S, Immelman EJ. Successful treatment of infected thoracoabdominal aortic graft by percutaneous catheter drainage. *J Vasc Surg.* 1991;13:513–515.

27. Schmitt DD, Bandyk DF, Pequet AJ, Towne JB. Bacterial adherence to vascular prostheses. *J Vasc Surg.* 1986;3:732–740.

28. Seabrook GR, Schmitt DD, Bandyk DF. Anastomotic femoral pseudoaneurysm: an investigation of occult infection as an etiologic factor. *J Vasc Surg.* 1990;11:629–634.

29. Calligaro KD, Westcott CJ, Buckley RM, Savarese RP, DeLaurentis DA. Infrainguinal anastomotic arterial graft infections treated by selective graft preservation. *Ann Surg.* 1992;216:74–79.

30. Jarret F, Darling RC, Mundth ED, Austen WG. The management of infected arterial aneurysms. *J Cardiovasc Surg.* 1977;18:361–366.

31. Ouriel K, Geary KJ, Green RM, DeWeese JA. Fate of the exposed saphenous vein graft. *Am J Surg.* 1990;160:148–155.

Chapter 10

In Situ Repair of Infected Aortic Grafts

D.L. Steed

Introduction

Infections in vascular grafts occur in approximately 1% to 2% of cases.[1-7] Though uncommon, they are a major cause of morbidity and mortality with a high incidence of limb loss. Infections in aortic grafts are a difficult problem in many ways. Infections may not become apparent for months to years after the initial graft placement. When infection does appear, it may lead to sepsis, pseudoaneurysm, gastrointestinal erosion, gastrointestinal hemorrhage, or graft thrombosis. Because of the deep-seated position of the graft, the diagnosis may not be suspected initially as there may be few, if any, findings on physical examination.

Infected grafts may occur as an isolated graft infection, a graft-enteric erosion, or a graft-enteric fistula.[8] Graft-enteric erosions occur less frequently than graft-enteric fistulae. Most graft-enteric erosions occur between the aortic graft and the duodenum. Less commonly, the graft communicates with the stomach, jejunum, ileum, or colon. The management of a graft-enteric communication may be different depending upon whether the body of the graft (graft-enteric erosion) or both the graft and anastomosis (graft-enteric fistula) communicate with the gastrointestinal tract.

There is uniform agreement that graft infections left untreated are fatal.[3,5,9-20] There are many examples in the literature where graft infections were not treated, most often because the diagnosis was not recognized or the patient was considered too ill to undergo an operation. These patients have died, usually from uncontrolled sepsis or exsanguinating gastrointestinal hemorrhage.

Standard therapy for a patient with an infected aortic graft has been complete removal of the infected graft with oversewing of the aortic stump usually with a monofilament nonabsorbable suture in several layers. Revascularization of the lower extremities is achieved by an extra-anatomic bypass either before or immediately following the graft removal. Occasionally, a patient may have apparent adequate arterial blood flow to the lower extremities through collateral channels and revascularization may not be necessary or, if needed, can be delayed until the patient's condition has improved. This is more likely to occur in patients in whom

From Bunt, TJ: *Vascular Graft Infections*. Armonk: Futura Publishing Co., Inc.; © 1994.

the initial aortic graft was placed for aorto-iliac occlusive disease or in patients with occluded grafts as opposed to grafts placed for aortic aneurysm. With this complex form of therapy, the morbidity and mortality are high with a significant incidence of limb loss. Graft replacement with extra-anatomic bypass may have a mortality rate greater than 50%, an amputation rate greater than 25%, and an aortic stump blowout rate greater than 33%.[1,8] Dissatisfaction with results of traditional or standard therapy has prompted surgeons to consider alternatives. Local therapy, graft excision alone, or replacement of the graft into the same vascular bed or in situ graft replacement has been considered as an alternative in selected patients.

Infected Grafts

Isolated graft infections usually occur months to years after the initial aortic repair. Local treatment of an infected graft has been attempted with some success. Often, local care has been considered when the patient was too ill to undergo a more aggressive approach such as graft removal, with or without bypass. More recently, local repair has been considered because of continued dissatisfaction with the outcome of graft removal and the possibility of a good outcome with local care with improvement in antibiotics and the use of omental or muscle flaps to cover the graft. A summary of the patients reported in multiple series shows that in 61 patients with isolated graft infections treated with local care only, there was only a 23% mortality rate (Table 1). The mortality rate seems low considering the seriousness of the problem. It seems likely that successes were more often reported than failures. The incidence of limb loss is difficult to determine as many series do not report amputation rates, but lower extremity amputation is not uncommon in patients treated with graft infections. In the largest series reported by Lorentzen et al. half of the patients treated with local care died.[15] The amputation rate among survivors was

Table 1
Graft Infections: Local Care

Study	Year	No. of Pts.	Died	Recovered
Javid[14]	1962	4		4
Carter[35]	1963	6		6
Vandewater[36]	1965	1	1	
Conn[2]	1970	4	2	2
Szilagyi[3]	1972	1		1
Bouhoutsos[37]	1974	3		3
Goldstone[4]	1974	2	1	1
Perdue[38]	1975	1		1
Liekweg[6]	1977	4		4
Yashar[7]	1978	1		1
Almgren[39]	1981	4		4
Kwaan[40]	1981	5		5
Lorentzen[15]	1985	18	9	9
Edwards[22]	1988	2	1	1
Calligaro[21]	1992	5		5
Total		61	14 (23%)	47 (77%)

Table modified from Bunt[1,8]

Table 2
Graft Infections: Graft Excision

Study	Year	No. of Pts.	Died	Recovered
Schramel[41]	1959	3	1	2
Javid[14]	1962	1	1	
Shaw[42]	1963	1	1	
Cohn[17]	1968	2	2	
Conn[2]	1970	5	2	3
Szilagyi[3]	1972	12	8	4
Bouhoutsos[37]	1974	3		3
Goldstone[4]	1974	18	3	15
Perdue[38]	1975	1		1
Jamieson[5]	1975	3	1	2
Crawford[43]	1977	4		4
Liekweg[6]	1977	3	3	
Casali[44]	1980	9	6	3
Lorentzen[15]	1985	6	1	5
Yeager[45]	1985	1	1	
O'Hara[26]	1986	11	10	1
Thomas[28]	1986	1	1	
Edwards[22]	1988	14	3	11
Quinones-Baldrich[46]	1991	9	4	5
Total		107	48 (45%)	59 (55%)

Table modified from Bunt[1,8]

22%. In a recent report by Calligaro et al., there were no deaths among five patients treated in this manner.[21]

There have been multiple reports of excision of an infected graft without revascularization of the lower extremity (Table 2). This technique has been used more commonly in patients with graft thrombosis or those patients who underwent aortic grafting for occlusive disease. A review of the literature reporting 107 patients suggests a mortality rate of 45%. When excision of an infected graft without revascularization is selected for a patient, revascularization may be performed at a subsequent operation if the lower extremities become ischemic. Szilagyi et al. reported that four patients treated with graft excision alone required subsequent amputation.[3] In contrast, Goldstone et al. treated 18 patients with graft excision alone.[4] Six of these patients lost their limbs while seven subsequently required revascularization with salvage of their limbs. In the series by Edwards et al. 14 of 16 patients who underwent graft excision later required revascularization for limb salvage.[22]

There have been reports of cases where in situ replacement was used successfully in managing an isolated graft infection (Table 3). If the blood supply to the lower extremities is judged to be inadequate without revascularization, excision of the infected graft with immediate in situ replacement has been used. The overall mortality rate in 14 patients in the series reviewed is only 14% (Table 3). However, the number of reported cases is small. It should also be noted, again, that surgeons are more likely to report successes than failures.

Bandyk et al. reported the use of in situ aortic graft replacement in four patients with infected aortic grafts.[23] The treatment involved removal of the infected graft mate-

Table 3
Graft Infections: In Situ Graft Replacement

Study	Year	No. of Pts.	Died	Recovered
Conn[2]	1970	1	1	
Szilagyi[3]	1972	3		3
Perdue[16]	1980	1		1
Yeager[45]	1985	1	1	
Thomas[28]	1986	1		1
Yeager[47]	1990	2		2
Bandy[23]	1991	4		4
Quinones-Baldrich[46]	1991	1		1
Total		14	2 (14%)	12 (86%)

Table modified from Bunt[1,8]

rial, excision of the inflamed perigraft tissue, parenteral antibiotics, and replacement with an expanded polytetrafluoroethylene graft. There were no deaths and no deep wound infections. There were no recurrent graft infections in follow-up of 5 to 50 months (mean 21 months). He suggested therefore that complications of perigraft infection could be eradicated by antibiotics, local debridement, and in situ graft replacement.

Graft-Enteric Erosions

Only a small number of graft-enteric erosion treated by a local repair has been reported (Table 4). The first aortoenteric communication to be repaired successfully occurred in 1957.[24] The repair was simple closure of the fistula without graft replacement. Since that time, several authors have reported success with local suture repair. A review of the 19 patients in the series re-

Table 4
Graft-Enteric Erosions: Local Repair

Study	Year	No. of Pts.	Died	Recovered
Deweese[48]	1962	1	1	
Long[49]	1962	1	1	
Vandewater[36]	1965	1		1
Sheil[50]	1969	1	1	
Elliott[9]	1974	3	1	2
O'Mara[25]	1977	7	6	1
Buchbinder[51]	1980	2	2	
Perdue[16]	1980	1		1
O'Mara[52]	1981	1	1	
Higgins[27]	1990	1		1
Total		19	13 (68%)	6 (32%)

Table modified from Bunt[1,8]

Table 5
Graft-Enteric Erosions: Graft Excision

Study	Year	No. of Pts.	Died	Recovered
Youmans[53]	1967	1	1	
Dass[54]	1968	1	1	
Elliott[9]	1974	3	2	1
Tagart[55]	1974	1	1	
O'Mara[25]	1977	4	2	2
Perdue[16]	1980	2		2
Total		12	7 (58%)	5 (42%)

Table modified from Bunt[1,8]

ported on graft-enteric erosions treated locally with closure of the bowel and without graft replacement suggests a mortality of 68%. O'Mara et al. reported that six of seven patients treated with local care died.[25] Thus, when local treatment including antibiotic therapy without revascularization has been used, the mortality rate has been quite high. Most vascular surgeons agree that local closure of the enteric erosion without graft excision and replacement or extra-anatomic bypass has an unacceptably high mortality rate and adequate treatment of this problem necessitates graft removal.

Even with excision of the infected graft, with or without revascularization, the mortality for graft-enteric erosion remains quite high. A review of the literature with only 12 patients suggests a mortality of 58% for graft excision without revascularization, although the number of patients is small (Table 5).

A handful of cases has been reported where a graft has been placed back into the same bed in patients with graft-enteric erosions. The mortality rate is 40% in the five reported cases (Table 6). The number of patients is too small to assess this form of treatment. This may suggest, however, that surgeons have found this management to be unsatisfactory, but have not reported poor results.

Graft-Enteric Fistula

A review by Bunt in 1983 summarized the reported literature on local treatment of

Table 6
Graft-Enteric Erosions: In Situ Graft Replacement

Study	Year	No. of Pts.	Died	Recovered
Elliott[9]	1974	1	1	
Tagart[55]	1974	1	1	
O'Mara[25]	1977	1		1
Perdue[16]	1980	1		1
Yeager[45]	1985	1		1
Total		5	2 (40%)	3 (60%)

Table modified from Bunt[1,8]

graft-enteric fistulae by closing the aorta with or without a patch and closure of the enteric defect with or without interposition of tissue between the bowel and the aorta.[8] Of the 62 reported cases, 55 patients had died representing a mortality rate of 88%. Based on these reports, many surgeons then advocated total excision of the aortic graft, closure of the involved bowel, and extra-anatomic bypass through uninvolved tissue planes. Optimal treatment also consisted of broad spectrum antibiotics chosen on the basis of culture results, debridement of the aortic bed with or without drainage, and coverage of the aortic stump with autogenous tissue such as omentum or anterior spinous ligament. Since that report, however, more cases of local repair have been reported, and the mortality rate for the combined series of 70 patients reviewed is 77% (Table 7). As with other series, the incidence of amputation is difficult to determine and many authors have not reported amputation rates. O'Mara et al. reported on three patients with aortoenteric fistulae who underwent suture repair.[25] All three died of a recurrent aortoenteric fistula. O'Hara et al. reviewed a 25-year experience of patients with infected aortic grafts and found no survivors among the nine patients who underwent local repair.[26] In contrast, Higgins et al. reported 2 cases of successful primary fistula closure without graft replacement.[27] Thomas et al. reported four direct repairs of an aortoduodenal fistula with one recurrent fistula and three patients alive and well.[28] Despite the several isolated reports of successful management of aortoenteric fistula with local repair without graft replacement, the extremely high mortality of 77% to 88% would suggest that this form of therapy should be avoided except in the most unusual circumstances. Repair of a graft-enteric fistula by closure of the bowel and excision of the graft without revascularization has been attempted in a number of cases (Table 8). In the series reviewed with 31 patients, the mortality was 71%, although, again, the number of patients reported is small. The

largest series reported by Kleinman et al. had an 80% mortality rate in five patients only.[20] In general, this treatment has been considered when the patient appears to have adequate circulation to the lower extremity.

Although local repair by suture closure of the aortic fistula has, in general, not been successful, there has been significant interest in the repair of aortoenteric fistulae using in situ graft replacement into the same vascular bed. By 1983, 66 cases had been reported where the treatment of a graft-enteric fistula had been performed by excising the involved graft and placing a new graft in situ into the same vascular bed.[8] Of the 66 cases, 37 patients had died (56% mortality rate). A more recent review of the literature now includes 102 patients with a 40% mortality rate (Table 9). The recent improvement is likely related to improvements in antibiotics, anesthesia, and critical care. Although only 60% of the patients survived, this option of in situ replacement now seems reasonable in selected cases.

Walker et al. treated 20 patients who had an aortoduodenal fistula following placement of an aortic graft.[29] They were treated with closure of the enteric fistula, excision of the old graft, and placement of a new graft in the same location. Three patients with erosion into the jejunum underwent a similar repair. Eighteen patients survived the repair and were followed for a mean of 5 years. Three patients had early recurrent rupture or false aneurysm formation, but 15 patients (83%) recovered. There was no limb loss. Fourteen of these patients had interposition of the greater omentum between the bowel and new aortic graft as a protective barrier. Higgins et al. reported on nine patients with aortoenteric fistulae.[27] Of four patients treated with in situ repair after graft excision, two patients survived. An omental wrap was placed over the grafts when possible. Vollmar et al. reported six of seven patients surviving with in situ graft replacement and Robinson et al. reported

Table 7
Graft-Enteric Fistula: Local Repair

Study	Year	No. of Pts.	Died	Recovered
Sharf[56]	1959	1	1	
Hagland[57]	1959	1	1	
MGH[58,59]	1959	2	1	1
Boyd[60]	1959	1	1	
Cordell[61]	1960	1	1	
Thistlewaite[62]	1960	1		1
Pollock[63]	1961	1	1	
Deweese[48]	1962	2	2	
Javid[14]	1962	3	3	
Humphries[18]	1963	7	7	
Ferris[64]	1965	1		1
Wierman[65]	1966	1	1	
Donovan[19]	1967	1	1	
Schramel[66]	1971	1	1	
Szilagyi[3]	1972	1		1
Tobias[67]	1973	1		1
Elliott[9]	1974	2	2	
Brenner[68]	1974	1		1
Ray[69]	1976	1		1
Mehta[70]	1978	1	1	
Dean[71]	1978	4	3	1
Yashar[7]	1978	1	1	
Kleinman[20]	1979	2	2	
Baird[72]	1979	2	2	
Busuttil[73]	1979	4	4	
Buchbinder[51]	1980	2	2	
Perdue[16]	1980	1	1	
Puglia[74]	1980	4	3	1
Puppala[75]	1980	1	1	
O'Mara[52]	1981	3	3	
O'Hara[26]	1986	9	9	
Thomas[28]	1986	4		4
Higgins[27]	1990	2		2
Total		70	55 (77%)	15 (23%)

Table modified from Bunt[1,8]

four of four patients were treated successfully.[30] Thomas et al. used in situ graft replacement in two patients with infected aortic grafts and both patients survived.[28] Based upon their experience, they suggested that a more conservative approach be considered for patients with aortoenteric fistulae, although the criteria by which patients can be chosen for this treatment remain unclear.

When in situ replacement of infected aortic grafts has been successful, treatment has involved not only graft replacement, but also debridement of infected tissues in the area of the graft, parenteral antibiotics chosen on the basis of cultures, and soft tissue coverage whenever possible. Omentum has been commonly used to cover aortic grafts, but muscle flaps can also be used, especially in the groin.[31,32]

Table 8
Graft-Enteric Fistula: Graft Excision

Study	Year	No. of Pts.	Died	Recovered
Crawford[77]	1960	2		2
Deweese[48]	1962	1	1	
Garrett[78]	1963	1	1	
Beach[79]	1966	1	1	
Youmans[53]	1967	2		2
Schramel[66]	1971	2	1	1
Szilagyi[3]	1972	1	1	
Elliott[9]	1974	1	1	
Busuttil[73]	1979	2	2	
Kleinman[20]	1979	5	4	1
Rosenthal[80]	1979	1	1	
Perdue[16]	1980	1	1	
Connelly[76]	1981	1	1	
O'Mara[52]	1981	1	1	
O'Hara[26]	1986	2	2	
Vollmar[30]	1987	2		2
Edwards[22]	1988	3	3	
Ricotta[81]	1991	2	1	1
Total		31	22 (71%)	9 (29%)

Table modified from Bunt[1,8]

Vetsch et al. examined the anastomotic tensile strength following in situ replacement of infected Dacron grafts in dogs.[33] He found that the anastomotic tensile strength at the site of the graft aortic anastomosis following in situ replacement was similar to that of noninfected control grafts. Aortitis, that is, an infection in the arterial wall, has been implicated as a major cause of aortic stump dehiscence following removal of infected grafts. The findings in this study suggest that a local repair provides better strength in the aorta in the region of the infection.

Using all these techniques, in situ replacement of aortic grafts in the management of graft-enteric fistulae is reasonable in selected cases. However, the morbidity and mortality rates still remain high. In most cases, standard therapy with complete graft excision and extra-anatomic bypass should still be used. The problem of aortic stump blowout and the significant mortality rate with this approach still exists. In situ graft replacement should not be considered unless local infection can be eradicated by wide debridement of the vascular bed.

It is reasonable, based on the existing reports in the literature to adopt the principles suggested by Robinson et al. in the management of patients with infected aortic grafts.[34] If pus and inflammation in the para-aortic and retroperitoneal tissues is widespread beyond the point where adequate debridement is possible, then the aortic stump should be closed and covered with autogenous tissue when possible. The retroperitoneum should be drained and an extra-anatomic bypass should be performed except in the circumstance where blood supply to the lower extremities is adequate. When technically possible, debridement of the aorta and para-aortic tissue should be performed with culture and histologic ex-

Table 9
Graft-Enteric Fistula: In Situ Graft Replacement

Study	Year	No. of Pts.	Died	Recovered
Mackenzie[24]	1958	1		1
Lawton[82]	1959	1		1
Erskine[83]	1960	2		2
Nevin[84]	1960	1		1
Thistlewaite[62]	1960	1	1	
Crawford[77]	1960	3		3
Javid[14]	1962	1		1
Sprout[85]	1962	1		1
Humphries[18]	1963	6	5	1
Garrett[78]	1963	10	2	8
Levy[10]	1965	1		1
Ferris[64]	1965	1		1
Rosato[86]	1967	1		1
Cohn[17]	1968	2	1	1
Conn[2]	1970	3	3	
Szilagyi[3]	1972	1		1
Pinkerton[87]	1973	1		1
Elliott[9]	1974	2	1	1
Dean[71]	1978	3	2	1
Yashar[7]	1978	1	1	
Rosenthal[80]	1979	5	4	1
Kleinman[20]	1979	2	2	
Busuttil[73]	1979	2	2	
Perdue[16]	1980	2	1	1
Puglia[74]	1980	4	2	2
O'Mara[52]	1981	3	3	
Thomas[28]	1986	1		1
Vollmar[30]	1987	7	1	6
Walker[29]	1987	23	7	16
Higgins[27]	1990	4	2	2
Robinson[34]	1991	4		4
Syme[88]	1992	1		1
Total		101	40 (40%)	61 (60%)

Table modified from Bunt[1,8]

amination of the tissues. In situ aortic reconstruction can then be used to restore blood flow to the lower extremities. Antibiotic irrigation of the retroperitoneum may be of benefit. The new graft should be separated from the intestine by autogenous tissue such as omentum. Intravenous antibiotics, and subsequently oral antibiotics, should be used for an extended period of time. Careful surveillance of the in situ graft with a computer tomography scan is then indicated.

Summary

In situ repair may be reasonable when graft infection is limited to a small portion of the graft or involves only the aortic graft anastomosis. Direct repair by simple suturing of the aortic fistula is unlikely to be successful, except in the most unusual circumstances. If the perigraft tissues can be debrided and all of the involved graft removed, in situ replacement may be successful without recurrent graft infection and may result in a lower morbidity and mortality rate including a lower incidence of limb loss. Coverage of the graft with living tissues such as omentum may increase the likelihood of success. However, the traditional approach of total graft excision with extra-anatomic bypass may still be needed in cases where the infection is extensive and a limited repair is unlikely to rid the aortic bed of infection.

References

1. Bunt TJ. Synthetic vascular graft infections: I: graft infections. *Surgery.* 1983;93(6):733–746.
2. Conn JH, Hardy JD, Chavez CM, Fain WR. Infected arterial grafts. *Ann Surg.* 1970;171:704–712.
3. Szilagyi DE, Smith RF, Elliott JP, Vrandecic MP. Infection in arterial reconstruction with synthetic grafts. *Ann Surg.* 1972;176:321–333.
4. Goldstone J, Moore WS. Infection in vascular prosthesis. *Am J Surg.* 1974;128:225–233.
5. Jamieson GG, DeWeese JA, Rob CG. Infected arterial grafts. *Ann Surg.* 1975;181:850–852.
6. Liekweg WG, Greenfield LJ. Vascular prosthetic infections: collected experience and results of treatment. *Surgery.* 1977;81:335–342.
7. Yashar JJ, Weyman AK, Burnard RJ, Yashar J. Survival and limb salvage in patients with infected arterial prostheses. *Am J Surg.* 1978;135:499–504.
8. Bunt TJ. Synthetic vascular graft infections: II: graft-enteric erosions and graft-enteric fistulas. *Surgery.* 1983;94(1):1–9.
9. Elliott JP, Smith RF, Szilagyi DE. Aortoenteric and paraprosthetic fistulas. *Arch Surg.* 1974;108:479–490.
10. Levy MS, Todd DB, Lillehei CW, Varco RL. Aortointestinal fistulas following surgery of the aorta. *Surg Gynecol Obstet.* 1965;120:992–996.
11. Garrett HE, Beall AC, Jordan GL, DeBakey ME. Surgical considerations of massive gastrointestinal tract hemorrhage caused by aortoduodenal fistula. *Am J Surg.* 1963;105:6–11.
12. O'Hara I, Nakano S. Rupture of arterial plastic prosthesis. *Arch Surg.* 1958;77:55.
13. Brown L, Essig H. Fatal rupture of Ivalon (polyvinol formalinized) sponge aortic graft into duodenum: a case report. *Arch Surg.* 1959;79:72–74.
14. Javid H, Julian OC, Dye WS, Hunter JA. Complications of abdominal aortic grafts. *Arch Surg.* 1962;85:142–153.
15. Lorentzen JE, Nielsen OM, Arendrup H, et al. Vascular graft infection: an analysis of 62 graft infections in 2411 consecutively implanted synthetic vascular grafts. *Surgery.* 1985;98(1):81–86.
16. Perdue GD, Smith RG, Ansley JD, Constantino MJ. Impending aortoenteric hemorrhage: the effect of early recognition on improved outcome. *Ann Surg.* 1980;192:237–243.
17. Cohn R, Angell WW. Late complications from plastic replacement of aortic abdominal aneurysms. *Arch Surg.* 1968;97:696–698.
18. Humphries AW, Young JW, DeWolfe VG, LeFevre FA. Complications of abdominal aortic surgery:I: aortoenteric fistulas. *Arch Surg.* 1963;86:43.
19. Donovan TJ, Bucknam CA. Aortoenteric fistula. *Arch Surg.* 1967;95:810–818.
20. Kleinman LH, Towne JB, Bernhard VM. A diagnostic and therapeutic approach to aortoenteric fistulas: clinical experience with 20 patients. *Surgery.* 1979;86:868–880.
21. Calligaro KD, Veith FJ, Schwartz ML, Savarese RP, DeLaurentis DA. Are Gram-negative bacteria a contraindication to selective preservation of infected prosthetic arterial grafts? *J Vasc Surg.* 1992;16:337–346.
22. Edwards MJ, Richardson JD, Klamer TW. Management of aortic prosthetic infections. *Am J Surg.* 1988;155:327–330.
23. Bandyk DF, Bergamini TM, Kinney EV, Seabrook GR, Towne JB. In situ replacement of vascular prostheses infected by bacterial biofilms. *J Vasc Surg.* 1991;13:575–583.
24. Mackenzie RJ, Buell AH, Pearson SC. Aneurysm of aortic homograft with rupture into the duodenum. *Arch Surg.* 1958;77:965–969.
25. O'Mara C, Embembo AL. Paraprosthetic-enteric fistula. *Surgery.* 1977;81:556–566.
26. O'Hara PJ, Hertzer NR, Beven EG, Krajewski LP. Surgical management of infected abdominal aortic grafts: review of a 25-year experience. *J Vasc Surg.* 1986;3:725–731.
27. Higgins RSD, Steed DL, Julian TB, Makaroun MS, Peitzman AB, Webster MW. The management of aortoenteric and paraprosthetic fistulae. *J Cardiovasc Surg.* 1990;31:81–86.
28. Thomas WEG, Baird RN. Secondary aortoenteric fistulae: towards a more conservative approach. *Br J Surg.* 1986;73:875–878.
29. Walker WE, Cooley EA, Duncan JM, Hallman GL, Ott DA, Reul GJ. The management of aortoduodenal fistula by in situ replacement of the infected abdominal aortic graft. *Ann Surg.* 1987;205(6):727–732.
30. Vollmar JF, Kogel H. Aortoenteric fistulas as a postoperative complication. *J Cardiovasc Surg.* 1987;28:479–484.

31. Goldsmith HS, de los Santos R, Vanamee P, Beattie EJ. Experimental protection of vascular prosthesis by omentum. *Arch Surg.* 1968; 97:872–877.

32. Mendes D, Kahn M, Ibrahim IM, Sussman B, Fox B, Dardik H. Omental protection of autogenous arterial reconstruction following femoral prosthetic graft infection. *J Vasc Surg.* 1985;2:603–606.

33. Vetsch R, Bandyk DF, Schmitt DD, Bergamini TM, Storey JD, Towne JB. Anastomotic tensile strength following in situ replacement of an infected abdominal aortic graft. *Arch Surg.* 1989;124:425–428.

34. Robinson JA, Johansen K. Aortic sepsis: is there a role for in situ graft reconstruction? *J Vasc Surg.* 1991;13:677–684.

35. Carter SC, Cohen A, Whelan TJ. Clinical experience with management of the infected dacron graft. *Ann Surg.* 1963;158:249–255.

36. Vandewater JM, Gaal PG. Management of patients with infected vascular prostheses. *Am Surg.* 1965;31:6511–6518.

37. Bouhoutsos J, Chavatzas D, Martin P, Morris T. Infected synthetic arterial grafts. *Br J Surg.* 1974;61:108–111.

38. Perdue GD. Antibiotics as an aid in the prevention of infections after peripheral arterial surgery. *Am Surg.* 1975;41:296–300.

39. Almgren B, Ericksson I. Local antibiotic irrigation in the treatment of arterial graft infections. *Acta Chir Scand.* 1981;147:33–36.

40. Kwaan JH, Connolly JE. Successful management of prosthetic graft infection with continuous povidone-iodine irrigation. *Arch Surg.* 1981;116:716–720.

41. Schramel RS, Creech O. Effects of infection and exposure on synthetic arterial prostheses. *Arch Surg.* 1959;78:102–108.

42. Shaw RS, Baue AE. Management of sepsis complicating arterial reconstructive surgery. *Surgery.* 1963;53:75–86.

43. Crawford ES, Manning LG, Keely TF. Redo surgery after operations for aneurysm and occlusion of the abdominal aorta. *Surgery.* 1977;81:41–52.

44. Casali RE, Tucker WE, Thompson BW, Read RC. Infected prosthetic grafts. *Arch Surg.* 1980;115:577–580.

45. Yeager RA, McConnell DB, Sasaki TM, Vetto RM. Aortic and peripheral prosthetic graft infection: differential management and causes of mortality. *Am J Surg.* 1985;150: 36–41.

46. Quinones-Baldrich WJ, Hernandez JJ, Moore WS. Long-term results following surgical management of aortic graft infection. *Arch Surg.* 1991;126:507–511.

47. Yeager RA, Moneta GL, Taylor LM, Harris EJ, McConnell DB, Porter JM. Improving survival and limb salvage in patients with aortic graft infection. *Am J Surg.* 1990;159:466–469.

48. DeWeese MS, Fry WJ. Small bowel erosion following aortic resection. *JAMA.* 1962;179: 882–884.

49. Long L, Hunter J, Dye WS. Migration of aortic prosthesis into the duodenum. *Ann Surg.* 1962;157:560–565.

50. Sheil AGR, Reese TS, Little JM, Coupland AE, Loewenthal J. Aortointestinal fistulas following operation on the abdominal aortic and iliac arteries. *Br J Surg.* 1969;53:840–842.

51. Buchbinder D, Leather R, Shah D, Karmody A. Pathologic interactions between prosthetic aortic grafts and the gastrointestinal tract. *Am J Surg.* 1980;140:192–196.

52. O'Mara CS, Williams GM, Ernst CB. Secondary aortoenteric fistula. *Am J Surg.* 1981;142: 203–209.

53. Youmans CR, Derrick JR. Gastrointestinal erosion after prosthetic arterial reconstructive surgery. *Am J Surg.* 1967;114: 711–715.

54. Dass T. Small bowel erosion after aortic replacement by synthetic graft. *Am J Surg.* 1968;116:460.

55. Tagart REB. Infection of an aortic prosthesis caused by duodenal erosion. *Proc R Soc Med.* 1974;67:1181.

56. Sharf AG, Acker ED. Surgical intervention in ruptured and thrombosed aortic homografts. *Arch Surg.* 1959;78:67–69.

57. Hagland L. Sweetman W, Wise R. Rupture of an abdominal aortic homograft with ileal fistula. *Am J Surg.* 1959;98:746–748.

58. Case records of the Massachusetts General Hospital. *N Engl J Med.* 1959;261:12–24, 1339–1341.

59. Case records of the Massachusetts General Hospital (case 45282). *N Engl J Med.* 1959;261: 292.

60. Boyd DP, Pastel H. Results of treatment of aneurysm of abdominal aorta. *Postgrad Med.* 1959;25:238–242.

61. Cordell AR, Wright RH, Johnston FR. Gastrointestinal hemorrhage after abdominal aortic operations. *Surgery.* 1960;48:997–999.

62. Thistlewaite JR. Spontaneous arteriovenous fistula between abdominal aorta and vena cava. *Arch Surg.* 1960;81:61–63.

63. Pollock AV, Pratt D, Smiddy FG. Aortic homograft replacement: a sequel. *Ann Surg.* 1961;153:472–476.

64. Ferris EJ, Koltay SMR, Sciammas FD. Abdominal aortic and iliac graft fistulae: unusual roentgenologic findings. *Am J Roentgenol Radiother Nucl Med.* 1965;94:416–418.

65. Wierman WH, Strahan RW, Spencer JR. Small bowel erosion by synthetic aortic grafts. *Am J Surg.* 1966;112:791.
66. Schramel A, Weisz GM, Erlik D. Gastrointestinal bleeding due to arterioenteric fistula. *Digestion.* 1971;4:103–108.
67. Tobias JA, Daicoff GR. Aortogastric and aortoileal fistulas repaired by direct suture. *Arch Surg.* 1973;107:909–912.
68. Brenner WI, Richman A, Reed GF. Roofpatch repair of an aortoduodenal fistula resulting from suture line failure in an aortic prosthesis. *Am J Surg.* 1974;127:762–764.
69. Ray R, McAfee RE, Hiebert CA, Hall WJ. Aortoduodenal fistula: primary repair with saphenous vein patch graft. *JAMA.* 1976;236: 2423–2425.
70. Mehta AI, McDowell DE, James EC. Treatment of massive gastrointestinal hemorrhage from aortoenteric fistula. *Surg Gynecol Obstet.* 1978;146:59–73.
71. Dean RH, et al. Aortoduodenal fistula: an uncommon but correctable cause of upper gastrointestinal bleeding. *Am Surg.* 1978;44: 37–43.
72. Baird RL, Slagle GW, Boggs HW. Arterioenteric fistulas. *Dis Colon Rectum.* 1979;187.
73. Busuttil RW, Rees WR, Baker JD, Wilson SE. Pathogenesis of aortoduodenal fistula: experimental and clinical correlates. *Surgery.* 1979;85:1–13
74. Puglia E, Fry PD. Aortoenteric fistulas: a preventable problem? *Can J Surg.* 1980;23:74–76.
75. Puppala AR, Munaswamy M, Doshi AM, Steinheber FU. Endoscopic diagnosis of aortoduodenal fistula. *Am J Gastroenterol.* 1980; 73:414–417.
76. Connolly JE, Kwaan JH, McCart PM, Brownell DA, Levine EF. Aortoenteric fistula. *Ann Surg.* 1981;194:402–412.
77. Crawford ES. Evaluation of late failures after reconstructive operations for occlusive lesions of the aorta, femoral, and popliteal arteries. *Surgery.* 1960;47:79–104.
78. Garrett HE, Beal AC, Jordan GL, DeBakey ME. Surgical considerations of massive gastrointestinal tract hemorrhage caused by aortoduodenal fistula. *Am J Surg.* 1963;105:6.
79. Beach PM, Risley THA. Aorticosigmoid fistulization following aortic resection. *Arch Surg.* 1966;92:805–807.
80. Rosenthal D, Deterling RA, O'Donnell TF, Callou AD. Positive blood culture as an aid in the diagnosis of secondary aortoenteric fistulae. *Arch Surg.* 1979;114:1040–1044.
81. Ricotta JJ, Faggioli GL, Stella A, et al. Total excision and extra-anatomic bypass for aortic graft infection. *Am J Surg.* 1991;162: 145–149.
82. Lawton RL, Peterson FR, Brenterall ES. Aortointestinal fistula following aortic homotransplantation. *Angiology.* 1959;10:85.
83. Erskine J, Thoshinsky M, Wilson J. Rupture of aortic homografts into the small intestine. *Ann Surg.* 1960;152:991–997.
84. Nevin I, Bump W, Thverer G. Preoperative diagnosis of rupture into the duodenum of an aortic homograft anastomosis. *N Engl J Med.* 1960;263:243.
85. Sprout G. Rupture of an infected aortic graft into jejunum: resection and survival. *JAMA.* 1962;182:1118.
86. Rosato FE, Barker C, Roberts B. Aortointestinal fistula. *J Thorac Cardiovasc Surg.* 1967;53: 511–514.
87. Pinkerton JA. Aortoduodenal fistula. *JAMA.* 1973;225:1196–1199.
88. Syme RG, Doobay BS, Gregor P, Franchetto A. Aortoenteric fistula 24 years after aortic endarterectomy. *Can J Surg.* 1992;35(1): 100–103.

Chapter 11

Muscle Flaps for Graft Infection

B.A. Perler

Introduction

At a time of dramatic advances in vascular diagnostic and therapeutic technology, arterial bypass graft infection continues to represent a difficult challenge for the surgeon and a potentially devastating complication for the patient. Infection of prosthetic bypass grafts (PGI) has been noted following 1% to 6% of peripheral arterial reconstructions, with an incidence of 1% to 2.5% in most large series.[1-8] The serious nature of this complication is reflected in mortality rates ranging from 25% to 75%, and in the reported incidence of significant morbidity, including limb loss, in 25% to 75% of patients.[1,3-7,9-11] The highest mortality rates have been associated with infection of aortoiliofemoral grafts, and the incidence of amputation is greatest when infection involves infrainguinal reconstructions.[2,6]

After more than 2 decades of experience, the optimal management of PGI remains unsettled. The dogma that infection involving a foreign body can be eradicated only by removal of that foreign body is the basis for the conventional surgical approach, namely, complete graft excision and revascularization, if necessary, through uninfected, clean, extra-anatomic tissue planes.[2,6] However, some of the highest morbidity and mortality rates have been reported in association with this conventional solution to PGI.[2,6,12] In view of this experience, alternative strategies have been pursued such as graft excision and in situ replacement with autogenous arteries or veins,[13] graft excision and replacement with cadaveric homograft veins,[14] and perhaps most radically, aggressive local wound care with preservation of the graft.[12,15,16]

Local Care

The local treatment of PGI is not a new concept. Nearly 30 years ago, Carter et al. first reported the successful treatment of 6/7 (86%) patients with infected Dacron grafts through aggressive soft tissue debridement, frequent wound irrigation and dressing changes, and the administration of systemic antibiotics, with healing achieved by secondary intention.[17] More recently, other researchers have reported successful eradication of graft infection in selected patients with modifications of this approach.[12,15,16]

The obvious appeal of the local treatment of PGI is its potential to avoid the substantial morbidity associated with complete graft excision. Conversely, this approach conveys other significant drawbacks. Achieving wound healing by secondary intention mandates a prolonged period of hospitalization with enormous financial costs. In addition, during this period the patient must undergo frequent uncomfortable dressing changes and remain relatively immobile. Furthermore, during this period of treatment, other complications of smoldering graft infection, such as acute anastomotic hemorrhage, or secondary infection by more virulent organisms may develop.[18]

The use of muscle flaps is a further and innovative refinement of the local therapy of graft infection, with several significant potential benefits. First, early coverage of the exposed graft with muscle should theoretically reduce the likelihood of secondary complications of hemorrhage or further bacterial contamination. Second, it can expedite wound healing and reduce the period of hospitalization. Finally, and perhaps most importantly, there is a growing body of experimental evidence suggesting that well-vascularized muscle possesses an inherent biologic potential to actually eradicate the underlying infection.

Muscle Flaps: Experimental Observations

Healing of an implanted prosthetic graft in humans involves the development of a thick, acellular, and relatively avascular capsule.[19] When infection develops, it has been postulated that this acellular tissue reaction may serve as a barrier to host immune function and eradication of infection.[20] This avascular capsule around the graft results in a relatively hypoxic local environment. It has been well demonstrated that hypoxia both predisposes to the development and can interfere with the eradication of infection through its inhibition of leukocyte function[21,22] Muscle flaps possess a rich capillary network. When placed in continuity with the infected graft, rapid ingrowth around the graft occurs and a high

level of antibiotics may be delivered to the local wound. Furthermore, by increasing oxygen delivery and wound oxygen tension in the infected tissues, muscle flaps may improve leukocyte function and expedite bacterial elimination.[20] These hypothetical speculations have been studied in a number of experimental models. Chang and Mathes developed a model of deep space *Staphylococcus aureus* infection in dogs, and compared the effects of rectus abdominis musculocutaneous flaps versus corresponding random pattern flaps. Significantly reduced bacterial counts were observed in the wounds closed with musculocutaneous flaps and conversely, significant bacterial proliferation and eventual necrosis was observed when random pattern flaps were used.[23] Furthermore, a significantly higher oxygen tension was noted in the musculocutaneous flap when compared to the random pattern flap.[23]

These findings have been confirmed in other studies. Calderon et al. performed similar experiments in which bacterial suppression in musculocutaneous and fasciocutaneous flaps inoculated within closed wound spaces was assessed. Both flaps remain viable, although significantly greater bacterial killing was achieved by musculocutaneous flaps.[24] In another study, paired musculocutaneous and fasciocutaneous flaps were performed in dogs, and wound cylinders created beneath the flaps were inoculated with *S aureus*. Significantly lower bacterial concentrations were detected on postoperative days 1, 3, and 6 in the musculocutaneous flaps when compared to the fasciocutaneous flaps ($P < 0.001$). Musculocutaneous flaps demonstrated a marked decrease in bacterial counts within the first 24 hours, dropping from a range of 10^7 to 10^3 bacteria per milliliter ($P < 0.0001$), whereas bacterial counts n the fasciocutaneous flaps dropped from a range of 10^7 to 10^5 bacteria per milliliter ($P < 0.05$). Between days 1 and 6 postoperatively, bacterial counts within the musculocutaneous flaps gradually declined to a range of 10^2 bacteria per milliliter, while counts in the fasciocutaneous flaps remained within a range of 10^5 bacteria per milliliter.[25] These investigators concluded that the rapid decline in bacterial counts beneath the musculocutaneous flaps resulted from the rapid increase in blood flow during the first 24 hours. Using radionuclide microspheres, they demonstrated that arterial flow to the muscle in musculocutaneous flaps increased rapidly during the first 24 hours, and then reached a plateau, whereas flow to the subcutaneous tissue and fascia in fasciocutaneous flaps demonstrated a gradual and steady increase during the 6 days of observation. Furthermore, at sacrifice on day 6, it was noted that wound cylinders within musculocutaneous flaps tended to be incorporated by the surrounding muscle.[25]

Other laboratory work has specifically addressed the potential of muscle flaps to treat infection involving prosthetic grafts. Dacey et al. studied unilateral carotid artery bypass performed in dogs with polytetrafluoroethylene (PTFE) grafts, after which the grafts were inoculated with *S aureus* at implantation. Three days later, the wounds were opened and the patent grafts were debrided, irrigated, and randomized to three treatment groups: 1) primary closure and oral antibiotics; 2) sternocephalicus muscle flap closure but no antibiotics; and 3) antibiotics and muscle flap closure. The animals were followed for 60 days or until anastomotic disruption occurred and at sacrifice the fluid and muscle around the graft was cultured. All dogs in groups 1 and 2 experienced anastomotic disruption whereas only 20% of group 3 dogs experienced this complication ($P < 0.05$). Furthermore, at sacrifice, less bacterial colonies were cultured from the muscle of group 3 than group 1 dogs ($P < 0.05$), suggesting the efficacy of muscle flap coverage and systemic antibiotic administration in the treatment of PGI.[26]

Mehran et al. replaced the abdominal aortas of pigs with PTFE and then inoculated the grafts with *S aureus*.[20] One week later, the animals were randomized to six treatment groups: 1) debridement of the retroperitoneum only; 2) debridement and placement of a new graft; 3) the infected graft was left in place and wrapped in a rectus abdominis flap; 4) the graft was left in place and wrapped with the seromuscular layer of the jejunum; 5) a new graft was placed and wrapped with a rectus abdominis muscle flap; and 6) a new graft was placed and wrapped with the seromuscular layer of the jejunum.

At reoperation 2 weeks later, graft patency was assessed and bacterial cultures obtained. The incidence of graft infection was significantly reduced in group 5 (0 of 10; $P < 0.01$) and 6 (1 of 10; $P < 0.02$) compared to group 1, and the incidence of graft thrombosis was significantly reduced in groups 5 (2 of 10) and 6 (1 of 10) versus group 1 (10 of 10; $P < 0.01$). Infection was also controlled in groups 3 (1 of 6) and 4 (2 of 6), but these grafts were thrombosed at reoperation.[20]

Cruz et al. placed PTFE interpositional grafts in the femoral arteries of 20 dogs; the wounds were inoculated with *S aureus* (1×10^4 or 1×10^5 organisms per mL). In 10 animals the graft was wrapped with a distally based sartorius muscle flap, and all wounds were then closed in two layers. No antibiotics were given. All animals were sacrificed 1 month later and quantitative wound cultures were obtained. At sacrifice, among the grafts inoculated with 1×10^4 organisms, 5 of 10 grafts without a sartorius wrap were infected versus 0 of 10 in which the graft had been wrapped with sartorius muscle ($P < 0.05$). Among the animals inoculated with 1×10^5 at implantation, 9 of 10 treated without a muscle flap were infected versus 6 of 10 in which a sartorius flap had been performed. This difference did not achieve statistical significance.[27]

Although these data suggest that well-vascularized muscle tissue may contribute to eradication of infection involving a prosthetic conduit, it does also emphasize that this biologic potential of muscle tissue may be limited by the quantitative degree of bacterial contamination.[27,28] Furthermore, since these experimental studies have all used models of acute graft infection, the relevance of these findings to the problem of chronic graft infection remains speculative and deserves further study.[28]

Clinical Experience with Nonvascular Muscle Flaps

For a number of years plastic surgeons have performed muscle flap procedures to close difficult wounds resulting from trauma, pressure sores, radiation injury, extensive tumor resection, and congenital anomalies.[29–31] Although these experimental studies provide a solid rationale for the use of muscle flaps to treat PGI, most clinical experience to date has been reported in the treatment of nonvascular surgical infection. A growing body of evidence has demonstrated the efficacy of muscle flaps in eradicating serious infection in the fields of thoracic, orthopedic, and cardiac surgery.

Thoracic Surgery

Numerous reports have examined the use of muscle flaps in the management of invasive infection after pulmonary or esophageal surgery.[32–37] In the largest series reported to date, Arnold et al. described 118 muscle transpositions, including 48 serratus anterior, 33 latissimus dorsi, 26 pectoralis major, and a variety of other muscles that were performed upon 87 consecutive patients with postthoracic surgical complications. Active infection was documented in 65 (75%) cases. Excellent results were documented in 65 (75%) patients at a mean follow-up of 28.3 months, including 45 (69%) of 65 patients with documented intrathoracic infection at the time of muscle flap closure.[38]

Latissimus dorsi, serratus anterior, and pectoralis major have been the most frequently used muscles in these series, both because of their anatomic proximity to the wounds and their size and bulk which provide for adequate closure of large thoracic defects.[39] Furthermore, in the presence of bacterial contamination, primary healing has been shown to be more common with these muscle flaps than with skin grafts, probably as a result of the rich arterial supply of these muscles.[39–42]

Orthopedic Surgery

The failure of bone debridement and antibiotic administration to consistently achieve healing of osteomyelitic bone has been well documented. In 1946, Stark reported the initial series of patients with osteomyelitis treated with muscle flap coverage. Eighty-four percent of wounds closed with muscle flaps remained healed versus only 43% of those treated by conventional means without the use of muscle flaps.[43] Subsequently, Ger reported 17 consecutive patients with lower extremity osteomyelitis who were successfully treated by debridement and coverage with local muscle flaps.[44] In a more recent report, 11 patients with chronic osteomyelitis (average duration of symptoms, 14 years) involving the distal tibia and foot were successfully treated with gracilis muscle transposition, and none developed recurrent infections with an average follow-up of 1.8 years.[45]

Perhaps even more relevant to the issue of PGI is infection of orthopedic endoprostheses since it has been a well-established principle in orthopedic surgery that open wounds over exposed endoprostheses should be treated by removal of the implant.[46] In view of the prolonged hospitalization and potential morbidity associated with this approach, and in light of the experience with osteomyelitis, interest has developed in using muscle flap coverage to salvage exposed endoprostheses. In a recent report from UCLA, by LeSavoy et al., four patients with exposed orthopedic endoprostheses were successfully treated with muscle flaps. In two patients, the gastrocnemius muscle was used to cover a knee and an exposed distal femoral endoprosthesis, respectively. The other two patients with exposed humeral endoprostheses were treated with latissimus dorsi and pectoralis major flaps, respectively.[47]

Cardiac Surgery

Mediastinal infection is seen following approximately 1% of cardiac surgical procedures and conveys the same degree of life-threatening morbidity as noted with PGI.[48-50] The traditional management of this problem has included sternal debridement, continuous closed mediastinal antibiotic irrigation, and delayed skin closure, and has mandated a prolonged and difficult hospital course.[51,52] Treatment was dramatically refined when Jurkiewicz reported excellent results in patients treated by aggressive sternal debridement and closure with muscle flaps. Six patients who did not respond to conventional therapy underwent muscle flap closure; all survived, all were cured, and the average duration of hospitalization was only 19 days after the infection was identified.[53] In a more recent report, infected sternotomy wounds were treated in 100 consecutive patients by Pairolero et al., including the use of 175 muscle flaps in 94 of these cases.[54] Among the 98 operative survivors, only 26 developed recurrent infection and 22 of these patients subsequently were successfully treated.[54] These observations have been confirmed in other series in which definitive cure has been achieved with muscle flap closure in approximately 90% of cases.[54-57] In fact, Pairolero has concluded that muscle flaps represent the most exciting development in the field of thoracic surgery in the last decade.[54]

The pectoralis major has been the most frequently used muscle to treat sternal infection in these reports. It has a dominant blood supply based on the thoracoacromial artery, and mobilization of the muscle allows an arc of rotation that reaches all of the anterior chest wall except the lower sternum.[55] The rectus abdominis and occasionally latissimus dorsi flaps have also been used in this setting.[58] The superb vascularity of these muscles has been felt to be paramount in their ability to achieve healing of this type of infected wound.[59] Furthermore, mobilization of these muscles to treat sternal infection has been associated with excellent long-term functional results.[58]

Muscle flaps have been used to treat other septic vascular complications in the chest. Schaff et al. reported a 54-year-old patient who presented with an infected pseudoaneurysm of the left ventricle 2 years following aneurysmectomy. He underwent successful resection of the pseudoaneurysm through a bed of purulent material, and the repair was closed with a pectoralis major muscle flap, with complete recovery.[60] In another series, 10 patients with postoperative infection involving the ascending aorta and aortic arch were successfully treated with muscle flaps and long-term oral antibiotics and all have remained infection-free with follow-up ranging to 6.5 years.[61]

Clinical Experience with Muscle Flaps for Prosthetic Graft Infection

Although experience to date using muscle flaps to treat PGI is somewhat limited when compared to other surgical infection problems, it is predicated upon sound biologic principles demonstrated in experimental studies, as well as an extensive clinical experience that has accumulated in other areas, as described above. Currently two types of muscle flaps have been performed to treat peripheral vascular graft infections; namely, local sartorius transfer and formal rotational muscle flap (RMF) procedures.

Local Sartorius Transfer

For a variety of reasons, the majority of graft infections develop in the groin. There may be contamination by local skin flora at the site of incision or from adjacent perineal organisms, as well as bacterial growth in inguinal lymph nodes or lymphatic channels secondary to infected distal extremity lesions. In addition, postoperative hematoma or lymphocele formation may provide a rich culture medium to promote bacterial growth. In some patients, extensive relatively avascular scar tissue secondary to previous surgery may also impede the healing process and predispose to wound breakdown and the development of infection.[1,2,4,62,63] Based upon its anatomic course therefore it is not surprising that local sartorius transfer has been a popular muscle flap to treat arterial graft infection.

The sartorius is the longest muscle in the body, arising from the anterior superior iliac spine and inserting on the upper medial shaft of the tibia. Furthermore, the sartorius has an extensive segmental arterial blood supply. The most cephalad aspect of the muscle is perfused by branches of the lateral femoral circumflex artery. Beyond the adductor canal, the distal extent of the muscle is fed by geniculate branches of the popliteal artery. However, the vast majority of the muscle blood supply is derived from 8 to 11 segmental branches of the superficial femoral artery (SFA).[64] Therefore, this muscle may be detached proximally, distally, or in its mid-portion for graft coverage at any site along the upper leg. Typically, the origin of the muscle is detached from the ileum, rotated medially, and reattached to the inguinal ligament for graft coverage in the groin. The distal muscle may be detached and mobilized medially for graft coverage in the lower thigh or it may be reflected superiorly to provide coverage in the groin. In the occasional case where the graft is exposed in the mid-thigh the middle portion of the sartorius may be mobilized medially to provide coverage while leaving the proximal and distal insertions undisturbed.[65]

Sartorius muscle transfer was first described in 1948 to cover exposed native femoral vessels after inguinal lymphadenectomy.[66] Subsequent reports documented the efficacy of local sartorius transfer in closing difficult groin wounds secondary to trauma or radiation injury.[32] In a recent prospective study by Scher, local sartorius transfer was performed prophylactically in 24 patients who required reexploration of the groin within 7 days of an arterial reconstruction, and routine primary closure was performed in a comparable group of 28 patients. Although wound complications occurred in more than 50% of the patients in both groups, graft exposure-infection developed in only 4.2% of the patients in whom local sartorius transfer had been performed, but in 28.6% of patients in whom the sartorius had not been used to cover the graft at reexploration ($P < 0.01$).[67]

Local sartorius transfer has also been performed in the face of groin infection involving native arteries, as well as autogenous saphenous vein and prosthetic bypass grafts. The experience reported to date demonstrates that excellent results have been achieved in treating infection involving native arteries and vein grafts. Meyer et al. reported successful healing of groin wounds in eight consecutive patients with infected infrainguinal saphenous vein grafts. Follow-up ranged from 6 to 30 (mean 16) months, without recurrent infection.[68] In another center, Kaufman et al. reported successful healing in four patients with native arterial and four patients with saphenous vein graft infections using local sartorius transfer.[65]

However, eradication of infection involving a prosthetic conduit is a more difficult challenge. Although reported clinical experience with local sartorius transfer for PGI is limited, early results have been encouraging (Table 1). Healing of the wounds reported in these series has been achieved either by primary closure, by the application of split thickness skin grafts to the muscle, or by secondary intention.[64,69–73] However, it is well recognized that indolent graft infection may smolder silently for extended

Table 1
PGI: Experience with Local Sartorius Transfer

Author	No. Grafts	Material	No. Healed (%)	No. Recurrent Infection (%)	Follow-Up Months
Kaufman[65]	6	Dacron (3) PTFE (3)	6 (100%)	1 (17%)	N/A
Soots[69]	5	Dacron	5 (100%)	1 (20%)	6–54
Mendez-Fernandez[70]	2	Dacron	2 (100%)	0 (0%)	24–132
Hejnal[71]	1	N/A	1 (100%)	N/A	N/A
Dagher[72]	2	PTFE	2 (100%)	0 (0%)	11–14
Bandyk[73]	7	PTFE	7 (100%)	0 (0%)	5–30

PGI = prosthetic graft infection; PTFE = polytetrafluoroethylene.

periods of time to only reappear clinically months or years later. In the largest series with long-term follow-up reported to date, recurrent infection has developed in 11% of cases.[64,69,73] Furthermore, some surgeons have expressed reservations about performing local sartorius transfer when there is anastomotic exposure.[18,68] Nevertheless, local sartorius transfer appears to be a useful adjunct to the management of selected patients with graft infection. Its major advantage lies in the technical simplicity of the procedure and its safety. In addition, local sartorius transfer leaves the patient with no functional deficit.

Conversely, for several reasons, the author believes that local sartorius transfer may not represent the optimal muscle flap procedure in the setting of PGI. Mobilization of the muscle may result in division or occlusion of some of its arterial supply. It has been previously demonstrated that interruption of more than three pedicles may result in ischemia and necrosis of a part of the flap, with subsequent wound breakdown.[64] Furthermore, since so many of these patients have extensive arteriosclerotic occlusive disease, often involving the SFA, the vascularity of the muscle may not be optimal, even prior to its mobilization. In addition, since the anatomic course of the sartorius is contiguous to the bed of the infected graft, it is reasonable to assume some degree of bacterial contamination of this muscle prior to its translocation.

Rotational Muscle Flaps

Background

In view of the potential drawbacks inherent in local sartorius transfer, as well as the experimental data and nonvascular clinical experience described above, it is my opinion that performance of a formal rotational muscle (RMF) procedure represents the optimal method of treating localized PGI. A RMF is defined by mobilizing a muscle from a clean, noninfected bed, which is separate from the site of graft infection and that is based upon a pedicled arterial blood supply.[74] The RMF conveys several theoretical advantages when compared to local sartorius transfer. Since the muscle is mobilized from an isolated bed, it can be assumed to be sterile at the time of placement around the infected graft. Selecting a muscle with an arterial supply that is independent of the site of infection and is not compromised by the process of mobilization ensures optimal vascularity of the translocated tissue. This normally perfused muscle will bring into the infected field a high level of antibiotics and immunocompetent cells and will maximally stimulate wound healing.[75] Furthermore, if the muscle is rotated with its overlying skin as a myocutaneous flap, primary closure is immediately achieved. If the muscle is rotated without its overlying skin, it provides a superb base to which a split thickness skin graft can be placed to complete the closure. In addition, the particular muscle used can be selected based upon the anatomic requirements of the wound being treated. A variety of muscles are available to treat PGI in the groin and upper thigh, its most frequent site of presentation (Table 2). The major advantage of the rectus abdominis is its bulk and length, which allows it to be wrapped circumferentially around an extended length of exposed graft in the groin and upper leg. It derives its blood supply from the deep inferior epigastric artery.[74] Division of the inguinal ligament allows easy translocation of the muscle to an infrainguinal location.[18] The muscle may be reliably transferred with a horizontal, vertical, or extended thoracoepigastric cutaneous component, or it may be translocated without its overlying skin.[18] Its long arc of rotation is another important advantage.[76] Although this muscle may be mobilized without significant functional deficit for the patient, in some cases it does result in abdominal wall laxity or hernia formation.[76]

Another useful muscle for graft coverage in the groin is the rectus femoris which is based upon the descending branch of the lateral femoral circumflex artery.[18] It may be mobilized with or without its overlying skin, and has a wide arc of rotation.[77] One disadvantage that some surgeons have noted when using the rectus femoris muscle is that this may result in loss of terminal extension of the knee.[32,77] Furthermore, significant arteriosclerotic disease of the profunda femoris artery may potentially compromise the viability of this flap.

The tensor fascia lata, which receives its blood supply from the lateral femoral circumflex artery, has also been used to close difficult groin wounds.[74,78,79] Although the muscle contributes to abduction and medial rotation of the thigh, it may be used in this setting without significant functional impairment,[78] although in an occasional patient some knee instability may result.[18] Furthermore, since the muscle is thin and flat, the donor site can usually be closed primarily.[19] Another option for graft coverage in the groin is the relatively small gracilis muscle, which is supplied by the medial femoral circumflex artery. Although it may be rotated with no residual functional deficit, its relatively small size and limited arc of rotation have limited its usefulness to closing small wounds.[18,80] The same principles and considerations that pertain to graft coverage in the groin apply to the selection of muscle flaps to cover exposed grafts in other anatomic sites throughout the body (Table 2).

Clinical Experience

Clinical experience with RMF procedures to treat arterial infection is somewhat limited when compared to the experience reported in treating other serious surgical infectious complications, as described above. Nevertheless, the early results have been quite favorable. More than 15 years ago, Ger reported on a case of a 26-year-old man who underwent repair of a traumatic arm injury with subsequent septic breakdown of the wound and exposure of a brachial artery suture line. The wound was debrided and closed with a brachioradialis

Table 2
Rotational Muscle Flaps

Groin	Axilla/Upper Arm
Rectus abdominis	Pectoralis major
Rectus femoris	Latissimus dorsi
Tensor fascia lata	*Forearm*
Gracilis	Latissimus dorsi
Popliteal Space	Flexor digitorum
Medial gastrocnemius	sublimis
Lateral gastrocnemius	*Mediastinum*
Soleus	Pectoralis major
Neck	Rectus abdominis
Pectoralis major	Latissimus dorsi
Sternocleidomastoid	
Latissimus dorsi	

muscle flap, and later a skin graft was placed to achieve complete wound healing.[75] Subsequently, Hodgkinson and Sheppard reported on a case of a 70-year-old man with an exposed, infected PTFE dialysis graft fistula in the arm. The wound was debrided and covered with a sublimis myocutaneous flap. The wound remained healed at follow-up 6 months later.[81] In a more recent report by Ammor et al., three patients with nonpurulent groin wound breakdown and exposed prosthetic grafts (Dacron in two and PTFE in the other case) were successfully treated with tensor fasciae latae myocutaneous flaps. All three patients' wounds have remained healed and they had no further complications on follow-up of 31, 37, and 68 months, respectively.[78] In no case was there anastomotic exposure and in each case the bacterial count was less than 10^5 organisms per gram of tissue.[77]

In the largest series reported to date, Mixter et al. reported on 20 cases of PGI, involving Dacron in 13, PTFE in 6, and both Dacron and PTFE grafts in 1 case. All of the patients underwent aggressive local wound care and coverage with rotational muscle flaps. Graft salvage was achieved in 19 (95%) cases. An additional patient with an exposed, infected saphenous vein graft was also successfully treated with a RMF procedure. Follow-up has ranged from 4 to 102 (mean 36) months, and no recurrent infections have been identified among the 20 patients.[82] It should be pointed out, however, that in one of these cases there was an anastomotic breakdown, which the authors considered to be a contraindication to the use of RMF procedures.[82] In fact, others have urged caution with respect to wound closure with RMF procedures when there is simply anastomotic exposure in the wound.[18]

The Johns Hopkins Experience

We have taken a more aggressive, or perhaps, more liberal approach with respect to the use of rotational muscle flaps for the treatment of PGI; specifically, we believe that anastomotic exposure and/or breakdown is not an absolute contraindication to this method of treatment.[83] Over a 5- and 1/2-year period, 11 RMF procedures have been performed upon patients ranging in age from 42 to 79 (mean 64) years at the Johns Hopkins Hospital[84] (Table 3). Infection involved 5 aortofemoral, 3 femoro-

---

Table 3
RMF Procedures for PGI: Johns Hopkins Experience

				Patient Characteristics			
Pt	Sex	Age	Graft	Material	Site	Signs	Time
1	M	58	ABF	Dacron	Groin	Abscess	Subacute
2	F	79	ABF	Dacron	Groin	Abscess	Chronic
3	M	69	ABF	Dacron	Groin	Hemorrhage	Acute
4	M	77	ABF	Dacron	Groin	Pur.drain	Chronic
5	F	61	ABF/F-pop	Dacron/PTFE	Groin	Hemorrhage	Acute
6	M	78	F-pop	PTFE	Groin	Hemorrhage	Acute
7	F	67	F/pop	PTFE	Groin	False An.	Acute
8	F	74	Fem-fem	Dacron	Groin	Pur.drain	Subacute
9	M	42	S-C-C	Dacron	Neck	Pur.drain	Acute
10	F	39	CC-IC	Dacron	Neck	Abscess	Chronic

RMF = rotational muscle flap; ABF = aortobifemoral; F-pop = femoropopliteal; Fem-fem = femorofemoral; S-C-C = subclavian-carotid-carotid; CC-IC = common carotid-internal carotid.

popliteal, 1 subclavian-carotid-carotid, and 1 common-internal carotid bypass and were composed of Dacron (8) or PTFE (3). Five infections were acute (less than 30 days after implantation), 2 were subacute (2 and 3 months after implantation), and 3 were chronic (12, 29, and 36 months after implantation). All patients presented with true Szylagyi grade III infections,[1] in the groin in 8, and in the neck in 2 patients. Clinical presentations included frank abscess and/or purulent drainage in 6 cases, acute hemorrhage in 3 cases, and an anastomotic false aneurysm in 1 patient (Table 3). There was anastomotic exposure in every case and all but 1 patient who had been taking oral antibiotics chronically presented with fever and/or leukocytosis. Positive bacterial cultures were confirmed in each case, including 18 isolates in these 10 patients. A single organism was cultured in 6 patients, two organisms in 2 patients, and four organisms in 2 patients (Table 4).

All patients were treated with organism-specific intravenous antibiotics; the duration of therapy ranged from 7 to 30 days. The RMF procedures, including rectus abdominis (1), rectus femoris (1) and pectoralis major (2), were performed at the time of the initial wound exploration and debridement procedure at our institution in 4 cases (No. 3,4,9,10) (Table 3), although 2 of these patients had undergone 2 (No. 10) and 4 (No. 4) previous incision and drainage procedures during previous hospitalizations and presented with persistent or recurrent infection. Three patients (No. 1,2,8) (Table 3) who presented with abscess and/or purulent drainage underwent an initial drainage and debridement procedure. Dressings were placed on the wounds and then closed with rectus abdominis (2) or tensor fascia lata (1) flaps 7, 30, and 3 days later, respectively. The use of a tensor fascia lata flap to close the wound of one patient (No. 2) is seen in Figure 1.

The most intriguing, and perhaps instructive group of cases was 3 patients (No. 5,6,7) (Table 3), who developed recurrent hemorrhage after initial repair and graft

Table 4
RMF Procedures for PGI: Johns Hopkins Experience

Bacteriology

Organism	No. Pts.
Pseudomonas aeroginosa	5
Staphylococcus epidermidis	4
Streptococcus D enterococcus	3
Staphylococcus aureus	1
Cornyebacterium	1
Proteus mirabilis	2
Streptococcus B	1
Escherichia coli	1
Total	18
Single organism Gram (+) 4 Gram (−) 2	6
Two organisms Mixed	2
Four organisms Mixed	2
Total	10

RMF = rotational muscle flap; PGI = peripheral graft infection.

coverage with local sartorius transfer. In each case the graft was again repaired and covered with rectus abdominis muscle flaps. The placement of the rectus abdominis flap in 1 case (No. 5) is seen in Figure 2. In 1 of these patients (No. 6), the inferior portion of the wound broke down secondary to necrosis of the distal portion of the rectus abdominis flap. Complete wound healing was achieved with a secondary gracilis muscle flap. There were no other complications of the RMF procedures in these 10 patients.

In summary, 11 RMF procedures were performed, using the rectus abdominis (6), pectoralis major (2), tensor fascia lata (1), rectus femoris (1), and gracilis (1), and wound healing was achieved in each patient. One patient (No. 3) expired 4 months later secondary to ischemic colitis. The 9 survivors have been followed for 2 to 60

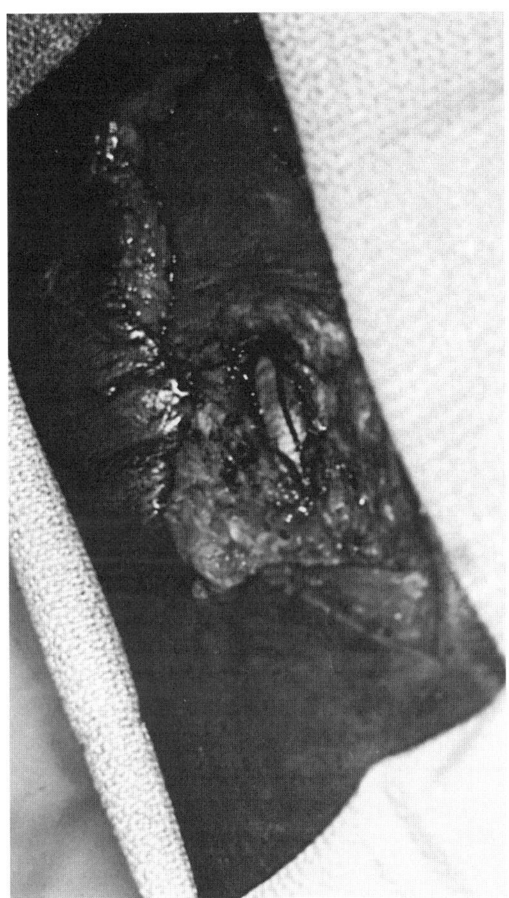

Figure 1A. An exposed limb of an aortofemoral Dacron graft after wide debridement of the groin wound.

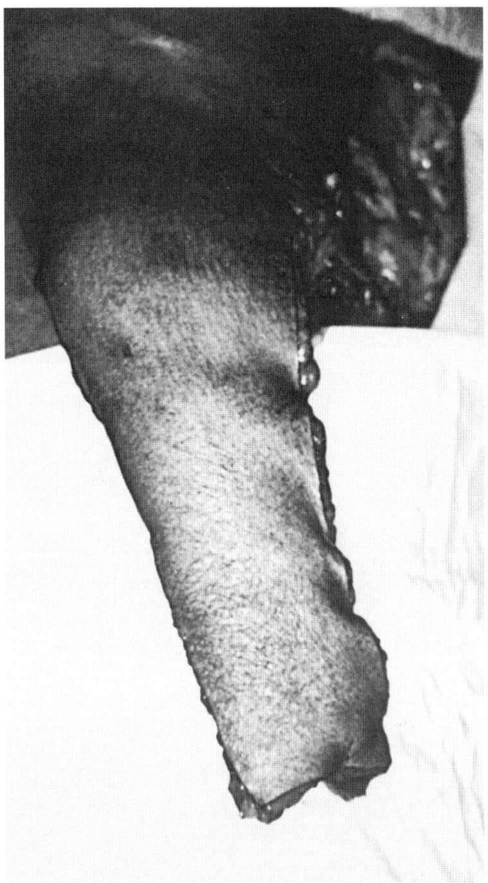

Figure 1B. A mobilized tensor fascia lata myocutaneous flap.

(mean 21) months. One patient (No.8) presented with recurrent infection of a femorofemoral Dacron graft 12 months after RMF closure. The graft had occluded in the interim and was removed without sequelae. The other 8 (88%) patients' wounds remain healed with patent grafts over a mean follow-up period of 21 months, including 6/7 (86%) patients treated for PGI in the groin, and including all 3 patients who underwent RMF procedures after failed local sartorius transfer.

Conclusion

In attempting to define the optimal treatment for PGI, one must recognize that no two patients with this complication are exactly the same. The graft material, anatomic site of presentation of the infection, the extent of soft tissue involvement, the specific organism(s) involved and quantitative concentrations, the patient's nutritional state, immunologic status, and other factors will collectively determine the successful local treatment of PGI.

Nevertheless, the preponderance of evidence available today suggests that RMF procedures are an important and highly efficacious refinement of the local treatment of PGI. In addition to providing mechanical coverage for the graft, expediting wound healing and consequently shortening the period of hospitalization, an abundant body

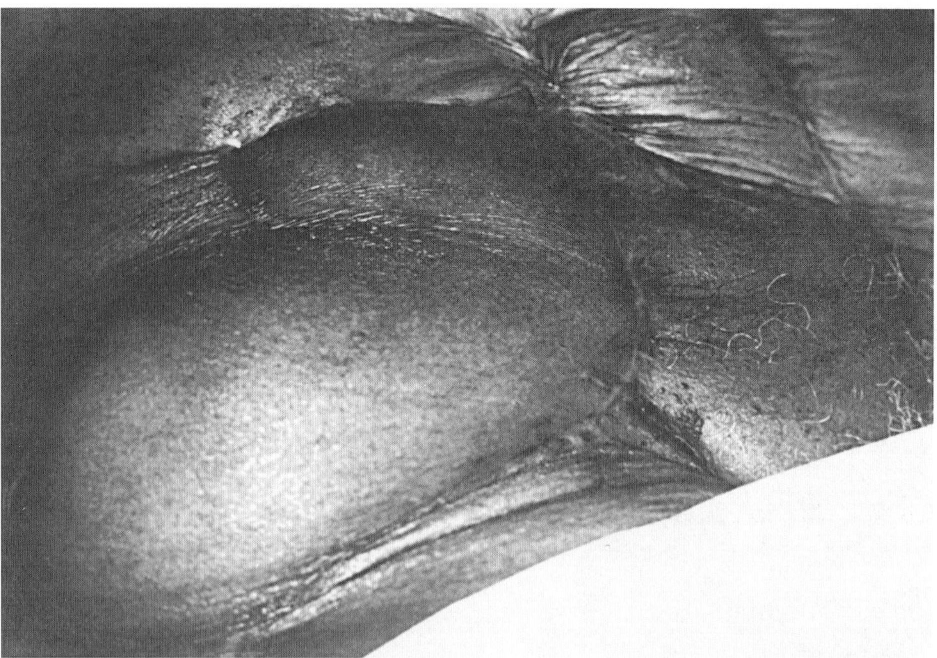

Figure 1C. A healed groin wound in this patient at discharge.

of both experimental and clinical evidence suggests that well-vascularized muscle tissue can actually promote eradication of the infection itself.

In order to perform a RMF procedure, there must be absolute physical and radiologic evidence that the infection is truly localized. Infection propagating along the entire extent of a prosthetic graft is a contraindication to this approach. Furthermore, the graft limb being covered should be patent. Although some have suggested that an intact anastomotic suture line is a prerequisite to attempting a RMF procedure,[82] we disagree. In the Hopkins series, there was anastomotic exposure in every case and in 30% of the cases there was actual anastomotic disruption, as manifested by hemorrhage or false aneurysm formation.[83,84]

The use of a RMF to treat PGI is no substitute for meticulous local wound care. Aggressive and extensive soft tissue debridement is a fundamental component of this approach. The advisability of immedi-

ate versus delayed flap coverage of the infected graft is essentially a clinical judgment. Certainly the patient who develops an extensive abscess should undergo an initial drainage procedure and cleansing dressing changes prior to definitive closure. Based upon the clinical experience reported to date, it is not possible to offer dogmatic recommendations regarding the optimal duration of these dressing changes when flap coverage is delayed. In addition, the duration of intravenous antibiotic administration and the necessity for long-term oral antibiotics remains unsettled.[62,82–84]

Nevertheless, there is mounting evidence that the use of muscle flap coverage may salvage some infected prosthetic grafts in properly selected patients. Although local sartorius transfer may be easily performed by the vascular surgeon to treat graft infection in the groin, I believe that it represents a suboptimal approach when compared to the formal rotation of a muscle flap from a separate and clean anatomic

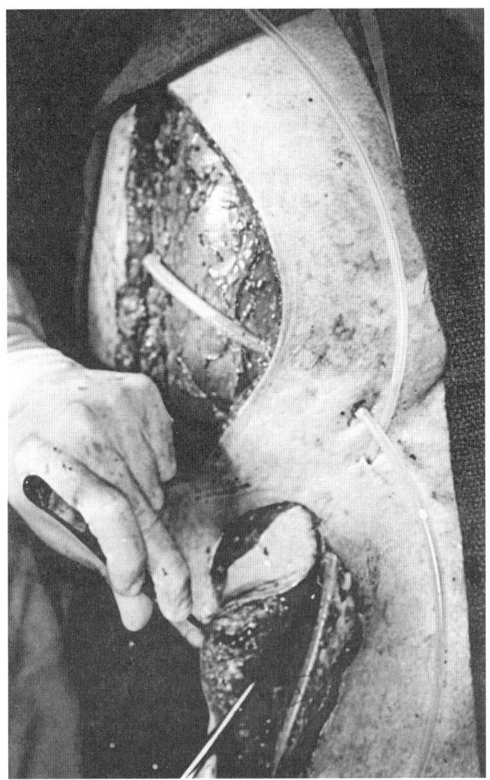

Figure 2A. A rectus abdominis myocutaneous flap being placed to close a left groin wound. Note the donor site superiorly.

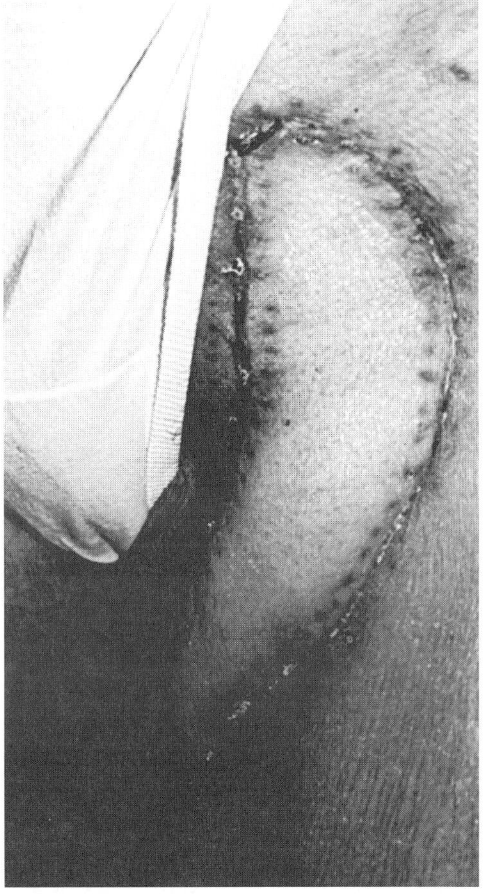

Figure 2B. A healed groin wound in this patient at discharge.

bed, and with a blood supply that is uncompromised and independent of the site of infection.

References

1. Szilagyi DE, Smith RF, Elliott JP, Urandecic MP. Infection in arterial reconstruction with synthetic grafts. *Arch Surg.* 1972;176: 321–333.
2. Bunt TJ. Synthetic vascular graft infections. I. Graft infections. *Surgery.* 1983;93:733–746.
3. Lindenauer SM, Fry WS, Schaub G, Wild D. The use of antibiotics in the prevention of vascular graft infections. *Surgery.* 1967;62: 487–492.
4. Goldstone J, Moore WS. Infection in vascular prostheses. *Am J Surg.* 1974;128:225–233.
5. Jamieson GG, DeWeese JA, Rob CG. Infected arterial grafts. *Ann Surg.* 1975;101:850–852.
6. Liekweg WC, Greenfield LJ. Vascular prosthetic infections: collected experience and results of treatment. *Surgery.*1977;81:335–342.
7. Yashar JJ, Weyman AK, Burnard RD, Yashar J. Survival and limb salvage in patients with infected arterial prostheses. *Am J Surg.* 1978; 135:499–504.
8. Reilly LM, Altman H, Lusby RJ, Kersh RA, Ehrenfeld WK, Stoney RJ. Late results following surgical management of vascular graft infection. *J Vasc Surg.* 1984;1:36–44.
9. Hoffert PW, Gensier SS, Haimovici H. Infection complicating arterial grafts. *Arch Surg.* 1965;90:427–435.
10. Najafi H, Javid H, Dye WS, Hunter JA, Julian OC. Management of infected arterial implants. *Surgery.* 1969;65:539–547.
11. Conn JH, Hardy JD, Chavez CM, Fain WR. Infected arterial grafts. *Ann Surg.* 1970;171: 704–712.

12. Knight CD Jr, Farnell MB, Hollier LA. Treatment of aortic graft infection with povidone-iodine irrigation. *Mayo Clin Proc.* 1983;58: 472–475.

13. Seeger JM, Wheeler JR, Gregory RT, Synder SO, Gayle RG. Autogenous graft replacement of infected prosthetic grafts in the femoral position. *Surgery.* 1983;93:39–45.

14. Snyder SO, Wheeler JR, Gregory RT, Gayle RG, Zirkle K. Freshly harvested cadaveric venous homografts as arterial conduits in infected fields. *Surgery.* 1987;101:283–291.

15. Kwann JHM, Connelly JE. Successful management of prosthetic graft infection with continuous povidone iodine irrigation. *Arch Surg.* 1981;116:716–720.

16. Popovsky J, Singer S. Infected prosthetic grafts: local therapy with preservation. *Arch Surg.* 1980;115:203–205.

17. Carter SC, Cohen A, Whelan TJ. Clincal experience with management of the infected Dacron graft. *Ann Surg.* 1963;158:249–255.

18. Budny PG, Fix RJ. Salvage of prosthetic grafts and joints in the lower extremity. *Clin Plast Surg.* 1991;18:583–591.

19. Sauvage LR, Berger DE, Wood SJ, et al. Interspecies healing of porous arterial prostheses. *Arch Surg.* 1974;109:698–705.

20. Mehran RJ, Graham AM, Ricci MA, Symes JF. Evaluation of muscle flaps in the treatment of infected aortic grafts. *J Vasc Surg.* 1992;15:487–494.

21. Hahn DC, MacKay RD, Halliday B, Hunt TK. Effect of O_2 tension on microbial function of leukocytes in wounds and in vitro. *Surg Forum.* 1976;27;18–20.

22. Hunt TK. Disorders of repair and their management In: Hunt TK, Dunphy JE, eds. *Fundamentals of Wound Management.* New York: Appleton-Century-Crofts; 1979:68–168.

23. Chang N, Mathes SJ. Comparison of the effect of bacterial inoculation in musculocutaneous and random-pattern flaps. *Plast Reconstr Surg.* 1982;70:1–9.

24. Calderon W, Chang N, Mathes SJ. Comparison of the effect of bacterial inoculation in musculocutaneous and fasciocutaneous flaps. *Plast Reconstr Surg.* 1986;77:785–792.

25. Grosain A, Chang N, Mathes S, Hunt TK, Vasconez L. A study of the relationship between blood flow and bacterial inoculation in musculocutaneous and fasciocutaneous flaps. *Plast Reconstr Surg.* 1990;86:1152–1162.

26. Dacey LJ, Miett TOC, Huntsman WT, Colen LB, Schneed AR, McDaniel MD. Efficacy of muscle flaps in the treatment of prosthetic vascular graft infections. *J Surg Res.* 1988;44: 566–572.

27. Cruz NI, Canario QM. Muscle flaps in the management of vascular grafts in contaminated wounds: an experimental study in dogs. *Plast Reconstr Surg.* 1988;82:480–483.

28. Mathes SJ, Canario QM. Discussion of: Muscle flaps in the management of vascular grafts in contaminated wounds: an experimental study in dogs. *Plast Reconstr Surg.* 1988;82:484–485.

29. Mathes SJ, McCraw JB, Vasconez LO. Muscle transposition flaps for coverage of lower extremity defects: anatomic considerations. *Surg Clin North Am.* 1974;54:1337–1354.

30. Mathes SJ, Vasconez LO, Jurkiewicz MJ. Extensions and further applications of muscle flap transposition. *Plast Reconstr Surg.* 1977; 60:6–13.

31. McCraw JB, Dibbell DG, Carraway JH. Clinical definition of independent myocutaneous vascular territories. *Plast Reconstr Surg.* 1977; 60:341–352.

32. Ramasastry SS, Liang MD, Hurwitz DJ. Surgical management of difficult wounds. *Surg Gynecol Obstet.* 1989;169:418–422.

33. Eggers C. The treatment of bronchial fistulae. *Ann Surg.* 1920;72:345–351.

34. Maier HC, Luomanen RKJ. Rectoral myoplasty for closure of residual empyema cavity and bronchial fistula. *Surgery.* 1949;25: 621–624.

35. Barker WL, Faber LP, Ostermiller WE Jr, Langston HT. Management of persistent bronchopleural fistulas. *J Thorac Cardiovasc Surg.* 1977;62:393–401.

36. Demos NJ, Timmes JJ. Myoplasty for closure of tracheobronchial fistula. *Ann Thorac Surg.* 1973;15:88–93.

37. Pairolero PC, Arnold PG. Bronchopleural fistula: treatment by transposition of pectoralis major muscle. *J Thorac Cardiovasc Surg.* 1980; 79:142–145.

38. Arnold PG, Pairolero PC. Intrathoracic muscle flaps: a 10-year experience in the management of life-threatening infections. *Plast Reconst Surg.* 1989;84:92–98.

39. Tobin GR, Marroudis C, Howe WR, Gray LA Jr. Reconstruction of complex thoracic defects with myocutaneous and muscle flaps: application of new flap refinements. *J Thorac Cardiovasc Surg.* 1983;85;219–228.

40. Pappas C, Goldrick G, Candy K, Wong W. Skin flaps vs. muscle flaps: coping with infection in the presence of a foreign body. *Plast Surg Forum.* 1980;3:133–135.

41. Arnold PG, Pairolero PC. Use of pectoralis major muscle flaps to repair defects of anterior chest wall. *Plast Reconstr Surg.* 1979;63: 205–213.

42. Arnold PG, Pairolero PC, Waldorf JC. The serratus anterior muscle: intrathoracic and extrathoracic utilization. *Plast Reconstr Surg.* 1984;73:240–248.

43. Stark WJ. The use of pedicled muscle flaps in the surgical treatment of chronic osteomyelitis resulting from compound fractures. *J Bone Joint Surg.* 1946;28:343–350.

44. Ger R. Muscle transposition for treatment of chronic posttraumatic osteomyelitis of the tibia. *J Bone Joint Surg.* 1977;59A:784–791.

45. Mathes SJ, Alpert BS, Chang N. Use of muscle flaps in chronic osteomyelitis: experimental and clinical correlation. *Plast Reconstr Surg.* 1982;69:815–828.

46. Ranawat CS. Future trends in knee Arthroplasty. In: Ranawat CS, ed. *Total Condylar Knee Arthroplasty: Technique, Results, and Complications.* New York: Springer-Verlag; 1985:268.

47. Lesavoy MA, Dubrow TJ, Wackym PA, Eckardt JJ. Muscle flap coverage of exposed endoprostheses. *Plast Reconstr Surg.* 1989;83:90–96.

48. Scully HE, Leclerc Y, Martin RD, et al. Comparison between antibiotic irrigation and mobilization of pectoral muscle flaps in treatment of deep sternal infections. *J Thorac CardiovascSurg.* 1985;90:523–531.

49. Brown AH, Brainbridge MV, Panagopoulos P, Sabar EF. The complications of median sternotomy. *J Thorac Cardiovasc Surg.* 1969;58:189–197.

50. Sanfellipo PM, Danielson GK. Complications associated with median sternotomy. *J Cardiovasc Surg.* 1972;63:419–423.

51. Shumaker HB, Mandelbaum I. Continuous antibiotic irrigation in the treatment of infection. *Arch Surg.* 1963;83:384–387.

52. Thurer RJ, Bognolo D, Vargas A, Isch JH, Kaiser GA. The management of mediastinal infection following cardiac surgery: an experience utilizing continuous irrigation with povodine-iodine. *J Thorac Cardiovasc Surg.* 1974;68:962–968.

53. Jurkiewicz MJ, Bostwick J III, Hester TR, Bishop JB, Craver J. Infected median sternotomy wound: successful treatment by muscle flaps. *Ann Surg.* 1980;191:737–744.

54. Pairolero PC, Arnold PG, Harris JB. Long-term results of pectoralis major muscle transposition for infected sternotomywounds. *Ann Surg.* 1991;213:583–590.

55. Gross EA, Culliford AT, Krieger KH, et al. A survey of 77 major infectious complications of median sternotomy: a review of 7949 consecutive operative procedures. *Ann Thorac Surg.* 1985;40:214–223.

56. Majure JA, Albin RE, O'Donnell RS, Arganese TJ. Reconstruction of the infected median sternotomy wound. *Ann Thorac Surg.* 1986;42:9–12.

57. Miller JI, Nahai F. Repair of the dehisced median sternotomy incision. *Surg Clin North Am.* 1989;69:1091–1102.

58. Kohman LJ, Auchincloss JH, Gilbert R, Beshara M. Functional results of muscle flap closure for sternal infection. *Ann Thorac Surg.* 1991;52:102–106.

59. Pairolero PC, Arnold PG, Piehler JM, McGoon DC. Intrathoracic transposition of extrathoracic skeletal muscle. *J Thorac Cardiovasc Surg.* 1983;86:809–817.

60. Schaff HV, Arnold PG, Reeder GS. Late mediastinal infection and pseudoaneurysm following left ventricular aneurysmectomy: repair utilizing a pectoralis major muscle flap. *J Thorac Cardiovasc Surg.* 1982;84:912–916.

61. Caselli JS, Crawford ES, Williams TW Jr. Treatment of postoperative infection of ascending aorta and transverse aortic arch, including use of viable omentums and muscle flaps. *Ann Thorac Surg.* 1990;50:868–881.

62. Bennion RS, Hiatt JR, Williams RA, Wilson SE. Surgical management of unilateral groin infection after aorto-femoralbypass. *Surg Gynecol Obstet.* 1983;156:724–728.

63. Newington DP, Houghton PWJ, Baird RN, Horrocks M. Groin wound infection after arterial surgery. *Br J Surg.* 1991;78:617–619.

64. Kaiser E, Genz KS, Habermeyer P, Mandelkow H. Die arterielle versorgung des musculus sartorius. *Chirurg.* 1984;35:731–732.

65. Kaufmann JL, Shah DM, Corson JD, Skudder PA, Leather RP. Sartorius muscle coverage for the treatment of complicated vascular surgical wounds. *J Cardiovasc Surg.* 1989;30:475–483.

66. Baronofsky I. Technique of inguinal lymph node dissection. *Surgery.* 1948;24:555–556.

67. Scher KS. Sartorius transposition to protect vascular grafts in the groin. *Ann Surg.* 1989;55:158–161.

68. Meyer JP, Durham JR, Schwartz TH, Sawchuk AP, Schuler JJ. The use of sartorius muscle rotation-transfer in the management of wound complications after infrainguinal vein bypass: a report of eight cases and description of the techniques. *J Vasc Surg.* 1989;9:731–735.

69. Soots G, Mikati A, Warembourg H Jr, Watel A, Noblet D. Treatment of lymphorrhea with exposed or infected vascular grafts in the groin using sartorius myoplasty. *J Cardiovasc Surg.* 1988;29:42–45.

70. Mendez-Fernandez MAM, Quast DC, Geist

RC, Henley WS. Distally based sartorius muscle flap in the treatment of infected femoral arterial prostheses. *J Cardiovas Surg.* 1980;21:628–631.

71. Hejnal J, Michal V, Firt P, Kocandrle V. The mobilized omentum and muscle flaps in the treatment of infectious complications in cardiovascular surgery. *Thorac Cardiovasc Surg.* 1990;38:244–246.

72. Dagher FJ, Stueber K. Use of muscle flaps to salvage prosthetic grafts. *Contemp Surg.* 1989; 35:31–34.

73. Bandyk DF, Bergamini TM, Kinney EV, Seabrook GR, Towne JB. In situ replacement of vascular prostheses infected by bacterialbiofilms. *J Vasc Surg.* 1991;13:575–583.

74. Mathes SH, Nahai F. *Clinical Applications for Muscle and Myocutaneous Flaps.* St. Louis: CV Mosby Co; 1982:3–137.

75. Ger R. The coverage of vascular repairs by muscle transposition. *J Trauma.* 1976;16: 974–978.

76. Guzman-Stein G, Fix RJ, Vasconez LO. Muscle flap coverage for the lower extremity. *Clin Plast Surg.* 1991;18:545–552.

77. Peters W, Cartotto R, Morris S, Jewett M. The rectus femoris myocutaneous flap for closure of difficult wounds of the abdomen, groin, and trochanteric areas. *Ann Plast Surg.* 1991; 26:572–576.

78. Ammar AD, Turrentine MW. Exposed synthetic vascular grafts of the groin; graft preservation by means of a tensor fasciae latae flap. *J Vasc Surg.* 1989;10:202–204.

79. Stair JM, Perry PM. Clinical uses of the tensor fascia lata myocutaneous flap. *J Arkansas Med Soc.* 1985;81:475–477.

80. McCraw JB, Dibbell DG, Carraway JH. Clinical definition of independent myocutaneous vascular territories. *Plast Reconst Surg.* 1977; 60:341–352.

81. Hodgkinson DJ, Shepard GTT. Coverage of exposed Gortex dialysis access graft with local sublimis myocutaneous flap.*Plast Reconstr Surg.* 1982;69:1010–1012.

82. Mixter RC, Turnipseed WD, Smith DJ Jr, Acher CW, Rao VK, Dibbell DG. Rotational muscle flaps: a new technique for covering infected vascular grafts. *J Vasc Surg.* 1989;9: 472–478.

83. Perler BA, Vander Kolk CA, Dufresne CA, Williams GM. Can infected prosthetic grafts be salvaged with rotational muscle flaps? *Surgery.* 1991;110:30–34.

84. Perler BA. Use of muscle flaps in the treatment of prosthetic graft infection. In: *Current Clinical Problems in Vascular Surgery.* St Louis: Quality Medical Publishing, Inc; 1990: 380–386.

Chapter 12

Local Treatment of Infected Extracavitary Arterial Grafts

K.D. Calligaro
D.A. DeLaurentis
F.J. Veith

Introduction

Traditional treatment of infected arterial grafts has included immediate and total graft excision regardless of the manner of presentation of the infection or patency status of the graft.[1-4] When infection involves the intra-abdominal portion of an aortic graft, we agree with others that the safest management is immediate graft excision.[2,5-7] However, Dr. Veith has demonstrated during the past 20 years that under certain well-defined circumstances, preservation of extracavitary infected arterial grafts can be safely accomplished in the majority of cases using aggressive, local treatment.[5,8-10] Our mortality and amputation rates compare quite favorably with other series when routine graft excision was carried out to treat these devastating complications. Management consisting of routine excision of infected extracavitary grafts has resulted in mortality rates of 10% to 22% and amputation rates of 27% to 79%.[1,2,11-14] We and others believe that if certain strict criteria are used,

selective graft preservation is a superior method of treatment compared to routine graft excision.[15-17]

Indications for Local Treatment and Graft Preservation

Local treatment and graft preservation of infected extracavitary grafts is indicated only if all of the following strict criteria exist:

1. The graft must be patent.
2. The infected anastomosis and body of the graft must be intact.
3. The patient cannot be systemically septic.

When these criteria are present, we have shown that successful graft preservation can be accomplished in the majority of cases for infections that involve not only the body but also the anastomosis of extracavitary arterial grafts,[5,6,8-10] infected autologous vein and prosthetic grafts,[18] and infections due to Gram-positive and most Gram-negative bacteria.[19] These aspects of selective graft preservation will be reviewed in detail.

Indications for Graft Excision to Manage Infected Arterial Grafts

Certain graft infections cannot be treated by local treatment and graft preservation. We agree with others that any occluded infected graft must be excised since bacteria are likely to propagate along the thrombus inside the graft.[1,2,5,6,8,9] However, we believe that a subtotal excision of an occluded graft, leaving an oversewn graft remnant on an underlying patent intact artery, can be a simpler, easier method to treat these cases than complete graft excision.[8–10] (Figs. 1,2).

Any patient presenting with an infected, disrupted anastomosis (infected pseudoaneurysm or frank bleeding) should be treated by excision of the infected part of the graft and not by local treatment only, since recurrent hemorrhage will commonly occur.[1,2,8–10] Excision of the infected segment of the graft and any surrounding infected soft tissue, and extension of a new graft from an uninfected part of the original, patent graft to a different segment of uninvolved artery, has been shown to be an acceptable and improved form of treatment

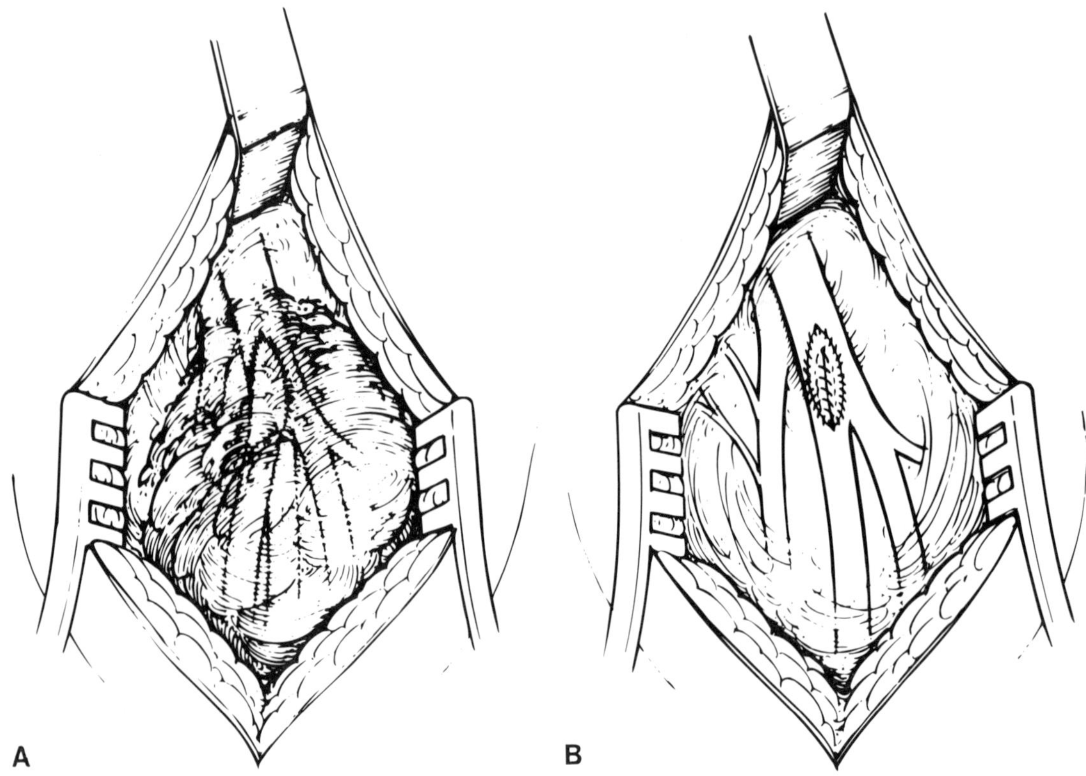

Figure 1. (A) Schematic representing an infected groin anastomosis of an occluded femorodistal polytetrafluoroethylene (PTFE) graft. (B) Schematic showing the groin wound after aggressive operative excision of all infected tissue and subtotal excision of the graft. A small remnant of the PTFE graft on the common femoral artery was oversewn to maintain flow through the underlying patent deep femoral artery.

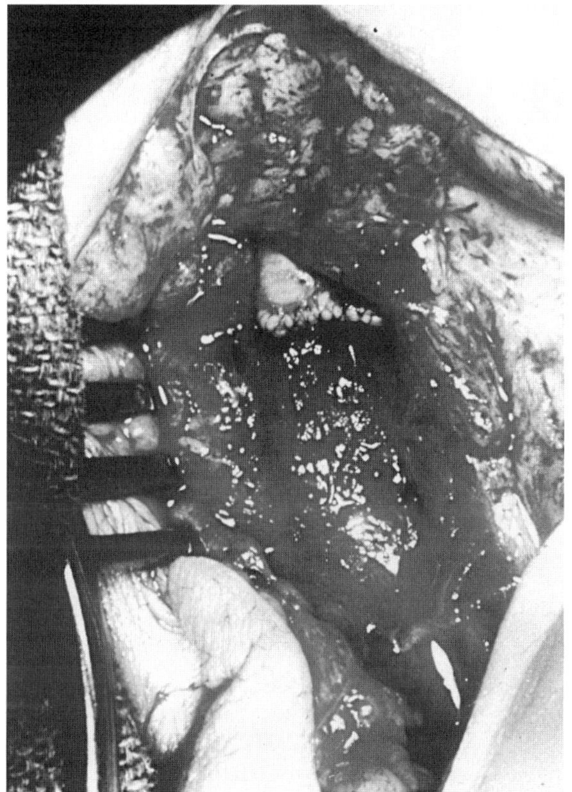

Figure 2A. Operative photograph of Figure 1B. The wound was debrided multiple times and healthy granulation tissue surrounds the oversewn polytetrafluoroethylene (PTFE) remnant attached to the femoral artery. Granulation tissue covers the involved artery by this time.

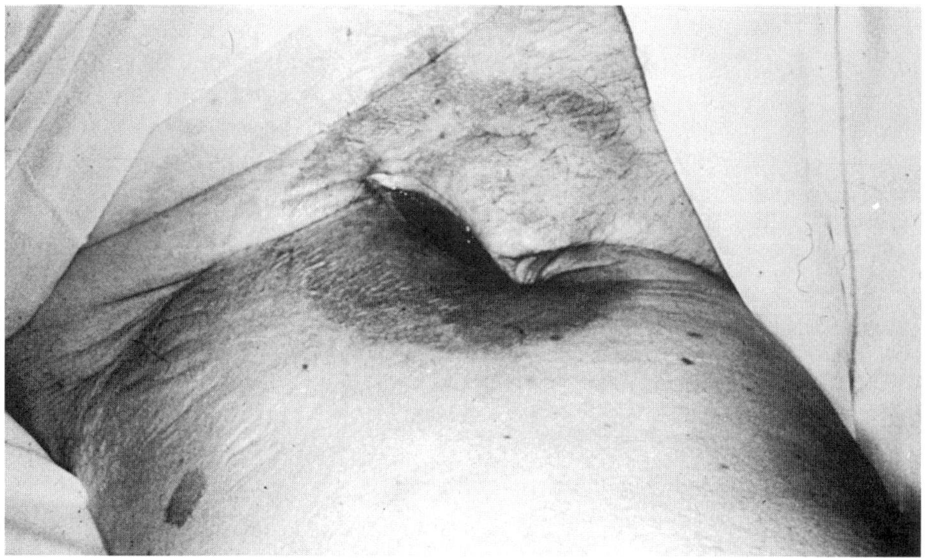

Figure 2B. Operative photograph of Figure 1B. After frequent wet-to-dry dressings and repeated operative debridements, the groin wound is almost healed and granulation tissue covers the polytetrafluoroethylene (PTFE) remnant.

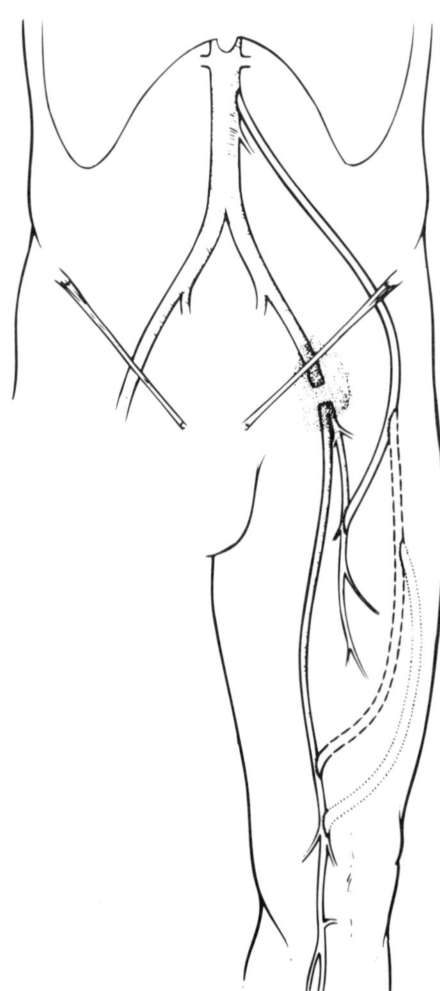

Figure 3. Schematic illustrating an infected groin wound after total excision of a femoropopliteal graft that presented with homorrhage of the femoral anastomosis. The infected segment of the common femoral artery was excised and the proximal and distal femoral arteries were oversewn. The surrounding infected soft tissues were excised. After isolation of the wound, inflow was reestablished by placing a polytetrafluoroethylene (PTFE) bypass from the infrarenal aorta to the deep femoral artery. The graft was tunneled lateral to the infected wound under the inguinal ligament. Additional potential outflow sites include the mid-superficial femoral and popliteal arteries.

compared to total graft excision.[5,6,8–10] (Fig. 3).

We believe that systemic sepsis mandates total graft excision because the graft is irreversibly seeded with virulent bacteria and that the infection will not respond to local treatment and intravenous antibiotics alone.[1,2,5,6,8–10] Finally, although a few reports suggest that in selected cases replacement of an infected aortic graft with a new graft placed in situ may represent an acceptable form of treatment, we still believe that infection involving the intra-abdominal portion of an aortic graft is best treated by graft excision.[5–7,13] Local treatment and complete graft preservation do not generally play a role in the above circumstances.

Advantages of Local Treatment and Graft Preservation

The advantages of local treatment with graft preservation to treat selected extracavitary graft infections are twofold. First, in most instances, difficult dissection in a scarred field is minimized and inadvertent injury to the artery or graft can be avoided. Second, successful graft preservation of a patent graft preserves flow to a threatened extremity and avoids the need for complex revascularization procedures. When routine graft excision is carried out, frequently a complex extra-anatomic or in situ bypass may have to be performed or an amputation may be necessary. We do not recommend placement of a prosthetic graft into a field that is already infected to restore arterial flow to a threatened extremity. Similarly, we have been disappointed with placement of an autologous tissue graft (either as a patch or as a bypass) into an infected field.[8,9] We believe that these latter options are hazardous since a new graft placed into an infected field is prone to develop anastomotic bleeding.

Local Care Adjuncts to Achieve Successful Graft Preservation

If a patient who is not systemically septic presents with a patent infected extracavitary graft with intact anastomoses, essential adjuncts must be carried out to achieve successful graft preservation and wound healing.

Repeated, aggressive debridement of all surrounding infected tissue must be performed in the operating room as often as necessary until healthy granulation tissue covers the graft or until an autologous tissue flap is placed on the exposed graft. Failure to treat infected arterial grafts using selective graft preservation in previous reports may in part have been due to a lack of an aggressive attitude regarding repeated operative excision of all infected tissue.

Another essential adjunct of local treatment and selective preservation of infected arterial grafts includes moist dressing changes 3 times a day using a dilute povidone-iodine solution (1 cc of 1% betadine mixed in 1 of liter normal saline).[8,9,17,20] This concentration has been shown to be toxic to bacteria but does not inhibit fibroblasts or impair wound healing.[20]

Once healthy granulation tissue is present, placement of autologous tissue such as a muscle flap onto the exposed graft can be performed to speed healing of the wound, although this may not be necessary.[21] We have demonstrated that when treating infected prosthetic grafts, successful graft preservation and wound healing is as likely whether the wound heals by delayed secondary intention or by placement of a muscle flap. Conversely, we have also shown that a successful outcome is more likely using an autologous tissue flap when treating infected vein grafts than when the wound is allowed to heal by secondary intention.[8,9,18]

When graft preservation is attempted, these patients must be observed in the intensive care unit until the graft is covered by autologous tissue. Since directly visualized local treatment and repeated operative debridements are critical aspects of our management plan, we are understandably reluctant to recommend attempted graft preservation when infection involves the intra-abdominal portion of an arterial graft since local treatment is usually not possible.

Prolonged administration of appropriate intravenous antibiotics is essential to achieve wound healing and graft preservation. We prefer giving intravenous antibiotics for a 6-week course, which usually requires placement of a Hickman catheter.[2-7] The relatively recent development of more efficacious antibiotics to treat particularly virulent organisms may also account for our high rate of successful selective graft preservation compared to older series.

Local Treatment of Graft Infections Involving an Intact Anastomosis

Bhat et al. showed that infection confined to the body of a prosthetic arteriovenous dialysis graft could be successfully treated by graft preservation.[22] We and others have shown that the majority of infected, patent, extracavitary grafts can be successfully preserved using this management protocol even when the infection involves an intact anastomosis. Ghosn noted that 10 of 13 aortofemoral prosthetic grafts were successfully preserved in patients who were seen with an infection confined to the groin.[16] Kwaan reported that local treatment of infections involving only the distal limb of aortofemoral prosthetic grafts was successful in 5 of 5 cases when wounds were continuously irrigated with povidone-iodine solution.[17] We have also shown that graft excision is only necessary for about a quarter of infections involving an intact anastomosis of a patent graft to a peripheral artery.[8-10] If there is any evidence of anastomotic disruption, the graft must be excised immediately.

Attempted Preservation of Infected Prosthetic versus Vein Grafts

Although autologous tissue conduits may be more resistant to infection than prosthetic grafts,[11] we have demonstrated that prosthetic grafts are more likely to be successfully preserved than vein grafts if involved with an infectious process.[8–10,18] A prosthetic graft has a thicker wall than a vein graft, does not represent living tissue, and therefore may not be as prone to develop complications such as dessication, graft thrombosis, or disruption.[18,23,24] Despite these potential reasons why selective preservation of infected vein grafts may not be successful, Ouriel et al. reported that many vein grafts can be salvaged, although complications frequently occurred.[24] We documented that 11 of 16 infected patent vein grafts of the lower extremity with intact anastomoses were successfully preserved using our previously described protocol.[18] As previously mentioned, placement of an autologous tissue flap onto an infected, exposed, intact vein graft is critical to achieve a high rate of successful graft salvage and wound healing.[18]

Effect of Bacteriology on Local Treatment and Graft Preservation

Gram-negative bacteria are generally believed to be more virulent than Gram-positive organisms.[4,15,23–27] In particular, *Pseudomonas* represents an extremely virulent pathogen. It has a mucopolysaccharide coating which is resistant to phagocytosis and complement-activated antibodies.[3] *Pseudomonas* produced proteases which can digest vascular tissue and cause arterial hemorrhage and prevent wound healing.[3,26,27] The organism also has minimal obligatory nutritional requirements, has a high adaptability to a wide variety of physi-

cal conditions, and often is resistant to antibiotics.[3]

However, mandatory graft excision for all graft infections due to Gram-negative bacteria is controversial. Kwaan has previously shown in a small series of patients that successful graft preservation can be accomplished in the presence of Gram-negative bacteria.[17] We recently reported an equivalent rate of successful graft preservation and wound healing in a larger group of patients whether Gram-positive or Gram-negative bacteria were cultured from the wound.[19] In a series of 42 infected, intact, patent extracavitary prosthetic grafts treated by attempted complete graft preservation, we documented a 70% (23/33) graft preservation rate when Gram positives were present versus a 73% (16/22) success rate when Gram negatives were cultured (many infections were polymicrobial in nature). We and others have confirmed that *Pseudomonas* is a particularly virulent organism.[19,23,24] However, we found that although successful graft preservation was accomplished in only 44% (4/9) of cases when *Pseudomonas* was present, a successful outcome was accomplished in 92% (12/13) of cases when any Gram-negative bacteria other than *Pseudomonas* were cultured from the wound.[19] Based on these results, we generally recommend that local treatment and graft preservation not be attempted if *Pseudomonas* is cultured from the wound. When this organism is isolated, graft preservation may be attempted if graft excision is particularly hazardous or if limb loss will almost certainly result. A successful outcome can be expected in about half of *Pseudomonas* infections. Conversely, we believe that Gram-negative bacteria other than *Pseudomonas* do not represent a contraindication for selective graft preservation.

Conclusion

We believe that aggressive local treatment of selected infected extracavitary arte-

Table 1
Clinical Results of Local Therapy and Graft Preservation to Treat
Extracavitary-Infected Arterial Grafts*

| | | | Technique | | Results** | | |
| | | Type of Graft† | Muscle Flap (No. Pts) | Dressing Changes | Successful Graft Preservation | Mortality | Limb Loss |
Author	No. Pts						
Liekweg[13]	21	P	0	—	81%	19%	0%
Ghosn[16]	13	P	0	—	60%	23%	8%
Kwaan[17]	10	P	2	50% Betadine	100%	0%	0%
Calligaro[18]	16	V	4	1% Betadine	69%	19%	8%
Calligaro[19]	42	P	7	1% Betadine	76%	10%	3%
Perler[21]	7	P	7	—	86%	0%	0%
Ouriel[24]	16	V	0	—	43%	19%	25%
Cherry[28]	11	P, V	5	—	100%	0%	0%
Joffe[29]	8	P	0	10% betadine	75%	0%	0%
Mixter[30]	19	P	19	10% Betadine	95%	0%	0%
Kaufman[31]	10	P, V	10	—	90%	0%	0%
Petrasek[32]	8	P, V	8	—	88%	0%	0%
Meyer[33]	8	V	8	—	100%	0%	0%

* Some of the details of the management and results of each series were not always included in the manuscripts.

    Generally only infected grafts that were patent with intact anastomoses in patients who were not systemically septic were treated by local therapy and attempted graft preservation. A few surgeons treated occasional patients with infected pseudoaneurysms by total graft preservation, although we do not agree with graft preservation in this setting.

    The infected grafts were excised and replaced with new in-situ grafts were not included in this summary since this represents a different form of treatment.

** Results include patients who died or required graft excision or a major amputation as a direct result of infection involving the graft during hospitalization or during long-term follow-up.

† P = prosthetic graft; V = autologous vein graft.

rial grafts represents an easier and more efficacious method of treatment compared to routine graft excision. A summary of the results of this treatment reported in the literature are listed in Table 1. Graft preservation should only be attempted when the graft is patent, the anastomosis is intact, and the patient is not septic. If any of these three criteria are not fulfilled, then local treatment and attempted preservation of infected arterial grafts should not be considered and graft excision should be carried out. Successful graft preservation can be accomplished only by repeated operative excision of all surrounding infected tissue. Wound healing can usually be accomplished by delayed secondary intention or by placement of a muscle flap onto the exposed graft and healthy granulation tissue. Prolonged intravenous antibiotics and frequent dressing changes are also mandatory adjuncts to achieve a successful outcome. Our extensive and long-term experience has demonstrated that local treatment and graft preservation is applicable for infections involving: 1) the body or intact anastomosis of an extracavitary arterial graft; 2) autologous vein and prosthetic grafts; and 3) Gram-positive and Gram-negative bacteria, with the possible exception of pseudomonal infections.

References

1. Szilagyi DE, Smith RF, Vrandecic MP. Infection in arterial reconstruction with synthetic grafts. *Ann Surg.* 1972;176:321–333.
2. Bunt TJ. Synthetic vascular graft infections I: graft infections. *Surgery.* 1983;6:733–746.

3. Pollack M. *Pseudomonas aeruginosa*. In: Mandell GL, ed. *Principles and Practice of Infectious Disease, 3rd ed.* New York: Churchill Livingstone Inc; 1990;1673–1691.

4. Threlkeld MG, Cobbs CG. Infectious disorders of prosthetic valves and intravascular devices. In: Mandell GL, ed. *Principles and Practice of Infectious Disease, 3rd ed.* New York: Churchill Livingstone Inc; 1990;706–715.

5. Veith FJ. Surgery of the infected aortic graft. In: Bergan JJ, Yao JST, eds. *Surgery of the Aorta and its Body Branches.* New York: Grune and Stratton; 1979;521–533.

6. Calligaro KD, Veith FJ. Diagnosis and management of infected prosthetic aortic grafts. *Surgery.* 1991;110:805–813.

7. O'Hara PJ, Hertzer NR, Beven EG, Drajewski LP. Surgical management of infected abdominal aortic grafts: review of a 25-year experience. *J Vasc Surg.* 1986;3:725–731.

8. Samson RH, Veith FJ, Janko GS, Gupta SK, Scher LA. A modified classification and approach to the management of infections involving peripheral arterial prosthetic grafts. *J Vasc Surg.* 1988;8:147–153.

9. Calligaro KD, Veith FJ, Gupta SK, et al. A modified method for management of prosthetic graft infection involving an anastomosis to the common femoral artery. *J Vasc Surg.* 1990;11:485–492.

10. Calligaro KD, Westcott CJ, Buckley RM, Savarese RP, DeLaurentis DA. Infrainguinal anastomotic arterial graft infections treated by selective graft preservation. *Ann Surg.* 1992;216:74–79.

11. Ehrenfeld WK, Wilbur BG, Olcott CN IV, Stoney RJ. Autogenous tissue reconstruction in the management of infected prosthetic grafts. *Surg* 1970;85:82–92.

12. Lorentzen JE, Nielsen OM, Arendrup H, et al. Vascular graft infection: an analysis of 62 graft infections in 2400 consecutively implanted synthetic vascular grafts. *Surgery.* 1985;98:81–86.

13. Liekweg WE, Greenfield L. Vascular prosthetic infections: collected experience and results of treatment. *Surgery.* 1977;81:335–342.

14. Kikta MJ, Goodson SF, Bishara RA, Meyer JP, Schuler JJ, Flanigan DP. Mortality and limb loss with infected infrainguinal bypass grafts. *J Vasc Surg.* 197;5:566–571.

15. Bandyk DF, Bergamini TM, Kinney EV, Seabrook G, Twone JB. In situ replacement of vascular prostheses infected by bacterial biofilms. *J Vasc Surg.* 1991;13:575–583.

16. Ghosn PB, Rabaat AG, Trudel J. Why remove an infected aortofemoral graft? *Can J Surg.* 1983;26:330–331.

17. Kwaan JHM, Connolly JE. Successful management of prosthetic graft infection with continuous povidone-iodine irrigation. *Arch Surg;* 1981;116:16–20.

18. Calligaro KD, Veith FJ, Schwartz ML, et al. Management of infected lower extremity autologous vein grafts by selective graft preservation. *Am J Surg.* 1992;164:291–294.

19. Calligaro KD, DeLaurentis DA, Schwartz ML, Savarese RP, Veith FJ. Are Gram-negative bacteria a contraindication to selective preservation of infected prosthetic arterial grafts? *J Vasc Surg.* 1992;16:337–346.

20. Lineaweaver W, Howard R, Soucy D, et al. Typical antimicrobial toxicity. *Arch Surg.* 1985;120:267–270.

21. Perler BA, VanderKolk CA, Dufresne CA, Williams GM. Can infected prosthetic grafts be salvaged with rotational muscle flaps? *Surgery.* 1991;110:30–34.

22. Bhat DJ, Tellis VA, Kohlberg WI, Driscoll B, Veith FJ. Management of sepsis involving expanded polytetrafluoroethyelene for hemodialysis access. *Surgery.* 1980;87:445–450.

23. Geary KJ, Tomkiewica AM, Harrison HN, et al. Differential effects of a Gram negative and a Gram positive infection on autogenous and prosthetic grafts. *J Vasc Surg.* 1990;11:339–347:

24. Ouriel K, Geary KJ, Green RM, DeWeese JA. Fate of the exposed saphenous vein graft. *Am J Surg.* 1990;160:149–150.

25. Baltimore RS, Mitchell M. Immunologic investigation of mucoid strains of *Pseudomonas aeruginosa*: comparison of susceptibility of opsonic antibody in mucoid and non-mucoid strains. *J Infect Dis.* 1980;141:23–47.

26. Rotschafer JC, Skikuma LR. *Pseudomonas aeruginosa* susceptibility in a university hospital: recognition and treatment. *Drug Intell Clin Pharm.* 1986;20:575–581.

27. Nicas TI, Iglewski BH. The contribution of exoproducts to virulence of *Pseudomonas aeruginosa. Can J Microbiol.* 1985;31:387–392.

28. Cherry KJ, Roland CF, Pairolero PC, et al. Infected femorodistal bypass: is graft removal mandatory? *J Vasc Surg.* 1992;15:295–305.

29. Joffe B, Mordechay I. Conservative treatment of polytetrafluoroethylene graft infection. *Vasc Surg.* 1989;464–469.

30. Mixter R, Turnipseed WD, Smith DJ, Acher CW, Rao VK, Dibbell DG. Rotational muscle flaps: a new technique for covering infected vascular grafts. *J Vasc Surg.* 1989;9:472–478.

31. Kaufman JL, Shah DM, Corson JD, Skudder PA, Leather RP. Sartorius muscle coverage

for the treatment of complicated vascular surgical wounds. *J Cardiovasc Surg.* 1989;30:475–483.

32. Petrasek PF, Kalman PG, Martin RD. Sartorius myoplasty for deep groin wound following vascular reconstruction. *Am J Surg.* 1990;160:175–178.

33. Meyer JP, Durham JR, Schwarz TH, Sawchuk AP, Shuler JJ. The use of sartorius muscle rotation-transfer in the management of wound complications after infrainguinal vein bypass: a report of eight cases and description of the technique. *J Vasc Surg.* 1989;9:731–735.

Chapter 13

Improving Results Treating Aortic Prosthetic Graft Infection: The Case for *Standard Excisional Therapy*

R. A. Yeager

Introduction

Prosthetic graft infection represents a difficult surgical problem that historically has been associated with a disappointing outcome as measured both in terms of mortality and limb salvage. Bunt's excellent review of this important topic identified an overall operative mortality for aortic prosthetic graft infection ranging from 20% to 38%, with optimal surgical management including total aortic graft excision and extra-anatomic revascularization.[1,2] Many patients with aortic prosthetic graft infection are poor candidates for extensive operative procedures since they typically are elderly, debilitated, and harbor multiple comorbid medical problems. Understandably, there has been renewed interest in the use of local therapy or in situ replacement and biologic coverage in selected patients with localized prosthetic graft infection.[3-11] These innovative approaches may indeed have a place in the management of graft infection and they are discussed elsewhere in this text. However, in the absence of prospective randomized trials, results using nonresectional and in situ approaches should be compared to similar patients concurrently treated by conventional means. The objective of this chapter, therefore, is to summarize current results treating aortic prosthetic graft infection using a standard surgical approach which includes excisional therapy and revascularization.

Improved Results with Standard Excisional Therapy

Numerous authors continue to advocate extra-anatomic revascularization and total aortic graft excision as the preferred treatment for aortic graft infection; historically, this constitutes *conventional* treatment.[12-18] (Fig. 1) It is noteworthy that a striking improvement in patient survival has been reported recently using this form of therapy. Undoubtedly, the improved outcome is due to a multitude of reasons

---

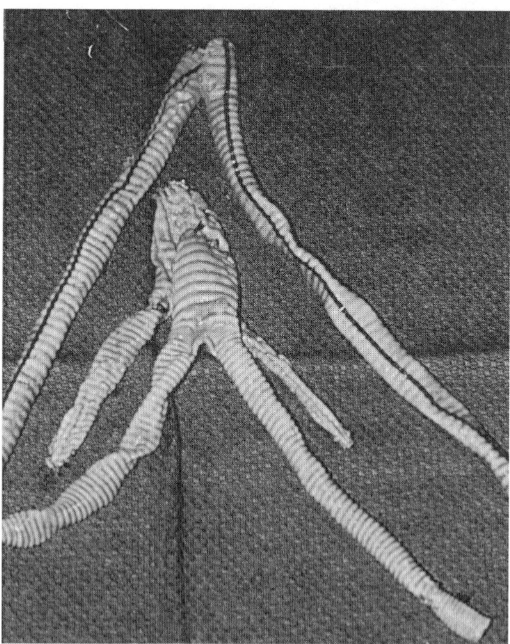

Figure 1. Three aortic grafts removed from a patient with an aortic prosthetic graft infection.

including advancements in diagnostic technology, more effective antibiotics, improved operative strategies, better anesthesia and monitoring techniques, and advancements in intensive care.

The largest published experience with aortic graft infection is that of Reilly et al.[12] who favor initial extra-anatomic bypass followed by total aortic graft excision. They reported a 16% perioperative mortality among 101 patients with aortic prosthetic graft infection. Our group at Oregon recently reported a 14% mortality for 22 patients managed with standard excisional therapy and revascularization during the 1980s, a notable improvement over the 44% mortality experienced by our group during the 1970s.[13] Bergeron[14] reported an exceptional 8% perioperative mortality in 13 patients treated conventionally for graft-enteric fistula during the 1980s. Fulenwider et al.[15] reported a 14% mortality rate in 21 aortic graft infection patients treated by conventional means. Four of their patients in

whom partial graft excision was attempted required early reoperation and total graft excision to control sepsis.

Extra-anatomic revascularization and total aortic graft excision with aortic stump closure is proving to be a durable surgical solution to the problem of aortic graft infection. A recent series reported by Ricotta[16] related outcome to treatment strategy in 32 patients with aortic graft infection. Late complications occurred only in those patients who underwent partial removal of their aortic graft. The best results were following total excision with revascularization. This group had a 17% mortality and no patient experienced a late infection or amputation during a mean follow-up of 34 months. Additionally, Schmitt et al.[17] have recently reported a perioperative mortality of 15% when treating 20 patients with aortic graft infection by total graft excision and extra-anatomic bypass. Mean follow-up was 44 months and late complications included only one patient who developed infection of the axillofemoral bypass and one patient who died from aortic stump sepsis. Reilly et al.[12] have recently described patients with a mean follow-up of 37 months. Late deaths related to the original graft infection occurred in 9% of those with periaortic graft infection and 24% of those with graft-enteric fistula.

Improvement in 1-year patient survival following conventional treatment of aortic graft infection is well documented. O'Hara[18] reported a 1-year survival rate of 31% before 1980 compared with 54% for patients treated since 1980. It is noteworthy that Reilly[12] recently reported a 72% 1-year patient survival following surgical treatment for aortic graft infection. Bandyk et al.[19] have reported a 66% survival at 1 year; our 1-year patient survival at Oregon since 1980 is 61%.[13] Death during the 1-month to 1-year postoperative interval is commonly due to cardiovascular complications such as myocardial infarction and stroke, although problems related to residual retroperitoneal sepsis including late aortic stump blowout are also reported.[13,14,17]

Advocates of in situ grafting emphasize that their approach obviates the problem of aortic stump closure.[4,5] Indeed, surgical management of the aortic stump following aortic graft excision has historically been a difficult problem.[20] O'Hara[18] reported that 32% (8/25) of deaths in patients with aortoenteric fistulae were caused by ruptured aortic closures. Ruptures occurred at a mean interval of 94 days after graft removal. Improved techniques in managing the aortic stump have been developed. A critical aspect of aortic stump management is adequate aortic wall debridement, which includes all grossly infected and devitalized tissue, prior to aortic stump closure. Renal artery bypass or relocation can be used to allow for adequate proximal aortic debridement. Macbeth[21] emphasized the importance of aortic wall and periaortic debridement and pointed out that when arterial wall cultures were positive, suture line disruption occurred 57% of the time compared with a zero disruption rate when cultures were negative. Optimally, the aortic stump is closed in two layers using large monofilament sutures. The omentum can also be used as vascularized tissue coverage for the aortic stump. Additionally, in cases with an associated perigraft abscess, extensive posterior drainage can be used.[22] By implementing these techniques, we believe aortic stump disruption can be avoided and patient survival further improved.

Deaths occurring beyond the first postoperative year are commonly due to the patient's coexisting medical conditions rather than to complications of graft infection or problems related to the aortic stump.[12] O'Hara[18] noted that 82% of their patients had died by 5 years after operation for aortic graft sepsis. More recent authors have, however, documented modest improvement in long-term survival following conventional surgical treatment. Quinones-Baldrich[23] reported a 5-year patient survival of 49%. In our experience, 5-year survival for all aortic graft infection patients was 52%, but for perioperative survivors, 5-year survival was 77%.[13] This follow-up information combined with the recently documented improvement in perioperative mortality, is cause for tentative optimism when discussing patient outcome following conventional surgical treatment for aortic graft infection.

Surgical Strategy

The sequencing and timing of the operative management of aortic graft infection is the source of ongoing controversy. The majority of authors agree that optimal treatment includes initial extra-anatomic bypass followed by total aortic graft excision.[12–14,16,18,24] The strategy of initial aortic graft excision and observation to determine if patients will manifest symptoms of lower limb ischemia is not currently recommended. In our earlier experience, all graft infection patients who underwent aortic graft excision required urgent lower limb revascularization to maintain lower limb viability, except the rare patient with a chronically occluded graft and viable lower extremities. Available information clearly indicates amputation rates are strikingly less frequent with preliminary revascularization as opposed to initial aortic graft excision followed by extra-anatomic bypass (11% versus 46%).[25] Interestingly, perioperative mortality, as well as late axillofemoral graft infection (18% to 23%), appears similar whether the bypass is performed prior to or after aortic graft excision.[25]

It is unclear whether staging the extra-anatomic bypass several days prior to aortic graft removal is advantageous compared to immediately removing the aortic graft during the same operation. Reilly[12] contends that there is less physiologic stress on the patient with a staged approach. We prefer combining the two procedures during the same operation often using two operative teams to conserve time.[13] Our surgical approach is described in detail in another section of this text.

Summary

Improved results managing prosthetic graft infection are due to several factors including improved knowledge of the pathophysiology of infection, earlier and more accurate diagnosis, and improved perioperative management, and intensive care. It is important to note that selected graft infection patients manifest an indolent course and appear initially to experience a favorable outcome regardless of the method of management. To attribute improved results solely to a new surgical approach or technique without comparison to similar patients currently treated by conventional surgical methods is invalid. The current encouraging results summarized herein using excisional therapy and extra-anatomic revascularization should serve as a benchmark for those investigators using nonresectional or in situ replacement techniques for the treatment of aortic prosthetic graft infection.

References

1. Bunt TJ. Synthetic vascular graft infections. *Surgery.* 1983;93:733–746.
2. Bunt TJ. Synthetic vascular graft infections II: Graft enteric erosions and graft enteric fistulas. *Surgery.* 1983;94:1–9.
3. Bandyk DF, Bergamini TM, Kinney EV, Seabrook GR, Towne JB. In situ replacement of vascular prostheses infected by bacterial biofilms. *J Vasc Surg.* 1991;13:575–583.
4. Walker WE, Cooley DA, Duncan JM, Hallman GL Jr, Ott DA, Reul GJ. The management of aortoduodenal fistula by in situ replacement of the infected abdominal aortic graft. *Ann Surg.* 1987;205:727–732.
5. Robinson JA, Johansen K. Aortic sepsis: is there a role for in situ graft reconstruction? *J Vasc Surg.* 1991;13:677–684.
6. Higgans RSD, Steed DL, Julian TB, Makaroun MS, Peitzman AB, Webster MW. The management of aortoenteric and paraprosthetic fistulae. *J Cardiovasc Surg.* 1990;31:81–86.
7. Jacobs MJHM, Reul GJ, Gregoric I, Cooley DA. In situ replacement and extra-anatomic bypass for the treatment of infected abdominal aortic grafts. *Eur J Vasc Surg.* 1991;5:83–86.
8. Kretschmer G, Niederle B, Huk I, et al. Groin infections following vascular surgery: obturator bypass (BYP) versus "biologic coverage" (TRP)–a comparative analysis. *Eur J Vasc Surg.* 1989;3:25–29.
9. Thomas WEG, Baird RN. Secondary aortoenteric fistulae: towards a more conservative approach. *Br J Surg.* 1986;73:875–878.
10. Ghosn PB, Rabbat AG, Trudel J. Why remove an infected aortofemoral graft? *Can J Surg.* 1983;26:330–331.
11. Francois F, Thevenet A. Conservative treatment of prosthetic aortic graft infection with irrigation. *Ann Vasc Surg.* 1991;5:199–201.
12. Reilly LM, Stoney RJ, Goldstone J, Ehrenfeld WK. Improved management of aortic graft infection: the influence of operation sequence and staging. *J Vasc Surg.* 1987;5:421–431.
13. Yeager RA, Moneta GL, Taylor LM Jr, et al. Improving survival and limb salvage in patients with aortic graft infection. *Am J Surg.* 1990;159:466–469.
14. Bergeron P, Espinoza H, Rudondy P, et al. Secondary aortoduodenal fistulas: value of initial axillofemoral bypass. *Ann Vasc Surg.* 1991;5:4–7.
15. Fulenwider JT, Smith RB III, Johnson RW, Johnson RC, Salam AA, Perdue GD. Reoperative abdominal arterial surgery: a ten year experience. *Surgery.* 1983;93:20–27.
16. Ricotta JJ, Faggioli GL, Stella A, et al. Total excision and extra-anatomic bypass for aortic graft infection. *Am J Surg.* 1991;162:145–149.
17. Schmitt DD, Seabrook GR, Bandyk DF, Towne JB. Graft excision and extra-anatomic revascularization: the treatment of choice for the septic aortic prosthesis. *J Cardiovasc Surg.* 1990;31:327–332.
18. O'Hara PJ, Hertzer NR, Beven EG, Krajewski LP. Surgical management of infected abdominal aortic grafts: review of a 25 year experience. *J Vasc Surg.* 1986;3:725–731.
19. Bandyk DF, Berni GA, Thiele BL, Towne JB. Aortofemoral graft infection due to *Staphylococcus epidermidis. Arch Surg.* 1984;119:102–108.
20. Martin-Paredero V, Busuttil RW, Dixon SM, Baker JD, Machleder H, Moore WS. Fate of aortic graft removal. *Am J Surg.* 1983;146:194–197.
21. Macbeth GA, Rubin JR, McIntyre KE, Gold-

stone J, Malone JM. The relevance of arterial wall microbiology to the treatment of prosthetic graft infections: graft infection vs. arterial infection. *J Vasc Surg.* 1984;1: 36–44.

22. Taylor LM Jr, Deitz DM, McConnell DB, Porter JM. Treatment of infected abdominal aneurysms by extra-anatomic bypass, aneurysm excision, and drainage. *Am J Surg.* 1988; 155:655–658.

23. Quinones-Baldrich WJ, Hernandez JJ, Moore WS. Long-term results following surgical management of aortic graft infection. *Arch Surg.* 1991;126:507–511.

24. Trout HH III, Kozloff L, Giordano JM. Priority of revascularization in patients with graft enteric fistulas, infected arteries, or infected arterial prostheses. *Ann Surg.* 1984;199: 669–683.

25. Yeager RA, Porter JM. Basic data concerning arterial and prosthetic graft infection. *Ann Vasc Surg.* 1992;6:485–491.

Chapter 14

Staging Remote Bypasses for Graft Infections, Graft-Enteric Fistulae, and Erosions

H. H. Trout, III

R. L. Feinberg

L. Kozloff

Introduction

The two main issues pertaining to staging of bypass grafts are 1) whether a remote bypass should be performed *before* or *after* removal of an infected graft or a graft involved with an enteric communication; and 2) whether the remote bypass and the graft removal should be performed at the same operation (combined) or should be separated by 24 or more hours (staged). Since graft-enteric communications present a different set of problems from those presented by prosthetic graft infections, the approaches for each will be addressed separately.

From experience and review of the medical literature two guiding principles become obvious. First, prosthetic grafts, when placed in previously contaminated areas, have a high incidence of becoming infected. Second, patients with complex aortic graft complications do not tolerate long periods of lower body ischemia, there-fore its avoidance is an important tenet of therapy.

Theoretical Objections to Constructing a Remote Bypass Before Removal of an Aortic Prosthetic Graft

The two theoretical objections to constructing a remote bypass are: 1) The remote bypass will become infected at the time the aortic graft is removed. Remote bypass infection is possible and has been reported,[1-3] though it appears to be relatively infrequent. Moreover, the incidence of infection of the remote bypass does not seem to be less when the remote bypass is placed after removal of an infected graft.[1] Even in these instances, however, most of the time treatment of the infected bypass is successful. Furthermore, the possibility of remote graft infection is overshadowed by the complications of prolonged ischemia associated with removal of the infected graft before placement of a remote bypass. These include distal gangrene, acidosis, hypothermia, bleeding disorders, compartment syndromes, myoglobinemia, renal failure, myocardial infarction, and death.

2) The competitive flow that exists for the few hours or days the remote bypass and the infected aortic graft are both functional will result in thrombosis of the remote bypass. Concerns about competitive flow are apparently not justified. Thrombosis in this setting has not occurred to our knowledge. This is probably because the arrival of the pulse wave at the groin from a remote bypass is almost certainly out of phase with the pulse wave from the in situ graft. Ernst reported a patient whose axillofemoral artery bypass remained patent until removal 123 days after insertion, despite the fact that it existed in parallel with a patent aortofemoral autogenous arterial system.[4] Moreover, in the unlikely event that a previously inserted remote bypass did thrombose during an operation to remove an infected graft, a thrombectomy of the remote bypass could be performed easily after the infected graft was removed.

Infected Aortic, Aortoiliac, or Aortofemoral Grafts

The issue whether to perform the remote bypass *before* or *after* removal of an infected graft is fairly straightforward. In 1984, all patients reported in the English medical literature who had a remote bypass performed before or after removal of an infected aortic graft were reviewed.[5] Of 13 patients reported who had a remote graft constructed *after* an infected aortic graft was removed, 10 died in the perioperative period for a mortality rate of 71%. Of 23 patients who had a remote bypass constructed *before* the infected graft was removed, 6 died for a mortality rate of 26%. Though management of critically ill patients has undoubtedly improved since that time, the survival disparity between these two treatment regimens surely has not narrowed sufficiently to justify removal of an infected graft before construction of a remote bypass. Indeed, there are now so few reports of patients treated with infected graft removal prior to remote bypass that it is impossible to derive a current mortality rate. Several subsequent reports, however, have also documented high mortality rates when graft removal preceded remote bypass construction.[1,2]

In summary, mortality and morbidity data strongly suggest that remote bypass should precede removal of an infected prosthetic aortic graft.

One Operation (Combined) Versus Two Operations (Staged)

Infected Aortic Graft Treated by Remote Bypass Followed by Graft Removal

Data supporting the staged approach over the combined method are scanty and cannot be regarded as statistically significant. One of the problems encountered in trying to answer this question is that several of the larger series group patients with aortic graft infections with those with aortoenteric fistulas.[1-3] These reports also obligatorily include patients treated in different eras with evolving management plans. For instance, treatment before 1980 was dominated by graft removal and remote bypass construction in varying order; treatment groups since 1980 have been composed mainly of remote bypass preceding graft removal. Staging, though not new,[6] has gained in popularity as well.[2,5]

Even though a statistically convincing argument cannot be made in favor of a staging approach, data suggest that staging is associated with a lower amputation rate,[3] is better tolerated by the surgical teams,[2] and may have a lower mortality rate.[2,5] Accordingly, despite reports that some surgeons achieve excellent results using the combined approach,[1] It is our view that the staged approach, when possible, is the better method.

In summary, when feasible, staging operations for treatment of infections of prosthetic aortic grafts will be tolerated better by patients as well as surgical teams, may lower amputation rates, and may be associated with a lower mortality rate.

Aortoenteric Communications

Because of recent or ongoing bleeding, the issue whether to perform the remote bypass before or after removal of an aortoenteric fistula is more complex than it is when considering treatment of an infected graft.

Patients with Active Bleeding

If the patient is bleeding actively, the treatment choices are to remove the aortic graft and then insert a remote bypass or to remove the aortic graft and insert a graft, either autogenous or prosthetic, in the same (in situ) position. In 1984, all patients reported in the English medical literature who had a remote bypass performed before or after removal of an aortoenteric fistula were reviewed.[5] Of 75 patients reported who had an aortoenteric fistula removed *before* a remote graft was constructed, 40 died in the perioperative period for a mortality rate of 53%. It should be noted that this did not include any patients who were bleeding acutely at the time of the operation. Though the data were not included in that paper, when those who were actively bleeding at the beginning of the operation were also included, the mortality was considerably higher. As a consequence, graft removal followed by remote bypass construction has a high morbidity and mortality and is not a good choice. The better approach would be to insert an in situ graft. On a theoretical basis, autogenous material is preferred but acquisition of enough autogenous material

of sufficient size in the limited time available is rarely possible. Accordingly, in the actively bleeding patient with an aortoenteric communication, the best treatment is aortic graft removal, wide debridement, and insertion of a prosthetic aortoiliac graft in the in situ position (avoiding the groins if possible). One would then treat such a patient with long-term antibiotics (probably for life). Careful monitoring would include interval magnetic resonance imaging (MRI) or computer tomography (CT) scans for evidence of aortic graft infection. At the first signs of graft infection, the patient should have a remote bypass (usually axillobifemoral) and removal of the aortic graft. Thus, the in situ bypass may be either a curative procedure or a temporizing one allowing patient survival and stabilization until a staged axillobifemoral bypass and aortic graft removal are performed for recurrent aortic graft contamination.

In summary, the best treatment probably is removal of the contaminated aortic graft, wide debridement, and replacement with a new prosthetic graft in the same (in situ) position. Subsequently, care should be taken to observe the patient carefully for evidence of recurrent graft infection.

Patients without Active Bleeding

In that same study,[5] of 29 patients reported who had an aortoenteric fistula (that was not actively bleeding at the time of the operation) treated by removal of the aortic graft *after* a remote graft was constructed, 5 died in the perioperative period for a mortality rate of 17% (in contrast to the 53% mortality when the order of the procedures was reversed). Others[2] have also reported success with this approach with satisfactory mortality rates (given the severity of the underlying problem).

In summary, in patients without active bleeding, the best treatment for an aortoenteric fistula is construction of a remote bypass (usually axillobifemoral) followed by removal of the aortic graft.

One Operation (Combined) Versus Two Operations (Staged)

Patients With an Aortoenteric Fistula Treated by a Remote Bypass and Graft Removal

The data for this category of patients are anecdotal and small. Nonetheless, it seems that patients with aortoenteric communications who have infection as their primary mode of presentation and those who have bled only a small amount and are stable can have a staged approach with good success.[2,5] Those who have had a recent major *herald* bleed are probably better managed with the combined approach.

In summary, a staged procedure for patients with aortoenteric fistulae is the preferred approach if there has been minimal or no bleeding. Combined approaches are probably best in those patients with a recent major *herald* bleed.

Summary

Attempts to avoid prolonged lower body ischemia should form the cornerstone of therapy both for patients with aortic graft infections and for those with aortoenteric fistulae since protracted ischemia results in a high rate of amputation and death.

Infected Aortic Graft

Mortality and morbidity data strongly suggest that a remote bypass should precede removal of an infected prosthetic aortic graft. When feasible, staging (remote bypass followed 1 or more days later by graft removal) operations for treatment of infections of prosthetic aortic grafts will be tolerated better by patients as well as surgical teams, may lower amputation rates, and

may be associated with a lower mortality rate.

Aortoenteric Fistula

In patients with active bleeding, the best treatment probably is removal of the contaminated aortic graft, wide debridement, and replacement with a new prosthetic graft in the same (in situ) position. Subsequently, great care should be taken to observe the patient carefully for evidence of recurrent graft infection.

In patients without active bleeding, the best treatment for an aortoenteric fistula is construction of a remote bypass (usually axillobifemoral) followed by removal of the aortic graft.

Staged procedures for patients with aortoenteric fistulae are the preferred approach if there has been minimal or no bleeding. Combined approaches are probably best in those patients with a recent major *herald* bleed.

References

1. Yeager RA, Moneta GL, Taylor LM Jr, Harris EJ Jr, McConnell DB, Porter JM. Improving survival and limb salvage in patients with aortic graft infection. *Am J Surg.* 1990;159:466–469.
2. Reilly LM, Stoney RJ, Goldstone J, Ehrenfeld WK. Improved management of aortic graft infection: the influence of operation sequence and staging. *J Vasc Surg.* 1987;5:421–431.
3. O'Hara PJ, Hertzer NR, Beven EG, Krajewski LP. Surgical management of infected abdominal aortic grafts: review of a 25-year experience. *J Vasc Surg.* 1986;3:725–731.
4. Ernst CB. Axillofemoral bypass graft patency without aortofemoral pressure differential: disuse atrophy of ipsilateral ileofemoral segment. *Ann Surg.* 1975;181:424–427.
5. Trout HH III, Kozloff L, Giordano JM. Priority of revascularization in patients with graft enteric fistulae, infected arteries, or infected arterial prostheses. *Ann Surg.* 1984;199:669–683.
6. Casali RE, Tucker WE, Thompson BW, Read RC. Infected prosthetic grafts. *Arch Surg.* 1980;115:577–580.

Chapter 15

Homografts: Alternative Treatment for Overtly Infected Prosthetic Grafts

E.M. Masuda

S.O. Snyder

Introduction

Prosthetic graft infection in vascular reconstruction undoubtedly represents one of the most challenging complications of vascular surgery. Infected grafts may be overtly infected and surrounded by frank purulence or may involve the presence of an infected false aneurysm. The traditional treatment for this formidable problem has been graft excision, and if collateral perfusion is inadequate, revascularization with either autologous vessel[1,2] or extra-anatomic prosthetic bypass.[3,4] Infection may be localized, may present with a draining sinus, or may involve an exposed graft which lacks coverage due to wound healing problems. Recent clinical experience suggests that local wound debridement and preservation of grafts in cases of limited infection or those involving less virulent bacteria such as *Staphylococcus epidermidis* may be a safe and effective alternative.[5]

Despite a recent renewed interest in graft retention in infected fields and in situ prosthetic replacement, results of these less aggressive therapeutic measures in overtly purulent fields remain largely unknown. Furthermore, although traditional management by graft excision and revascularization has been effective for these major infections, dissatisfaction with thrombosis and infection of long extra-anatomic prosthetic bypass grafts[6] and frequent lack of sufficient autologous material for direct replacement has prompted a search for an alternative vascular conduit.

In 1987, we reported the first series[7] of patients with prosthetic graft infections who underwent complete graft excision and revascularization with venous homografts placed directly into infected fields. In this pilot study of six patients, all demonstrated grafts immersed in purulent fluid and all involved groin wounds. Successful clinical eradication of infection was achieved in all cases, and there was only one case of early limb loss.

This chapter provides a summary of our experience over a 9-year period and the literature regarding the indication, procurement, preparation, and clinical results of venous homografts used as arterial substitutes in the management of prosthetic graft infections. Homografts may be implanted directly in contaminated wounds when an autogenous vein graft is not available or when direct replacement of infected grafts is required. Since it is generally known that vascular homografts invariably occlude with time,[8] they should be applied as a temporizing measure to maintain limb perfusion while the infection is eradicated by appropriate antibiotics and aggressive wound care.

Background

Homografts have been used experimentally for replacement of blood vessels since the early part of this century. In 1912, Alexis Carrel[9] reported the successful replacement of a thoracic aorta in a healthy dog, using the jugular vein of a second dog. The venous allograft had been preserved in cold storage for 24 hours prior to transplantation and the animal survived 2 years until she expired from an acquired infection. The aortic graft was described as patent but minimally dilated and composed primarily of connective tissue. Following this remarkable accomplishment, studies involving vascular homografts did not reappear until the late 1940s. Early work in humans was as performed using arterial homografts for aortic replacement in noninfected cases.[10] The major problem encountered with arterial grafts was an alarmingly high rate of late mural degeneration, aneurysm formation, and rupture. In 1970, Szilagyi and colleagues[11] showed that arterial homografts were associated with a significant incidence of aneurysm formation (14 of 53 aortic grafts) when followed for 6 to 15 years after implantation. Furthermore, infrainguinal grafts showed poor patency over the long term (8 of 9 occluded). Interest in the general use of arterial homografts for revascularization declined and they were essentially abandoned.

In an effort to avoid the problems of aneurysm formation observed with arterial grafts, investigators examined homologous veins as a source for arterial replacement. Several experimental studies[12-14] showed that homologous veins demonstrated a lower propensity for degeneration and aneurysm formation than did homologous arteries; however, long-term patency rates were similar to arteries and were disappointingly low.

Application of Homografts in Infected Fields: Experimental Work

The initial work of Moore et al.[15] using fresh arterial homografts as arterial substitutes in infected tissues provided a major stimulus for our present work. They compared the results of fresh arterial homografts, arterial autografts, and Dacron synthetic grafts implanted into the femoral arteries of dogs, which were subsequently infected with *Staphylococcus aureus*. At 3 months following implantation, infection was successfully eliminated in 11 out of 12 autografts and 10 out of 12 allografts, whereas 7 out of 8 Dacron grafts remained infected. The evidence demonstrated that fresh homografts could be used as vascular conduits in grossly infected fields. Furthermore, fresh homografts remained patent long enough to allow eradication of infection. Clinical application of arterial homografts, however, remained restricted because of the tendency for mural degeneration and aneurysm formation.

The Norfolk Experience

The concept obtained from Moore's experimental work using fresh homografts was coupled with reports by Ochner and others[12-14] indicating lower rates of aneurysm formation with venous homografts as opposed to arterial sources. By merging these two concepts, we developed an approach to overtly infected prosthetic bypasses, and began using freshly harvested and eventually cryopreserved venous homografts for replacement of infected grafts.

In 1987 we reported favorable clinical

results with freshly harvested venous homografts as arterial substitutes in infected fields.[7] All patients had had previous multilevel prosthetic grafts. All six demonstrated graft infection of the entire conduit with involvement of the distal graft at the femoral anastomoses, and proximal graft at the axillary artery (5 cases), and infrarenal aorta (1 case). To achieve control of infection, complete graft excision was required. Freshly harvested vena cava, iliac, femoral, and saphenous veins were procured during multiple organ donor procedures and joined to create a new conduit which was inserted directly into the infected field after removal of the prosthetic graft. In all cases, grafts remained patent long enough to allow complete elimination of infection. Although there were two cases in which a secondary revascularization procedure was required due to thrombosis of the grafts, the newly inserted prostheses were not associated with recurrent infection. There were no cases of limb loss or death in this early report.

Recently we reported our overall experience using homografts over a period of 9 years.[16] There were 16 prosthetic graft infections in 12 patients with groin infections and frank purulence surrounding the prostheses. Cryopreserved vascular grafts became more readily available from tissue banks after 1987, and subsequently, cryopreserved venous homografts were used instead of fresh conduits. Following complete removal of prosthetic grafts and replacement with a homograft, eradication of infection was achieved in 11 (92%) of 12 cases. Mean follow-up was 20 months. There was one death related to uncontrolled infection and early limb loss occurred in 2 (16%) of 12 patients. All grafts remained patent long enough for elimination of infection and in 4 cases, replacement was required with new prosthetic grafts and no recurrent infection when followed from 14 to 50 months.

Since our initial report, several recent studies have corroborated our findings and support the use of homografts as interim

conduits while infection is eliminated. There are basically three series with reasonable numbers and one case report.

In a study published in 1992 that closely resembled ours, Fujitani et al.[17] reported encouraging results in 10 lower extremity reconstructions using cryopreserved saphenous vein homografts. They demonstrated control of infection in all cases and limb salvage rate of 89%. Of 10 homografts, 7 remained patent during follow-up with no evidence of graft degeneration or aneurysm formation, and one patient died with a patent graft 1 month postoperatively. There were only two grafts that occluded during follow-up, one of which was salvaged after thrombectomy.

In the most recent series reported by Kieffer et al. in 1992,[18] 37 patients with infected infrarenal aortic prosthetic grafts underwent in situ replacement with homografts obtained from cadavers during multiorgan transplant retrieval. They showed that there were no early or late amputations, and this approach was associated with a low incidence of infection and vascular-related complications. Mean follow-up was 13.5 months. Of four deaths following operation, only one death was directly related to persistent infection.

Donaldson and Ross,[19] in a slightly different but related clinical setting, reported their successful results of using a homograft aortic root for replacement of prosthetic valve endocarditis. Although benefits of lowering operative mortality were not demonstrated, the procedure did provide complete cure of infection in 19 of 20 survivors.

Finally, Bahnini et al.[20] described the use of a fresh allogenic aortic graft to replace an infected prosthetic graft and demonstrated complete eradication of infection, graft patency, and no signs of graft degeneration at 18 months after surgery. The potential for aneurysmal development of arterial homografts was discussed and a more optimistic outlook was presented. Further work would be needed to support their observations regarding the safety of arterial as opposed to venous homografts in contaminated wounds.

Surgical Indications

The use of venous homografts should be reserved for select cases of overt prosthetic graft infections in which autogenous material is not available for direct replacement in infected fields, or when extra-anatomic bypass with prosthetic graft is not desirable. This includes cases of infection involving the femoral anastomosis of an aortofemoral, axillobifemoral, or infrainguinal bypass graft. When femoral limbs of aortofemoral grafts are infected, one approach is to excise the prosthesis and revascularize with autogenous material by axillofemoral bypass or by direct, in situ replacement of the aortic graft. Because of the enormous quantity of autogenous vessels that would be needed, this is not always possible. Freshly harvested or, more recently, cryopreserved venous homografts can serve as an alternative conduit without the supply limitations encountered with autologous material.

Extra-anatomic bypass with prosthetic material can be achieved by axillary to popliteal or superficial femoral artery bypass to circumvent femoral wounds. However, long, circuitous grafts are associated with poor long-term patency. In a recent series by Taylor et al.,[6] high failure rates led to graft revision in 63% of cases. The use of homografts and their placement directly into contaminated wounds may provide a more preferable alternative.

Homografts can also be combined with autogenous material to create a composite conduit. Our early results with this method have proved favorable. Although autogenous grafts will likely remain patent longer than homografts, both are subject to eventual occlusion and will probably need replacement with a more definitive procedure once infection is cleared.

Since homografts may potentially deteriorate and become aneurysmal, they should probably not be implanted directly in the aortic position in case of bleeding into the retroperitoneum. Homografts are best used in the nonretroperitoneal position as in axillofemoral or infrainguinal bypasses, where they can be monitored serially by clinical assessment or by duplex scanning.

In the event of aneurysm formation, the homograft may be replaced electively with new prosthetic material without a significant risk for reinfection.

Homograft Procurement and Preparation

Fresh Homografts

Prior to 1987 fresh venous homografts were obtained from the Virginia Tissue Bank, Virginia Beach, Virginia. Vena cava, iliac, superficial femoral, and saphenous veins were harvested from preheparinized cadaver donors after confirming ABO and Rh compatibility. Prior to implantation all grafts and donors were screened for routine viral and bacterial transmittable diseases. Harvested veins were stored in 1-40 C McCoy's 5A medium containing 400 units/mL streptomycin and 10,000 units of heparin. Fresh veins were implanted no sooner than 3 days after harvest to assure negative donor cultures and no later than 7 days after harvest to avoid losing graft sterility. The surgical procedure consisted of two teams working simultaneously. While one team excised the infected prosthesis, the other prepared the homograft on a side table by ligating branches, repairing holes, and joining segments to create a conduit of sufficient length. Five millimeters was the minimal diameter accepted.

Cryopreserved Homografts

After 1987 cryopreserved venous homografts as opposed to fresh veins became available through the tissue banks. Veins were prepared by standard cryopreservation methods. Venous homografts were cryopreserved in 10% fetal calf serum and 10% dimethylsulfoxide (DMSO). Tissues were treated by slow freezing and thawing methods. Grafts were frozen with liquid nitrogen at a controlled rate of 1°C per minute until a temperature of −40°C was reached. They were then stored in a vapor phase of liquid nitrogen of 150 to 175°C.

Cultures

Virulent pathogens such as *Staphylococcus aureus* and *Pseudomonas aeruginosa* are associated with a higher risk of sepsis, limb, and life-threatening complications.[21,22] Homograft replacement would seem most useful in cases of major infections with virulent bacterial strains. The most common organism cultured in our series[16] was *S aureus* which was present in 58% of cases. According to recent investigations,[5] treatment of infections involving less virulent species such as *S epidermidis* may be successfully controlled with less aggressive measures such as debridement and antibiotics with or without muscle flap coverage, although long-term results are still pending.

Fresh versus Cryopreserved Grafts in Infected Fields: Experimental Work

In recent canine experiments performed in our laboratory, a comparative study was conducted between cryopreserved and fresh venous homografts implanted into wounds infected with *S aureus*. Canine jugular veins were cryopreserved in 10% or 15% DMSO using either rapid or slow freezing and thawing methods. The groups with fresh homografts and those with cryopreserved grafts treated by 10%

DMSO with slow freezing and thawing rates of 1°C per minute showed clearly superior results with no aneurysm formation during a 30-day postoperative period. Occlusion rates were also comparable. This was in contradistinction to results of homografts prepared with 15% DMSO and rapid freezing and thawing rates, in which 30% were associated with aneurysm development.

Although the behavior of fresh and 10% DMSO-prepared cryopreserved homografts in infected fields was similar, they demonstrated some differences in histologic features. The degree of plasma cell and macrophage infiltration was greater in the fresh as opposed to cryopreserved grafts, supporting the observations by others that fresh homografts are more antigenic than cryopreserved vessels. In both, the adventia were greatly thickened by large numbers of fibroblasts and vasa vasorum. Fresh homografts appeared more viable than cryopreserved veins and demonstrated a well-organized layer of smooth muscle cells and collagen in the media. In contrast, the media of cryopreserved veins were clearly less cellular and collagen appeared more dispersed.

Based on these results in the canine model, it appeared that use of cryopreserved vein grafts prepared with 10% DMSO using slow freezing and thawing techniques proved equally effective as fresh homografts when used in contaminated wounds. Histologic changes suggested that fresh homografts showed a higher degree of viability and antigenicity than cryopreserved specimens, although aneurysm and occlusion rates did not differ.

These findings supported our use of cryopreserved veins in infected fields in humans. Because of the obvious advantage and ease of procuring cryopreserved veins as opposed to fresh vessels, most investigators have resorted to cryopreserved venous homografts taken from human cadavers stored in tissue banks.

Homologous Arteries versus Veins

Venous homografts have been preferred over arterial vessels because of studies suggesting lower aneurysm formation rate[23,24] and lower graft antigenicity with venous homografts. Most studies leading to these conclusions were observed in noninfected clinical situations.

The higher incidence of graft disruption observed with arterial homografts has been attributed to the dual blood supply of the arterial wall. Arteries normally depend on two sources of blood—the vessel lumen and the vasa vasorum that penetrate from the adventitia into the outer third of the media. Since a larger portion of the arterial wall is dependent on the vasa vasorum the artery, when excised for implantation, is essentially devascularized. According to Ochsner,[12] the arterial wall undergoes ischemic degeneration and change from a large fibromuscular layer to a hypocellular layer which lacks significant secondary fibrosis and is thought to be more prone to dilation or disruption. In contrast, veins do not depend on vasa vasorum, primarily receiving nutrition from the lumen. Furthermore, the lower antigenicity of veins when compared to arteries is believed to account for the greater cellularity and fibroblast formation in venous homografts which may be important in maintaining wall strength. In general, problems with degeneration and aneurysm formation appear to be less frequent with venous conduits as opposed to arterial grafts.

Although aneurysm formation is reduced by the use of venous grafts, disappointingly low long-term graft patency remains a severe limitation. The largest clinical experience using venous homografts in noncontaminated cases was reported by Ochsner et al.[8] They implanted 129 homologous vein grafts in 91 patients for arterial bypass at different levels with a mean follow-up of 22.4 months. Seventy-five grafts were inserted at the femoropopliteal or tibi-operoneal level, and by 1 year 50% of grafts occluded and by 5 years the cumulative patency rate was only 30%.

Homograft Antigenicity and the Role of Immunosuppressive Treatment

Despite early reports describing the low antigenicity of venous homografts,[25] their high propensity for thrombosis was postulated to be the result of an immunologic process. This led to studies examining various methods of host immunosuppression and graft preservation in order to reduce the immunologic response to the transplanted vessel.

Initial work by Schwartz et al.[25] indicated that homograft veins were weakly antigenic. This observation was supported by the lack of accelerated skin graft rejection in the recipient animal, and the persistence of viable donor cells in the graft based on sex chromatin studies. However, use of a mongrel model in this study was later found to be an unreliable model for allograft studies as a result of random histocompatibility matching; subsequent studies[8,26–28] have suggested that both fresh and frozen veins elicited humoral and cellular immune response leading to early graft thrombosis.

The concept that homograft rejection was related to eventual graft occlusion was first emphasized by Williams and associates.[28] They showed that graft rejection and patency rates improved with low-dose Imuran.® Histologic changes were found in the transplanted vessel with heavy infiltration of inflammatory cells most notably in the adventitia as opposed to the intima. Matching for ABO was therefore recommended by Oschner,[8] but only minimally improved patency rates.

Treatment was then aimed at either reducing or abolishing the immunogenicity of the graft or treating the host with immunosuppressants. Cryopreservation and preservation of grafts with glutaraldehyde have been tried, with little improvement in patency rates over fresh homografts.[26,29] The addition of a cryoprotectant such as DMSO to freezing methods has shown variable benefits in reducing antigenicity.[26,30] Although the addition of cryopreservation to homograft preparation may not show clear benefits over fresh conduits, at least no significant detrimental effect is observed. Undoubtedly, access to cryopreserved homografts for use when needed from tissue banks is clearly more convenient and desirable than procuring fresh specimens.

There has been some evidence to suggest that treatment of the host with immunosuppressive agents such as cyclosporine A may improve graft patency[31,32] in noninfected cases. The dosage used by most studies, however, is moderate and not desirable for use in patients with serious graft infections. Low-dose Imuran® has been advocated[28] and has not been found to be associated with acceleration of infection when used as adjuvant treatment with implantation of homografts in the presence of infection.[7]

Finally, there has been some evidence that antiplatelet drugs such as aspirin and dipyridimole have been associated with longer homograft patency.[33,34] Low-dose aspirin has been empirically added to the regimen in our patients to reduce the tendency of thrombosis following the expected loss of endothelial cells and subsequent exposure of the underlying thrombogenic surface.

In general, results of altering either the graft or host to reduce the immunologic effect and improve patency remain controversial and further studies are needed to elucidate the value of these methods.

Summary

In summary, vascular graft infection continues to pose a clinical challenge. The concept of implanting a biologic graft such as a homograft into an overtly infected field is appealing since the graft demonstrates resistance to infection and serves as a temporizing measure to permit extremity perfusion while infection is eradicated. This provides an attractive alternative when more conventional approaches are not preferable and may be a useful addition to the vascular surgeon's armamentarium when prosthetic graft infection is encountered.

References

1. Seeger JM, Wheeler JR, Gregory RT, Snyder SO, Gayle RG. Autogenous graft replacement of infected prosthetic grafts in the femoral position. *Surgery*. 1983;93:39–45.
2. Ehrenfeld WK, Wilbur BG, Olcott CN, Stoney RJ. Autogenous tissue reconstruction in the management of infected prosthetic grafts. *Surgery*. 1979;85:82–92.
3. Liekweg WG, Greenfield LJ. Vascular prosthetic infections: collected experience and results of treatment. *Surgery*. 1977;81:335–342.
4. Bunt TJ. Synthetic vascular graft infections. I: graft infections. *Surgery*. 1983;93:733–746.
5. Bandyk DF. Retention of vascular prostheses in infected fields. In: Veith FJ, ed. *Current Critical Problems in Vascular Surgery*. Vol. 3. St. Louis: Quality Medical Pub, Inc; 1991: 368–373.
6. Taylor SM, Mills JL, Fujitani RM, Robison JG. The influence of groin sepsis on extra-anatomic bypass patency in patients with prosthetic graft infection. *Ann Vasc Surg*. 1992;6:80–84.
7. Snyder SO, Wheeler JR, Gregory RT, Gayle RG, Zirkle PK. Freshly harvested cadaveric venous homografts as arterial conduits in infected fields. *Surgery*. 1987;101:283–291.
8. Ochsner JL, Lawson JD, Eskind SJ, Mills NL, DeCamp PT. Homologous veins as an arterial substitute: long-term results. *J Vasc Surg*. 1984;1:306–313.
9. Carrel A. Ultimate results of aortic transplantations. *J Expt Med*. 1912;15:389–392.
10. Szilagyi DE, McDonald RT, Smith BF, Whitcomb JG. Biologic fate of human arterial homograft. *Arch Surg*. 1957;75:506–529.
11. Szilagyi DE, Rodriguez FJ, Smith RF, Elliott JP. Late fate of arterial allografts. *Arch Surg*. 1970;101:721–733.
12. Ochsner JL, DeCamp PT, Leonard GL. Experience with fresh venous allografts as an arterial substitute. *Ann Surg*. 1971;173:933–939.

13. Field P, Mata A, Agrama H. An assessment of allograft veins for arterial grafting. *Circulation* 1969;XL(suppl III):79.

14. Barner HB, DeWeese JA, Schenk EA. Fresh and frozen homologous venous grafts for arterial repair. *Angiology.* 1966;17:389.

15. Moore WS, Swanson RJ, Campagna G, Bean B. The use of fresh tissue arterial substitutes in infected fields. *J Surg Res.* 1975;18:229–233.

16. Masuda EM, Snyder SO, Adcock GA, et al. 9-year experience with venous homografts in infected fields. Presented at the 17th Annual Southern Assoc. *Vasc Surg.* 1993. (Submitted for publication).

17. Fujitani RM, Bassiouny HS, Gewertz BL, Glagov S, Zarins CK. Cryopreserved saphenous vein allogenic homografts: an alternative conduit in lower extremity arterial reconstruction in infected fields. *J Vasc Surg.* 1992;15:519–526.

18. Kieffer E, Bahnini A, Koskas F, Plissonnier D. In situ allograft replacement of infected infrarenal aortic prosthetic grafts: results in 37 patients. *J Vasc Surg.* 1992;15:1077. Abstract.

19. Donaldson RM, Ross DM. Homograft aortic root replacement for complicated prosthetic valve endocarditis. *Circulation.* 1984; 70(suppl I):178–181.

20. Bahnini A, Ruotolo C, Koskas F, Kieffer E. In situ fresh allograft replacement of an infected aortic prosthetic graft: 18-month follow-up. *J Vasc Surg.* 1991;14:98–102.

21. Martin LF, Harris JM, Fehr DM, et al. Vascular prosthetic infection with Staphylococcus epidermidis: experimental study of pathogenesis and therapy. *J Vasc Surg.* 1989;9: 464–471.

22. Geary KJ, Tomkiewicz ZM, Harrison HN, et al. Differential effects of a Gram-negative and a Gram-positive infection on autogenous and prosthetic grafts. *J Vasc Surg.* 1990; 11:339–347.

23. Barner JB, DeWeese JA, Schenk EA. Fresh and frozen homologous venous grafts for arterial repair. *J Angiol.* 1966;17:389–401.

24. Sauvage LR, Harkins HN. Experimental vascular grafts: an evaluation relating to types, means of preservation, and methods of suture in the growing pig. *Surgery* 1953;33:587.

25. Schwartz SI, Kutner FR, Neistadt A, Barner H, Resnicoff S, Vaughan J. Antigenicity of homografted veins. *Surgery.* 1967;61: 471–477.

26. Axthelm SC, Porter JM, Strickland S, Bauer GM. Antigenicity of venous allografts. *Ann Surg.* 1978;189:290–293.

27. Stephen M, Sheil AGR, Wong J. Allograft vein arterial bypass. *Arch Surg.* 1978;113: 591–593.

28. Williams GM, Hoar A, Krajewski C, Parks LC, Roth J. Rejection and repair of endothelium in major vessel transplants. *Surgery.* 1975;78:694–706.

29. Weber TR, Lindenauer SM, Dent TL, Allen E, Salles CA, Weatherbee L. Long-term patency of vein grafts preserved in liquid nitrogen in dimethyl sulfoxide. *Ann Surg.* 1976; 184:709–712.

30. Weber TR, Dent RL, Lindenauer SM, et al. Viable vein graft preservation. *J Surg Res.* 1975;18:247.

31. Vermassen F, Degrieck N, De Kock L, et al. Immunosuppressive treatment of venous allografts. *Eur J Vasc Surg* 1991;5:669–675.

32. Bandlien KO, Toledo-Pereyra LH, MacKenzie GH, Choudbury SP, Cortez JA. Immunosuppression with cyclosporine: a new approach to improve patency of venous allografts. *Arch Surg.* 1983;118:829–833.

33. Ricotta JJ, Schaff HV, Gadacz TR. The effect of aspirin and dipyridamole on the patency of allograft veins. *J Surg Res.* 1979;26: 262–269.

34. Sitzmann JV, Imbembo AL, Ricotta JJ, McManama GP, Hutchins GM. Dimethyl-sulfoxide-treated, cryopreserved venous allografts in the arterial and venous systems. *Surgery.* 1984;95:154–159.

Chapter 16

Remote Bypasses for Graft Infections

H.H. Trout III
R.L. Feinberg
L. Kozloff

Introduction

For effective treatment of patients with infected prosthetic grafts or with graft-enteric communications, the vascular surgeon must have a thorough understanding of specific management principles. Prior consideration of the complex issues involved and derived treatment approaches based on rational algorithms will yield substantively better results than otherwise possible when confronted with the acute problem. Though surgeons pride themselves on a rigorously logical approach, many graft infection problems do not respond to treatment in the way *logic* would predict. For instance, on the surface it appears illogical that in situ insertion of a prosthetic aortoiliac bypass can be successful with a low incidence of infection as treatment for a primary aortoduodenal fistula caused by an abdominal aortic aneurysm. Nor does it seem logical that one can place a remote axillobifemoral bypass and subsequently excise a grossly contaminated aortoiliac bypass graft with a low incidence of infection of the axillobifemoral bypass. These two improbable treatments, however,

are appropriate and effective. Graft infection problems are complex, require urgent action, and are technically perilous. Best treatment does not always follow the rules that logic would seem to dictate. As a consequence, surgeons should have reasoned and well-organized management plans before encountering these often devastating problems in the acute setting.

There are no prospective randomized studies to guide therapy. These infectious problems are infrequent, exhibit a myriad of presentations, and require careful analysis during each stage of treatment. Many different methods of treating infected prosthetic grafts, including local and topical measures[1-8] have been reported as successful. Generally, methods providing distal arterial perfusion through conduits placed in uncontaminated planes along with complete removal of the infected graft have yielded the best results.[9-11] It is reasonable, though often not wise, to treat infected prosthetic grafts with local measures if the consequences of treatment failure are restricted mainly to a longer hospitalization and more operative procedures. In contrast, when the

---

consequence of treatment failure is loss of life or limb, aggressive therapy, often including use of a remote bypass, is usually best.

Though the term extra-anatomic is frequently used in describing arterial bypasses which traverse pathways that are not in the normal anatomic location for the artery being bypassed, the literal meaning of the term suggests a bypass outside the body. We therefore prefer the term remote to describe such bypasses. Remote bypasses have been of enormous benefit in reducing morbidity and mortality in the treatment of prosthetic graft infections; these bypasses, however, are not without their own liabilities. As a rule, they do not have as good a patency rate as bypasses in the anatomically correct position; remote bypass operations frequently take longer to perform, particularly when an infected prosthetic graft is removed during the same operation. Finally, the remote bypass itself is subject to infection. In spite of these limitations, however, remote bypasses are invaluable adjuncts in treating patients with infected prosthetic grafts.

This chapter discusses:

1. indications for remote bypasses;
2. preferred locations for the remote bypasses; and
3. choices of bypass material.

The issue of staged operations will be discussed in Chapter 14.

Discussion

Indications for Remote Bypasses

Use of autogenous tissue has been successful,[12–15] but in general, the best approach to a patient with an infected prosthetic graft includes use of a remote bypass. Exceptions to this dictum will be discussed below under each of the infectious problems reviewed. There are three situations in which in situ reconstruction seems feasible, based on a number of reports from different institutions. These are:

1. infected abdominal aortic aneurysms[16]
2. primary aortoenteric fistulae[16–18]
3. prosthetic grafts infected by *Staphylococcus epidermidis* with biofilm production.[19]

Also, some[16,20] advocate in situ replacement for secondary (communication between a prosthetic graft and the bowel) aortoenteric fistula. Though this might be a reasonable approach, remote bypass followed by complete graft removal is probably the better option, as explained below when the patient is not bleeding perceptibly when the operation begins.

Preferred Locations for Remote Bypass

The location and extent of the infection determine available options. The principles, however, are simple: the inflow must be well proximal and remote from the site of infection; the distal anastomosis should be constructed distal to and, once again, remote from the site of infection. The following options have been described; axillobifemoral grafts,[21] bilateral axillosuperficial femoral or axillopopliteal grafts,[22] axilloprofunda femoris grafts,[23] retroperitoneal aortoiliac or aortofemoral grafts,[24] supraceliac aortoiliac or aortofemoral grafts, descending thoracic aortoiliac or aortofemoral grafts,[25,26] ascending thoracic aortoiliac grafts,[27] obturator bypasses,[28,29] direct approaches to the profunda femoris artery,[23] cross-over ilioprofundal bypasses through the obturator foramen,[32] femorofemoral bypasses,[33,34] femorofemoral cross-perineal infrascrotal bypasses,[35,36] and lateral approaches to the popliteal artery.[37,38] Brief descriptions of the techniques of the obturator bypass and of the axillopopliteal are included below.

The reader is referred to each appropriate reference for technical details of performance of other bypasses.

Obturator Bypass

The obturator bypass is extremely useful in providing a clean, alternate route for infrainguinal revascularization in the presence of infection in the groin. The reader is referred to two other excellent descriptions for a more comprehensive account of the technical considerations.[39,40] As emphasized above, in discussing the general principles of remote bypass construction, inflow for the obturator bypasses must be from a proximal vessel which is uninvolved in the infectious process; in most cases this will be either the common or external iliac artery or an uninfected aortofemoral graft limb (either ipsilateral or contralateral). Occasionally, the aorta itself may be the most suitable inflow source, though this is an infrequent circumstance. We prefer to gain access to the pelvic aspect of the obturator foramen by means of an abdominal incision along the lateral border of the rectus sheath, with exposure of the pelvic vessels and the obturator internus muscle by means of an entirely extraperitoneal dissection. Through a posteromedial incision in the thigh, the intermuscular plane deep to the adductor longus muscle is entered, and blunt dissection with the fingertip along this plane enables contact with the external muscular covering of the obturator foramen, the obturator externus. Care must be taken to remain deep to the adductor longus muscle as this will prevent accidental entry into the femoral triangle and the contamination which will invariably result. From within the pelvis, an opening in the obturator membrane should be made sharply under direct vision, at a distance anteromedially from the point of entry of the obturator vessels and nerve so as to avoid injury to these structures. Because of an economy of space within the pelvic field it is best to pass the tunneling instrument from the thigh toward the pelvis meeting the surgeon's fingertip, which is positioned at the opening in the obturator membrane within the pelvis.

As is the case with all of these infectious situations, the choice of a distal anastomotic site is primarily a function of the extent of infection and the distribution of occlusive lesions. Most commonly, either the distal superficial femoral or the popliteal artery will serve as the recipient of the distal anastomosis, although the profunda femoris artery may, on occasion, serve this purpose. The choice of conduit for performing obturator bypass is a function of availability as well as of the precise location of anastomosis. For most cases, we have found externally reinforced expanded polytetrafluoroethylene (ePTFE) to be quite suitable; although for bypasses to the popliteal artery, autogenous saphenous vein may be preferable.

Axillopopliteal Bypass

The technique of axillopopliteal bypass grafting has been well described.[22,41] Nevertheless, emphasis on certain technical aspects of the performance of these procedures bears repeating. The general technical principles underlying the performance of axillofemoral bypass grafting apply to the performance of axillopoplital bypass as well. The creation of a long, oblique anastomosis to the axillary artery, as well as the avoidance of tension on this anastomosis, are essential in order to reduce the incidence of kinking, thrombosis, and false aneurysm formation. We have tended, in recent years, to favor the use of externally supported ePTFE as the graft material of choice. If at all possible, every effort should be made to use either the common femoral artery or the profunda femoris artery as the recipient of the long axillary limb in creating a sequential axillofemoral-popliteal bypass, in view of the significantly higher long-term patency of such sequential bypasses compared with that of straight axillopopliteal grafts.[22]

In the presence of significant infection in the groin precluding the creation of such a sequential bypass, the choice of the site for distal anastomosis is a function of both the localization of the infectious process and the pattern of the infrainguinal arterial occlusive disease. In such cases, the graft is tunneled along the midaxillary line, coursing lateral to the anterior superior iliac spine and along the lateral aspect of the upper thigh. If either the distal superficial femoral or the popliteal artery is to be the recipient of the bypass, the graft is gradually curved anteromedially along the distal thigh, enabling access to the normal anatomic route of the popliteal artery. If, in the event of scarring or extended infection, the standard medial approach to the popliteal artery is inaccessible, then the graft tunnel is continued along the lateral aspect of the distal thigh, allowing access to either the above or below knee segment of the popliteal artery through a lateral approach.[38] Although a direct approach to the distal profunda femoris artery in mid-thigh may be possible, we have found that groin infection often precludes this approach and risks inadvertently entering infected tissue planes.

Choices of Bypass Material

Bypass materials include autologous artery[13] or vein,[15,42] cadaver arterial allografts,[43] cryopreserved saphenous vein allogenic homografts,[44] xenografts such as a bovine graft, heterologous material such as human umbilical vein, or prosthetic graft material such as Dacron or polytetrafluoroethylene.[45] (The use of saphenous vein, however, should be avoided in the in situ position when the graft infection is caused by Gram-negative organisms.)[46]

Experimental data in dogs suggest that when prophylactic antibiotics are not used Dacron grafts better demonstrate fewer clinically evident infections induced by intravenous bolus injections of *Staphylococcus aureus* than polytetrafluoroethylene grafts.[47]

Similarly, investigative studies in dogs show a superiority of knitted and velour Dacron grafts over woven Dacron grafts when challenged with percutaneous *S aureus* 1 month after insertion.[48]

In contrast, no persuasive human clinical data exist demonstrating substantial differences among woven, knitted, velour, or ePTFE grafts in their propensity to become infected. Anecdotal clinical reports exist concerning infected and exposed ePTFE grafts healing with local treatment;[49,50] while this is only occasionally reported with Dacron.

In the future, bonding of antibiotics or bacteria-resistant surfaces to prostheses may prove beneficial.[51-55] At present, in all likelihood, choice of graft material at the primary operation should be based on patency data[56] rather than concerns about possible subsequent graft infection.

Specific Problems

Infected Hemoaccess Grafts

This is one of the few situations in which local therapy consisting of topical irrigation,[57] skin grafting,[58] or muscle flaps[59-61] can succeed. Moreover, the penalty for failure is not life threatening, but rather persistence of a local infection. Once local measures (described more fully in Chapter 12) have been deemed inadvisable or have been attempted and failed, the choices are: 1) removal of the infected portion of the graft and insertion of an entirely new graft in another location, or 2) bypass of the infected portion of the graft. If the later option is chosen, the treatment algorithm should be as follows:

1. Give preoperative antibiotics appropriate to the previously cultured organism.
2. Paint the skin around the draining infected graft with benzoin and cover the draining area with a plastic adhesive (Tegaderm®, Op Site®,

etc.) making sure it is securely adherent around the entire periphery. (Note: If the skin is intact over an erythematous area, the infection has often spread proximally or distally more than surface examination might indicate. Accordingly, incisions for the bypass should be made well away from the erythematous area if possible).

3. Prepare the skin and the adhesive overlying the draining area.

4. Make incisions proximal and distal to the infected area, expose and control the arteriovenous (AV) graft in both areas.

5. Administer heparin; clamp and divide the graft both proximal and distal to the infected area (instill 5–10 cc of a 100 unit per cc solution of heparin into the venous side of the graft). (Note: One can also insert a No. 5 French embolectomy balloon catheter with an attached stopcock and inflate this in the old graft at the level of the previous graft arterial anastomosis. This maneuver avoids the presence of a column of blood within the thrombogenic prosthetic graft while the revised graft is constructed).

6. Pass a new graft in an uncontaminated plane around the contaminated graft and construct end-to-end anastomoses at both ends.

7. Excise 1–3 cm of the remaining graft segments in both incisions and close both incisions, being sure to obliterate the subcutaneous tunnels toward the infected graft so that the revised bypass will not become contaminated when the infected graft segment is removed.

8. Close the wounds and place occlusive dressings over each of the incisions.

9. Remove the infected graft through an incision overlying the contaminated area; leave this wound open and treat with local measures until secondary wound healing is achieved.

Infected Aortic, Aortoiliac or Aortofemoral Grafts

Prosthetic Infection Involving Aortic Tube Grafts or Aortoiliac Bifurcation Grafts

These can be treated in one or two stages by remote bypass followed by aortic graft removal with careful attention to closure of the stump of the aorta. The absence of a previous groin anastomotic site simplifies management considerably.

Aortobifemoral Grafts—Infection Restricted to the Groin

When a single groin infection is seen in a patient with an aortobifemoral graft, the question arises as to whether the infection is restricted solely to the groin or whether it extends up the iliac limb to the tube portion of the graft. If a draining sinus is present, the question may be answered by a gentle sinogram. When the graft limb is thrombosed or if both groins are infected, then it is likely that the entire graft is infected. When only one groin is involved with no obvious extension above the inguinal ligament (after thorough testing with appropriate imaging and nuclear scans), then one approach would be local or topical therapy primarily using local irrigation. Results with this method have been mediocre with limited control of the infection and with occasional catastrophe. Another much better option is the use of groin debridement and coverage with a muscle flap.[59,61–68]

Remote bypasses probably have a higher success rate and perhaps an even shorter hospitalization. This consists of walling off the infected area with plastic adhesive drapes and making a suprainguinal curvilinear incision, similar to that used for kidney transplants, to expose the limb of the graft retroperitoneally at about the level of the internal iliac artery. This incision should be positioned so that if perigraft infection is found at this level the incision can be promptly closed and an axillodistal superficial femoral artery bypass can still be constructed in an uncontaminated field (as discussed in the following section on infection involving an entire aortobifemoral prosthesis). Provided the tissue surrounding the graft appears healthy and well incorporated into the graft interstices, another incision should be made in the distal thigh and an obturator bypass[28,29,69] or a lateral subcutaneous bypass,[30,31] should be constructed, bypassing the contaminated area. Proximally, the graft–graft anastomosis should be end-to-end. The site of distal anastomosis requires prior arteriographic demonstration. This may be the superficial femoral artery or sometimes the profunda femoris artery or popliteal artery distally. The divided distal end of the original graft is trimmed and oversewn and healthy autogenous tissue is closed over this stump, separating it from the newly constructed bypass. All incisions are then carefully closed in multiple layers using running sutures of synthetic absorbable suture and occlusive dressings are applied. A groin incision can then be made to remove the infected graft completely, including the recently oversewn covered stump. Any infected tissue is debrided, the femoral arteriotomy site oversewn, and the wound is left open and drained. If the iliac portion of the graft was not involved with infection and care was exercised in all of the steps outlined, relatively prompt and uncomplicated wound healing should be anticipated.

Prosthetic Infection Involving Suprainguinal Portions of Aortofemoral Bifurcation Grafts

The diagnosis of infection restricted to the suprainguinal portion of an aortobifem-

oral graft is often difficult. When the diagnosis is certain, bilateral groin incisions can be used. If no infection is found, then an axillobifemoral bypass can be connected end-to end to the short distal stumps of the previously inserted graft. The proximal limbs of the old aortobifemoral graft are then trimmed, oversewn, tucked beneath the inguinal ligament into the suprainguinal area, and covered with autogenous tissue. All wounds are closed. Several days later, the infected graft can be removed through a midline incision. The extent of the lower incision should be limited to avoid contaminating the femorofemoral portion of the newly inserted axillobifemoral graft. Great care is required when closing and reinforcing the aorta to prevent aortic stump disruption.

When the diagnosis of an infected graft cannot be made preoperatively, abdominal exploration may be necessary. The diagnosis is then confirmed by direct inspection of the graft, the area of infection is irrigated thoroughly, and the incision is closed without abdominal or wound drains. High doses of appropriate systemic antibiotics should be administered and all instruments, gowns, gloves, and drapes changed. An axillobifemoral graft is promptly constructed. Several days later, the abdominal incision can be reopened and the graft removed as previously outlined.

Allographs or autogenous tissue grafts are useful alternatives in contaminated fields.[13–15,28,42–44] Difficulties in obtaining adequate size and length of autogenous material and the incidence of later thrombotic complications,[14] however, probably make remote bypassing with prosthetic material the preferred procedure when feasible. Nevertheless, autogenous tissue reconstruction fulfills the goals of reducing recurrent infection, preventing prolonged distal ischemia, and preventing aortic stump disruption. This technique can be used when remote bypassing seems difficult or contraindicated.

Prosthetic Infection Involving the Tube Portion and One Groin in an Aortobifemoral Graft

When the prosthetic limb to the infected groin is thrombosed and that distal extremity is viable, one approach that can be used is a contralateral axillofemoral bypass followed by complete removal of the infected bifurcation graft. When both prosthetic limbs are patent, however, a useful treatment plan is a unilateral axillofemoral bypass on the uninfected side opposite the groin infection (the groin incision should be made first to confirm absence of apparent infection on that side), closure of the incisions, and application of occlusive dressings. The prosthetic limb to the infected groin should then be ligated. If collateral circulation is adequate and no distal limb ischemia occurs, the operation should be terminated. Several days later, the entire aortic bifurcation prosthesis should be removed. If the distal extremity becomes ischemic with ligation of the involved prosthetic limb, all gowns and instruments should be changed, the patient should be prepared and draped, and an immediate revascularization procedure performed. Options for this procedure include: 1) a remote ipsilateral axillary distal superficial femoral or popliteal artery bypass,[70,71] or 2) an autogenous femorofemoral bypass from the previously inserted contralateral axillofemoral bypass to the femoral artery on the infected side.[13,14] Several days later, the entire aortic bifurcation prosthesis can then be removed.

Prosthetic Infection Involving an Entire Aortobifemoral Graft

In this case, the choice is an autogenous bypass[13,14] or bilateral axillary distal superficial femoral or popliteal bypass.[22,23] Though bilateral axillary popliteal bypasses may seem quite tenuous in this setting, results with these procedures are not dismal.[71] In the presence of severe distal occlusive dis-

ease, an autogenous bypass is probably preferable. Otherwise, bilateral axillary popliteal bypasses should be considered for the period needed to clear the infection. Then another more direct bypass could be inserted if necessary.[72]

Though many authors have described that techniques other than remote bypass can be successful, careful review of collected reports consistently reveal the overall advantages of remote bypasses. Two caveats exist: 1) the remote bypass must be constructed *before* the infected graft is removed since the major advantage of remote bypass is that prolonged ischemia is avoided but this is achieved only if the remote bypass precedes removal of the infected graft, and 2) in cases of graft-enteric communications the rate of hemorrhage must not be so great that time is not available for construction of a remote bypass.

Nothing is more frustrating for surgeons nor more dangerous for patients than for an unanticipated event to foreclose important options. Satisfactory results in the management of graft infections is greatly enhanced by thorough familiarity with the various combinations and permutations of treatment options. Equally important in such instances is the need to formulate specific diagnostic and management algorithms for rational treatment. Contaminated prosthetic graft problems are too complex and the consequences of poor decision making are too severe to justify any but the most reasoned and careful approaches. Good to excellent results can be achieved with meticulous planning and well-executed operations.

References

1. Nielsen OM, Noer HH, Jorgensen LG, Lorentzen JE. Gentamycin beads in the treatment of localized vascular graft infection: long-term results in 17 cases. *Eur J Vasc Surg.* 1991; 5:283–285.
2. Quick CR, Vassallo DJ, Colin JF, Heddle RM. Conservative treatment of major aortic graft infection. *Eur J Vasc Surg.* 1990;4:63–67.

3. Kwaan JH, Connolly JE. Successful management of prosthetic graft infection with continuous povidone-iodine irrigation. *Arch Surg.* 1981;116:716–720.

4. Popovsky J, Singer S. Infected prosthetic grafts: local therapy with graft preservation. *Arch Surg.* 1980;115:203–205.

5. Francois F, Thevenet A. Conservative treatment of prosthetic aortic graft infection with irrigation. *Ann Vasc Surg.* 1991;5:199–201.

6. Calligaro KD, Veith FJ, Schwartz ML, Savarese RP, DeLaurentis DA. Are Gram-negative bacteria a contraindication to selective preservation of infected prosthetic arterial grafts? *J Vasc Surg.* 1992;16:337–345.

7. Moran KT, Jewell ER. Local antiseptic treatment of infected prosthetic vascular grafts in the groin. *Br J Surg.* 1988;75:1037–1038.

8. Knight CD Jr, Farnell MB, Hollier LH. Treatment of aortic graft infection with povidone-iodine irrigation. *Mayo Clin Proc.* 1983;58:472–475.

9. Bunt TJ. Synthetic vascular graft infections I: graft infections. *Surgery.* 1983;93:733–746.

10. Bunt TJ. Synthetic vascular graft infections II: graft enteric erosions and graft enteric fistulas. *Surgery.* 1983;94:1–9.

11. Trout HH III, Kozloff L, Giordano JM. Priority of revascularization in patients with graft enteric fistulas, infected arteries, or infected arterial prostheses. *Ann Surg.* 1984;199:669–683.

12. Nevelsteen A, Suy R. Autogenous venous reconstruction in the treatment of aortobifemoral prosthetic infection. *J Cardiovasc Surg (Torino).* 1988;29:315–317.

13. Ehrenfeld WK, Wilbur BG, Olcott CN, Stoney RJ. Autogenous tissue reconstruction in the management of infected prosthetic grafts. *Surgery.* 1979;85:82–92.

14. Seeger JM, Wheeler JR, Gregory RT, Snyder SO, Gayle RG. Autogenous graft replacement of infected prosthetic grafts in the femoral position. *Surgery.* 1983;93:39–45.

15. Lorentzen JE, Nielsen OM. Aortobifemoral bypass with autogenous saphenous vein in treatment of paninfected aortic bifurcation graft. *J Vasc Surg.* 1986;3:666–668.

16. Robinson JA, Johansen K. Aortic sepsis: is there a role for in situ graft reconstruction? *J Vasc Surg.* 1991;13:677–682.

17. Daugherty M, Shearer GR, Ernst CB. Primary aortoduodenal fistula: extra-anatomic vascular reconstruction not required for successful management. *Surgery.* 1979;86:399–401.

18. Pfeiffer RB Jr. Successful repair of three primary aortoduodenal fistulae. *Arch Surg.* 1982;117:1098–1099.

19. Bandyk DF, Bergamini TM, Kinney EV, Seabrook GR, Towne JB. In situ replacement of vascular prostheses infected by bacterial biofilms. *J Vasc Surg.* 1991;13:575–583.

20. Walker WE, Cooley DA, Duncan JM, Hallman GL Jr, Ott DA, Reul GJ. The management of aortoduodenal fistula by in situ replacement of the infected abdominal aortic graft. *Ann Surg.* 1987;205:727–732.

21. Harris EJ Jr, Taylor LM Jr, McConnell DB, Moneta GL, Yeager RA, Porter JM. Clinical results of axillobifemoral bypass using externally supported polytetrafluoroethylene. *J Vasc Surg.* 1990;12:416–420.

22. Ascer E, Veith FJ, Gupta S. Axillopopliteal bypass grafting: Indications, late results, and determinants of long-term patency. *J Vasc Surg.* 1989;10:285–291.

23. Nunez AA, Veith FJ, Collier P, Ascer E, Flores SW, Gupta SK. Direct approaches to the distal portions of the deep femoral artery for limb salvage bypasses. *J Vasc Surg.* 1988;8:576–581.

24. Peck JJ, McReynolds DG, Baker DH, Eastman AB. Extraperitoneal approach for aortoiliac reconstruction of the abdominal aorta. *Am J Surg.* 1986;151:620–623.

25. Constantino MJ. Recurrent aortic graft infection following descending thoracic aorta to femoral artery bypass: a case report and review. *J Cardiovasc Surg (Torino).* 1991;32:477–481.

26. Criado E, Johnson G Jr, Burnham SJ, Buehrer J, Keagy BA. Descending thoracic aorta-to-iliofemoral artery bypass as an alternative to aortoiliac reconstruction. *J Vasc Surg.* 1992;15:550–557.

27. Yared SF, Masri ZH, Melo JC, Lansing AM, Norman JC. A unique inlet (the ascending aorta) for extra-anatomic bypass of infected arterial prostheses. *J KY Med Assoc.* 1991;89:274–276.

28. Panetta T, Sottiurai VS, Batson RC. Obturator bypass with nonreversed translocated saphenous vein. *Ann Vasc Surg.* 1989;3:56–62.

29. Erath HG Jr, Gale SS, Smith BM, Dean RH. Obturator foramen grafts: the preferable alternate route? *Am Surg.* 1982;48:65–69.

30. Leather RP, Karmody AM. A lateral route for extra-anatomical bypass of the femoral artery. *Surgery.* 1977;81:307–309.

31. Trout HH III, Smith CA. Lateral iliopopliteal arterial bypass as an alternative to obturator bypass. *Am Surg.* 1982;48:63–64.

32. Atnip RG. Cross-over ilioprofunda reconstruction: an expanded role for obturator foramen bypass. *Surgery.* 1991;110:106–108.

33. Ricco JB. Unilateral iliac artery occlusive dis-

ease: a randomized multicenter trial examining direct revascularization versus crossover bypass. Association Universitaire de Recherche en Chirurgie. *Ann Vasc Surg.* 1992; 6:209–219.

34. Sanchez LA, Gupta SK, Veith FJ, et al. A 10-year experience with 150 failing or threatened vein and polytetrafluoroethylene arterial bypass grafts. *J Vasc Surg.* 1991;14: 729–736.

35. Johnson HA, Mehrez IO, Vittimberga F, Kasparian A, Bartlett F. Femorofemoral crossperineal infrascrotal bypass. *Ann Vasc Surg.* 1988;2:425.

36. Lawrence PF, Albo D Jr. Femorofemoral bypass with an infrascrotal perineal approach for the patient with an infected groin wound. *J Vasc Surg.* 1985;2:485–487.

37. Padberg FT Jr. Lateral approach to the popliteal artery. *Ann Vasc Surg.* 1988;2:397–401.

38. Veith FJ, Ascer E, Gupta SK, Wengerter KR. Lateral approach to the popliteal artery. *J Vasc Surg.* 1987;6:119–123.

39. DePalma RG. Obturator foramen bypass grafts in groin sepsis. In: Ernst CB, Stanley JC, eds. *Current Therapy in Vascular Surgery.* Toronto: Decker; 1991;353–356.

40. Schwartz RA, Baue AE. Bypass grafts using the obturator foramen. In: Haimovicie H, ed. *Vascular Surgery: Principles and Techniques.* Norwalk: Appleton & Lange; 1989;539–545.

41. Keller MP, Hoch JR, Harding AD, Nichols WK, Silver D. Axillopopliteal bypass for limb salvage. *J Vasc Surg.* 1992;15:817–822.

42. Cimochowski GE, Rutherford WE, Blondin J, Harter H. Use of the spiral vein graft as an arterial substitute for secondary access. *Am J Nephrol.* 1991;11:64–66.

43. Bahnini A, Ruotolo C, Koskas F, Kieffer E. In situ fresh allograft replacement of an infected aortic prosthetic graft: 18-month follow-up. *J Vasc Surg.* 1991;14:98–102.

44. Fujitani RM, Bassiouny HS, Gewertz BL, Glagov, Zarins CK. Cryopreserved saphenous vein allogenic homografts: an alternative conduit in lower extremity arterial reconstruction in infected fields. *J Vasc Surg.* 1992;15:519– 526.

45. Feliciano DV, Mattox KL, Graham JM, Bitondo CG. Five-year experience with PTFE grafts in vascular wounds. *J Trauma.* 1985;25: 71–82.

46. Ouriel K, Geary KJ, Green RM, DeWeese JA. Fate of the exposed saphenous vein graft. *Am J Surg.* 1990;160:148–150.

47. Moore WS, Malone JM, Keown K. Prosthetic arterial graft material: influence on neointimal healing and bacteremic infectibility. *Arch Surg.* 1980;115:1379–1183.

48. Weber TR, Lindenauer SM, Miller TA, Salles CA, Ramsburgh S. Focal infection of aortofemoral prostheses. *Surgery.* 1976;79: 310–312.

49. Butler HG III, Baker LD Jr, Johnson JM. Vascular access for chronic hemodialysis: polytetrafluoroethylene (PTFE) versus bovine heterograft. *Am J Surg.* 1977;134:791–793.

50. Tellis VA, Kohlberg WI, Bhat DJ, Driscoll B, Veith FJ. Expanded polytetrafluoroethylene graft fistula for chronic hemodialysis. *Ann Surg.* 1979;189:101–105.

51. Chervu A, Moore WS, Chvapil M, Henderson T. Efficacy and duration of antistaphylococcal activity comparing three antibiotics bonded to Dacron vascular grafts with a collagen release system. *J Vasc Surg.* 1991;13: 897–901.

52. Greco RS. Utilizing vascular prostheses for drug delivery. *J Vasc Surg.* 1991;13:753–755.

53. Shue WB, Worosilo SC, Donetz AP, Trooskin SZ, Harvey RA, Greco RS. Prevention of vascular prosthetic infection with an antibiotic-bonded Dacron graft. *J Vasc Surg.* 1988;8: 600–605.

54. Chervu A, Moore WS, Gelabert HA, Colburn MD, Chvapil M. Prevention of graft infection by use of prostheses bonded with a rifampin-collagen release system. *J Vasc Surg.* 1991;14: 521–524.

55. Haverich A, Hirt S, Karck M, Siclari F, Wahlig H. Prevention of graft infection by bonding of gentamycin to Dacron prostheses. *J Vasc Surg.* 1992;15:187–193.

56. Pevec WC, Darling RC, L'Italien GJ, Abbott WM. Femoropopliteal reconstruction with knitted, nonvelour Dacron versus expanded polytetrafluoroethylene. *J Vasc Surg.* 1992;16: 60–65.

57. Bhat DJ, Tellis VA, Kohlberg WI, Driscoll B, Veith FJ. Management of sepsis involving expanded polytetrafluoroethylene grafts for hemodialysis access. *Surgery.* 1980;87:445–450.

58. Tellis VA, Weiss P, Matas AJ, Veith FJ. Skin-flap coverage of polytetrafluoroethylene vascular access graft exposed by previous infection. *Surgery.* 1988;103:118–121.

59. Perler BA, Vander Kolk CA, Dufresne CR, Williams GM. Can infected prosthetic grafts be salvaged with rotational muscle flaps? *Surgery.* 1991;110:30–34.

60. Budny PJ, Fix RJ. Salvage of prosthetic grafts and joints in the lower extremity. *Clin Plast Surg.* 1991;18:583–591.

61. Mixter RC, Turnipseed WD, Smith DJ Jr, Acher CW, Rao VK, Dibbell DG. Rotational muscle flaps: a new technique for covering

infected vascular grafts. *J Vasc Surg.* 1989;9:
472–478.

62. Dougherty M, Shearer GR, Ernst CB. Primary aortoduodenal fistula: extra-anatomic vascular reconstruction not required for successful management. *Surgery.* 1979;86: 399–401.

63. Goldsmith HS, de los Santos R, Beattie EJ, Vanamee P. Experimental protection of vascular prosthesis by omentum. *Arch Surg.* 1968;97:8872–8888.

64. Fry WJ, Lindenauer SM. Infection complicating the use of plastic arterial implants. *Arch Surg.* 1967;94:600–609.

65. Roy A, Hayes DF. Closure of an aortic stump. *Am J Surg.* 1983;145:403–404.

66. Shah DM, Buchbinder D, Leather RP, Corson J, Karmody AM. Clinical use of the seromuscular jejunal patch for protection of the infected aortic stump. *Am J Surg.* 1983;146: 198–202.

67. Reilly LM, Ehrenfeld WK, Goldstone J, Stoney RJ. Gastrointestinal tract involvement by prosthetic graft infection. *Ann Surg.* 1985;202:342–348.

68. Laustsen J, Bille S, Christensen J. Transposition of the sartorius muscle in the treatment of infected vascular grafts in the groin. *Eur J Vasc Surg.* 1988;2:111–113.

69. Pearce WH, Ricco JB, Yao JS, Flinn WR, Bergan JJ. Modified technique of obturator bypass in failed or infected grafts. *Ann Surg.* 1983;197:344–347.

70. Kwaan JHM, Connolly JE. Extended axillopopliteal-axillotibial bypass: valuable adjunct to limb revascularization. *Arch Surg.* 1983; 118:25–28.

71. Gupta SK, Veith FJ, Ascer E, et al. Five-year experience with axillopopliteal bypasses for limb salvage. *J Cardiovasc Surg.* 1985;26: 321–324.

72. Reilly LM, Ehrenfeld WK, Stoney RJ. Delayed aortic prosthetic reconstruction after removal of an infected graft. *Am J Surg.* 1984; 148:234–239.

Chapter 17

The Neoaortic Iliac System Operation for Infected Aortic Prostheses

G.P. Clagett

Introduction

The most commonly used treatment for the dreaded complication of aortic prosthetic infection is extra-anatomic bypass coupled with removal of the aortic prosthesis. In data pooled from major series reported since 1980, the overall mortality with this approach is 19.2% (95% CI, 14.6% to 23.8%) and the amputation rate is 13.6% (95% CI, 8.1% to 19.1%).[1–13] Furthermore, in analyzing variations on this approach, the mortality and morbidity remain at high levels whether or not prosthesis excision precedes or follows extra-anatomic bypass or whether these operations are staged or performed together. Despite the lack of clear-cut differences in major outcomes, most experts prefer the staged approach with extra-anatomic bypass preceding removal of the infected prosthesis by 2 to 3 days.[3]

In addition to high mortality and morbidity, extra-anatomic bypass and aortic prosthesis removal are subject to the infection of the new extra-anatomic prosthesis and aortic stump blowout. In pooled data from contemporary reports, the incidence of infection of the extra-anatomic prosthesis is 15.6% (95% CI, 10.0% to 21.2%) and the incidence of fatal aortic stump blowout is 8.5% (95% CI, 5.4% to 11.6%).[1–7,11,13,14] An alternative approach recently reported is that of in situ replacement of infected aortic prostheses with venous and aortic homografts.[15,16] However, even with this approach recurrent infection and fatal homograft rupture have occurred and late deterioration may be expected.

One of the most disappointing features of extra-anatomic bypass is the high rate of acute thrombosis. In our experience this is often sudden, catastrophic, and leads to major amputation. This often occurs in patients with extensive multilevel vascular disease who have complex extra-anatomic bypasses such as axillary unilateral profunda or popliteal bypasses. In one recently reported large series of patients with extra-anatomic bypasses for aortic prosthetic infection, the primary patency was 43% at 3 years with one third of all survivors coming to major amputation.[6]

Dissatisfaction with extra-anatomic prosthetic bypass has led us to develop an in situ autologous reconstruction from venous autografts. We term this a neoaortoiliac system (NAIS). Ehrenfeld et al. originally advocated the autogenous approach and reported reconstructing the aortoiliac system by endarterectomizing occluded aortoiliac segments combined with arterial and venous autografts.[17] Our approach differs in that the NAIS is fashioned exclusively from superficial and deep lower extremity veins.

The Neoaortic Iliac System Operation

Successful NAIS reconstruction depends on large caliber venous autografts. We use duplex ultrasonography preoperatively to assess the size of lower extremity greater saphenous veins (GSV) and the superficial femoral-popliteal systems or deep veins (DV). As experience has accrued, it is apparent that only large GSVs which are at least 8 millimeters in diameter perform satisfactorily in this position. Smaller GSVs are prone to the development of focal stenoses and diffuse neointimal hyperplasia (see experience detailed below). This has led to the need for multiple revisions and replacement procedures. In contrast, DVs maintain excellent patency and, in our experience to date, none have developed focal stenoses or intimal hyperplasia. In some NAIS reconstructions, GSV and DV segments have been used; in such cases, an effort is made to preserve one or the other in each lower extremity to prevent limb edema.

The operation begins with vein harvest and this is considered a *clean* portion of the procedure. Groin sinuses and infected wounds are excluded from the field by placement of adherent, iodine-impregnated plastic sheets (Ioban®) over grossly infected areas. The operative time can be reduced to

under 5 hours using a two-team approach with one team harvesting veins while the other removes the infected prosthesis. With the two-team approach, cross-contamination of the vein harvest wounds is minimized by using separate surgical instruments and scrub teams.

To harvest DV autografts, the lateral border of the sartorius is exposed from the upper thigh (below the infected groin wounds, if present) to the knee. The sartorius muscle is mobilized along its lateral border and reflected medially in order to preserve its blood supply which enters the muscle belly from its inferomedial aspect. Care is also taken to preserve the saphenous nerve, major collateral branches of the superficial femoral and popliteal arteries, and the greater saphenous vein. The adductor canal is opened by incising the tendon of the adductor magnus muscle and multiple branches of the superficial femoral-popliteal vein are carefully ligated and divided; large branches are doubly ligated or suture ligated. A key feature in preventing excessive venous hypertension is to preserve the profunda femoris vein. The junction of the profunda femoris and the common femoral vein is identified, and the proximal superficial femoral vein is transected and oversewn flush with this junction. Distally, the popliteal vein is mobilized until a length adequate for NAIS reconstruction is achieved. This most often requires mobilization to the knee joint or just below.

Venous autografts are distended with chilled whole blood or a cold solution consisting of Ringer's lactate (1 liter), heparin (5000 units), albumin (25 gm), and papaverine (60 mg) and venous valves are fractured by retrograde passage of a Mills-Leather valvulotome. Autografts are stored in these solutions and kept at 40° C, until they are required for NAIS reconstruction. Vein harvest incisions are liberally irrigated with solutions containing antibiotics and closed completely.

All infected prosthetic material is removed and the aorta and periaortic tissues

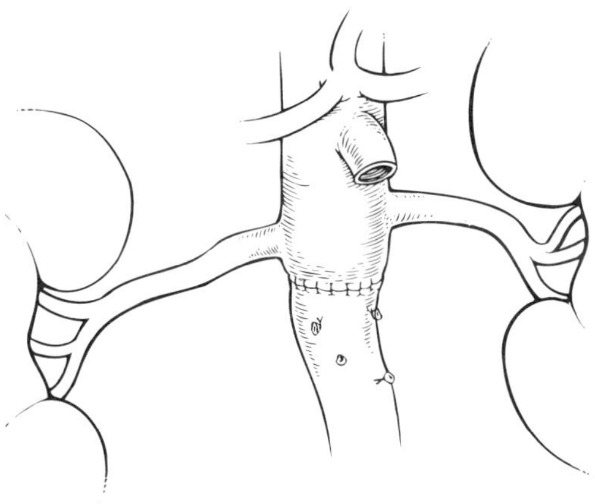

Figure 1. A neoaortoiliac system proximal anastomosis. A deep vein autogaft sewn end-to-end to the infrarenal aorta.

are liberally debrided in order to achieve a a clean proximal anatomotic site and bed for the venous autograft. Aortic debridement is often facilitated by suprarenal aortic control either by intraluminal balloon or cross-clamp. Our preferred proximal anastomotic technique involves simply suturing the DV autograft end-to-end to the aorta (Fig. 1). The proximal end of the DV autograft is the largest and this is usually selected for anastomosis. We have also used conjoined GSVs sewn together in a pantaloon configuration and anastomosed end-to-end to the aorta or end-to-side to the anterior aorta after oversewing the aortic stump. However, conjoined GSV autografts at the proximal anastomosis are prone to kinks and other unfavorable hemodynamic conditions which, in our experience predispose to failure. We no longer anastomose GSVs to the aorta and rely solely on sewing the DV autograft end-to-end to the aorta. Standard, continuous polypropylene (4–0) suture technique is used, with care being taken to make slightly more advancement on the aorta than the venous autograft because of the greater circumference of the aorta. Because of the close size match usually found between the proximal DV autograft and the aorta, undue advancement and other techniques to com-

pensate for size discrepancy are usually unnecessary to achieve a comfortable anastomosis.

Infected femoral wounds are then opened, debrided, and all prosthetic material is removed from below. The retroperitoneal tunnels are irrigated with antibacterial solution and mechanically debrided by pulling opened gauze sponges through them. Venous autografts are brought through the old tunnels and anastomosed to the femoral vessels.

Preferred configurations for NAIS reconstructions are illustrated in Figures 2 and 3. In Figure 2, a DV autograft is sutured to the proximal aorta and to the left femoral artery with a femoral cross-over bypass

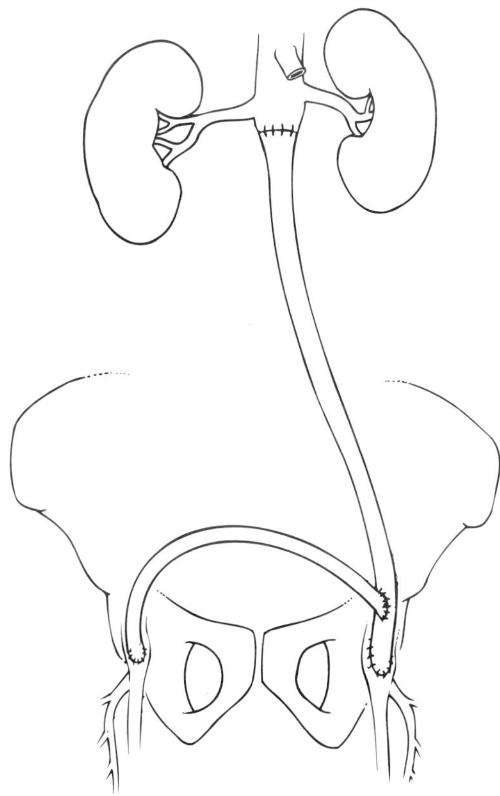

Figure 2. A neoaortoiliac system reconstruction: unilateral aortofemoral bypass fashioned with a deep vein autograft and a femoral cross-over bypass constructed from deep vein or greater saphenous vein.

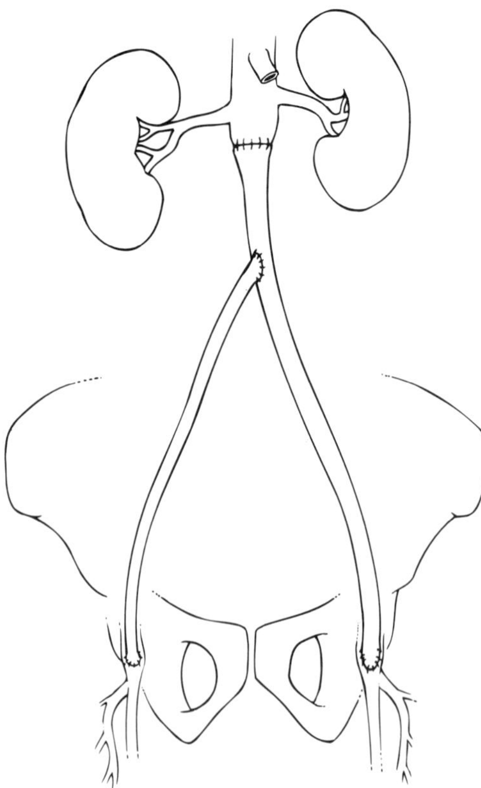

Figure 3. A neoaortoiliac system reconstruction: left aortofemoral bypass from DV autograft and right femoral limb (either deep vein or greater saphenous vein) anastomosed end-to-side to the proximal deep vein graft.

fashioned from DV or GSV (if of adequate caliber). The other configuration is similar except that the right femoral limb, constructed of either GSV or DV, is sewn end-to-side to the proximal DV autograft. These limbs are placed in the tunnels remaining after removal of the infected prosthesis.

At the completion of NAIS reconstruction, the subcutaneum of the femoral wounds is closed over the venous autografts and the skin left open. It has not been necessary to cover the venous autografts with muscle flaps. Drainage is rarely used and antibiotics are discontinued within 5 to 7 days postoperatively. Intermittent pneumatic compression stockings and low-dose heparin prophylaxis have been liberally used, especially in patients in whom DV autografts are harvested. Long-term anticoagulation is not used.

Experience

Our 5-year experience with the NAIS procedure has been detailed in a recent publication.[18] Twenty-one patients have undergone this operation at the University of Texas Southwestern Medical Center. Eighteen patients underwent NAIS reconstruction because of aortic prosthetic infection (16 infected aortofemoral bypasses (AFBs), 1 aortoenteric erosion, and 1 aortoenteric fistula). Sixteen patients had paninfected AFBs or aortoiliac prostheses with pus surrounding the body and limbs of the prostheses, and 2 patients had single AFB limb involvement. Most patients had the original aortic operation performed for occlusive disease. The mean interval between the original aortic operation and diagnosis of prosthetic infection was 68 ± 54 months (range: 4–192 months) and modes of presentation included femoral abscesses, chronic draining groin sinuses, infected femoral anastomotic aneurysms, fever, anemia and gastrointestinal bleeding. Almost all patients complained of malaise and chronic fatigue. Risk factors for prosthetic infection included multiple femoral reoperations after initial aortic procedure (mean = 3 ± 2, range: 0–10) usually for anastomotic aneurysms, limb thromboses, or wound complications.

Before undertaking NAIS reconstruction, at least half of these patients had failure of more conservative, local procedures. These included excision of single AFB limb with an extra-anatomic bypass (obturator bypass, axillofemoral bypass, and axillopopliteal bypass), continuous irrigation with antibiotic solution coupled with multiple debridements, muscle flap coverage, and debridement with in situ limb replacement with expanded polytetrafluoroethylene (ePTFE). One patient had infection of a prosthetic secondary AFB 1 year after removal of an infected primary AFB and placement of an axillobifemoral bypass that failed because of multiple, recurrent thromboses. All of these patients were treated with prolonged oral or parenteral antibiotics and had healing before developing signs of recurrent, more extensive infections. Organisms cultured from excised prosthetic material or pus surrounding prostheses are tabulated in Table 1. Consistent with other contemporary reports, Gram-positive organisms, especially *Staphylococcus epidermidis*, predominated; however, there were also Gram-negative prosthetic infections that included *Pseudomonas aeruginosa* and *Proteus mirabilis.*

Veins harvested for NAIS reconstruction included bilateral GSV (n = 7 patients), bilateral DV (n = 3 patients), GSV and DV from opposite limbs (n = 3 patients), and single limb DV (n = 8 patients). The mean operative time was 6.5 ± 1.8 hours (range 4.5–10 hours) and intraoperative blood transfusion requirement was 4 ± 3 units (range 0–9 units) with additional fluid (Ringer's lactate and colloid) requirement being 7 ± 2 liters. Suprarenal aortic control was required in 4 patients.

There were no immediate operative deaths; however, 2 patients died at prolonged intervals (28 days and 35 days after operation) from peritonitis, sepsis, and multisystem organ dysfunction. There were also 2 amputations in survivors for an overall mortality and amputation rate of 10%. Other major morbidity included severe gastrointestinal complications in 4 patients and a single case of deep vein thrombosis and pulmonary embolus that came from the side of DV harvest. The 4 cases of peritonitis were of interest because they demonstrated the ability of these vein grafts to resist infection. Peritonitis developed in these patients from a perforated duodenal diverticulum with pancreatitis, ischemic small bowel necrosis, acute cholecystitis, and gangrene of the gallbladder. Three of these patients had diffuse peritonitis with DV autografts being bathed in polymicrobial pus. Vein grafts were inspected when these patients were reexplored on multiple occasions and NAIS vein grafts and anastomoses remained intact and uninfected.

The mean follow-up time has been approximately 2 years (range 3–60 months) and there has been one death from myocardial infarction in a patient who also required a below-knee amputation for progression of distal disease. An interesting finding was the difference of behavior between GSV and DV autografts. Three patients with GSV NAIS developed total occlusion within 1 year from progressive diffuse, neointimal hyperplasia documented by angiography and biopsy at reexploration. One of these patients underwent secondary prosthetic AFB and the remaining two had noncritical lower extremity ischemia with severe claudication but desired no further intervention. Four patients developed focal stenoses in GSV autografts (Figure 4) and three required reoperation with patch angioplasty or femoral crossover limb replacement. Small saphenous veins were particularly prone to failure. However, large saphenous veins had sustained patency. Focal stenoses were likely to develop at areas of kinking and at valve

Table 1
Bacteriology of Infected Aortic Prostheses
Corrected with NAIS Reconstruction

Organism	No. of Pts.
S epidermidis	7
S aureus	4
Pseudomonas aeruginosa	2
β hemolytic Streptococcus	1
Enterobacter aerogenes	1
Bacteroides bivius	1
Proteus mirabilis	1
Propionibacterium acnes	1
Candida albicans	1
Multiple organisms	4
No growth	4

S = Staphylococcus.

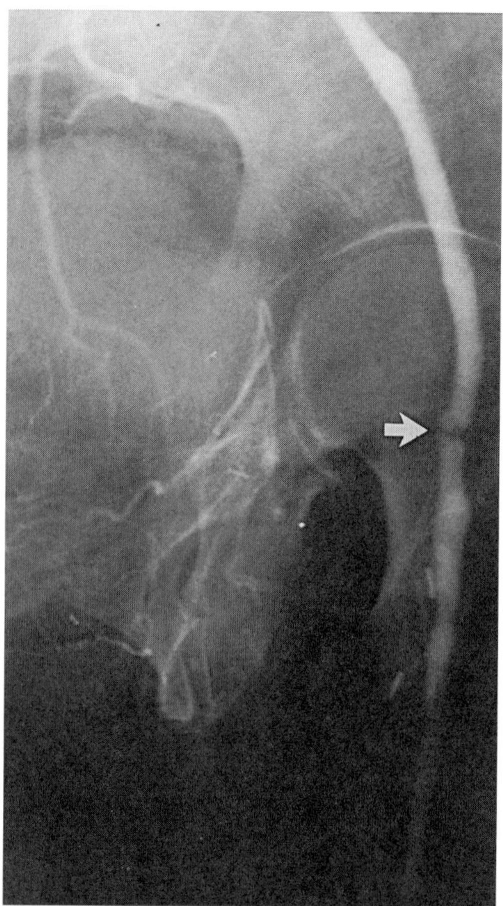

Figure 4. Focal stenosis that developed 3 months after a neoaortoiliac system procedure in a patient who developed left lower extremity intermittent claudication and a falling left ankle pressure index. The patient underwent reexploration and a vein patch angioplasty of the stenotic area which proved to be a neointimal hyperplasia at a venous valve site.

deterioration has not occurred. The overall failure rate (defined as occlusion or stenosis requiring reintervention) of GSV NAIS was 64% in comparison to 0% for DV NAIS ($P = 0.01$). Of the 14 patients who had unilateral or bilateral DV harvest, only 2 have had significant chronic limb edema requiring compression stockings. One was the patient who had ipsilateral venous thrombosis who presumably had valvular injury and the other patient had the ipsilateral GSV used for a distal bypass.

Because of the propensity of GSV autografts used for NAIS reconstructions to de-

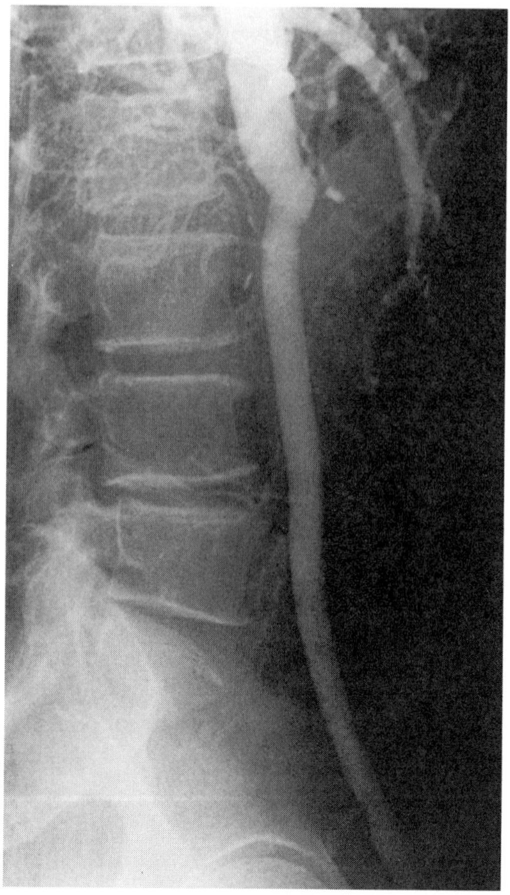

Figure 5. Lateral view of a neoaortoiliac system reconstruction using a deep vein anastomosed end-to-end to the aorta. Note the good size match between the native aorta and the deep vein autograft.

sites, and aortic anastomoses with GSV were also prone to develop problems. All failures were apparent within the first year and were manifested by falling ankle pressure indices, changes on duplex surveillance, and onset of intermittent claudication. Despite the high failure rate of GSVs, no amputations have been required.

In contrast, all NAIS from larger caliber DV autografts have remained patent and nonstenotic Figures 5 and 6. Aneurysmal

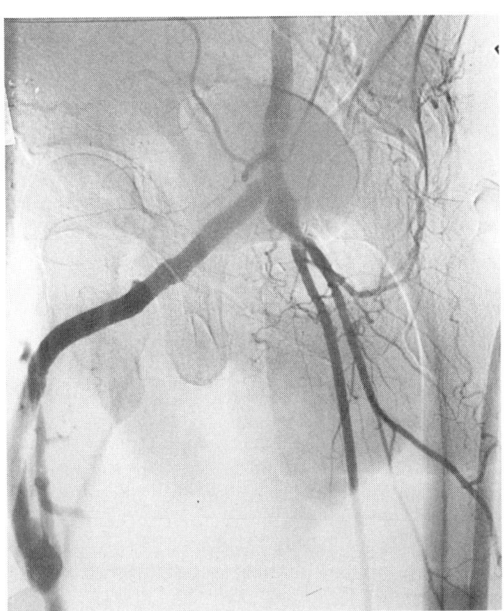

Figure 6. Oblique view of the distal portion of a neoaortoiliac system reconstruction. Deep vein autografts were used to fashion a left aortofemoral bypass and a femoral cross-over bypass to the midright superficial femoral artery.

velop diffuse intimal hyperplasia and focal stenoses, it is important to monitor these vein grafts with frequent duplex ultrasound examinations and clinical assessment, especially in the first year after placement. Focal stenoses can be corrected by timely reoperation. In spite of this limitation, GSV NAIS occlusion is more gradual than the sudden thrombotic occlusion experienced by patients with extra-anatomic prosthetic bypasses who, in our experience, frequently present with profound, irreversible limb ischemia. The slowly progressive occlusion in our patients with GSV NAIS reconstructions has allowed for early detection, intervention, and, possibly, development of collateral circulation.

We currently favor DV autografts for NAIS reconstructions and use GSV grafts only if they are large ($\geq$ 8 mm in diameter). We have not observed focal or diffuse intimal hyperplasia in DV or large GSV autografts. The superficial femoral-popliteal vein has a diameter of 1.0–1.5 cm and this allows end-to-end anastomosis to a normal caliber aorta with relative ease. Another advantage of the DV autograft is that minor kinks and areas of intimal hyperplasia at valve sites do not produce hemodynamic disturbances and compromise flow to the degree that similar size defects would produce in smaller caliber GSV grafts. A potential problem with the DV autograft is the possibility of development of mural thromboembolism. Shulman reported that DV autografts greater than 1.2 cm in diameter used for femoropopliteal bypass were particularly prone to failure because of this problem.[19] We have not observed this and predict that it will not occur because of the better size match between the aortoiliac femoral system and DV autografts.

The absence of significant limb edema has been gratifying. This has also been the experience of others who have used the DV autograft for femoral-popliteal and other peripheral grafts. Schanzer et al. reported a mild but persistent calf enlargement along with a pattern on strain-gauge plethysmography indicative of venous outflow obstruction in the majority of patients who had DV harvest or femoropopliteal bypass.[20] Despite these observations, clinically significant edema requiring compression stockings was rare and there was no functional disability in these patients. This is in agreement with the findings of Masuda et al. who studied the long-term hemodynamic and clinical outcomes in patients who had ligation of the superficial femoral vein.[21] These investigators concluded that there was no correlation between physiologic obstruction of this vein and the clinical status of the patient, and that obstruction is well tolerated when the profunda femoris and ipsilateral GSV are intact. Although Shulman et al. did not find significant edema in limbs from which both GSV and DVs were removed, we would caution against this. We also feel that preservation of the profunda femoris vein is critical in preserving sufficient venous collateral flow to prevent excessive venous hypertension.

Conclusions

We conclude that venous autografts resist infection in this position and that relatively small GSVs are prone to failure from the development of focal stenoses and intimal hyperplasia. In contrast, DVs perform well, anastomose comfortably with the proximal aorta, and have sustained patency. Furthermore, DV harvest is well tolerated with no functional disability and minimal problems with limb edema as long as the profunda to common femoral venous junction remains intact and the ipsilateral GSV is preserved. Finally, we believe that NAIS reconstruction is a successful option in patients with aortic prosthetic infections.

References

1. Bacourt F, Koskas F. French University Association for Research in Surgery. Axillobifemoral bypass and aortic exclusion for vascular septic lesions: a multicenter retrospective study of 98 cases. *Ann Vasc Surg.* 1992;6: 119–126.
2. Ricotta JJ, Faggioli GL, Stella A, et al. Total excision and extra-anatomic bypass for aortic graft infection. *Am J Surg.* 1991;162: 145–149.
3. Reilly LM, Stoney RJ, Goldstone J, Ehrenfeld WK. Improved management of aortic graft infection: the influence of operation sequence and staging. *J Vasc Surg.* 1987;5: 421–431.
4. O'Hara PJ, Hertzer NR, Beven EG, Krajewski LP. Surgical management of infected abdominal aortic grafts: review of a 25-year experience. *J Vasc Surg.* 1986;3:725–731.
5. Trout HH, Kozloff L, Giordano JM. Priority of revascularization in patients with graft enteric fistulas, infected arteries, or infected arterial prostheses. *Ann Surg.* 1984;6:669–682.
6. Quinones-Baldrich WJ, Hernandez JJ, Moore WS. Long-term results following surgical management of aortic graft infection. *Arch Surg.* 1991;126:507–511.
7. Yeager RA, Moneta GL, Taylor LM, Harris EJ Jr, McConnell DB, Porter JM. Improving survival and limb salvage in patients with aortic graft infection. *Am J Surg.* 1990;159: 466–469.
8. Schellack J, Stewart MT, Smith RB, Perdue GD, Salam A. Infected aortobifemoral prosthesis: a dreaded complication. *Am Surg.* 1988;54(3):137–141.
9. Lorentzen JE, Nielsen OM, Arendrup H, et al. Vascular graft infection: an analysis of 62 graft infections in 2411 consecutively implanted synthetic vascular grafts. *Surgery.* 1985;98(1):81–86.
10. Casali RE, Tucker WE, Thompson BW, Read RC. Infected prosthetic grafts. *Arch Surg.* 1980;115:577–580.
11. Yeager RA, McConnell DB, Sasaki TM, Vetto RM. Aortic and peripheral prosthetic graft infection: differential management and causes of mortality. *Am J Surg.* 1985;150: 36–43.
12. Olah A, Vogt M, Laske A, Carrell T, Bauer E, Turina M. Axillofemoral bypass and simultaneous removal of the aortofemoral vascular infection site: is the procedure safe? *Eur J Vasc Surg.* 1992;6:252–254.
13. Schmitt DD, Seabrook GR, Bandyk DF, Towne JB. Graft excision and extra-anatomic revascularization: the treatment of choice for the septic aortic prosthesis. *J Cardiovasc Surg.* 1990;31:327–332.
14. Turnipseed WD, Berkoff HA, Detmer DE, Acher CW, Belzer FO. Arterial graft infections: delayed vs. immediate vascular reconstruction. *Arch Surg.* 1983;118:410–414.
15. Bahnini A, Ruotolo C, Koskas F, Kieffer E. In situ fresh allograft replacement of an infected aortic prosthetic graft: 18-months' follow-up. *J Vasc Surg.* 1991;14:98–102.
16. Snyder SO, Wheeler JR, Gregory RT, Gayle RG, Zirkle PK. Freshly harvested cadaveric venous homografts as arterial conduits in infected fields. *Surgery.* 1987;101(3):283–291.
17. Ehrenfeld WK, Wilbur BG, Olcott CN, Stoney RJ. Autogenous tissue reconstruction in the management of infected prosthetic grafts. *Surgery.* 1979;85(1):82–92.
18. Clagett GP, Bowers BL, Lopez-Viego MA, Rossi MB, Valentine RJ, Myers SI, Chervu A. Creation of a neoaortoiliac system from lower extremity deep and superficial veins. *Ann Surg.* In press.
19. Schulman ML, Badhey MR, Yatco R. Superficial femoral-popliteal veins and reversed saphenous veins as primary femoropopliteal bypass grafts: a randomized comparative study. *J Vasc Surg.* 1987;6:1–10.
20. Schanzer H, Chiang K, Mabrouk M, Peirce EC. Use of lower extremity deep veins as arterial substitutes: functional status of the donor leg. *J Vasc Surg.* 1991;14:624–627.
21. Masuda EM, Kistner RL, Ferris EB III. Long-term effects of superficial femoral vein ligation: 13-year follow-up. *J Vasc Surg.* 1992;16: 741–749.

Graft-Enteric Fistulae and Erosions

Honest surgeons make mistakes; intelligent surgeons learn from them . . .

Chapter 18

Overview of Graft-Enteric Fistulae and Erosions

T.J. Bunt

Introduction

The most feared infectious complication of aortic surgery is the development of a secondary graft-enteric fistula (GEF), due to its recognized high mortality rate either from exsanguination or prolonged sepsis. This highly morbid complication was initially recognized soon after introduction of aortic homografting by Oudot in 1951, with Schramel and then Brock reporting cases in 1953.[1–3] Its management has fallen into two basic camps, those favoring total graft resection with EAB, and those favoring in situ repair and reconstruction. Unlike the improving results with graft infection (GIF), the mortality and morbidity of this complication has not changed materially in the 40 years since its recognition.

Two major classification schemes have been proposed. Szylagyi first used the terms aortoenteric fistula (AEF) (Figs. 1,2) and paraprosthetic fistula (Fig. 3). Youmans later introduced the term of graft-enteric fistula.[4–5] We prefer the overall classification scheme of graft infection, graft-enteric fistula (GEF), and graft-enteric erosion (GEE) (Fig. 4). The terms are related in their acronym spelling, and the terms are all inclusive and usefully simple. A GEF or GEE may have any portion of the graft (shaft, limb, proximal or distal anastomosis) and any viscera (duodenum, jejunum, sigmoid) without requiring a change in nomenclature.

Literature Review

It is worthwhile to review the past 40 years of surgical experience with GEF. There were many highly competent and perceptive surgeons dealing with this challenging problem, who observed potential causes and devised potential preventative measures. Most of the 565 cases presented have been either single case reports or very small (less than 5) patient experiences with the problem. These are summarized in Table 1, which total the varied and widespread experience to arrive at some reasonable conclusions as to presentation, diagnostic workup, and optimal management. In addition, a number of authors presented larger series on which they based theories of both etiology as well as treatment.

From Bunt, TJ: *Vascular Graft Infections*. Armonk: Futura Publishing Co., Inc.; © 1994.

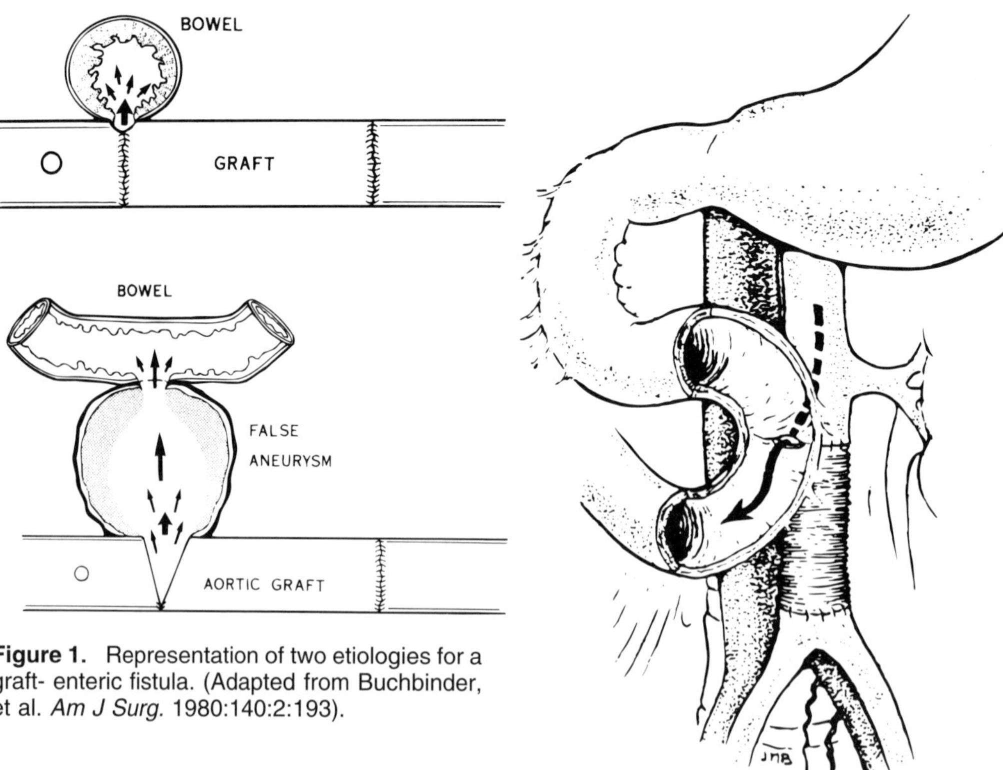

Figure 1. Representation of two etiologies for a graft- enteric fistula. (Adapted from Buchbinder, et al. *Am J Surg.* 1980:140:2:193).

Figure 2. Schematic representation of herald bleed into the duodenum from an acute graft-enteric fistula.

Intra-abdominal vascular surgery began with homograft aortic reconstruction by Oudot in 1951 and aortic aneurysmorrhaphy by DuBost in 1952. Due to intrinsic structural problems with the homograft, only a year passed when problems with aortoenteric fistulae were encountered.[1,6]

The first GEF was presented by Brock in 1953; the case is of interest as a microcosm of possible etiologies that would be echoed by numerous subsequent authors. A 44-year-old patient underwent homograft aortic replacement for LeRiche syndrome. It was noted that the proximal aorta was *tenuous* postthromboendarterectomy, and that a short graft dictated that the anastomosis be done under *tension*. A follow-up angiogram 10 days later revealed a small pseudoaneurysm at the left common iliac and possibly also at the proximal anastomosis.

The patient expired of upper gastrointestinal hemorrhage (UGIH) 6 months postoperatively, and at autopsy was found to have a proximal aortic pseudoaneurysm

eroding into the duodenum.[3]Three years later the first GEF from a synthetic graft was reported by Claytor (1956); the patient expired without any attempted therapy.[7]

Mackenzie (1958) reported the first successful management of GEF. A 70-year-old patient presented with UGIH after aortic homografting, and at surgery was found to have a 1-mm fistula into the duodenum from a proximal aortic pseudoaneurysm. In situ replacement with a nylon graft was performed with at best a short-term success.[8]

O'Hara (1958) presented a fatal GEF 13 months following nylon aortic grafting; the graft dilated and its anterior surface eroded into the duodenum. Histologic examination showed disappearance of the duodenal musculature, with the submucosa in direct continuity with the graft sheath.[9]

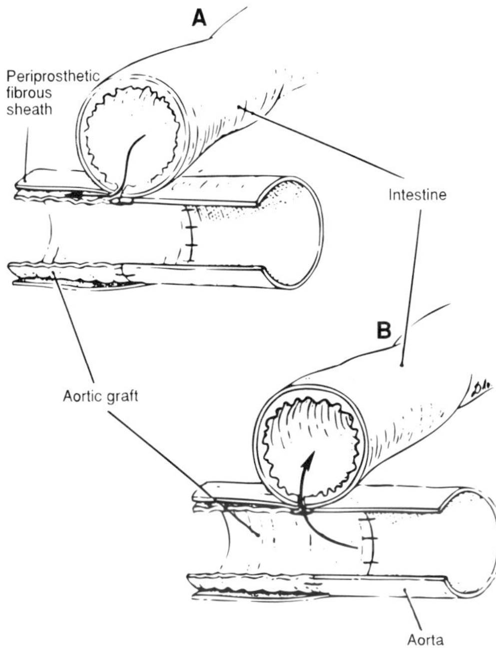

Figure 3. Representation of the progressive stages of a graft-enteric erosion resulting in periprosthetic graft infection (A) which then results in secondary communication with the aortic anastomosis (B). (Adapted from Buchbinder, et al. *Am J Surg.* 1980;140:1.192).

Lawton (1959) reported on three patients who presented with acute fatal UGIH at 7, 18, and 36 months following homograft aortic replacement. He theorized that the grafts eroded mechanically into the duodenum due to lack of adequate retroperitoneal tissues, that the bleeds were sporadic because duodenal spasm caused a local tamponade of the bleeding, and this spasm caused the usual acute pain syndrome.[10]

Sharf and Acker (1959) reported on two fatal GEFs 14 months following onlay homografting and 17 months following nylon aortic grafting with early anastomotic rupture leading to both free intraperitoneal bleeding and an acute GEF. They theorized a mechanical etiology and suggested placing an Ivalon sponge between the duodenum and the proximal anastomosis to provide an interposed tissue layer between the two.[11]

Table 1.
Chronology of Graft-Enteric Fistulae-Erosions

Brock (1953)	First case report
Claytor (1956)	First case from a synthetic graft
MacKenzie (1958)	First successful operation by in situ operation
Gryska (1959)	First graft-enteric erosion
Crawford (1960)	Advocated urgent laparotomy for herald bleed including thorough dissection of duodenum from the graft
Donovan (1967)	Differentiated between a GEF and a GEF with associated GIF, advocating EAB for the latter situation, performing successful thoracofemoral graft
Mirmadjelassi (1967)	First endoscopy diagnosis
Ehrenfeld (1968)	Advocated total excision and EAB
Pinkerton (1972)	Advocated intra-aortic balloon control of fistula
Elliott (1973)	First description of aortic stump sepsis
Kleinmann (1979)	Provided algorithm for management of gastrointestinal bleeding in patients with aortic graft
Martin (1980)	Advocated staged rather than sequential operations

GEF = graft-enteric fistula; GIF = graft infection; EAB = extra-anatomic bypass.

Sheranian (1959) presented the long-term results of 110 aortic homografts, and noted that 3 patients died of GEF. Boyd (1959) noted 2 fatalities from GEFs and suggested that mechanical factors might be ameliorated by a thorough retroperitonealization of the graft, and by avoiding any disparity between the graft and the proximal cuff.[12–13]

Humphries (1956) noted 3 GEFs in 120 aortic cases (2.6% incidence), all fatal, without intervention and occurring at 15, 16, and

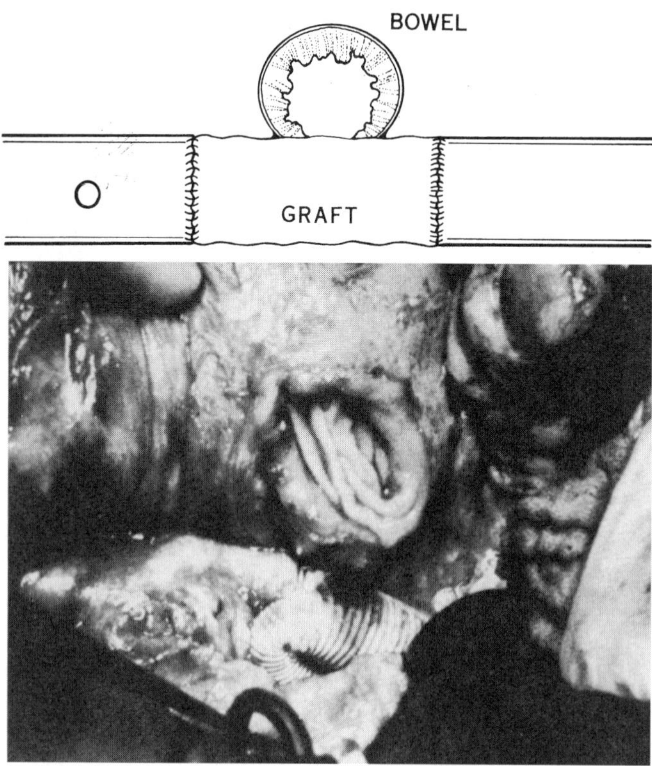

Figure 4. Graft-enteric erosion. (Adapted from Buchbinder, et al. *Am J Surg.* 1980;140:1.192).

122 days. He noted that all 3 cases involved suprarenal aneurysms in which infrarenal grafting to dilated aortic cuffs had been performed.[14]

Erskin (1960) reported on two successfully managed GEFs occurring at 13 and 17 months, and noted that no retroperitonealization had been performed in either case. Both cases were remarkable for primary homograft failure as the precipitant cause.[15]

Cordell (1960) reported one acute fatal GEF occurring one week following an anastomotic bleed which had been locally repaired at first reexploration on the seventh postoperative day; the case was all the more remarkable for being an aortic thromboendarterectomy without any synthetic patching. Histology of the fistula noted fibrotic fixation of the duodenum to the aortic suture line.[16]

Crawford (1960) reviewed a series of 1225 patients treated with aortic reconstruction for occlusive disease over a 6-year period, and noted 6 GEFs among the 16% of patients noted to have late graft failures. He stressed that most patients presented with exsanguinating hemorrhage within hours of initial herald bleed, and that the diagnosis was best made by exploratory laparotomy which specifically included reflection of the duodenum from the aortic suture line. As a technical measure, he recommended preliminary dissection for supracoeliac aortic control prior to fistula visualization.[17]

Carter (1961), in a paper detailing the supposedly successful local management of graft infections (Section IV), noted a case of *Salmonella* mycotic aneurysm treated with in situ Dacron grafting. That patient developed a GEF at 19 months, which was then treated by repeat in situ replacement. Three months later, the patient returned with an aortoiliac fistula and distal pseudoaneurysm. Without learning from the first two errors, Carter and his group again performed in situ replacement and noted the patient to be "well at 3 months," if such a statement can be made. Such cases amply illustrate the hazards of leaving synthetic foreign bodies in a Gram-negative infected field, and perhaps even more so the complications patients sometimes have to endure when their physicians are committed to a *one size fits all* management regimen.[18]

Sproul (1962) reported the development of a GEF 8 weeks post-Dacron aortic reconstruction complicated by a *Staphylococcus aureus* GIF. This case, along with those of Carter and O'Hara, illustrated early on the potential for early postoperative GEF if an acute aortic GIF occurred.[19]

Deweese (1962) reported on two cases (as well as two GEEs) all, however, with fatal results, one from a recurrent GIF and aortic stump sepsis (ASS) after in situ Dacron replacement. He characterized the presentation of GEFs as being of two types: type I being a direct communication from the duodenal lumen to the aortic suture line, and type II, a communication from bowel surface or lumen to the perigraft space. He also noted that retroperitonealization did not per se prevent GEF, as this technical detail was noted in the original operative notes, and also made the observation that synthetic grafts did not disrupt or degenerate as had homografts, and so were a preferable graft. He lastly described a two-layer closure of the retroperitoneum as a technique to aid in the prevention of GEF.[20]

Humphries (1963) reported on the first large series of GEF and presented the first literature review, noting 20 cases in 850 consecutive aortic cases for a 5% incidence. The average time of onset was 2 years for homografts but only 6 months for synthetic grafts. Eighty percent of the homografts involved a degeneration of the graft midshaft, and

25% formed acute pseudoaneurysms, whereas 75% of synthetic cases involved the proximal aortic suture line. Thirteen of the 20 cases presented within 2 months of original surgery, suggesting infection and/or graft disruption as major etiologies.[21]

Vasko (1963) also presented a review of the literature to date, noting an 80% mortality with 10 cases of local repair, 43% with 7 in situ, and 34% with 3 graft excisions. He advocated not only an early operative approach, but also that antibiotics be used for 6 weeks postoperatively to decrease the incidence of secondary septic complications which were often the cause of delayed mortality.[22]

Garrett (1963) presented another large series, noting 13 cases in 3000 abdominal aortic operations for a 4.1% incidence; onset was from 2 months to 3 1/2 years; the overall mortality was 40%, with actual surgical mortality of 31%. Those results were far better than all other authors of his time, and would stand up well against current therapeutic standards. This is all the more remarkable for the technique selected; five of seven cases treated with in situ replacement survived for 3 to 6 years. He further pointed out, in contrast to earlier authors, that 75% of his cases were seen with more than 6 hours of symptoms, sufficient to allow preparation for surgical correction.[23]

Ferris et al. (1965) reported on the first series from a radiologists's point of view, noting positive upper gastrointestinal series findings in three cases, and classifying the positive radiologic findings as an intraluminal graft, obstruction of the third portion of the duodenum, or actual visualization of the fistula. Although they did not review the literature for the sensitivity of radiologic studies, the paper did demonstrate textbook examples of the positive findings that may occur.[24]

Beach (1966) reported a case of GIF with associated GEF between the sigmoid colon and the iliac suture line; the patient died of pelvic ischemia after graft resection. He noted that local replacement of synthetic material in an infected field would be a futile procedure leading to recurrent infection and advocated, for the first time, that optimal management would be total graft excision with a *rerouted* revascularization.[25]

Donovan (1967) noted the development of 5 GEFs after 119 abdominal aortic aneurysmorrhaphies, for a 4.2% incidence. All presented with herald bleeds, and 3 were due to aortic pseudoaneurysms (PAs). He stated that the rate of GEF was 6.6% for woven but 0% for knitted Dacron grafts, 80% of GEFs in his series occurred prior to 1962 during a time when silk sutures had been routinely used, and there was a 14% incidence of GEF when silk sutures had been used versus 1% with braided Dacron suture.

However, he also noted that there had not been an observed suture breakdown in any of those 5 cases. Lastly, he made the differentiation between the locally infected-contaminated GEF versus a GEF occurring within a noninfected field, and suggested that extra-anatomic reconstruction be considered for the former situation to avoid further potentiation of the infection. Most importantly, he used an extra-anatomic bypass (EAB) reconstruction for the first time successfully, performing thoracofemoral grafting in 2 cases.[26]

Ehrenfeld (1968) reported on three cases that were successfully managed with EAB, and stated that "control requires that all infected synthetic graft be removed."[27] With Donovan's and now Ehrenfeld's experience, the tide was turned toward more complete excision and revascularization. However, a number of authors would still report less complete procedures over the next decade.

Unusual causes of GEF were then successively reported. Lise (1968) presented the first GEF from an aortic Dacron patch angioplasty, which was seen 4 months postoperatively, with a GEF without either a PA or GIF. Sheil (1969) reported four cases, all of which occurred following aortic endarterectomy and saphenous vein patching. Cerny

(1972) reported two cases of aortorenal grafts causing GEF: one an infected and thrombosed renal graft stump postnephrectomy for failure of that bypass that eroded into the duodenum, and a second from fixation of the duodenum to the site of aortic closure after autologous graft failure and removal. Both cases therefore involved GEF from adherence of the duodenum to an aortic suture line.[28–30]

Pinkerton (1972) detailed successful management of a single GEF case by approaching the fistula directly and using balloon catheter tamponade for aortic control. This useful technique for proximal aortic control was not widely appreciated.[31]

The first reported case of endoscopy used to diagnose GEF was by Mir-Madjelessi (1963). He described the endoscopic findings during herald hemorrhage, which were not recognized at the time but have subsequently become the diagnostic hallmarks of the endoscopic diagnosis: a pulsatile posterior wall of the distal duodenum, with a mass effect of extrinsic compression, often with a nipplelike protrusion (representing the fistula), as well as blood restricted to the distal duodenum without visualization of a distinct more proximal positive etiology.[32]

Elliott (1974) described a large series including 11 GEFs and 8 GEEs; 12 of these occurred as in-house complications of 2085 aortic surgeries for a 4.5% incidence. These occurred after 1.7% of emergency aortic aneurysmorrhaphy, 0.7% of elective abdominal aortic aneurysmorrhaphy (AAA), and 0.2% of aortic reconstructions. They associated the development of GEF with duodenal injury at the time of primary operation in many cases, especially following dissection of the duodenum in inflammatory aneurysms. They theorized that mechanical erosion of the duodenum occurred first, with secondary digestion of the aortic suture line causing final fistulization. Conversely, they clearly described the syndrome of GEE. In their GEF series, 5 UGIHs were sudden and 6 were preceded by herald bleeds. Finally, they described the problem with aortic stump sepsis (ASS), relating 3 delayed deaths from this complication. Total operative mortality for their series was 43% (6/14) with an additional 14% (2/14) late mortality from ASS.[33]

Spanos (1976) presented three cases, two of which offer instructive insight. In one, a graft infection led to acute GEF which was resected with EAB; however, the patient succumbed within 2 months to ASS with recurrent GEF. In the second, the duodenum was entered at attempted aneurysmorrhaphy, which was aborted until 3 months later. However, an acute GEF developed within the year, with fatal results. Such cases underscore the malignancy of local infections in causing recurrent ASS despite graft removal; in the second case, it would now be preferable to perform aneurysmorrhaphy via a retroperitoneal approach to obviate repeat duodenal exposure.[34]

Jackson (1976) in a report from the radiology department at Duke, stated that radiologic findings were usually helpful in the diagnosis of GEF. He noted 16 GEFs seen within a 7-year period, with 11 of the 16 being diagnosed radiologically. Positive studies were noted in 4 of 7 upper GIs, 6 of 11 angiograms, and 1 of 6 barium enemas. Seventy-five percent of cases could be diagnosed preoperatively and 75% of cases reported symptoms for more than 24 hours, allowing such diagnostic procedures.[35]

Dean (1978) presented a series of nine patients with presumed GEF, although the description of erosion in four and the septic presentation in three indicates that some may have been GEEs. Seventy percent had a herald bleed, however, preoperative studies were unrewarding including endoscopy which was negative in four of four and misleading in two of these. Four of the patients had documented duodenal injury or multiple mobilizations for redo aortic surgery to indicate an underlying mechanical etiology for their fistula; only one had a graft infection.[36]

Mehta (1978) reported an interesting case of a primary aortoduodenal fistula being repaired locally and resulting in recurrent secondary GEF 15 days postoperatively; this in contrast to the usual dictum that primary aortoduodenal fistulae may be safely repaired with an in situ technique.[37]

Busuttil et al. (1979) reported the UCLA experience with 11 patients over 18 years in a paper that also detailed a laboratory exploration of mechanical versus infectious etiologies. The only good results were obtained with total graft excision and extra-anatomic grafting. They suggested that the primary etiologic problem was low-grade graft infection that led secondarily to fistulization, and discounted a purely mechanical etiology. Two thirds of the series had undergone primary grafting for aortic aneurysm; two had clinical GIFs and seven were culture positive. They suggested a diagnostic trial for GEF on endoscopy that included negative endoscopy to the second portion of the duodenum, in a patient with UGIH and known aortic grafting.[38]

Kleinman et al. (1979), speaking for the Milwaukee group (and a paper that would give Vic Bernhard virtual rights to book chapters on this topic) reported the largest experience to date—20 cases in 20 years. Review of prior operative records revealed inadequate reperitonealization in 3 cases and redo aortic surgery in 5 cases. The presentation included two PAs and one GIF. Nineteen of the 20 patients gave preliminary signs of bleeding with 16/17 actual herald bleeds, 10 with hematemesis, 4 with melena, 2 with hematochezia, and 4 with occult anemia. Diagnostic studies were variably important. Angiograms showed PAs in 2 of 6, and endoscopy was diagnostic in 1 of 6, but was normal to the distal duodenum in the other five cases. The overall mortality for the series was 65%, which decreased to 22% in 6 cases done with EAB. Aortic stump sepsis, with or without GEF, was the major complicating factor, occurring in 5 patients (20% incidence).

They outlined an algorithm (Table 2)

Table 2.
Recommended Evaluation of Gastrointestinal Bleeding in a Patient with an Aortic Graft

1. Massive UGIH	Immediate laparotomy required, mandatory dissection duodenum/jejunum for graft supracoeliac or balloon catheter aortic control Sequential operation
2. Herald bleed	Endoscopy in operating suite a. If gastroduodenal source found—treat b. If negative to 3rd portion of duodenum, or c. If signs of GEF—immediate staged surgery
3. Low grade UGIH	Workup to include angiography, endoscopy, CAT scan, and other tests for other source of UGIH if desired.
4. Hematochezia	Endoscopy first, angiography second, and barium enema third.
5. Anemia and Fever	Complete workup for GEF/GIF/GEE to include EGD, CAT, leukocyte scan, and angiography.

GEF = graft-enteric fistula; CAT = computer axial tomography; UGIH = upper gastrointestinal bleeding; EGD = esophagogastroduodenoscopy.
(Modified from Kleinman et al.[39])

with five clinical situations for the management of the patient with UGIH and aortic grafting.

1. Massive UGIH: laparotomy required for fistulacontrol
2. Low grade UGIH: perform UGI and angiography, although results may be misleading; then perform esophagogastroduodenoscopy (EGD) to rule out other lesions. This is best performed in the operating room with laparotomy following negative EGD to the second portion of the duodenum.
3. Hematochezia: perform angiography and BAE if a preliminary EGD was negative.
4. Anemia and fever: complete evaluation with EGD, angiogram, BAE, UGI. (Editor's note: to this would now be added a CAT and/or MRI).
5. UGIB with a PA: angiogram first to delineate the anatomy, then to the operating room for correction. EGD can be done in the OR prior to laparotomy.

They furthermore emphasized that the operative exploration must be thorough and include complete dissection and reflection of the duodenum and jejunum from the graft. In their experience, preliminary gastrotomy to find a proximal source was unwarranted and prolonged the hemorrhage. They further recommended proximal aortic control prior to visualization of the fistula. All of these recommendations still stand as a primer of how to manage the patient with suspected GEF[39] (Table 2).

Martin (1980) for the first time raised the question of sequential versus staged resection. Previous authors had reported cases done either way, but their smaller series specifically addressed the question of improved results with sequential (0/2 mortalities) versus staged (1/2). The ability to perform staged resection is dependent on an understanding of the natural history; that many GEFs are seen with herald bleeding symptoms well in advance of exsanguination, thus allowing time for staged excision.[40]

Puglia (1980) reported an extensive series from Vancouver with 22 cases occurring after 1500 aortic procedures, 14 of these following AAA. Half of the cases were seen with herald bleeds, the remainder as acute UGIBs. There were two PAs in the group and no GIFs. Their operative mortality was 47%. The paper is interesting for the first recorded use of the vascular stapler for control of the aortic stump, with TA_{55} or $TA_{30} V_2$ vascular staples being used successfully.[41]

Perdue et al. (1980) reported the Emory experience with 22 aortic complications over 7 years, of which 10 were GEFs and 6 GEEs without clear-cut differentiation between the two as to results and/or symptoms. Only one patient presented with an acute UGIH, the remainder with herald bleeds. A variety of diagnostic measures were used with variable results. The paper described the use of gallium scanning for the first time to demonstrate GIF, which was positive in 5 of 5 cases. Similarly, the use of a CAT scan was first described and also highly useful with 4 of 4 being positive. Since the paper also describes 6 clinical GIF cases without GEF/GEE, the exact usefulness of these tests for the latter situation is unclear.

The etiology of these cases was also thoroughly addressed. Four of 16 had initial grafts greater than 22 mm in size; 2 had presented with PAs and 3 with GIFs. A multitude of corrective operative approaches were used, but the best results were seen with EAB reconstruction in which there were no mortalities or amputations in 13 of 14 patients. They recommended EAB, complete local debridement with buttressing of the aortic stump with prevertebral fascia, and also recommended stomal decompression of the involved viscera.[42]

Connolly et al. (1981) provided the experience at Irvine with 29 cases from six hospitals over 15 years, with an overall 51% mortality. They classified GEF into four types:

I. Spontaneous
II. Communication between graft and gut following aortoiliac aneurysm treatment, which may or may not be to the suture line.
III. Similar to type II, but following aortic reconstruction.
IV. Similar to type II, but following excision of GIF or mycotic aortic aneurysm and EAB, with the fistula being between the aortic stump and the gut.

I would suggest that this categorization is confusing and not particularly useful. The differentiation between type II and type III is superfluous, and the terms GEF, GEE, ASS more accurately represent the clinical situations seen, (with subscripts 1 and 2 for primary and secondary GEF).[43]

Champion (1982) detailed 22 cases, representing a 1.6% incidence in 1376 aortic cases seen over 11 years. The distribution of sites was quite unusual, with only 60% to the duodenum, 12% to the jejunum, 18% to the ileum, 8% the cecum, and 4% to the appendix. This would indicate that many of these cases were actually GEE. The most useful diagnostic test was endoscopy with 8/11 being positive, 3 of these showing an intraluminal graft. Overall mortality was 77%.[44]

Gozzeti (1984) noted six GEF and one GEE over 22 years, representing a 1.1% incidence in 172 AAAs and 0.6% of 582 aortic reconstructions (AR). Five presented with herald bleeds; one was due to GIF and three to PA.[45]

Shah (1983) writing for the Albany group, reported two cases and suggested the clinical use of a jejunal seromuscular patch to provide a viable pedicled blood supply to the aortic stump. The pedicle was raised as a seromuscular flap from an adjacent loop jejunum and used as a secondary buttress to aortic closure. Although both patients subsequently died, autopsy examination of their aortic closures revealed intact vascularized pedicles with no evidence of aortic infection or disruption.[46]

Flye (1983) reported the experience with 19 GEFs, all from Dacron grafts. Fourteen of the 19 presented with herald bleeds, and 8 with abdominal pain. A variety of operative procedures were used with an overall 74% mortality; best results were a 30% mortality with 10 EABs. Causes of death were 3 recurrent GEFs, shock in 8, and sepsis in 4.[47]

Paaske (1983) speaking for the Illinois group, noted remarkably good results with eight GEF, noting one mortality only. Four were managed by synthetic (3) or autologous (1) in situ repair, all uneventfully; the only death was after local repair.[48]

O'Donnell (1985) presented 13 patients seen over 2 arbitrary time frames in Boston. Prior grafts were woven Dacron in 6 and knitted Dacron in 7; proximal anastomosis was equally split between end-to-side and end-to-end. Repair was by total graft resection and EAB in 11 of the 13; the overall mortality was 65% (8/13), but improved from 86% (6/7) to 33% (2/6) over the 15-year time frame. The authors attributed their improving results to earlier diagnosis and treatment, as well as more aggressive intraoperative hemodynamic monitoring. They furthermore indicated that a left retroperitoneal approach could be used to obtain aortic control.[49]

The largest and most completely detailed series was presented for the USF group by Reilly (1985 and 1987) with 111 GIFs over 20 years, of which 43 were GEFs. Bleeding episodes were acute in 14, herald in 9, and chronic occult in 10; 15 showed no clinical evidence of blood loss. Within the scope of the article, they addressed the issue of what role endoscopy played in correctly diagnosing the cause of hemorrhage, which is reviewed later in this section. The preferred management was excision and EAB. In a series of combined GIF and GEF, the overall mortality was 49%.[50,51]

O'Hara (1986) presented the Cleveland Clinic experience with 33 GEFs, representing a 0.36% incidence (13/3 652) of cases originating at that institution. The 30-day operative mortality was 51% and was heavily weighted by an excessive (8/9) mortality with local or in situ therapy. Operative mortality for EAB was 36% (8/22); 21 of these were done as a combined procedure. The authors specifically noted that this was a significantly higher ($P < .01$) mortality than that seen for GIFs at their institution (14%). Thirty-two percent of all the GEF deaths

were secondary to either/or ASS and aortoduodenal fistual (ADF). Pertinent to this point is the notation that 25 of the 33 patients with GEFs were dead within 1 year due to these recurrent complications, placing the real mortality for the series at 76%.[52]

Hanning (1986) reported an unusual case of GEF occurring by duodenal fistulization into the fibrotic site of an excised aortofemoral graft following GIF, with fatal presentation by bleeding sinus tracts at the groins.[53]

Moulton (1986) presented the Harborview experience with 20 GEFs and GEEs. Seventeen of the 25 followed redo aortic surgery; 92% presented with bleeding, 20 of these with herald bleeds. The overall mortality was 40% at first hospitalization plus a 32% additional mortality from further complications, so that only 28% of the series survived the year. Fifty-five percent of the survivors of initial surgery developed anastomotic suture line problems, including six GEF and two PAs of which six resulted in death despite routine omental pedicle buttressing of the aortic stump. Additional analysis showed that 80% (4/5) of GEEs developed new GEFs, significantly more ($P < .05$) than 20% (2/10) of GEFs.[52] This paper represents one in a genre of brutally honest papers from Kaj Johansen's group on a variety of topics. Although perhaps not as well received by traditional surgeons, these *the emperor has no clothes* papers clearly delineate the highly lethal nature of this problem, and underscore the high complication rate seen by experienced surgeons practicing all the standard tricks of the trade. As such, it inevitably raises the question of the total veracity of other institutional reports touting superb cure rates.[54]

D'Souza et al. (1987) presented five unusual cases to illustrate the utility of a newly described technique for the acute management of the exsanguinating GEF (Fig. 5). They recommended simply stapling off the involved viscus on either side of the fistula to tamponade the hemorrhage. This maneuver allows a less hurried dissection for prox-

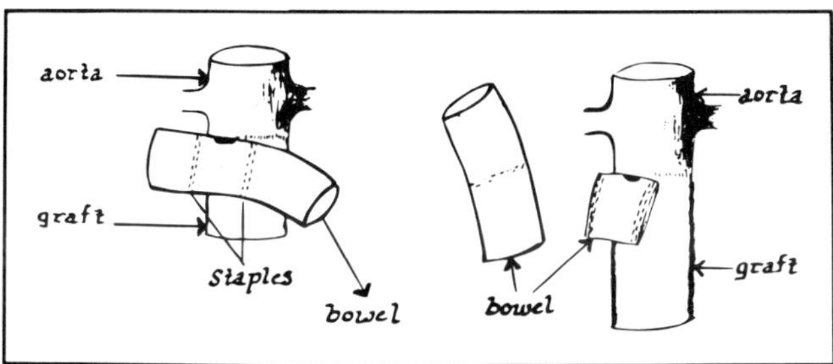

Figure 5. Schematic illustration of acute central hemorrhage by stapling off a segment of bowel. (Adapted from D'Souza.[55])

imal aortic control, even the possibility of performing EAB first, or transfer of the patient to another institution for definitive therapy. This novel and intuitive technique certainly should be added to the general surgeon's armentarium, since most cases are indeed seen by surgeons with limited experience with this problem.[55]

In addition, the paper described the first case of a thoracofemoral graft causing GEF, as well as a case of an umbilical tape ligation of a renal pedicle at nephrectomy causing later erosion into the duodenum.

Tillanus (1988) presented the experience from Rotterdam with 14 cases, most of which presented patients with herald bleeds. The mortality was (9/14) 64%, with a high (70%) mortality for EAB cases.[56] More sanguine experiences were, however, reported by other more recent authors.[54]

Walker (1987) reported a 14-year experience from Houston with 20 patients who had been treated with in situ replacement of their GEE/GEF with a 22% overall mortality, 6% in the last 18 patients. Follow-up averaged 5.2 years and was more than 1 year for all survivors. All postoperative deaths were due to sepsis, two with PAs and one with recurrent fistula. Although it was stated that there was no graft complication on long-term follow-up, there was an 11% additional mortality with two fatal episodes of ASS, so that the real mortality for the series was 33%. The authors routinely placed an omental pedicle between the (replaced) graft and required viscus, which they felt was integral to their success.[57] In discussion of this paper, Lord also extolled omental plication, noting (unpublished) a decrease from 3 GEFs in 141 aortic cases from 1953–1966 to zero in 177 cases done from 1967–1983 with omental plication.[58]

At face value, the results for in situ replacement appear extremely good and surpass those obtained with EAB; however, recalculation of the data shows that they had 23 patients with 4 immediate deaths, all associated with sepsis (4) and recurrent fistula (1) or pseudoaneurysm (2). This was followed by 3 late deaths due to aortic stump sepsis (2) or PA (1). Thus, all 7 deaths were due to recurrent and/or unmanaged sepsis at the aortic graft, which hardly speaks to in situ method as the optimal management modality, since all deaths were the direct responsibility of the surgeon in selecting that technique.

Umbleby (1987) presented 10 cases; 1 patient died preoperatively and 1 of 9 others died after excision and EAB. However, of the operative survivors, 2 later died of ASS (6 weeks and 2 years) and 1 of recurrent GEF to the aortic stump (12 weeks). Four of the 5 remaining axillofemoral grafts occluded. Two of 3 patients receiving EAB at intervals following graft excision had compartment syndromes with foot drops.[57] This rather dismal series underscores the long-term problems even if successful operative management is attained.[59]

Harris (1987) presented the experience at Sydney with GEFs in 24 years. Three cases resulted from thromboendarterectomy sites, overall mortality was 51%.[60] England (1990) presented a single case of recurrent GEF 10 months after successful EAB of the first GEF, and suggested that the best way to prevent such recurrences was to resect the distal duodenum and perform a duodenojejunal anastomosis with fresh tissue anatomically well removed from the aortic stump.[61]

Bergeron (1991) presented an interesting series in which GEEs (17) far outweighed GEFs (3), with both complications representing 0.7% of 2877 aortic procedures. The operative mortality for the series was 30% (6/20) with 3 additional deaths from ASS within the year for a total 45% mortality. The best results were obtained with EAB with 2/13 immediate and 4/13 total mortality.[62]

Low (1991) representing the USF group discussed the diagnostic role of CAT scanning, noting that in 23 GEFs and 12 GIFs that the CAT was correct in 33/35 situations for a 94% sensitivity and 85% specificity.[63]

Higgins (1990) presented the Pittsburgh experience, noting nine GEFs and six GEEs over 10 years. Seven presented with bleeding and eight with pain and septic symptoms. Local or in situ repair was successful in their hands with one mortality in seven cases, although two then had recurrent GEFs.[64] Haiart (1991) presented nine GEFs after 709 AAAs and 393 ARs within a series of 50 long-term aortic complications. Five underwent surgery, with three deaths.[65] Sailley (1991) presented ten cases over an 18-year time frame. The overall mortality for the series was 50%; five done as EAB, three local repair, and three by in situ grafting.[66]

Quinones-Baldrich (1991) summarized the UCLA experience with both GEF and GIF, noting routine total excision and EAB in all cases. Seven of the 45 patients presented with GEFs, which were not separately delineated from the entire series mortality of 24% (11/45).[67]

Ricotta (1991) noted eight GEFs in a multi-institutional, multi-year experience. Two underwent excision alone, one with fatal ASS and the other with an above-knee amputation. One of six additional patients treated with EAB also died for an overall (3/8) mortality.[68]

Graft-Enteric Erosions

The first GEE was reported erroneously as a GEF by Gryska (1959), resulting from a Dacron-Teflon graft that eroded into the duodenum with fatal results.[69] Hagland (1959) reported the second case, noting erosion of the midshaft of an aortic homograft into the ileum. In situ replacement led to a secondary fatal GIF. Subsequent cases were reported by both Deweese and Szylagyi within small series of GEFs.[4,20,69,70]

Youmans (1967) specifically addressed the concept of GEE for the first time. He reviewed the extant literature and stated that there had been 61 GEFs but only 3 GEEs (although my review as above does not corroborate those numbers). He described 3 cases of his own within a series of 250 aortic cases over 6 years, for an incidence of 1.2%. Two of these were diagnosed on UGI series by the characteristic coiled spring sign which represented a visible intraluminal graft.[5] Neither of these are, however, specific for GEE, being reported equally frequently with GEF.

Ng (1970) presented two cases to illustrate the radiologic signs of GEE; one showed the coiled spring sign of an intraluminal prosthesis, and the other, obstruction of the third portion of the duodenum.[71]

Elliott et al. (1974) described eight cases of GEE among a series of 19 GEF/GEE cases. They divided such cases into paraprosthetic enteric fistula and aortoenteric fistula; the former term seems both phonetically cumbersome and incompletely descriptive of the actual pathology. They described the occult septic presentation characteristic of GEE and theorized that this was due to intermittent bacteremia from the gut lumen via the directly exposed synthetic fabric.[33]

Skibba (1975) reported both the first endoscopic visualization of an actual intraluminal graft (although the radiographic signs on UGI series had been previously reported), and the first successful reconstruction with staged thoracofemoral EAB followed by graft excision. Furthermore, where Elliott had noted signs of occult sepsis as evidence for a GEE, Skibba specifically described transitory noninfected lower extremity (knee/ankle) effusions as being an indicator for GEE. These were noted to disappear following graft excision and appeared to represent subperiosteal osteopathy rather than sympathetic effusion or metastatic joint infection.[72]

Hobson (1976) reported a case of an intraluminal renal artery bypass graft seen at endoscopy, representing an unusual cause of GEE.

Kleinman (1977), speaking for the Milwaukee group, reported 3 GEEs within a series of 20 GEFs/GEEs seen over 20 years. Such experience could indicate that the incidence of GEE is actually much higher, being artificially deflated by the tendency of authors to report any bleeding episode from a graft as a GEF and not making the diagnostic differentiation.[39]

Puppula (1980) noted the erosion of a proximal aortic cuff into the duodenum 9 months following incomplete aortic graft resection for GIF; there was recurrent ASS/GIF resulting in a fatal duodenal GEE. Such cases underscore the importance of total graft excision when the aortic shaft is involved.[73]

Perdue (1980) presented a similar large experience to Kleinman, with 14 GEFs and 6 GEEs over 7 years; all GEE patients presented with herald bleeds and/or signs of graft sepsis, so that semielective workups could be obtained. Gallium scanning and CAT scanning for diagnosis of occult GIF were first described with uniform success. The authors recommended total graft excision and EAB and demonstrated no mortality or amputation in 5 cases so handled.[42]

Criado (1981) presented three cases, two of which were to unusual locations (sigmoid colon and appendix). Local therapy failed in one, leading to urgent EAB with fatal results; of the other two treated primarily with EAB, one died postoperatively of acute myocardial infarction. The failure of EAB after two successful resections underlines the variability of each institution's/individual's approach, even within the constraints of a generic classification, and therefore brings up the point of adequate aortic debridement control of local infection by wide debridement, closure of the aortic stump, and long-term antibiotic suppression of aortic stump infection.[74]

Paaske (1985) noted an unusual case of a superior mesenteric arterial graft eroding into the jejunum.[48]

Moulton (1986) for Harborview noted a disconcerting incidence of recurrent GEF following control of five GEEs with four of the five doing so after two local, one excisional, and two EABs. The most common problem in their series of GEE/GEFs was recurrent ASS/ADF (aortoduodenal fistula) with 55% of initial survivors returning with these problems, of which 75% then succumbed. Routine omental plication was used but did not prevent the problem.[54]

Vollmar (1987) presented 15 patients with GEE, representing a 0.2% incidence in AAA and 1.1% for AR totaling 1257 aortic cases. The mean onset was 34 months (1.73 months) with a mean delay in diagnosis of 9.5 days. Seven were to the duodenum, 3 to the jejunum, and 1 to the sigmoid colon. Nine of 11 patients presented with septic symptoms. The mortality was 5 of 6 for EAB but 1 of 8 for either local or in situ therapy, with 1 recurrent GEF at 3 years. They therefore recommended local measures rather than formal EAB.[75]

Harris (1987) presented 5 GEEs with 9 GEFs from the experience over 24 years at Sydney, with 2 to the duodenum, 2 to the jejunum, and 1 to the sigmoid colon.[60]

Bergeron (1991) presented a curious series representing an apparent reversal of the incidences, with 17 GEEs but only 3 GEFs over 19 years, representing 0.7% incidence in 2877 aortic operations. Eight presented with septic symptoms and 12 with hemorrhage; all 20 were duodenal in origin. They recommended sequential axillofemoral bypass and noted only two mortalities in 13 attempts; however, there were 3 additional late deaths from ASS within the year, for a total mortality of 45% (9/20).[62]

Higgins (1990) presented the experience at Pittsburgh with six GEEs treated with EAB, with only two mortalities.[64]

Discussion

The complete literature review just given reviews many aspects of the diagnosis and management of GEE/GEF, and emphasizes the variable surgical management that has been used. A few points of interest warrant further discussion.

Classification and Treatment

There have been 564 GEFs and 157 GEEs now reported; twice as many GEFs as found in my 1983 review, and four times as many GEEs.

We believe that the GEE-GEF-ASS classification most clearly denotes the anatomic presentation. Furthermore, it is of some clinical importance to differentiate GEE from GEF because the clinical manifestation tends to be different and the management certainly is so. Graft-enteric erosion tends to present as occult sepsis due to direct bacteremias from the small segment of intraluminal graft lying within the visceral lumen; bleeding is from the mucosal edge and therefore is low grade, with exsanguinating hemorrhage being rare. Sepsis is indeed a frequent symptom of GEF also, but it is of different variety, representing a frank GIF (with or without PA) that occurs early postoperatively and also progresses rapidly to major hemorrhage from GEF. Bleeding is the major symptom of a chronic (presumably mechanical) GEF, and characteristically involves a herald bleed followed within days to hours by exsanguination.

Treatment is therefore much different. The time course of GEE allows more complete workup, particularly measures (MRI, CAT, and leukocyte scans) that seek to prove or disprove a GIF. In contrast, the evaluation of GEF must be rapid, and the operative management decided on in a more urgent manner.

Finally, GEEs, when well described, are characteristic for being extremely localized processes, without surrounding necrotic tissue or widespread infection, and the graft is usually well incorporated at all other areas, indicating no spread of infection (Figs. 6,7). Obviously, this limited local process lends itself to local or in situ resections without requirement for formal and complete resection. This does not per se violate the cardinal rules of GIF management and indeed is parallel to the management of a single infected limb GIF by resection and local EAB.

The statistics to corroborate this perspective are admittedly a little difficult to come by because many series do not adequately differentiate between GEE and GEF, and the degree of therapy is sometimes unclear.

Etiology

In the first decade of reports on GEF, predominant causes that were recognized included the use of homografts or silk sutures at initial operation, and the role of expanding aneurysmal proximal cuffs and/or pseudoaneurysms. Graft infection as an etiology was uncommon.

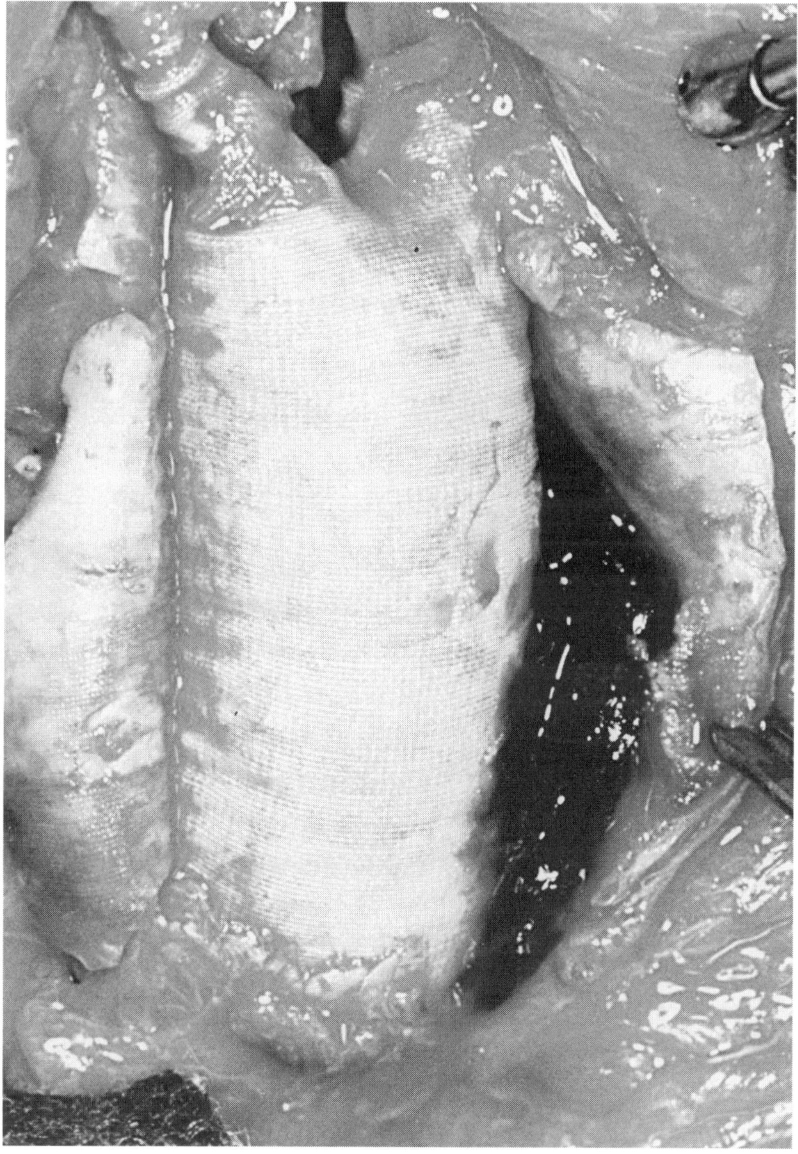

Figure 6. Operative photograph of a chronic graft-enteric erosion, demonstrating the chronic dense incorporation of the graft and the limited bile staining of its anterior surface.

Homografts were the first aortic replacement available, but in the original commercial form were soon noted to have problems with degeneration and either aneurysm or pseudoaneurysm formation at areas of weakness in the main aortic shaft. As synthetic grafts were introduced, it was rapidly noted that such graft degeneration was not a problem; however, the problem of synthetic graft infection with secondary aortic wall degeneration and pseudoaneurysm was substituted in its place. Multiple authors have addressed the theoretic etiology of GEF; the arguments basically come

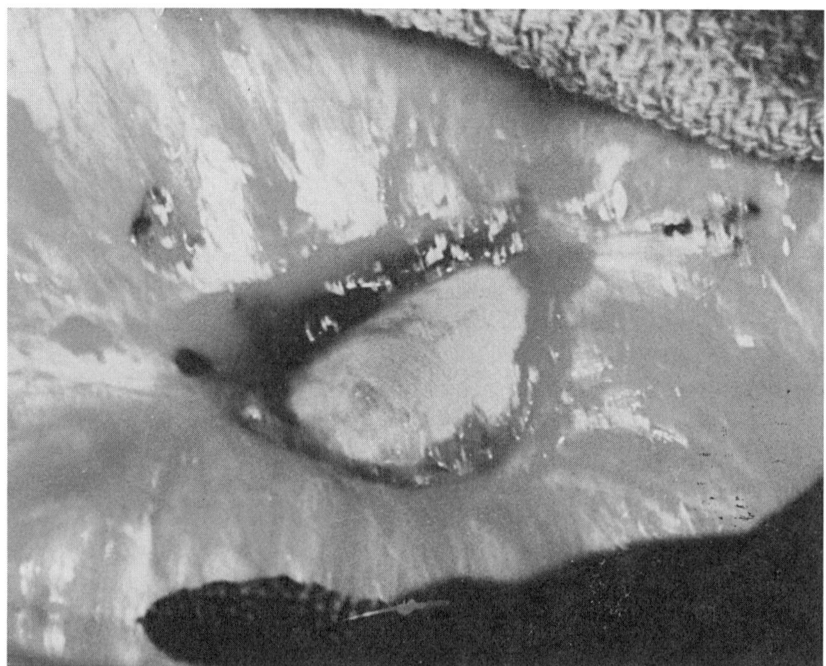

Figure 7. Operative photograph of a chronic graft-enteric erosion, demonstrating the chronic dense incorporation of the graft and the limited bile staining of its anterior surface.

down to the mechanical versus the infectious.

Mechanical

The basic concept to the mechanical model is that repetitive pulsation of graft foreign body against an immobile fibrotically fixed overlying viscus will eventuate in erosion of the latter. The evaluation and confirmation of the etiologic role of the mechanical model is important because it would therefore entail the surgeon having a distinct role in reducing GEF incidence by various techniques that minimize or eliminate visceral attachment to the graft, either by interposition of viable tissue (retroperitonealization, omental pedicle) or by visceral reflection away from the graft, most applicable as duodenal reflection from the proximal anastomosis.

Initial erosion then is perceived to re-sult in secondary graft contamination, which works its way to the suture line where proteolytic digestive enzymes work in synergy with the infection, causing arterial dissolution and hemorrhage (Fig. 3). Evidence for the mechanical model includes:

1. Observation that lack of retroperitonealization and/or redo aortic surgery, especially if duodenal injury is noted, is associated with GEF.

2. Observation that factors which magnify the pulsatile force of the aorta or graft are associated with GEF; for example, an increased incidence of GEF following AAA as opposed to AR, an association with aneurysmal cuff or use of a large (> 20 mm) graft at first operation, and later formation of a pseudoaneurysm. It is of interest that review of the literature demonstrates specific notation of a pseudoaneurysm in 41 cases

and of an aneurysmal cuff in an additional 7 cases.

3. Observation of GEEs, which by definition do not involve the anastomosis at all, but clearly involve simple mechanical erosion of the graft into the bowel lumen. Initially, GEEs were not specifically differentiated, but their recognized incidence has markedly increased in the past decade and currently they represent 25 to 35% of all cases.

4. Observation that thrombosed aortic grafts, or such nonaortic grafts as renal or mesenteric bypasses, and suture materials have all eroded into bowel, indicating that it may be a nonpulsatile mechanical interaction with the bowel.

5. Observation that GEFs have occurred in situations where there was no graft at all, for example, thromboendarterectomy sites. There are seven such reported cases.

Infectious Model

The infectious model postulates that a primary GIF either acutely or occultly festers in the graft, eventually causing increased fibrosis-surrounding reaction that fixes the viscus to the graft. In addition, the smoldering infection causes dissolution of the suture line, which then communicates via the paraprosthetic infected space to the eroded bowel lumen.

Evidence for the infectious model includes:

1. The incidence of *clinical* graft infection at presentation of GEF. There have been 28 such cases noted for GEF and 11 for GEE. This is to be clearly differentiated from occult sepsis (fevers, leukocytosis, migratory distal septic sites) that are caused by GEEs and potentially by GEFs when there is direct bacteremia from a small section of graft bathed in succus entericus, but the graft itself is otherwise incorporated and not infected; and also from the ability to culture organisms from the small visceral-exposed section of graft, which rate approaches 75%.

Clinical graft infections are early postoperative problems and have a marked propensity to result in classic GEF within days to weeks of initial surgery; acute PAs are not an uncommon accompaniment.

2. The observation that ASS or local sepsis frequently supervenes if local measures (local or in situ repairs) are used without graft removal. In our literature review, 23% (46/199) GEFs and 46% (18/41) of GEEs managed locally or by in situ repairs resulted in ASS, GEF, or GIF compared to 16% (36/230) of GEFs and 9% (4/47) GEEs managed by complete graft excision with EAB ($P < 0.05$).

Busuttil (1979) attempted to look at this problem with a canine model, as is completely described in Section II. He used the data from his lab model to suggest that an infectious etiology was most likely the cause. I would disagree. The model nicely duplicates the recognized clinical situation of acute GIF following aortic surgery, and in that respect does duplicate in the laboratory a recognized infectious etiology. However, the mechanical etiology model (noninfected PA) gave a high rate (33%) of GEF even at this early juncture. The fact that group 1 dogs did not form fistulae is a function of time only. Six weeks is not sufficient for that model. This is consistent with the observed delay (2 to 5 years) for the development of noninfected clinical GEFs.

It is obvious that the problem of arterial-visceral-graft pathologic interactions is variable in its etiology, just as it is variable in its clinical presentation. Patients presenting in the first few months postoperatively and with clinically recognized GIF, have an obviously predominantly infectious etiology that should be recognized so that complete graft excision can be used to appropriately and adequately deal with the problem. In contrast, patients presenting with GEE or GEF years following initial revascularization and without evident spread of the infection along the graft must represent a predominantly mechanical etiology. By extension of this logic, there is more logical room for considering an in situ approach if local contamination is minimal and Gram- negative bacteria are not evident.

Incidence

The incidence of GEF-GEE was reported as 3% to 7% in early papers and then said to decrease to incidences of 0.5% to 2.0% in papers from 1980 and beyond.[74] Few of these papers, however, calculate the incidence as the number of GEF-GEE occurring as a long-term complication of a set number of performed aortic operations, and those that do may underestimate the incidence due to the reality of patient follow-up loss, as well as the possibility that late deaths were not recognized as being due to the problem.

The number of reported cases per decade has not decreased.By 1980 there were 264 GEFs and 47 GEEs, and since 1980, there was an additional 296 GEFs and 110 GEEs being reported. Interestingly, many more GEEs are now being reported, indicating a confusion among earlier authors, as well as perhaps a reason for many supposedly successful local repairs and some institutional reports of decreased mortality, since they were dealing with less urgent situations. Since many more primary aortic grafts are (presumably) being performed in this decade, a small decrease in incidence is indeed possible, but the absolute numbers do not as yet reflect this.

It would be heartwarming to conclude that the incidence was decreasing due to prosetylization and therefore increased utilization of the preventative measures listed in Section II. However, much as we would like to suggest this, the data do not show such a palpable impact.

Diagnostic Methods

Review of all diagnostic measures used is summarized in Table 3. The various diagnostic tests used have ranged from none to a series of radiologic investigations, usually

Table 3.

Literature Review of Diagnostic Studies for Graft-Enteric Fistula

	No. of Studies	No. Positive
UGI	85	21 (25%)
BE	20	2 (10%)
Angiography	119	40 (34%)
CAT	10	6 (60%)
EGD	135	52 (39%)
Colonoscopy	0	4 (0)

UGI = upper gastrointestinal, CAT = computer axial tomography, EGD = esophagogastroduodenoscopy.

dependent on the time frame available. Most patients present with some occult hemorrhage, of which roughly half will additionally give a classic herald UGI (or uncommonly LGI) bleed. Of the 552 patients with GEF, only 36 were specifically noted to present with exsanguination while 215 had occult and/or herald bleeds. Seventy-one patients were seen with sepsis and 27 with abdominal pain.

A subset will present with clinical sepsis, usually defined as a fever with or without abdominal pain. Peculiar but highly suggestive presentations are migratory extremity cellulitis, septic emboli, osteomyelitis of a long bone, or osteoarthropathy, with joint pain and sterile effusions that resolve after correction of the graft sepsis. Of the 546 cases of GEE/GEF, 72 were specifically noted to present with sepsis, and 27 with abdominal pain.

The actual yield of the diagnostic tests overall was 25% (21/85) for UGI series, 20% (2/20) for barium enema, and 60% (6/10) for CAT scans. Thirty-four percent of angiograms were positive, with the diagnostic finding being a pseudoaneurysm in the majority, evidence of graft kink or angulation in a few, but only two cases of frank visualization of a fistula.

The Role of Endoscopy

Endoscopy is considered the standby diagnostic test. Thirty-two percent (52/149) were actually positive, but many authors considered EGD to be negative if the fistula per se was not somehow visualized, which is not an accurate condemnation of the study. Rather, positive findings on EGD have been predominantly exclusion of another source, combined with visualization of blood in the distal duodenum. In 10% or 15%, there may be a more direct visualization of an intraluminal mucosal defect with or without the diagnostic nipple (representing the fistula), and in about 20 cases direct visualization of the intraluminal graft actually has been documented.

Most authors suggest EGD in the operative suite as a preliminary to formal laparotomy, since a number of cases have been reported where sudden exsanguination from the fistula was precipitated by nonoperative EGD. However, the exact role of EGD in ruling GEF/GEE in or out is in some question. Traditionally, it was used to exclude other causes of UGIH, in which case formal laparotomy was then performed. However, a number of authors commented on false-positive EGDs, particularly the finding of gastritis as the presumed source; however, this hardly precludes a further set of diagnostic tests to elucidate a GEF/GEE as the underlying septic source. We would feel that the algorithm outlined by Kleinman et al.[40] is still the most appropriate management (Table 2).

The exact role of endoscopy in determining the source of UGIH in a patient with an aortic graft is hotly debated. Original authors advocated laparotomy to rule out the GEF. Subsequent authors suggested that EGD could be used adequately for differential diagnose. EGD is frequently stated to be normal or misleading because the definitive diagnosis of GEF was not made. In this regard, the overall success rate was 39% (52/135). However, the findings as previously described by Mir-Madjelessi, are not per se visualization of the intraluminal graft, but rather are the more indirect findings of distal duodenal bleeding without an obvious proximal source.

Pabst (1988) described the Arizona experience in following 253 aortic grafts for a mean of 46 months. Twenty-one percent of patients had a subsequent bleeding episode from 1 to 108 (mean 29) months postoperatively; however, only one of these 74 bleeding episodes was actually due to a GEF, an incidence of 1.4% of episodes and 0.4% of grafts. Thirty-eight of the 74 cases were intensively evaluated, 30 of whom had intrinsic gastrointestinal pathology; the remainder had no or incomplete evaluation but were not noted to develop a GEF at a mean follow-up of 26 months. Formal laparotomy was performed in 6 patients, 1 with preoperative evidence of GEF was demonstrated to have same, the other 5 did not (3 gastrointestinal lesions, 2 negative laparotomies). They concluded that the statistical risk of a UGIH in a patient with a known aortic graft actually being due to GEF/GEE was quite small, and that diagnostic workup for either another lesion or for more concrete evidence pointing toward GEF was definitely warranted.[76]

The largest series was by Reilly with 43 GEFs among 111 GIFs. She specifically addressed the issue of what role endoscopy played in correctly diagnosing the etiology.

She noted that there was no absolute correlation between the symptom of UGIH and the actual existence of a GEF, and that conversely endoscopic visualization of another source of UGIH did not rule out a GEF. The percentage of patients who were shown to have another source for the UGIH was 9.4%. Reilly et al. therefore disputed the heretofore accepted concepts that UGIH in face of aortic graft indicated a GEF, or that no bleeding meant no fistula, or conversely that you could rely on EGD to tell you the source of bleeding.[77]

The problem with this highly publicized and disconcerting conclusion is that it is based on a misleading variety of included clinical situations. For example, there were 11 GEEs within the series, and 10 did not have bleeding—certainly no endoscopic diagnosis would be expected. The series also included 71 GIFs, 18 of which were peripheral and not aortic, making delineation of the denominators confusing. Furthermore, it is not clearly stated if the diagnosis of a graft complication could have been made (especially for GIF and GEE) on clinical grounds or tests aimed at GIF detection (CAT and leukocyte scans).

Finally, the authors stated that their cases of GIF had UGI hemorrhage indistinguishable from GEF, while the predominant site of hemorrhage with GEF was stated to be the lower GI tract. The site of bleeding in GIF patients was not graft related in all cases, being gastritis or peptic ulcer in all five. I find this paper less helpful than obfuscating. My retabulation of the information provided would give the following:

1. 28 of 39 patients with GEF or GEE showed bleeding
2. 10 of 14 GEFs had acute exsanguinations
3. GIFs may also be associated with UGIH; of 53 aortic GIFs, 5 presented with peptic ulcer-gastritis-induced UGIH
4. EGD was therefore diagnostic (5/5) for GIF, but variable for GEF (7/17).
5. 15 of 39 GEE/GEF patients showed no bleeding, including 10 of 20 GEE patients.

Presented in this fashion, the data are similar to those of prior authors. Furthermore, the concept advanced in the article that EGD misleads the clinician is inappropriate, since it is based on the five GIF patients with documented gastroduodenal pathology requiring treatment and should not have diverted attention from the underlying GIF which had other obvious identifying clinical features.

Treatment

The management of GEE-GEF has become widely recognized, so that one sees few cases of *no therapy*, as had often occurred in earlier years (Table 4). The major remaining problem, and that which seems to be the basic cause of the higher mortality still seen with GEF/GEE as opposed to a steadily declining rate with GIF, is continued local sepsis. This results in recurrent ADF and/or ASS, or in persistent sepsis and multisystem organ failure, leading to death.

The management of GEF is as Yeager outlines it. We believe that there is little to theoretically recommend a local or in situ replacement, since of necessity that entails suturing the new prosthesis to a clearly contaminated prosthesis which in most situa-

Table 4.
Literature Review Summary of Graft-Enteric Fistula Treatment

Therapy	No.	Mortality	GIF	PA	GEF	ASS	Local failure
None	96	96 (100%)	—	—	—	—	—
Excise	38	24 (63%)	2	—	2	6	10/38 (36%)
In situ	104	49 (47%)	4	4	9	9	26/104 (25%)
Local	96	58 (80%)	2	—	13	5	20/95 (21%)
EAB	230	93 (40%)	—	1	16	19	36/230 (16%) ($P < .05$)
Total	564	320 (57%)					
Total Surgeries	468	224 (48%)					

GEF = graft enteric fistula, GIF = graft infection, PA = pseudoaneurysm, ASS = aortic stump sepsis, EAB = excision and extra-anatomic bypass.

tions is a clearly contaminated field, and in the presence of Gram-negative bacteria. None of these bode well for success. One does not recommend in situ grafts for infected aneurysm, for aortic GIFs, or even placement of a synthetic graft at primary operation when there has been visceral injury with spillage. It is difficult to justify an in situ reconstruction for the much more technically difficult and life-threatening situation of GEF.

Much of the opposition to more formal resection and EAB come from the perceived poor long-term performance of EAB. As we suggested in the section on GIF, the patency rate of axillofemoral grafts has improved in centers that use it frequently, suggesting that it all too often hasn't been done properly by the occasional surgeon. Furthermore, there is good theoretical reason to suggest either retroperitoneal supracoeliac or formal thoracofemoral bypass grafting as the preferred long-term reconstruction. Whether this could safely be done at first surgery, or should be done at a delayed (1-year) interval remains an important controversial point to be determined.

It is apparent that although EAB cannot be shown on total case summary to have a significantly lower mortality rate for GEF—46% (59/127) versus 49% (91/176) for in situ or for local therapy—it clearly provides better control of the local sepsis. There was a 23% (39/176) incidence of problems indicating lack of control of local sepsis (GIF, PA, GEF, or ASS) for cases managed by local or in situ technique, versus 16% (20/127) for EAB. Mortality rates for EAB for GEE appear somewhat better at 34% (16/47) versus 49% (20/39) for local and in situ therapy, with again the marked reduction in local recurrent septic phenomena; 48% (18/41) versus 9% (4/47) for EAB (P < 0.05). It would seem best on theoretical grounds, review of all cases in the literature, and the results reported in recent years by groups such as that at Portland, that the optimal control of the situation for both the

short and the long term, is complete graft excision and EAB.

The cardinal principles of management include an aggressive debridement of all infected and nonviable tissues to provide a less contaminated and optimally clean environment in which healing may occur. This entails complete resection of the fibrotic portions of the viscera and of the fibrous aortic bed-graft sheath. If this cannot be done safely, then in situ reconstruction certainly should not be done.

There is a distinct tendency to do less than optimal debridement. These are stressful cases, and it is all too easy to do less than adequate aortic debridement or duodenal mobilization to decrease operative time, presumed chance of further dissection injury, or precipitation of the need for splenorenal and/or hepatorenal bypass. However, the development of sepsis, GEF or ASS, is often a fatal event with the full onus placed on the surgeon to be certain all necrotic, contaminated tissue is excised, the aortic closure is secure within normal tissue, and the duodenal closure is also secure.

Treatment Recommendations

Graft-enteric fistula: Tables 5 and 6 detail the English literature experience with these problems, and bear summarizing.

1. No therapy. This results uniformly in death (96 of 96 cases), which is hardly a surprise. Patients have survived for up to 2 years with presumed GEF without treatment, but eventually all die of exsanguination.

2. Excision. Excisional therapy alone has predominantly been applied to the clinical situation of either a thrombosed graft, or a short (e.g., tube) graft, or an onlay graft with intact aortoiliac flow. Excisional therapy was attempted in 38 cases, with 63% (24/38) mortality, and 36% (10/38) further complications—two recurrent GEF, 6 ASS and 2 GIFs.

Table 5.
Large Series of Graft-Enteric Fistula-Graft Enteric Erosion

Author-Year	Pts.	Mortality	EAB mortality
Jackson (1976)	16	69%	—
Kleinman (1979)	20	65%	22% (6)
Puglia (1980)	22	47%	—
Perdue (1980)	16		7% (14)
Connolly (1981)	21	51%	—
Champion (1982)	22	77%	—
Flye (1983)	19	74%	30% (10)
Reilly (1985)	39	49%*	49% (31)
O'Hara (1986)	33	51%	36% (22)
Moulton (1986)	25	72%*	—
Volmar (1987)	15	—	—
Tilanus (1988)	20	64%	70%
Walker (1989)	23	33%*	—
Bergeron (1991)	20	30%	30% (13)

* Denotes my correction to include long-term mortality.
EAB: excision and extra-anatomic bypass.

These statistics do not lead one to a generic recommendation for this therapy. Most patients are going to require some variety of formal revascularization. Although often used as a *lesser* operation for an onlay aortic graft in an acutely ill patient, the reality is that a synthetic graft had been deemed necessary at the primary operation. There can be expectations of progression of the disease in the native vessels over the interim, and the whole marginal perfusion situation only will be aggravated, perhaps to threshold stage, by accompanying sepsis, hemorrhage, and hypotension. We would recommend excision only as a reasonable therapy for thrombosed grafts.

3. Local. Local therapy has been used 96 times, with 60% (58/96) mortality and 21% (20/95) subsequent graft complications, including 13 GEFs, 5 ASS and 2 GIFs. Such a management plan violates the basic concepts of GIF management in that the infected or contaminated graft is left in place. As such, it is not surprising that so many patients return with ongoing septic complications at the aortic stump. As discussed earlier, there is a higher incidence of recurrent local septic problems (GEF, GIF, PA, ASS) if grafts are left in situ; 23% (39/176) versus 16% (36/230) ($P < .05$). On theoretical grounds, surgeons appear more liable for continued local sepsis if they leave a potentiating foreign body at the site.

4. In Situ. In situ replacement with a new graft has been performed 104 times with 47% (49/104) mortality and 25% (26/104) secondary complications, including 9 GEFs, 9 ASSs, 4 GIFs, and 4 PAs. Our reservations with this technique are the same as for local

Table 6.
Literature Review Summary of Graft-Enteric Erosion Treatment

Therapy	No.	Mortality	GIF	PA	GEF	ASS	Local failure
None	5	5 (100%)	—	—	—	—	—
Excise	7	4 (47%)	—	—	2	2	4/7 (57%)
Local	27	16 (59%)	7	—	3	2	12/27 (46%)
In situ	18	5 (27%)	1	1	2	2	6/18 (33%)
EAB	54	17 (31%)	—	—	1	3	4/54 (7%) (p < .004)
Total	101	47 (47%)					
Total Surgery	96	42 (45%)					

GIF = graft infection, PA = pseudoaneurysm, GEF = graft-enteric fistula, ASS = aortic stump sepsis.

therapy. In addition, I suspect that many successful cases so handled were actually GEEs, which may better lend themselves to this modality due to extremely limited contamination.

5. EAB. Total graft excision with EAB reconstruction remains the preferred method on theoretical and clinical grounds. This management was followed in 230 cases with 40% (93/230) mortality and 16% (36/230) secondary complications, including 16 GEFs, 19 ASSs, and 1 PA. The relatively high rate of ASS/GEF, however, underscores the surgeon's responsibility to thoroughly and completely debride and drain the periaortic space.

Summary

Graft-Enteric Fistula

The overall mortality rates for the different modes of management of GEF are similar, ranging from 60% (58/96) for local, 47% (49/104) for in situ, 63% (24/38) for excision, and 40% (93/230) for excision with EAB. Subsequent local problems (ASS, GEF, PA, GIF), however, occur at statistically significantly higher ($P < .05$) levels in cases in which the graft is left in place (local and/or in situ) 23% (46/199) versus those in which it is excised for EAB—16% (36/230).

Graft-Enteric Erosion

For GEE, the overall mortality rates are also similar, ranging from 59% (16/27) for local, 27% (5/18) for in situ, 57% (4/7) for excision, and 31% (17/54), for excision and EAB. However, there is an even more significant reduction in secondary graft problems from 40% (18/45) if the graft remains, and only 7% (4/54) with excision and EAB ($P < .004$). The higher rate of local recurrent sepsis seems to us to argue for excision and EAB as the procedure of choice for both GEF and GEE.

Management of Acute Exsanguination

The optimal management will consist of acute intraoperative EGD to rule out a source proximal to the ampulla of Vater that might of itself require gastrotomy. This will be followed by a rapid laparotomy.

Control of the hemorrhage is best obtained by the novel technique described by D'Souza (1987),[53] with mobilization of the duodenum-jejunum proximal and distal to the presumed fistula and staples placed across. This stops the acute hemorrhage, allowing time for more meticulous dissection, preliminary EAB, or even transfer of the patient to a more experienced facility. If the fistula is inadvertently entered prior to good aortic control, balloon catheters inserted into the fistula (if large) or finger tamponade (if small) can provide the additional time to obtain formal aortic control. The surgeon does not want to have to try to rapidly obtain juxtarenal aortic control in the face of intraperitoneal exsanguination!

References

1. Oudot J, Beaconsfield P. Thrombosis of aortic bifurcation treated by resection and homograft replacement: a report of five cases. *Arch Surg.* 1953;66:3:365–370.
2. Schramel RJ, Creach O. Effects of exposure and infection on synthetic arterial prostheses. *Arch Surg.* 1959;78:271.
3. Brock RC. Aortic homografting: a report of six successful cases. *Guy's Hosp Rep* 1953;102:204–208.
4. Szylagyi DE, Smith RF, Elliott JP, et al. Infection in arterial reconstruction with synthetic grafts. *Ann Surg.* 1972;176:3:321–333.
5. Youmans CR, Derrick JR. Gastrointestinal erosion after prosthetic arterial reconstructive surgery. *Am J Surg.* 1967;114:711–715.
6. Dubost C, Allary M, Deconomos N. Resection of aneurysm of abdominal aorta: reestablishment of continuity by preserved human arterial graft with result after 5 months. *Arch Surg.* 1952;64:3:405–410.
7. Claytor H, Birch L, Cardwell ES, et al. Suture line rupture of a nylon aortic bifurcation

graft into the small bowel. *Arch Surg.* 1956;
73:947–949.

8. Mackenzie DJ, Buell AH, Pearson SC. Aneurysm of aortic homograft with rupture into the duodenum. *Arch Surg.* 1958;77:6: 965–968.

9. O'Hara I, Nakana S. Rupture of arterial plastic prosthesis (amylon-polyethylene tube). *Arch Surg.* 1958;77:1:55–58.

10. Lawton RL, Peterson FR, Britnoll ES. Aortointestinal fistula following aortic homotransplantation. *Angiology.* 1959;10:85–89.

11. Short AG, Acker ED. Surgical intervention in ruptured and thrombosed aortic homografts. *Arch Surg.* 1959;78:1:67–70.

12. Sheranian LO, Edwards JE, Kirklin JW. Late results in 110 patients with abdominal aortic aneurysm treated by resectional placement of aortic homograft. *SGFOB.* 1959;9:309–314.

13. Boyd DP, Pastel H. Results of treatment of aneurysm of the abdominal aorta. *Postgrad Med.* 1959;25:3:238.

14. Humphries AW, Dewolf VG, LeFevre FA. Analysis of 120 consecutive cases of major arterial grafts. *JAMA.* 1956;161:953.

15. Erskine JM, Thoshinsky M, Wilson JW. Rupture of aortic homografts into the small intestine. *Ann Surg.* 1960;152:6:991–997.

16. Cordell AR, Wright RH, Johnston FR. Gastrointestinal hemorrhage after abdominal aortic operations. *Surgery.* 1960;48:6: 997–1004.

17. Crawford ES, Debakey ME, Morris GC, et al. Evaluation of late failures after reconstructive operations for occlusive lesions of the aorta and iliac, femoral, and popliteal arteries. *Surgery.* 1960;47:1:79–104.

18. Carter SC, Cohen A, Whelan TJ. Clinical experience with management of the infected Dacron graft. *Ann Surg.* 1963;158:2:249–255.

19. Sproul G. Rupture of an infected aortic graft into jejunum: resection and survival. *JAMA.* 1962;182:11:143–145.

20. Deweese MS, Fry WJ. Small bowel erosion following aortic resection. *JAMA.* 1962;179: 882.

21. Humphries AW, Young JR, Dewolf VG, et al. Complications of abdominal aortic surgery: part I aortoenteric fistula. *Arch Surg.* 1963;86: 1:43–50.

22. Vasko JS, Spencer FC, Bahnson HF. Aneurysm of aorta treated by excision: review of 237 cases followed up to 7 years. *Am J Surg.* 1963;105:793–801.

23. Garrett HE, Beall AC, Jordan GL, et al. Surgical considerations of massive gastrointestinal tract hemorrhage caused by aortoduodenal fistula. *Am J Surg.* 1963;105:1:6–12.

24. Ferris EJ, Koltay MRS, Koltoy OP, et al. Abdominal aortic and iliac graft fistulae: unusual roenterographic findings. *Am J Roetgen.* 1965;94:2:416.

25. Beach PM, Risley TS. Aorticosigmoid fistulization following aortic resection. *Arch Surg.* 1966;92:5:805–807.

26. Donovan TJ, Buckman CA. Aortoenteric fistula. *Arch Surg.* 1967;95:5:810–819.

27. Ehrenfeld WK, Lord RSA, Stoney RJ, et al. Subcutaneous arterial bypass grafts in the management of fistulae between the bowel and plastic arterial prostheses. *Ann Surg.* 1968;168:1:29–35.

28. Lise M, Yacoub MH. Aortoduodenal fistula: a complication of abdominal aortic grafts. *J Thorac Cardiovasc Surg.* 1969;10:172–175.

29. Sheil AGR, Reeve TS, Little JM, et al. Aortointestinal fistulas following operations on the abdominal aorta and iliac arteries. *Br J Surg.* 1969;56:11:840–846.

30. Cerny JC, Fry WJ, Gamble J, et al. Aortoduodenal fistula. *J Urol.* 1972;107:1:12–16.

31. Pinkerton JA. Aortoduodenal fistula. *JAMA.* 1973;225:10:1196–1199.

32. Mir-Madjelessi SH, Sullivan BH, Farmer RG, et al.Endoscopic diagnosis of aortoduodenal fistula. *Gastrol Inf Endo.* 1973;19:4:187–188.

33. Elliott JR, Smith RF, Szylagyi DE. Aortoenteric and paraprosthetic-enteric fistulas. *Arch Surg.* 1974;108:4:479–490.

34. Spanos P, Gilsdorf RB, Sako Y, et al. The management of infected abdominal aortic grafts and graft enteric fistulas. *Ann Surg.* 1976;183:4:397–402.

35. Jackson DC, Thompson WM, Johnsrude IS. Aortic and iliac graft fistulae. *Vasc Surg.* 1977;11:291–298.

36. Dean RH, Allen TR, Foster JH, et al. Aortoduodenal fistula: an uncommon but correctable cause of upper gastrointestinal bleeding. *Am Surg.* 1978;44:1:37–41.

37. Mehta AI, McDowell DE, James EC. Treatment of massive gastrointestinal hemorrhage from aortoenteric fistula. *Surg Gynecol Obstet.* 1978;146:1:59–62.

38. Busuttil RW, Rees W, Baker JD, et al. Pathogenesis of aortoduodenal fistula: experimental and clinical correlates. *Surgery.* 1979;85:1: 1–8.

39. Kleinman LH, Towne JB, Bernhard VM. A diagnostic and therapeutic approach to aortoenteric fistulae: clinical experience with 20 patients. *Surgery.* 1979;86:6:868–880.

40. Martin J, Diconstanzo J, Cano P, et al. Four cases of gastrointestinal bleeding with abdominal aortic prostheses: endoscopic changes and therapeutic approach. *IV Euro-*

pean Congress of Gastrointestinal Endoscopy. Hamburg: June 13–14,1980.

41. Puglia E, Fry PD. Aortoenteric fistulae: a preventable problem? *Can J Surg.* 1980;23:1: 74–77.

42. Perdue GD, Smith RB, Ansley JD, et al. Impending aortoenteric hemorrhage: the effect of early recognition on improved outcome. *Ann Surg.* 1980;192:2:237–244.

43. Connolly JE, Kwaan JHM, McCort PM, et al. Aortoenteric fistula. *Ann Surg.* 1981;194:4: 402–411.

44. Champion MC, Sullivan SN, Coles JC, et al. Aortoenteric fistula: incidence, presentation, recognition and management. *Ann Surg.* 1982;195:3:314–318.

45. Gozzetti G, Poggioli G, Spolaore R, et al. Aortoenteric fistulae: spontaneous and after aortoiliac operations. *J Cardiovasc Surg.* 1984;25: 420–424.

46. Shah DM, Buchbinder D, Leather RP, et al. Clinical use of the seromuscular jejunal patch for protection of the infected aortic stump. *Am J Surg.* 1983;146:2.198–202.

47. Flye MW, Thompson WM. Aortograft enteric and paraprosthetic enteric fistulae. *Am J Surg.* 1983;146:2:183–187.

48. Paaske WP, Hansen HJB. Graft enteric fistulas and erosions. *Surg Gynecol Obstet.* 1985; 161:2:160–163.

49. O'Donnell TF, Scott G, Shepard A, et al. Improvement in the diagnosis and management of aortoenteric fistula. *Am J Surg.* 1985; 149:4:481–485.

50. Reilly LM, Altman H, Lusby RJ, et al. Late results following surgical management of vascular graft infection. *J Vasc Surg.* 1984;1: 1:36–41.

51. Reilly LM, Stoney RS, Goldstone S. Improved management of aortic graft infection: the influence of operation sequence and staging. *J Vasc Surg.* 1987;5:3:421–429.

52. O'Hara PS, Hertzer NR, Beven EG, et al. Surgical management of infected abdominal aortic grafts: review of a 25-year experience. *J Vasc Surg.* 1986;3:5:725–730.

53. Hannig E, Allpayer B, Disch M, et al. Duodenal fistula: a rare complication following the removal of an infected aortic graft: case report. *Cardiovasc Intervent Radiol.* 1986;9: 33–36.

54. Moreton S, Adams M, Johansen K. Aortoenteric fistula: a 7-year urban experience. *Am J Surg.* 1986;151:5:607–610.

55. D'Souza CR, Hebert RJ, Trautman AF, et al. Aortoentric fistula: case review and a new surgical technique. *Can J Surg.* 1987;30:6: 415–417.

56. Thomas WEG, Baird RN. Secondary aortoenteric fistulae: towards a more conservative approach. *Br J Surg.* 1986;73:11:875–880.

57. Walker WE, Cooley DA, Duncan JM, et al. The management of aortoduodenal fistula by in situ replacement of the infected abdominal aortic graft. *Ann Surg.* 1987;205:6: 727–732.

58. Lord. Commentary on: Moreton S, Adams M, Johansen K. Aortoenteric fistula: a 7-year urban experience. *Am J Surg.* 1986;151:5: 607–610.

59. Umbleby HC, Brittan DC, Turnbull AR. Secondary arterioenteric fistulae: a surgical challenge. *Br J Surg.* 1987;74:4:256–259.

60. Harris JP, Sheil AGR, Stephen MS, et al. Lesson learned in the management of aortoenteric fistulae. *J Cardiovasc Surg.* 1987;28: 449–452.

61. England DW, Simms MH. Recurrent aortoduodenal fistula: a final solution? *Eur J Vasc Surg.* 1990;4:427–429.

62. Bergeron P, Espinoza H, Rudondy P, et al. Secondary aortoduodenal fistulae: value of initial axillofemoral bypass. *Ann Vasc Surg.* 1991;5:1:4–7.

63. Low RN, Wall SD, Brooke JR, et al. Aortoenteric fistula and perigraft infection: evaluation with CT. *Radiology.* 1990;175:4:157–162:

64. Higgins RSD, Steed DL, Julian TB, et al. The management of aortoenteric and paraprosthetic fistulae. *J Cardiovasc Surg.* 1990;31: 81–86.

65. Haiart DC, Callam MJ, Murie JA, et al. Reoperations for late complications following abdominal aortic operation. *Br J Surg.* 1991;78: 2:204–206.

66. Saillen P, Mosimann F, Friedlender J. Fistulas aortoenteriques: rapport de 12 observations. *J Chir (Paris).* 1991;128:6:290–293.

67. Quinones-Baldrich WJ, Hernandez JJ, Moore WS. Long-term results following surgical management of aortic graft infection. *Arch Surg.* 1991;126:4:507–510.

68. Ricotta JJ, Faggioli GL, Stella A, et al. Total excision and extra-anatomic bypass for aortic graft infection. *Am J Surg.* 1991;162:2: 145–149.

69. Gryska. Case Records MGH #45522. 1959; 261:26:1339–1341.

70. Hagland LA, Sweetman WR, Wise RA. Rupture of an abdominal aortic homograft with ilial fistula. *Am J Surg.* 1959;98:5:746–748.

71. Ng E, Cooperman LR. Erosion of the small intestine with hemorrhage following aortic resection: roentgen findings. *Clin Radiol.* 1970;21:87–89.

72. Skibba RM, Greenberger NJ, Hardin CA.

Paraprosthetic enteric fistula: role of preoperative endoscopy. *Diag Dis.* 1975;20:11: 1081–1082.

73. Puppula AR, Monaswamy M, Doshi AM. Endoscopic diagnosis of aortoduodenal fistula. *Am J Gastroenterol.* 1980;73:414–417.

74. Criado FJ, Classen JN, Wilson TH. Secondary aortoenteric fistulas prosthetic and paraprosthetic. *Ann Surg.* 1981.47:1:313–321.

75. Vollmar JF, Kogel H. Aortoenteric fistulae as postoperative problems. *J Cardiovasc Surg.* 1987;28:479–484.

76. Pabst TE, Bernhard VM, McIntyre KE, et al. Gastrointestinal bleeding after aortic surgery: the role of laparotomy to rule out aortoenteric fistula. *J Vasc Surg.* 1988;8:3: 280–286.

77. Reilly LM, Ehrenfeld WK, Goldstone J, et al. Gastrointestinal tract involvement by prosthetic graft infection: the significance of gastrointestinal hemorrhage. *Ann Surg.* 1985; 202:3:342–348.

Additional Reports in Summary

Baird RL, Slagle GW, Boggs AW. Arterioenteric fistulas. *Dis Colon Rectum.* 1979;187–188.

Baker MS, Fisher JH, Van der Reis L, et al. The endoscopic diagnosis of an aortoduodenal fistula. *Arch Surg.* 1976;111:3:304–305.

Becker RM, Blundell PE. Infected aortic bifurcation grafts: experience with 14 patients. *Surgery.* 1976;80:5:544–549.

Brady PG. Aortoduodenal fistula: role of endoscopy in diagnosis. *Am J Gastroentol.* 1978;69: 6:705–707.

Brand EJ, Sivak MV, Sullivan BH. Aortoduodenal fistula: endoscopic diagnosis. *Diag Dis Sci.* 1979;24:12:940–942.

Brenner WI, Richman H, Reed GE. Roofpatch repair of an aortoduodenal fistula resulting from suture line failure in an aortic prosthesis. *Am J Surg.* 1974;127:6:762–764.

Brown L, Essig H. Fatal rupture of an Ivalon polyvinyl formalinized sponge aortic graft into the duodenum. *Arch Surg.* 1959;79:72–73.

Campbell HC, Ernst CB. Aortoenteric fistula following renal revascularization. *Am Surg.* 1978; 3:155–158.

Case records of MGH #45282. *N Engl J Med.* 1959;261:92–96.

Cranston D, Voyles KDJ. Aortoduodenal and subsequent aortocolonic fistula following operation for ruptured aortic aneurysm. *Br J Surg.* 1980;67:649–650.

Dass T. Small bowel erosion after aortic replacement by synthetic graft. *Am J Surg.* 1968; 116:460–463.

Florendo FT, Harmon HC. Aortoenteric fistula: a mandatory early operative diagnosis. *South Med J.* 1979;72:12:1516–1519.

Kukora JS, Rushton FW, Cranston PE. New computed tomographic signs of aortoenteric fistula. *Arch Surg.* 1984;119:3:1073–1075.

Lamerton AJ. Iliacoappendiceal fistula complicating endarterectomy alone. *Br J Surg.* 1984; 71:501.

Levy MS, Todd DB, Lillehei CW, et al. Aorticointestinal fistulas following surgery of the aorta. *Surg Gynecol Obstet.* 1965.120:5:992–997.

Long L, Hunter JA, Dye WS. Migration of aortic prosthesis into duodenum: case report and review. *Ann Surg.* 1963;137:4:560–564.

Martin-Paredo V, Busuttil RW, Dixon SM, et al. Fate of aortic graft removal. *Am J Surg.* 1983; 146:2.194–198.

Nevin IN, Bump WS, Theurer GR. Preoperative diagnosis of rupture into the duodenum of an aortic homograft anastomosis. *N Engl J Med.* 1960;263:5:243–245.

O'Mara C, Imbenubo AL. Paraprostheticenteric fistula. *Surgery.* 1977;81:5:556–567.

Pollock AV, Pratt D, Smiddy FG. Aortic homograft replacement: a sequel. *Ann Surg.* 1961; 153:3:427–476.

Ray R, McAfee RE: Hiebert R, et al. Aortoduodenal fistula: primary repair with saphenous vein patch graft. *JAMA.* 1976;236:21:2423–2425.

Rosato FE, Barker C, Roberts B. Aortointestinal fistula: three cases of successful management. *J Thorac Cardiovasc Surg.* 1967;53:4: 511–515.

Rosenthal D, Deterling RA, O'Donnell, et al: *Arch Surg.* 1979;114:3:1040–1044.

Salo J, Verkkala K, Ketonen P et al. Graft enteric fistula and erosions: complications of synthetic aortic grafting. *Vasc Surg.* 1986;2:88–92.

Schramek A, Weise GM, Erlik D. Gastrointestinal bleeding due to arterioenteric fistula. *Digestion.* 1971;4:103–108.

Scribner RG, Baker MS, Tawes RL, et al. Recurrent aortoduodenal fistula. *Arch Surg.* 1977; 112:1265.

Shaigany A, Gillespie L, Mock JP, et al. Aortoenteric fistula: a complication of renal artery bypass graft. *Arch Intern Med.* 1976;136:930.

Smiley K. Aortoduodenal fistula: a complication of synthetic grafts. *J Fl Med Assoc.* 1975; 62:24.

Tagart REB. Infection of an aortic prosthesis caused by duodenal erosion. *Proc Royal Soc Med.* 1974;67:11:1181–1182.

Tobias JA, Daicoff GR. Aortogastric and aortoilieal fistulae repaired by direct suture. *Arch Surg.* 1973;107:6:909–910.

Trout HH, Kozloff L, Giordana JM. Priority

of revascularization in patients with graft enteric fistulas, infected arteries, or infected arterial prostheses. *Ann Surg.* 1984;199:6:669–683.

Turnipseed WD, Berkoff HA, Detmer DE, et al. Arterial graft infections: delayed vs. immediate vascular reconstruction. *Arch Surg.* 1983;118:4:410–414.

Tyson RR, Maier WP, Dipietrantonio S. Iliacoappendiceal fistula following Dacron aortic graft. *Am Surg.* 1969;35:4:241–243.

Weirman WH, Strahon RW, Spencer JR. Small bowel erosion by synthetic aortic grafts. *Am J Surg.* 1966;112:5:791.

Wilson SE, Owens ML. Aortocolic fistula: a lethal cause of lower gastrointestinal bleeding. *Dis Colon Rectum.* 1976;19:614.

Chapter 19

Aortic Graft-Enteric Fistula: Diagnosis and Treatment

R.A. Yeager

Introduction

Aortic graft-enteric fistula remains a serious clinical problem extraordinarily difficult to manage successfully. During the 1980s, there was a disappointing 46% surgical mortality rate for this surgical complication, in contrast to a 21% surgical mortality rate associated with primary aortic prosthetic graft infection without bowel involvement.[1] The high mortality associated with graft-enteric fistula is significantly related to the associated gastrointestinal hemorrhage and hypovolemic shock which frequently requires emergency surgical correction under adverse circumstances. Reilly et al. reported that 36% of their patients with graft-enteric fistulae presented with acute gastrointestinal hemorrhage and hemodynamic instability precluded any preoperative evaluation in 18% of patients.[2]

Presentation and Classification

Graft-enteric fistulae are distinctly uncommon with fewer than 1% of aortic graft patients ever developing a prosthesis-bowel communication.[3–8] Despite the low incidence, maintenance of a high index of suspicion is essential to enable early diagnosis and prompt surgical correction, both of which clearly improve patient survival.[9] Without question, any patient with an aortic prosthetic graft who presents with gastrointestinal bleeding should be considered to have a graft-enteric fistula until proved otherwise.

While some patients require emergent surgery to control bleeding, most are able to undergo an urgent workup, which must critically include upper endoscopy to rule out another source for bleeding. Additionally, upper endoscopy may confirm a diagnosis of graft-enteric fistula.[10,11] In the experience of Reilly et al., upper endoscopy successfully visualized the fistula site in a surprising 24% of patients studied with acutely bleeding graft-enteric fistulae.[2]

Those patients with a graft-enteric fistula who are not acutely bleeding may present with other suggestive symptoms, including chronic gastrointestinal bleeding, abdominal or back pain, low-grade fever, leukocytosis, malaise, and/or weight loss.[12]

From Bunt, TJ: *Vascular Graft Infections.* Armonk: Futura Publishing Co., Inc.; © 1994.

In one series, 38% of graft-enteric fistula patients had no evidence of gastrointestinal blood loss, either acute or chronic.[2]

Authors have classified graft-enteric fistulae according to whether there is anastomotic suture line involvement (graft-enteric fistula) or bowel communication limited to the prosthesis (graft-enteric erosion or paraprosthetic fistula).[3,13,14] In our opinion, the clinical relevance of this classification system is limited, due to overlap between the two categories in terms of symptomatology, clinical presentation, and management recommendations.[13] In this discussion, the term graft-enteric fistula will be used to encompass any case involving an aortic prosthesis-bowel communication.

The presence of gross purulence in the perigraft region is extremely important and directly affects management decisions relative to retroperitoneal drainage and the potential for subsequent aortic stump or retroperitoneal sepsis.[14,15] It is important to remember that all graft-enteric fistula patients, including those without perigraft purulence, have by definition an infected aortic graft.[16] Investigators have suggested that prosthetic graft infection is the major underlying cause for graft-enteric fistula.[7,17] Others have emphasized the importance of mechanical factors.[18] Clearly, those patients with a proximal aortic pseudoaneurysm are at increased risk for a graft-enteric fistula.[6]

Diagnosis

The modalities used to diagnose primary graft infection are also used in patients suspected of graft-enteric fistula. Unfortunately, there are important limitations to all available tests. According to one recent review, computer tomography (CT) scanning has only a 57% sensitivity for diagnosing aortic graft infection, thus producing a disappointing number of false-negative exams.[1] Positive scan findings limited to perigraft fluid or gas remote to the performance of surgery are, however, highly specific for late graft infection.[19,20] Perigraft fluid that is noted on CT scanning can be needle aspirated and cultured, which is the next logical step.[21] This approach allows for a definitive preoperative diagnosis including perioperative antibiotic coverage aimed specifically at the offending organisms. Perigraft gas noted on CT scanning is virtually pathognomonic of graft-enteric fistula, although a gas-producing bacterial graft infection without bowel involvement may rarely be the explanation[19] (Fig. 1). Therefore, upper endoscopy and CT scanning are unquestionably the two most useful tests available for the preoperative detection of graft-enteric fistulae.

Unlike CT scanning, indium labeled white blood cell scans are overly sensitive (low specificity), resulting in a number of false-positive exams[22] (Table 1). In addition, leukocyte scans require at least 24 hours to perform and therefore are frequently not feasible in the acutely bleeding patient. Other tests used in patients suspected of having aortic graft infections include magnetic resonance imaging and immunoglobulin scans. Magnetic resonance imaging is quite sensitive to the presence of perigraft fluid, although gas images black with magnetic resonance, which makes it difficult to discriminate gas from calcific aortic

Table 1
Sensitivity and Specificity of Testing for Prosthetic Graft Infection*

Test modality	% Sens	% Spec
CT scan†	57	100
Indium-labeled WBC scan	96	85
MRI scan	85	100
Indium-labeled immunoglobulin G scan	88	100

CT = computer tomography; WBC = white blood cell; MRI = magnetic resonance imaging.
* Compiled from patients with clinical suspicion of late prosthetic graft infection.[23–31]
† Positive scan defined by presence of perigraft gas or fluid (From Yeager[1]).

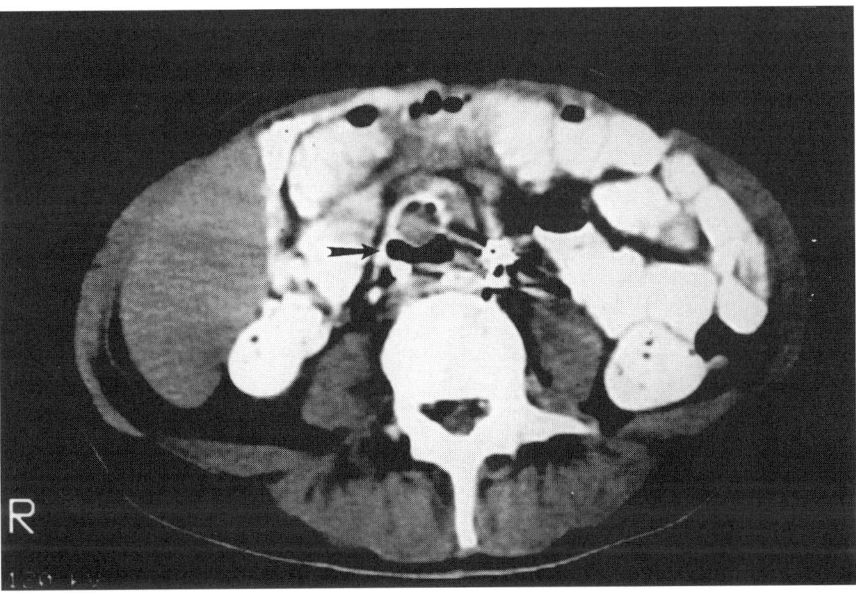

Figure 1. Computer tomography scan demonstrating perigraft gas (depicted by arrow) in patient with graft-enteric fistula.

plaque.[30] Limited data are available on immunoglobulin scans, although preliminary results suggest a high sensitivity for detection of aortic graft infection.[31] As with leukocyte scanning, however, additional experience may prove that this high sensitivity is associated with a low specificity. Arteriography is of limited use in the diagnosis of graft-enteric fistula, although it may be quite useful in the patient with gastrointestinal bleeding of uncertain etiology. Additionally, perioperative arteriography may be quite helpful in patients with graft-enteric fistulae in defining arterial anatomy and aiding in surgical planning. Documentation of renal artery patency and location is especially important prior to aortic graft excision.

Management Strategy

Clearly, the ideal management of graft-enteric fistula is prevention. Preventative measures used at the time of initial aortic grafting include those aimed at reducing graft infection rates as well as assuring complete coverage of the prosthetic graft with autogenous tissue, which helps prevent a mechanical origin for graft-enteric fistula.[16,32]

Optimal surgical management of graft-enteric fistula includes an initial extra-anatomic bypass, followed by aortic graft excision.[33-39] Authors have recommended staging the two operative procedures with an intervening interval of 2 to 6 days.[33,34,38] This approach avoids the cumulative physiologic stress of two synchronous procedures, but obviously requires two anesthetics and places the patient at risk for hemorrhage during the intervening period. Our preference is to perform both procedures during the same operation (sequential operations), often using two operating teams to reduce total operative time requirements.[36] In our opinion and that of others, initial extra-anatomic bypass followed by graft excision, when possible, is distinctly preferable to initial aortic graft excision followed by bypass because limb salvage rates are improved by performing the extra-anatomic bypass first

Table 2
Surgical Results for Management of Aortic Graft Infection According to Sequence and Staging of Extra-Anatomic Bypass and Aortic Graft Excision*

	% Mortality	% Amputation	% Extra-anatomic Bypass Graft Sepsis
Extra-anatomic bypass followed by graft excision	21	11	18
Graft excision followed by extra-anatomic bypass	26	46	23

* Data based on selected reports since 1980[35-39] and includes patients with graft-enteric fistula (From Yeager.[1])

(Table 2). It is, of course, arguable that such results may be skewed, since cases were not prospectively randomized and selected unstable patients required emergent aortic graft excision in order to control bleeding.

Some authors have recommended in situ aortic replacement grafting in selected patients with graft-enteric fistulae.[15,40] Walker et al. reported a 30% mortality with in situ grafting in this setting.[15] Those patients with perigraft purulence, however, had a 60% mortality including significant graft-related morbidity. These results suggest to us that while there may be a limited role for in situ grafting in carefully selected patients without perigraft purulence, this procedure certainly cannot be recommended generally at this time.

Patient Evaluation

Our perioperative evaluation of aortic graft patients with acute gastrointestinal bleeding includes upper endoscopy and CT scanning in all hemodynamically stable patients. In addition, colonoscopy is performed if lower gastrointestinal bleeding is suspected. If the diagnosis of graft-enteric fistula is confirmed, angiography is performed, followed by sequential axillary-bifemoral bypass and immediate aortic graft excision. If there is doubt concerning the diagnosis after angiography and the patient shows evidence of ongoing bleeding, we proceed with diagnostic laparotomy, which includes total duodenal dissection from the aortic graft. In one series of aortic graft patients with gastrointestinal bleeding, 26% were ultimately found at laparotomy to have a graft-enteric fistula.[41] If at laparotomy the fistula is identified but not disrupted and there is no current hemorrhage, then the abdominal incision is closed and the extra-anatomic bypass is performed. A negative diagnostic laparotomy is complete only after all bowel is surgically reflected away from the underlying prosthetic graft.

The nonbleeding patient suspected of having a graft-enteric fistula may undergo preoperative indium labeled white blood cell scanning. A nondiagnostic but suspicious CT scan in conjunction with a positive leukocyte scan is sufficient to warrant preliminary extra-anatomic bypass in many patients. In addition, the aortic graft patient with persistent or recurrent gastrointestinal bleeding of uncertain etiology in spite of a complete workup including a negative CT and leukocyte scan may require laparotomy as a final diagnostic maneuver to exclude graft-enteric fistula.[42,43] Once graft-enteric fistula is definitively excluded, management is simplified and further diagnostic and therapeutic efforts can focus on other causes for gastrointestinal bleeding.

Surgical Technique

Patients with aortoiliac grafts undergo a standard axillobifemoral bypass grafting to the common femoral arteries. The graft of choice is an 8 mm externally supported polytetrafluoroethylene (PTFE) prosthesis, which in our experience has a 75% 5-year primary patency.[44] The axillary artery supplying the arm with the highest brachial systolic pressure is the preferred site of inflow, usually the right. Our preference is to construct the femorofemoral component first and then insert the graft from the axillary artery onto the femorofemoral bypass in proximity to one of the femoral anastomoses.[44] This configuration maximizes flow through the entire length of the axillofemoral graft.

Patients with aortofemoral grafts require a more complex extra-anatomic revascularization. The axillary limb of the graft is routed lateral to the anterior superior iliac spine thereby avoiding the groin. When the superficial femoral artery is occluded, the distal profunda femoris artery is isolated lateral to the sartorius muscle, obviating a reoperative groin dissection[45] (Fig. 2). The femorofemoral segment of the graft is routed medial to the groin sites of the previous operation and often is tunneled in the subcutaneous tissues inferior to the pubic bone. Rarely an autogenous vein is used for the cross-pubic portion of the bypass if by necessity it courses within a region of infection.[12,46] Alternatively, in selected cases, bilateral axillary distal grafts may be performed.[47]

Once the extra-anatomic bypass is completed, the graft-enteric fistula can be approached in an unhurried and deliberate fashion. Supraceliac aortic control may be required.[48] Following division of the fistula, the bowel defect is repaired preferably by lateral closure. Complete excision of the aortic graft and involved tissues with drainage of purulence and debridement of the aortic wall is of utmost importance.[36,49] Rarely, renal artery bypass or relocation may be required to permit adequate proximal aortic debridement. When possible, circumferential dissection of the infrarenal aorta facilitates a secure closure without tension. Optimally, aortic stump closure is performed in two layers using a large mo-

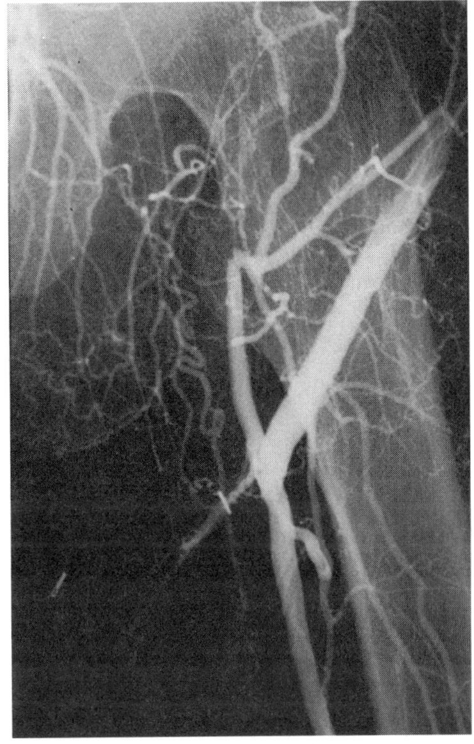

Figure 2. Arteriogram demonstrating axillofemoral bypass to profunda femoris artery exposed by a lateral approach.

nofilament suture. The omentum is often used as vascularized tissue coverage for the aortic stump.[50] Posteriorly placed, retroperitoneal drains are used in those patients with periaortic purulence.[49]

Current Surgical Mortality and Long-Term Survival

Historically, the surgical correction of graft-enteric fistula has been associated with poor results. Recent authors, however, have reported more encouraging mortality rates generally ranging from 15% to 20%.[38,39] The 5-year survival by life-table analysis approximates 50%, which is a manifestation of the coexisting medical problems present in these patients.[36]

Summary

Despite our best efforts to minimize graft-enteric fistulae, a few will inevitably occur. A high index of suspicion is key to a prompt diagnosis and surgical correction. Optimal treatment includes extra-anatomic prosthetic bypass through clean tissue followed by aortic graft excision. Results with this surgical approach are improving. Nonetheless, graft-enteric fistula remains a difficult surgical problem to treat successfully, and new management innovations deserve careful consideration and analysis including extended follow-up.

References

1. Yeager RA, Porter JM. Basic data concerning arterial and prosthetic graft infection. *Ann Vasc Surg.* 1992;6:485–491.
2. Reilly LM, Ehrenfeld WK, Goldstone J, Stoney RJ. Gastrointestinal tract involvement by prosthetic graft infection: the significance of gastrointestinal hemorrhage. *Ann Surg.* 1985;202:342–348.
3. Elliott JP, Smith RF, Szilagyi DE. Aorto-enteric and paraprosthetic-enteric fistulae: problems of diagnosis and management. *Arch Surg.* 1974;108:479–490.
4. Champion MC, Sullivan SN, Coles JC, Goldbach M, Watson WC. Aortoenteric fistula: incidence, presentation, recognition, and management. *Ann Surg.* 1982;195:314–317.
5. Puglia E, Fry PD. Aortoenteric fistulas: a preventable problem? *Can J Surg.* 1980;23:74–76.
6. Connolly JE, Kwaan JHM, McCart PM, Brownell DA, Levine EF. Aortoenteric fistula. *Ann Surg.* 1981;194:402–412.
7. Paaske WP, Hansen HJB. Graft-enteric fistulas and erosions. *Surg Gynecol Obstet.* 1985;161:161–164.
8. Vollmar JF, Kogel H. Aorto-enteric fistulas as postoperative complication. *J Cardiovasc Surg.* 1987;28:479–484.
9. Perdue GD Jr, Smith RB III, Ansley JD, Costantino MJ. Impending aortoenteric hemorrhage: the effect of early recognition and improved outcome. *Ann Surg.* 1980;192:237–243.
10. Bunt TJ, Doerhoff CR. Endoscopic visualization of an intraluminal Dacron graft: definitive diagnosis of aortoduodenal fistula. *South Med J.* 1984;77:86–87.
11. Schmitt DD, Seabrook GR, Bandyk DF, Towne JB. Graft excision and extra-anatomic revascularization: the treatment of choice for the septic aortic prosthesis. *J Cardiovasc Surg.* 1990;31:327–332.
12. Yeager RA, McConnell DB, Sasaki TM, Vetto RM. Aortic and peripheral prosthetic graft infection: differential management and causes of mortality. *Am J Surg.* 1985;150:36–43.
13. Bunt TJ. Synthetic vascular graft infections. II: Graft-enteric erosions and graft-enteric fistulas. *Surgery.* 1983;94:1–9.
14. Higgins RSD, Steed DL, Julian TB, Makaroun MS, Peitzman AB, Webster MW. The management of aortoenteric and paraprosthetic-fistulae. *J Cardiovasc Surg.* 1990;31:81–86.
15. Walker WE, Cooley DA, Duncan JM, Hallman GL Jr, Ott DA, Reul GJ. The management of aortoduodenal fistula by in situ replacement of the infected abdominal aortic graft. *Ann Surg.* 1987;205:727–732.
16. Bunt TJ. Synthetic vascular graft infections, I: graft infections. *Surgery.* 1983;93:733–746.
17. Busuttil RW, Rees W, Baker JD, Wilson SE. Pathogenesis of aortoduodenal fistula: experimental and clinical correlates. *Surgery.* 1979;85:1.
18. Kiernan PD, Pairolero PC, Hubert JP Jr, Mucha P Jr, Wallace RB. Aortic graft-enteric fistula. *Mayo Clin Proc.* 1980;55:731–738.
19. Low RN, Wall SD, Jeffrey RB Jr, Sollitto RA, Reilly LM, Tierney LM Jr. Aortoenteric fistula and perigraft infection: evaluation with CT. *Radiology.* 1990;175:157–162.
20. Qvarfordt PG, Reilly LM, Mark AS, et al. Computerized tomographic assessment of graft incorporation after aortic reconstruction. *Am J Surg.* 1985;150:227–231.
21. Katz BH, Black RA, Colley DP. CT-guided fine needle aspiration of a periaortic collection. *J Vasc Surg.* 1987;5:762–764.
22. Gilbert BR, Cerqueira MD, Vea HW, Nelp WB. Indium-111 labeled leukocyte uptake: false-positive results in noninfected pseudoaneurysms. *Radiology.* 1986;158:761–763.
23. Mark AS, McCarthy SM, Moss AA, Price D. Detection of abdominal aortic graft infection: comparison of CT and In-labeled white blood cell scans. *AJR.* 1985;144:315–318.
24. Williamson MR, Boyd CM, Read RC, et al. 111 In-labeled leukocytes in the detection of prosthetic vascular graft infections. *AJR.* 1986;147:173–176.
25. Olofsson PA, Auffermann W, Higgins CB, Rabahie GN, Tavares N, Stoney RJ. Diagnosis of prosthetic aortic graft infection by magnetic resonance imaging. *J Vasc Surg.* 1988;8:99–105.

26. Lawrence PF, Dries DJ, Alazraki N, Albo D Jr. Indium 111-labeled leukocyte scanning for detection of prosthetic vascular graft infection. *J Vasc Surg.* 1985;2:165–173.

27. Brunner MC, Mitchell RS, Baldwin JC, et al. Prosthetic graft infection: limitations of indium white blood cell scanning. *J Vasc Surg.* 1986;3:42–48.

28. Berridge DC, Earnshaw JJ, Frier M, et al. 111 In-labelled leucocyte imaging in vascular graft infection. *Br J Surg.* 1989;76:41–44.

29. Reilly DT, Grigg MJ, Cunningham DA, Thomas EJ, Mansfield AO. Vascular graft infection: the role of indium scanning. *Eur J Vasc Surg.* 1989;3:393–397.

30. Auffermann W, Olofsson PA, Rabahie GN, Tavares NJ, Stoney RJ, Higgins CB. Incorporation versus infection of retroperitoneal aortic grafts: MR imaging features. *Radiology.* 1989;172:359–362.

31. LaMuraglia GM, Fischman AJ, Strauss HW, et al. Utility of the indium 111-labeled human immunoglobulin G scan for the detection of focal vascular graft infection. *J Vasc Surg.* 1989;10:20–28.

32. Yeager RA, Moneta GL, Taylor LM Jr, McConnell DB, Porter JM. Can prosthetic graft infection be avoided? If not, how do we treat it? *Acta Chir Scand Suppl.* 1990;555: 155–163.

33. Trout HH III, Kozloff L, Giordano JM. Priority of revascularization in patients with graft enteric fistulas, infected arteries, or infected arterial prostheses. *Ann Surg.* 1984;199: 669–683.

34. Ricotta JJ, Faggioli GL, Stella A, et al. Total excision and extra-anatomic bypass for aortic graft infection. *Am J Surg.* 1991;162: 145–149.

35. O'Hara PJ, Hertzer NR, Beven EG, Krajewski LP. Surgical management of infected abdominal aortic grafts: review of a 25-year experience. *J Vasc Surg.* 1986; 3:725–731.

36. Yeager RA, Moneta GL, Taylor LM Jr, Harris EJ Jr, McConnell DB, Porter JM. Improving survival and limb salvage in patients with aortic graft infection. *Am J Surg.* 1990;159: 466–469.

37. Quinones-Baldrich WJ, Hernandez JJ, Moore WS. Long-termresults following surgical management of aortgic graft infection. *Arch Surg.* 1991;126:507–511.

38. Reilly LM, Stoney RJ, Goldstone J, Ehrenfeld WK. Improved management of aortic graft infection: the influence of operation sequence and staging. *J Vasc Surg.* 1987;5: 421–431.

39. Bergeron P, Espinoza H, Rudondy P, et al. Secondary aortoduodenal fistulas: value of initial axillofemoral bypass. *Ann Vasc Surg.* 1991;5:4–7.

40. Robinson JA, Johansen K. Aortic sepsis: is there a role for in situ graft reconstruction? *J Vasc Surg.* 1991;13:677–684.

41. Yeager RA, Sasaki TM, McConnell DB, Vetto RM. Clinical spectrum of patients with infrarenal aortic grafts and gastrointestinal bleeding. *Am J Surg.* 1987;153:459–461.

42. Freimanis IE, Kozak B, Taylor LM Jr, Porter JM. Failure of CT scanning to diagnose aortic graft infection. *J Vasc Surg.* 1987;5:779–780.

43. Pabst TS III, Bernhard VM, McIntyre KE Jr, Malone JM. Gastrointestinal bleeding after aortic surgery: the role of laparotomy to rule out aortoenteric fistula. *J Vasc Surg.* 1988;8: 280–285.

44. Harris EJ Jr, Taylor LM Jr, Moneta GL, Yeager RA, Porter JM. Extra-anatomic bypass: a new look. In: Cameron JL, ed. *Advances in Surgery, Vol. 26.*. St. Louis: Mosby Year Book; 1992.

45. Naraynsingh V, Karmody AM, Leather RP, Corson JD. Lateral approach to the profunda femoris artery. *Am J Surg.* 1984;147:813–814.

46. Seeger JM, Wheeler JR, Gregory RT, Snyder SO, Gayle RG. Autogenous graft replacement of infected prosthetic grafts in the femoral position. *Surgery.* 1983;93:39–45.

47. Ascer E, Veith FJ, Gupta S. Axillopopliteal bypass grafting: indications, late results, and determinants of long-term patency. *J Vasc Surg.* 1989;10:285–291.

48. Veith FJ, Gupta S, Daly V. Technique for occluding the supraceliac aorta through the abdomen. *Surg Gynecol Obstet.* 1980;151: 427–429.

49. Taylor LM Jr, Deitz DM, McConnell DB, Porter JM. Treatment of infected abdominal aneurysms by extra-anatomic bypass, aneurysm excision, and drainage. *Am J Surg.* 1988; 155:655.

50. Iliopoulos JI, Pierce GE, Thomas JH, Hermreck AS. Transmesocolic omentoplasty. *Surg Gynecol Obstet.* 1983;157:283–284.

Chapter 20

In-Situ Interposition Grafting for Aortic Sepsis

K. Johansen

Introduction

The catastrophic nature of bacterial infection of the aorta, whether primary or consequent to prosthetic graft involvement, scarcely requires emphasis. Mortality rates as high as 75% and lower extremity amputation rates of equivalent levels have been documented in such patients.[1-3] Operative therapy for aortic sepsis is complicated and prolonged, and may not solve the problem. Aortic stump blowout has been reported in as many as 60% of survivors of operative therapy for aortic sepsis,[3] and frequent complications associated with attempts at extra-anatomic bypass to the lower extremities have been recorded as well.[1-4]

All factors considered, optimal therapy for aortic disease would involve in-situ interposition aortic replacement with a suitable prosthetic graft. However, performing such a procedure in the presence of bacterial contamination or infection obviously risks immediate graft infection and sepsis. Standard practice since the 1960s for managing aortoiliac sepsis, either primary or in the presence of prosthetic grafts, has mandated aortic or graft excision, aortic ligation, and extra-anatomic bypass.[1,2,5]

Recently we have reported a successful experience, in carefully selected cases, of in-situ graft replacement for aortic sepsis;[6] others have reported similar successes.[3,7-12] There are reasons one would consider such a *radical* approach, and clinical settings which might be appropriate to pursue.

Clinical Settings

Aortic sepsis manifests itself in several different scenarios:

1. bacterial aortitis,[13] mycotic aortic aneurysm,[14] or secondarily infected aortic aneurysm[15]
2. primary aortoenteric fistula (AEF)[16]
3. aortic graft infection with or without erosion into the gut (secondary AEF or prosthetic enteric erosion).[1-3,5,17,18]

Clinical presentation, bacteriology, and appropriate diagnostic maneuvers in patients harboring various forms of aortic sepsis are discussed elsewhere in this monograph. The current discussion will focus on

From Bunt, TJ: *Vascular Graft Infections.* Armonk: Futura Publishing Co., Inc.; © 1994.

the indications for and techniques of in situ operative management options for this catastrophic problem.

Natural History

Aortic sepsis with or without the presence of a prosthetic graft is a potential disaster. If aneurysm formation and rupture does not result in massive hemorrhage (generally in an elderly patient with both cardiovascular disease and sepsis), septic emboli or aortic thrombosis may supervene. Since operations performed to treat infected aortic prostheses must remove the entire graft because attempts to save residual graft lead predictably to further infection,[18,19] the patient is left at substantial risk of lower extremity ischemia, especially if the original graft was placed for aneurysmal disease. Grafts placed to treat aortoiliac occlusive disease can sometimes be removed, counting upon endarterectomy and/or previously developed collaterals to maintain distal perfusion until infection is eradicated and wounds are healed.[20] While we have reported a case of spontaneous healing of a mycotic aortic aneurysm,[21] and successful treatment of a perigraft abscess by percutaneous catheter drainage has been reported,[22] infectious processes involving the aorta more often mandate operative intervention in virtually all circumstances.

Traditional Approach

Aortic infection in the form of aortitis[13] or mycotic aneurysm[14] (occurring frequently in patients with contiguous sepsis, bacterial endocarditis, or depressed immune competence), was considered uniformly lethal as late as 1967.[23] Early in the development of vascular surgery, it became evident that prosthetic grafts in the vascular tree were particularly prone to infection and, once infected, they required removal in their entirety. New grafts placed in the previously contaminated bed inevitably became reinfected. Through the 1950s and early 1960s, aortic infection, whether primary or following graft procedures, was tantamount to a death sentence.

Introduction of the concept of extra-anatomic bypass grafting through remote tissue planes by Louw[24] and Blaisdell[25] in the early 1960s offered, for the first time, a rational and feasible solution to the previously certain catastrophe of aortic sepsis. Use of the thoracic aorta or the axillary artery as a donor site to reperfuse the lower extremities via prosthetic grafts tunneled through remote (and presumably uninfected) tissue planes was a clinical revelation.[26] While the mortality rate associated with aortic sepsis remained high, primarily because of the triple-negative impact of sepsis, blood loss, and emergency operation in a systemically compromised elderly host, selected patients with mycotic aneurysm, AEF, or aortic graft infection now survived. Axillofemoral bypass grafting, either bilateral or unilateral with a femorofemoral cross-pubic graft, now could provide predictable survival in patients with aortic sepsis, especially if the diagnosis could be made prior to the onset of septic shock or massive blood loss.

Unfortunately, extra-anatomic bypass was found to have major shortcomings. While axillofemoral bypass itself proved minimally invasive, the extra time required to perform this revascularization procedure, when combined with an extensive aortic resection to treat mycotic aneurysm or aortic graft infection, frequently prolonged the overall procedure unacceptably.[27] In addition, axillofemoral grafts were prone to thrombosis, cutaneous erosion, infection, and other such complications, leading to overall 5-year success rates as low as 60%.[4,28] In addition, the presumption of safety in *remote* tissue planes proved to be illusory: the extra-anatomic graft can be subject to (secondary blood-borne?) infection.[21] Finally, a disquieting observation was that a frequent cause of later demise in patients who had undergone aortic resection for sepsis was rupture of a pseudoaneurysm of the oversewn aortic stump, either into the retroperitoneum or as a recurrent aortoenteric fistula.[3,19] While such aortic stump blowout resulted in some cases from residual aortitis in the oversewn aorta,[29] the conclusion was inescapable that aortic ligation risks further lethal complications.

Furthermore, whereas extra-anatomic bypass may be effective for revascularizing the lower body following resection of the infrarenal aorta, sepsis involving the ascending or transverse thoracic aorta or suprarenal abdominal aorta, provides a much greater challenge for reconstruction. Not only does distal revascularization need to be accomplished, but restoration of blood flow to the large branch arteries—the great vessels of the head and neck, or the visceral and renal arteries—needs to be assured. There are ways in which in situ reconstruction can be used in such a setting.

In Situ Reconstruction for Aortic Sepsis

As previously noted, attempts to perform aortic reconstruction in an infected bed had generally proven unsuccessful. Recurrent infection of the new graft was predictable. In 1978, however, we were confronted by three consecutive patients with isolated, nonruptured mycotic aortic aneurysms. In each case the aneurysmal process, while extensive, was circumscribed and isolated to the aorta and the periaortic retroperitoneal tissues. It seemed intuitive that radical local excision combined with in situ aortic interposition grafting and long-term parenteral antibiotics might be a reasonable alternative[14] (Fig.1) Subsequently in situ aortic reconstruction was extended to selected patients with secondary aortoenteric fistula and secondarily infected bland aortic aneurysms. Among 11 such patients treated in this fashion no recurrent graft complications have occurred during follow-up ranging from 1 to 12 years.[6]

Others, working with the thorny dilemma of sepsis involving the upper thoracic or juxtarenal aorta, have demonstrated similar success. Atnip presented a well-documented case of a supraceliac aortic mycotic aneurysm managed by radical excision

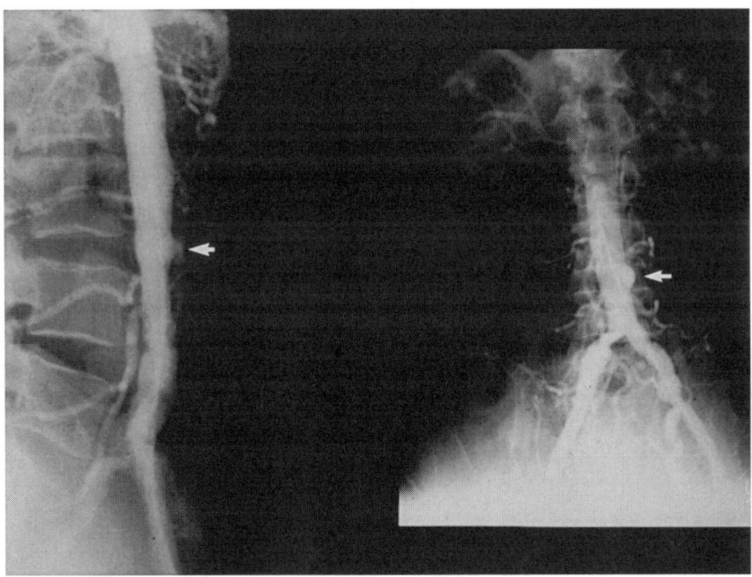

Figure 1. An aortogram in a middle-aged alcoholic man with streptococcal bacteremia (A) shows saccular outpouching consistent with a mycotic aortic aneurysm.

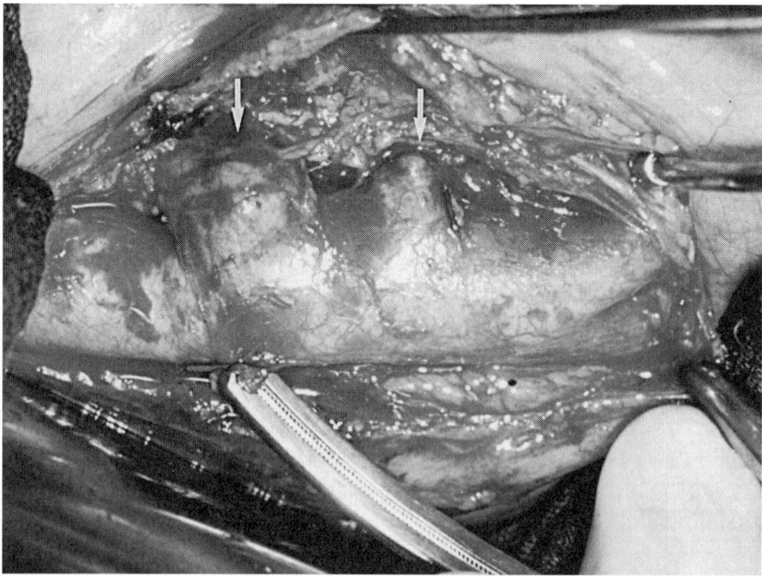

Figure 1B. An aortogram in a middle-aged alcoholic man with streptococcal bacteria. Operative view from the patient's right side shows two, well-circumscribed mycotic aortic aneurysms without evidence of suppuration or extravasation.

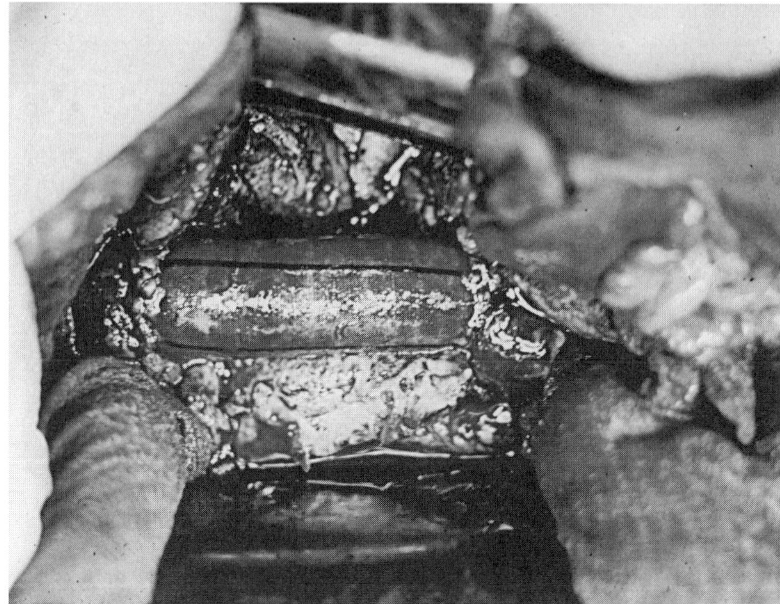

Figure 1C. An aortogram in a middle-aged alcoholic man with streptococcal bacteremia. Radical local excision of the aorta bearing the mycotic aneurysms, followed by in situ interposition aortic reconstruction.

of the aorta and graft interposition, with visceral artery reimplantation.[8] Walker et al. demonstrated excellent results with in situ reconstruction of the ascending and transverse thoracic aorta for mycotic processes,[9] and Chan et al., from the same Houston group, reported 22 patients with in situ thoracic or supraceliac abdominal aortic reconstruction. Patients undergoing such procedures were followed up for as much as 14 years, with only a 12% complication rate.[10]

Cardinal principles underlying these successful results with in situ aortic reconstruction in our hands,[6,14] and those of others[7-12] revolve around initial patient selection and operative technique. Patients who are actively bacteremic, or who have widespread suppuration or other evidence for uncontrolled infection at the time of exploration, would undergo *conventional* management—excision of the infectious process, aortic oversew, and extra-anatomic bypass Table 1). Patients with Gram-negative aortic involvement have unusually virulent infections[30] and also should probably be treated with aortic excision and remote bypass.

When the septic process is circumscribed, such as a nonruptured mycotic aortic aneurysm[14] or a localized erosion between a graft and the intestinal tract,[2,3] and where radical local excision back to uninvolved tissue planes can be accomplished, in situ reconstruction seems a rational alternative. We propose at least 6 weeks of parenteral antibiotics. Crawford's group suggests that lifelong antibiotics may be warranted.[10,11] In addition, serial surveillance of these patients, probably by computerized tomographic scanning,[31] is prudent to herald the development of pseudoaneurysms or other suture line complications.

Infection of aortic prosthetic grafts generally has been felt to require total resection of the involved graft, ligation of the aorta, and extra-anatomic bypass, an approach believed warranted because of the diffuse suppuration generally involving infected grafts. Emboldened by the observation that local resection and in situ aortic graft interposition was performed successfully in several cases of AEF,[32] Bandyk et al. have demonstrated early success with in situ replacement of aortic grafts infected by coagulase-negative staphylococcal biofilms.[33] This approach has not yet been widely adopted, and should probably be restricted to patients whose pre- and intraoperative evaluations demonstrate localized rather than generalized graft involvement.

Technical Considerations

Recently reported reviews of large experiences with axillofemoral bypass grafts suggest that technological advances involving extra-anatomic bypass grafting may have sharply improved the likelihood of long-term success. Both Porter's group in Portland[34] and Sauvage and his colleagues in Seattle[35] report 5-year patency rates exceeding 75% with axillofemoral bypass grafting. These advances, primarily involving external support of these grafts with plastic rings, may prevent compression of the graft by the weight of the patient during sleeping, thereby reducing the risk of acute thrombosis. If these results are borne out in other series, the previously unacceptable high-complication and failure rate of axillofemoral bypass grafting will be a less compelling justification for using the alternate therapy of in situ graft interposition for aortic sepsis.

Table 1
Treatment of Aortic Graft Infection with In Situ Graft Replacement

Indications	Contraindications
Nonruptured mycotic aneurysm	Systemic sepsis
Circumscribed infection	Widespread suppuration
Graft-enteric erosion	Uncontrolled infection
	Gram-negative infection

There may be better or worse choices for the optimal prosthetic graft to use in a potentially infected or contaminated site. Experiences growing out of the need for readily available arterial graft materials in contaminated traumatic wounds has suggested, both experimentally and clinically, that polytetrafluoroethylene (PTFE) grafts may be relatively infection-resistant in comparison to Dacron prostheses.[36-38] While autogenous reconstruction (either by vein, arterial autografts, endarterectomy, or simple reperfusion of previously existing collaterals) may be feasible in certain circumstances,[20,39] the optimal choice when prosthetic graft is mandated may well be PTFE.

Summary

Aortic sepsis is a medical and surgical catastrophe whose outcome is predictably lethal unless diagnosis and treatment are timely and effective. Total excision of involved aortic tissue and prosthetic grafts, oversew of the aorta, and distal revascularization through remote extra-anatomic tissue planes is a *conventional* approach, recently validated by newer, externally reinforced graft materials. In carefully selected patients whose septic aortic processes are relatively circumscribed, the technically more straightforward procedure of radical aortic debridement and in situ graft interposition appears to be a safe, effective, and durable alternative. In either case, long-term antibiotic administration and serial postoperative surveillance for recurrent complications involving the ligated or reconstructed aorta seem prudent.

References

1. Bunt TJ: Synthetic vascular graft infections. I: graft infection. *Surgery.* 1983;93:733–746.
2. Bunt TJ. Synthetic vascular graft infections. II: graft- enteric erosions and graft-enteric fistulas. *Surgery.* 1983;94:1–9.
3. Moulton S, Adams M, Johansen K. Aortoenteric fistula: a 7-year experience. *Am J Surg.* 1986;151:607–611.
4. Vaccaro PS, Harvey B, Fanning WJ, Smead WL. Axillofemoral bypass graft: the outcome of 66 procedures. *Vasc Surg.* 1986;11:157–160.
5. Schmitt DD, Seabrook GR, Bandyk DF, Towne JB. Graft excision and extra-anatomic revascularization: the treatment of choice for the septic aortic prosthesis. *J Cardiovasc Surg.* 1990;31:327–332.
6. Robinson JA, Johansen K. Aortic sepsis: is there a role for in situ graft reconstruction? *J Vasc Surg.* 1991;13:677–684.
7. Brown SL, Busuttil RW, Baker JD, Machleder HI, Moore WS, Barker WF. Bacteriologic and surgical determinants of survival in patients with mycotic aneurysms. *J Vasc Surg.* 1984; 1:541–547.
8. Atnip RG. Mycotic aneurysms of the suprarenal abdominal aorta: prolonged survival after in situ aortic and visceral reconstruction. *J Vasc Surg.* 1989;10:635–641.
9. Walker WE, Cooley DA, Duncan JM, Hallman GL, Ott DA, Reul GJ. The management of aortoduodenal fistula by in situ replacement of the infected abdominal aortic graft. *Ann Surg.* 1987;727–732.
10. Chan FY, Crawford ES, Coselli JS, Safi HJ, Williams TW. In situ prosthetic graft replacement for mycotic aneurysm of the aorta. *Ann Thorac Surg.* 1989;47:193–203.
11. Coselli J, Crawford ES, Williams TW, et al. Treatment of postoperative infection of ascending aorta and transverse aortic arch, including use of viable omentum and muscle flaps. *Ann Thorac Surg.* 1990;50:868–881.
12. Jacobs MJHM, Reul GJ, Gregoric I, Cooley DA. In situ replacement and extra-anatomic bypass for the treatment of infected abdominal aortic grafts. *Eur J Vasc Surg.* 1991;5: 83–86.
13. Bardin JA, Collins GM, Devin JB, Halasz NA. Nonaneurysmal suppurative aortitis. *Arch Surg.* 1981;116:954–956.
14. Johansen K, Devin J. Mycotic aortic aneurysm: a reappraisal. *Arch Surg.* 1983;118: 583–588.
15. Rogers AJ, Rowlands BJ, Flynn TC. Infected aortic aneurysm after intra-abdominal abscess. *Tex Heart Inst J.* 1987;14:208–214.
16. Sweeney MS, Gadacz TR. Primary aortoduodenal fistula: manifestation, diagnosis, and treatment. *Surgery.* 1984;96:492–497.
17. Busuttil RW, Rees W, Baker JD, Wilson SE. Pathogenesis of aortoduodenal fistula: experimental and clinical correlates. *Surgery.* 1979;85:1–12.
18. Bergqvist D, Alm A. Secondary aortoenteric

fistula: an analysis of 42 cases. *Eur J Vasc Surg.* 1987;1:11–18.

19. O'Hara PJ, Hertzer NR, Beven EG, Krajewski LP. Surgical management of infected abdominal aortic grafts: review of a 25-year experience. *J Vasc Surg.* 1986;3:725–731.

20. Ehrenfeld WK, Wilbur BG, Olcott CN, Stoney RJ. Autogenous tissue reconstruction in the management of infected prosthetic grafts. *Surgery.* 1979;85:82–92.

21. Johansen KH, Devin J. Spontaneous healing of mycotic aortic aneurysms: a case report. *J Cardiovasc Surg (Torino).* 1980;21:625–627.

22. Katz BH, Black RA, Colley DP. CT-guided fine needle aspiration of a periaortic collection. *J Vasc Surg.* 1987;5:762–764.

23. Bennett DE, Cherry JK. Bacterial infection of aortic aneurysms: a clinicopathological study. *Am J Surg.* 1967;113:321–327.

24. Louw JH. The treatment of combined aortoiliac and femoropopliteal occlusive disease by splenofemoral and axillofemoral bypass grafts. *Surgery.* 1963;81:33–38.

25. Blaisdell FW, Hall AD. Axillary-femoral artery bypass for lower extremity ischemia. *Surgery.* 1963;54:563–568.

26. Shaw RS, Baue AE. Management of sepsis complicating arterial reconstructive surgery. *Surgery.* 1963;53:78–86.

27. Reilly LM, Stoney RJ, Goldstone J, Ehrenfeld WK. Improved management of aortic graft infection: the influence of operation sequence and staging. *J Vasc Surg.* 1987;5:421–431.

28. Inahara T, Geary GL, Mukherjee D, et al. The contrary position to the nonresective treatment of abdominal aortic aneurysm. *J Vasc Surg.* 1985;4:42–50.

29. Malone JM, Lalka SG, McIntyre KE, et al. The necessity for long-term antibiotic therapy with positive aortic wall cultures. *J Vasc Surg.* 1988;8:262–267.

30. Geary KJ, Tomkiewicz ZM, Harrison HN, et al. Differential effects of a Gram-negative and Gram-positive infection on autogenous and prosthetic grafts. *J Vasc Surg.* 1989;9:665–670.

31. Brown OW, Stanson AW, Pairolero PC, et al. Computerized tomography following abdominal aortic surgery. *Surgery.* 1982;91:716–722.

32. Thomas WEG, Baird RN. Secondary aortoenteric fistulae: towards a more conservative approach. *Br J Surg.* 1986;73:875–878.

33. Bandyk DF, Bergamini TM, Kinney EV, Seabrook GR, Towne JB. In situ replacement of vascular prostheses infected by bacterial biofilms. *J Vasc Surg.* 1991;13:575–583.

34. Harris EJ, Taylor LM, McConnell DB, Moneta GL, Yeager RA, Porter JM. Clinical results of axillobifemoral bypass using externally supported polytetrafluoroethylene. *J Vasc Surg.* 1990;12:416–421.

35. El-Massry S, Saad E, Sauvage LR, et al. A 12-year follow-up of axillofemoral grafts. *J Vasc Surg.* (in press).

36. Shah PM, Ito K, Clauss RH, Babu SC, Reynolds BM, Stahl WM. Expanded microporous polytetrafluoroethylene (PTFE) grafts in contaminated wounds: experimental and clinical study. *J Trauma.* 1983;23:1030–1033.

37. Stone KS, Walshaw R, Sugiyama GT, Dean RE, Dunston RW. Polytetrafluoroethylene versus autogenous vein grafts for vascular reconstruction in contaminated wounds. *Am J Surg.* 1984;147:692–695.

38. Rosenman JE, Pearce WH, Kempezinski WE. Bacterial adherence to vascular grafts after in vitro bacteremia. *J Surg Res.* 1985;38:648–655.

39. Quinones-Baldrich WJ, Moore W. Autogenous tissue reconstruction in the management of aortoiliac graft infection. *Ann Vasc Surg.* 1990;4:223–228.

Chapter 21

Management of Aortoenteric Communications

H.H. Trout, III
R.L. Feinberg
L. Kozloff

Introduction

Primary aortoduodenal fistula is not strictly related to infection of existing grafts, but it is worth noting that closure of the duodenal defect, aneurysm resection, and in situ placement of a prosthetic graft is successful and without an inordinate infection rate. Preplacement of a remote bypass does not seem to give better results than primary grafting in the aorta.[1-3]

Graft-Enteric Communication with Active Bleeding

Regardless of whether the diagnosis has been confirmed, active bleeding at a rate that would likely require multiple blood transfusions within hours does not allow time for a thorough evaluation. If the diagnosis of a graft-enteric communication is certain in this situation, immediate celiotomy is necessary. When the diagnosis is suspected but not confirmed, prompt celiotomy is still necessary due to active bleeding. In either setting, time does not permit remote bypass prior to interruption of the graft-enteric communication. As a consequence, the bowel defect should be repaired and an in situ aortobiliac prosthetic graft should be inserted.[3] An aortobifemoral graft should not be placed if it can be avoided. Even if the graft being replaced is an aorto-bifemoral graft, the femoral portions of the graft are rarely, if ever, infected in aortoenteric communications. When possible, it is important to leave the groins undisturbed at this time, thus preserving the option of dividing the old limbs in the groins for a newly constructed axillobifemoral graft should this later become necessary.

The complications associated with in situ graft insertion are usually recurrent graft infection or development of a pseudoaneurysm at the proximal anastomosis. The major complication rate with this approach is around 15%[4,5] and the mortality rate is about 30%.[4-6] The complications associated with construction of a remote bypass after repair of the bowel and removal of the old graft are myoglobinemia, acidosis, limb loss, or death secondary to the prolonged lower limb ischemia necessitated by the bowel repair and graft removal. The mortality with this approach is about 50% and the morbidity is substantial.

Because the in situ approach allows earlier lower limb revascularization and apparent lower morbidity and mortality rates (at least in the short term), this approach seems preferable for the patient who is actively bleeding. Careful postoperative monitoring of the patient's temperature and white blood count, as well as repeat magnetic resonance imaging (MRI) examinations (to reduce the radiation exposure that would occur if multiple computer tomography (CT) examinations were used) are important, especially for the first year postoperatively. When graft complications appear likely, an axillobifemoral bypass graft can then be constructed followed by removal of the reinfected in situ prosthetic graft.

In summary, in the patient with active bleeding, preferred treatment of a graft-enteric communication is in situ graft replacement. This approach has a lower mortality rate than the procedure of construction of a remote bypass after repair of the bowel and removal of the old graft. The option of remote bypass followed by repair of the graft-enteric communication is not available because of the active bleeding. In situ repair of an actively bleeding graft-enteric fistula allows earlier revascularization of the lower extremities. It preserves the option of later remote bypass followed by removal of the in situ graft if required.

Suspected Graft-Enteric Communication Without Active Bleeding

The presence of a graft-enteric communication is sometimes uncertain despite aggressive attempts to confirm the diagnosis. In this setting, the approach most likely to provide the best result is a celiotomy and exposure of the prosthetic graft distal to the proximal anastomosis. Usually the tissue covering the graft at a level uninvolved with the aortoenteric fistula will be thick and densely adherent to the graft. With patience and persistence, however, the space between the graft and this thick, covering layer can be identified. Once the distal graft is exposed, the overlying tissue covering the graft is divided longitudinally toward the proximal anastomosis. When a graft-enteric communication is present, an erosion in the midportion of the graft or bile staining of the graft will be detected before the communication is uncovered. At this point, the diagnosis is established and the aortic dissection should cease. The abdominal skin is stapled closed, the surrounding skin painted with benzoin, and a plastic adhesive dressing applied, isolating the abdominal incision. The patient should then be reprepared and draped, and an axillobifemoral graft inserted. These incisions are then covered with occlusive dressings; the abdomen is reopened, the bowel is repaired, and the old graft is removed.

Collected mortality with this technique of remote bypass constructed prior to repair of a graft-enteric fistula or erosion was reported to be only 17% in 1984[3] and is probably even lower now. Though in situ replacement has been advocated[4,5] in this setting, it is highly improbable that an approach which places a new prosthesis in an area of possible contamination and is associated with at least a moderate amount of distal limb ischemia (because of the time required to remove the old graft and insert a new one) will have as low a mortality rate (reported to be 56% in 1983 and 35% in 1987) and morbidity rate as that associated with a procedure (remote bypass first) that has minimal lower limb ischemia and entirely avoids the area of contamination.[2,3] The major advantage to the in situ approach is that late aortic stump blowout (with remote bypass and oversewing of the aorta) may occur more frequently than suture line breakdown with in situ repair. Although either approach (in situ or remote) may yield acceptable results (given the magnitude of the problem), the procedure of remote bypass followed by bowel repair and graft removal will give the better result.

Confirmed Graft-Enteric Communication Without Active Bleeding

Remote bypass followed by bowel repair and graft removal has a mortality rate of 17%. As a consequence, this is the procedure of choice since this is less than the mortality rate of 35% associated with in situ replacement and the mortality rate of 53% associated with graft removal followed by remote bypass.[1-6]

Algorithm of Treatment

1. Construct an axillobifemoral graft. If the previously inserted aortic graft was aortobifemoral, divide the graft and sew the new graft into the distal prosthetic limbs end-to-end. Close all wounds and cover with plastic adhesive dressing.

2. Open the abdomen from the xiphoid to the pubis; do not attempt to expose the proximal aortic suture line at first.

3. Expose the graft at one of the limbs of the graft if it is a bifurcation graft, otherwise at the distal end of the tube graft.

4. If the previous graft is an aortobifemoral bifurcation graft, pull the distal limbs of the aortic bifurcation graft into the abdomen (they will have been divided in the groins at the time of the remote bypass) and obliterate the graft tracts from the abdomen to the groins with monofilament or absorbable sutures.

5. Dissect the duodenum until it becomes markedly adherent to the pseudocapsule covering the aortic graft, then stop.

6. Have the anesthesiologist undertake whatever renal protective measures deemed appropriate (low dose dopamine, mannitol, etc.) to protect the kidneys.

7. Slowly cut the pseudocapsule along the graft from the distal point of exposure toward the proximal anastomosis until hematoma or modest bleeding is encountered.

8. Control any bleeding with direct pressure, make a small incision in the graft distally, insert a 30 cc balloon catheter in the small opening in the graft, advance the catheter to just proximal to the aortograft anastomosis, and inflate the balloon.

9. Continue to dissect the pseudocapsule away from the graft and expose the proximal suture line and fistula. If the proximal anastomosis of the aortic graft was constructed in an end-to-end fashion, disconnect the aortic graft and then dissect along both sides of the aorta just below the left renal vein, place a clamp on the aorta as the balloon is removed, and close the aorta and duodenum carefully. A major cause of failure of this approach is blowout of an infected aortic stump 5-to-21 days after the procedure. As a consequence, successful closure of the aortic stump is particularly important. Techniques which have been advocated to secure this closure include using monofilament sutures, staples, omentum, prevertebral fascia, reshaping the distal aorta by means of an inverted V closure, or covering the aortic stump with a jejunal patch. The critical component seems to be adequate removal of all contaminated tissue, including aortic wall.

When the proximal anastomosis of the aortic graft is constructed end-to-side and only modest contamination is found, another option for treatment is to debride the aorta around the edges where the graft was attached. The aortic wall defect can then be closed using autogenous patch material such as an endarterectomized segment of a previously thrombosed superficial femoral artery harvested at the time of insertion of the remote bypass.

10. If the proximal anastomosis of the aortic graft was constructed in an end-to-side fashion, dissect the duodenum away,

insert another 30 cc balloon into the aorta distal to the end-to-side anastomosis to control back bleeding, disconnect the aortic graft and then dissect down both sides of the aorta just below the left renal vein, place a clamp on the aorta as the balloon is removed, and close the aorta proximally and distally, using whatever technique seems most appropriate.

References

1. Bunt TJ. Synthetic vascular graft infections I: graft infections. *Surgery.* 1983;93:733–746.

2. Bunt TJ. Synthetic vascular graft infections II: graft enteric fistulae and erosions. *Surgery.* 1983;94:1–9.

3. Trout HH III, Kozloff L, Giordana M. Priority of revascularization in patients with graft enteric fistulae, infected arteries, or infected arterial prostheses. *Ann Surg.* 1984;199:669–683.

4. Robinson JA, Johansen K. Aortic sepsis: is there a role for in situ graft reconstruction? *J Vasc Surg.* 1991;13:677–682.

5. Pfeiffer RB Jr. Successful repair of 3 primary aortoduodenal fistulae. *Arch Surg.* 1982;117: 1098–1099.

6. Walker WE, Cooley DA, Duncan JM, et al. The management of aortoduodenal fistula by in situ replacement of the infected abdominal aortic graft. *Ann Surg.* 1987;205:727–732.

SECTION VII

Long-Term Results

The severity of your complications is inversely related to the quality of your operative indications.

Chapter 22

Overview of Long-Term Follow-up

T.J. Bunt

Introduction

Initial reviews of institutional series and the majority of smaller case studies of graft infection tended to focus on the immediate mortality and morbidity associated with treatment. Few authors specifically addressed the concept of long-term survival of those who survived the initial carnage.

Literature Review

The first researchers to make any comment on long-term effects were Fry and Lindenauer (1966). In reviewing 12 cases at Michigan they noted gloomily not only a 75% operative mortality, but that only 1 of 3 survivors remained asymptomatic at 5 years; of the other 2, 1 had severe claudication, and 1 was a bilateral amputee.[1]

Urdaneta (1969) reported on a single patient following extra-anatomic bypass (EAB) who was working and asymptomatic at 35 months. Spanos (1976) reported long-term follow-up on the five survivors of their seven graft infection, graft-enteric fistula (GIF/GEF) series. All were treated with resection and EAB. One died of recurrent aortoduodenal fistula-aortic stump sepsis (ADF/ASS) at 7 months, and two had recurrent retroperitoneal abscesses at 2 and 8 months but went on to survive 3.5 and 4 years. Two others were alive and well at 2.5 and 3.5 years. There were no late thromboses of axillofemoral grafts and no late amputations. The paper did underscore the tendency for persistent retroperitoneal sepsis, occurring in three of the five initial survivors.[2,3]

A decade later, authors were more sanguine about both initial mortalities and the long-term survivals. Fulenwider (1983) noted in the Emory series of 10 GIF and 11 graft-enteric erosions GEE/GEF that there were 4 late amputations in the 29 survivors. In 3 patients, in situ tertiary aortofemoral grafts were placed uneventfully for problems with EAB patency.[4]

Reilly (1984), in two related articles, detailed the USF experience. Eighty-eight percent of survivors (67 of 76) had no further problems. Of the GIF survivors, 83% had long-term cures (10% operative mortality plus 7% persistent sepsis, although 25% suffered major amputation). For GEF, the figures were less enthusiastic; an initial 21% mortality rate was compounded by an additional 28% delayed but related mortality, including 5 ASS, 2 GEF, and 2 cases of clinical sepsis. The 18 survivors were alive at a mean 42 months (8–104) with an additional 24% amputation rate. Of the total 59 survi-

337

vors of either GIF/GEF, 24 of the 59 required reoperation for subsequent ischemia, and 4 developed infection of that EAB. In 7 patients, tertiary reconstruction was performed with 1 mortality but no new GIF. The procedures included 5 retroperitoneal supracoeliac and 2 infrarenal in situ reconstructions.

Reilly's data may be summarized as showing that 83% of the survivors of GIF will do well as compared to only 51% of GEF, although that survival rate was achieved for both groups at a 25% amputation rate and the realization that half of the patients would require further thrombectomies of their EABs.[5,6]

O'Hara (1986) presented a similar experience from the Cleveland Clinic with 51 GIFs and 33 GEFs, but with disparate findings. Only 18% of patients were alive at 5 years, with an interval 27% amputation rate. The initial survival rate was different for GIF versus GEF; 30-day survival rate was 49% for GEF versus 86% for GEF ($P < .01$) but the long-term survival curves from thereon were similar (Fig. 1). Similarly, they noted an improvement with increased institutional experience (Fig. 2), with the 1-year survival rate being 31% prior to 1980 but 54% post-1980 ($P < .05$).[7]

Yeager (1990) described the mean 3.7 year (1–125 month) course of 28 survivors of 15 GEFs and 23 GIFs at Oregon. Thirty-two percent died during follow-up—3 of cardiac causes, 2 from carcinoma, and 1 each of 1 stroke, ASS, diverticulitis, and unknown causes. The cumulative 5-year survival rate was 77% with a 76% limb salvage rate. Subsequent EAB GIF occurred in 22%; 43% (3/7) Dacron grafts versus 13% (2/16) polytetrafluoroethylene (PTFE) ($P = .142$); and 24% (4/17) staged EABs versus 17% (1/6) sequential grafts ($P = 1$). Only 1 of 5 EAB GIFs occurred as a delayed phenomenon at 16 months; curiously, 3 of 6 were due to *Staphylococcus epidermidis*.[8]

Secondary EAB-GIF represented a problem, since it led to 7 of the 10 late limb amputations, whereas only 1 of 35 limbs at risk without an EAB-GIF came to amputa-

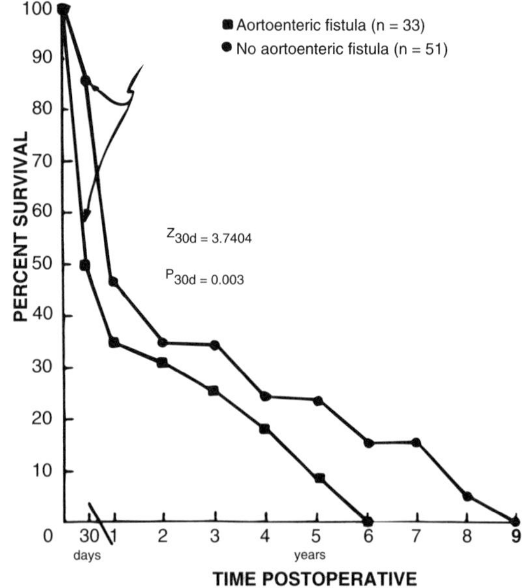

Figure 1. Comparative 5-year survivals in the Cleveland Clinic series, comparing aortoenteric fistulae (squares) to aortic graft infections (circles).

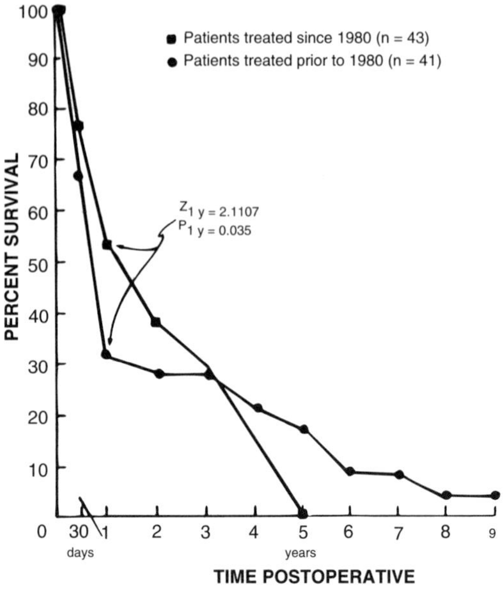

Figure 2. Comparative 5-year survivals in the Cleveland Clinic series, comparing the overall results for patients treated prior to 1980 (circles) and post-1980 (squares).

tion ($P < .001$). There were no episodes of retrograde aortic thrombosis and only 1 delayed ASS. Yeager's series clearly points out the potential for amputation if the EAB also becomes infected; however, this is clearly due to the fact that 80% occurred as an early complication of the original GIF excision surgery, in which circumstance it would indeed be difficult to provide a new EAB. Delayed onset of EAB-GIF is less common but should be easier to manage due to the availability of other tertiary reconstructions. It should be noted that both Reilly and Yeager report relatively high incidences of EAB-GIF, which is not the universal experience.[5,6,8]

Quinones-Baldrich (1991) detailed the experience at UCLA, noting that there were 30 survivors for long-term evaluation. All were treated with EAB; when this was done as a combined procedure, there was GIF of the EAB in 15%. When revascularization was delayed (to demonstration of such a need postgraft excision), 1 of 3 became infected (NSS). At an average 35-month follow-up (2–144), there had been a 22% new amputation and 20% new infection rate. Conservative therapy of new onset EAB-GIFs usually failed, necessitating either amputation or a new EAB. Only 63% of the survivors were asymptomatic. The 3-year survival rate was 55% and the 5-year rate 49% (including operative mortality). Limb salvage was 75% at 3 years and 66% at 5 years (Fig. 3). Primary patency of the EAB

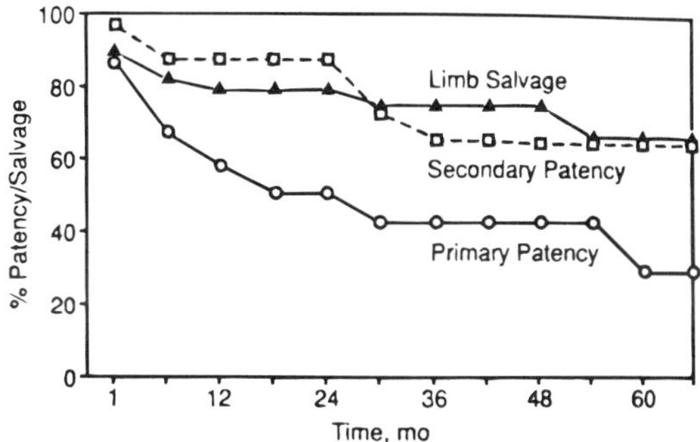

Figure 4. Summary of the UCLA experience with patency of extra-anatomic revascularization and limb salvage after successful total graft excision and bypass.

was 43% at 3 years and 30% at 5 years; secondary patency 65% and 65%. However, primary patency of a secondary thrombectomy was only 29% at 3 years and 21% at 5 years, indicating that those EABs which thrombosed tended to do so recurrently[9] (Fig. 4).

Discussion

Despite the decreasing mortality of initial treatment of GIF, and a stable mortality for GEE/GEF, the long-term survival and possibility of uneventful convalescence is not uniformly optimistic. About 10% to 15% of GEF patients and perhaps 3% to 5% of GIF patients will have recurrent retroperitoneal sepsis. Approximately, 25% of both series will come to amputation, either at primary graft excision or during subsequent failure of EAB, and between 30% and 50% will have recurrent problems with EAB, either infection in 5% to 15% or thrombectomy in a third. Certainly those who have thrombotic problems should be considered for tertiary reconstruction, since rethrombosis is the rule rather than the exception.

Philosophically, it should be realized that these *long-term* results are really 3- to 5-year follow-ups, that the more enthusiastic reports of 60% to 80% *cures* reflect the shorter follow-ups. O'Hara's 5-year data

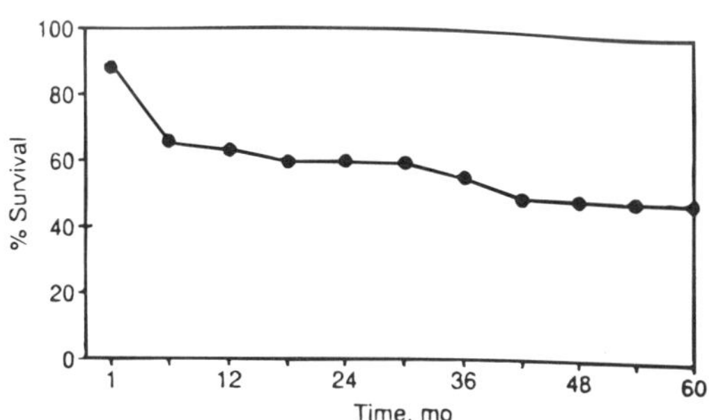

Figure 3. Summary of the UCLA experience with long-term survival of successfully treated aortic graft infections.

unfortunately may more realistically delineate the course of events. Certainly survival through graft excision and EAB does not entail guarantee of a further uneventful asymptomatic existence. Many patients will continue to suffer ill effects. If one considers that a quarter to a third die, another quarter undergo amputation, and a third of all survivors have EAB problems, it doesn't leave room for many totally satisfied customers!

References

1. Fry WJ, Lindenauer SM. Infection complicating the use of plastic arterial implants. *Arch Surg.* 1967;94:5:600–609.
2. Urdaneta LF, Visudh-Arom K, Delaney JP, et al. Use of bilateral axillofemoral bypass prosthesis for the management of infected aortic bifurcation grafts: report of a case with extended follow-up. *Surgery.* 1969;65:5:753–756.
3. Spanos SK, Gilsdorf RB, Sako Y, et al. The management of infected abdominal aortic grafts and graft enteric fistulae. *Ann Surg.* 1976;183:4:397–400.
4. Fulenwider JT, Smith RB, Johnson RW, et al. Reoperative abdominal arterial surgery: a 10-year experience. *Surgery.* 1983;93:1:20–27.
5. Reilly LM, Ehrenfeld WK, Stoney RJ. Delayed aortic prosthetic reconstruction after removal of an infected graft. *Am J Surg.* 1984;148:8: 234–238.
6. Reilly LM, Altman H, Lusby RS, et al. Late results following surgical management of vascular graft infection. *Surgery.* 1984;1:1:36–44.
7. O'Hara PJ, Hertger NR, Beven EG, et al. Surgical management of infected abdominal aortic grafts: review of a 25-year experience. *J Vasc Surg.* 1986;3:5:725–731.
8. Yeager RA, Moneta GL, Taylor LM, et al. Improving survival and limb salvage in patients with aortic graft infection. *Am J Surg.* 1990; 159:5:466–469.
9. Quinones-Baldrich WJ, Hernandez JJ, Moore WS. Long-term results following surgical management of aortic graft. infection. *Arch Surg.* 1991;126:4:507–511.

Chapter 23

Tertiary Thoracofemoral Grafting

E. Criado

Introduction

The descending thoracic aorta has been used as an inflow source for aortoiliac reconstruction for over 3 decades. However, the popularity gained by the technically more simple subcutaneous extra-anatomic bypasses limited interest in aortoiliac reconstruction based on the descending thoracic aorta. For this reason, the experience accumulated in the world literature with thoracofemoral bypass is limited, with less than 200 cases reported to the present. Furthermore, the experience at only a handful of institutions throughout the world accounts for a sizable series of these procedures.[1-5] The majority of the reported thoracic aorta to femoral artery bypasses have been performed for remedial aortic reconstruction in patients with previous aortic graft failure or to avoid the abdominal approach in patients with problems contraindicating repeated transabdominal aortic reconstruction. A minority of these procedures (16%) have been performed following removal of an infected aortic graft.[1] Therefore, the reported experience with the use of thoracic aorta to femoral artery bypass for aortic reconstruction following removal of an infected graft is limited. In this chapter we will try to discern those situations most suitable for the use of bypass from the descending thoracic aorta, the sequencing and staging of surgery, and the technical aspects of the procedure in the management of patients with aortic graft infection.

Infection of an abdominal aortic graft poses a significant threat to the limbs and the life of the patient; in one large series, the 1-year patient survival rate following treatment of aortic graft infection was 42% and the amputation rate was 41%.[6] The principles of treatment of aortic graft infection are an eradication of the infectious process and preservation of blood flow to the territories supplied by the infected graft. The type of arterial reconstruction and surgical staging in the management of aortic graft infection depends on the extent of graft involvement by the infectious process and the anatomic requirements for revascularization. The presence of an infected pseudoaneurysm involving the proximal anastomosis or a secondary aortoenteric fistula is a potentially life-threatening situation that requires emergency graft excision and aortic stump closure with extra-anatomic bypass in most cases. On the other end of the spectrum, patients with infection confined to one limb of an aortobifemoral graft may be treated in

From Bunt, TJ: *Vascular Graft Infections*. Armonk: Futura Publishing Co., Inc.; © 1994.

some cases with local groin wound debridement and muscle flap rotation, while others will also require unilateral graft limb replacement.[7] When removal of the infected graft is indicated, immediate revascularization is required in most cases to avoid limb loss. However, because of the risk of recurrent graft infection, extra-anatomic reconstruction should be done exclusively in those patients in whom graft removal threatens lower extremity viability. Patients with infected grafts that are occluded or were placed for severe arterial occlusive disease are less likely to require immediate limb revascularization after graft removal because they have developed collateral circulation. Patients with patent infected grafts placed for aneurysm repair will predictably have poor collateral circulation to the lower extremities and will require immediate revascularization in most instances.

The principles of extra-anatomic grafting in the management of aortic graft infection include the use of noninfected inflow and outflow anastomotic sites and placement of the new graft through a route that avoids contamination of the new graft. These principles have recently been challenged by the use of immediate in situ graft replacement in selected cases of aortoenteric fistula.[8,9] This approach produced excellent long-term limb salvage, but at the expense of a combined in-hospital and early mortality rate of 35% due to recurrent infection.[9] Using delayed in situ graft replacement, Reilly[10] reported no evidence of recurrent graft infection in seven patients during a mean follow-up period of 57 months. The in situ aortic graft replacement was performed 6 to 12 months after removal of an infected aortic graft, following failure of a subcutaneous bypass performed at the time of infected graft removal. The potential advantage of in situ graft replacement is avoidance of extra-anatomic grafting and aortic closure with preservation of a good inflow source from the abdominal aorta rather than from an axillary artery. These potential advantages are shadowed by a

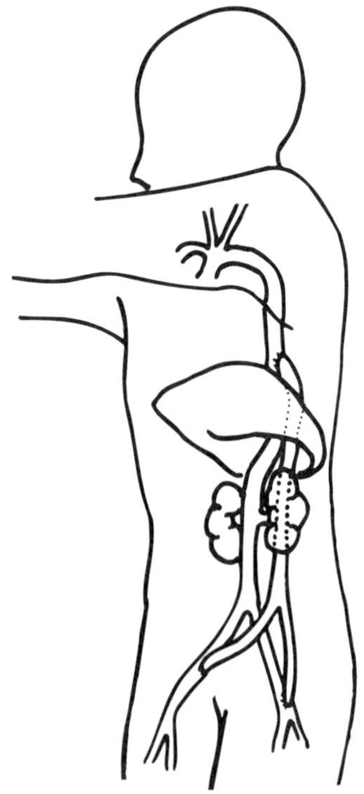

Figure 1. A descending thoracic aorta to femoral artery bypass. The graft is routed retroperitoneally posterior to the left kidney. The proximal anastomosis is separated from the abdomen by the diaphragm and the distal limbs of the graft are routed extraperitoneally to the femoral vessels. (From Criado,[14] with permission.)

high mortality rate and recurrent graft infection rate when performed simultaneously with removal of an infected graft. Bypass from the descending thoracic aorta also offers an excellent inflow source and places the graft remote to the potentially infected field, possibly reducing the risk of recurrent infection (Fig. 1).

Subcutaneous bypasses using the axillary artery as the inflow source have been the favored extra-anatomic reconstructions used during the last 2 decades in the management of infected abdominal aortic grafts. In retrospective reviews, extra-anatomic axillofemoral bypass performed prior to removal of the infected abdominal aortic graft has been shown to yield significantly lower amputation rates than graft removal prior to extra-anatomic bypass.[6,11] However, the long-term failure rate of subcutaneous bypasses using the axillary artery as an inflow source exceeds 50%,[10,12] with half of these being salvaged by secondary procedures. The descending thoracic aorta to femoral artery bypass has the advantage of offering primary patency rates of 98% at 1 year, 78% at 3 years, and 70% at 5 years, significantly higher than those of axillofemoral bypass.[1] Therefore, the use of the descending thoracic aorta as an inflow source for extra-anatomic arterial reconstruction in patients with infected abdominal aortic grafts has the potential to place the body of the new graft and anastomotic sites remote from the infected field, while offering excellent long-term patency. However, because of the risk of recurrent graft infection with simultaneous revascularization and the poor long-term patient survival rate, it is advisable to delay this procedure until after the infectious process has been cleared and the patient's life expectancy appears reasonable. Using this approach, McCarthy reported 12 patients who underwent delayed bypass from the descending thoracic aorta 7 months to 4 years after removal of an infected abdominal aortic graft with simultaneous axillofemoral or axillopopliteal bypass.[2] Half of these patients were converted to a bypass from the thoracic aorta while their subcutaneous bypasses were still patent, whereas the other half had failed grafts at the time of surgery. However, prior to conversion to thoracic aorta to femoral artery bypass, a total of 13 procedures had been performed to revise the subcutaneous axillofemoral bypasses in these patients. After a mean follow-up period of 45 months there was no evidence of recurrent graft infection in any of the 12 patients.

Despite the delayed staging of surgery, recurrent graft infection has been reported in a patient who underwent elective conversion from axillofemoral bypass to thoracofemoral bypass 18 months after excision of an infected aortic graft.[13] To my knowledge, there is no significant reported experience using bypass from the descending thoracic aorta immediately before or after removal of an infected aortic graft. Therefore, it is impossible to estimate the incidence of recurrent graft infection using this strategy. However, due to the potentially devastating consequences of recurrent infection in a bypass graft from the descending thoracic aorta, it seems advisable to delay this procedure until long after the original infected graft has been removed and the infectious process cleared. When immediate revascularization is necessary at the time of abdominal aortic graft removal, a subcutaneous bypass originating in the axillary artery would be the procedure of choice. The low patency rate of axillofemoral bypass grafts and the limitations that they impose on physically active patients, however, justify the rationale for converting to a thoracic aorta to femoral bypass in a delayed fashion, once the original infection is cleared and the patient's survival is estimated long enough to warrant a more durable arterial reconstruction. In those situations where immediate lower extremity revascularization is deemed necessary and in the absence of other adequate sources of arterial inflow, it would be reasonable to perform a bypass from the descending thoracic aorta prior to or immediately after removal of an infected abdominal aortic graft.

Technical Considerations

The procedure is performed under general anesthesia. Optimal exposure of the descending thoracic aorta is achieved with double lumen endotracheal intubation that allows collapse of the left lung during surgery. The use of an epidural catheter in these patients is helpful in the management of postoperative pain. First generation cephalosporins are administered for perioperative antibiotic prophylaxis; however, antibiotics covering the organisms involved in the original graft infection may be more ap-

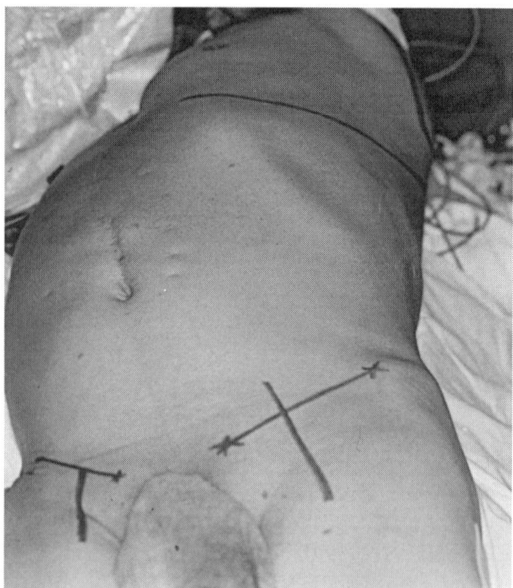

Figure 2. The patient is positioned in the right lateral decubitus position, with the pelvis as flat as possible to allow access to both femoral regions. The groin lines show the placement of the incisions in relation to the inguinal ligament. The thoracotomy incision is planned through the eighth intracostal space.

propriate, depending on the time since the removal of the infected graft and the clinical status of the patient. Positioning of the patient on the operating table is an important part of the procedure. The left chest has to be accessible to perform a full thoracotomy incision if so required. For this purpose, the left scapula has to be included in the field. Simultaneously, both groins need to be laid as flat as possible, so that the iliac or femoral vessels can be adequately exposed (Fig. 2). When the superficial femoral or popliteal arteries are selected for placement of the distal anastomosis, the lower extremities have to be included in the operative field as required for access. A vacuum bean bag placed under the patient is helpful to maintain the position. The left hemithorax is elevated approximately 60°, and the left arm is placed on a support with extreme care to avoid tension on the brachial plexus or pressure over the brachial artery or upper

extremity nerves. The skin preparation and draping should be generous and include the entire left hemithorax from the sternum to the spine and from the axilla to the thighs or calves. The use of adhesive plastic draping to prevent contact of the graft with the skin is recommended.

A double surgical team approach for simultaneous exposure of both femoral or iliac vessels may reduce the operative time required for the procedure. The distal anastomotic sites are exposed first through standard incisions. When the common femoral arteries are the selected distal anastomotic sites, the left groin incision is carried 5 cm proximal to the inguinal ligament, the external oblique muscle is divided in the direction of its fibers, and internal oblique and transversus muscles are transected with electrocautery. The left preperitoneal pelvic space is entered using blunt dissection, just anterior and lateral to the left iliac vessels. A plane is bluntly created posterior to the left kidney up to the level of the insertion of the left diaphragm. Another tunnel is created between the left preperitoneal suprainguinal space and the right groin, posterior to the rectus muscles and anterior and superior to the bladder. The right inguinal ligament has to be partially divided to allow passage of the graft without compression. Umbilical tape is left in the tunnel to allow later routing of the graft. Once dissection of the femoral vessels and tunnels is completed, the wounds are packed with sponges soaked with antibiotic solution, the table is rotated towards the right, and the eighth intercostal space is entered through an anterolateral thoracotomy. Alternatively, the left pleural space can be approached through the seventh or ninth intercostal spaces without major difference in the exposure. The pleural space is entered, and the left lung is selectively deflated. The left retrorenal tunnel is completed by dividing the insertion of the left diaphragm in the posterior medial aspect of the chest and bluntly detaching it from the thoracoabdominal wall (Fig. 3). Inserting one hand

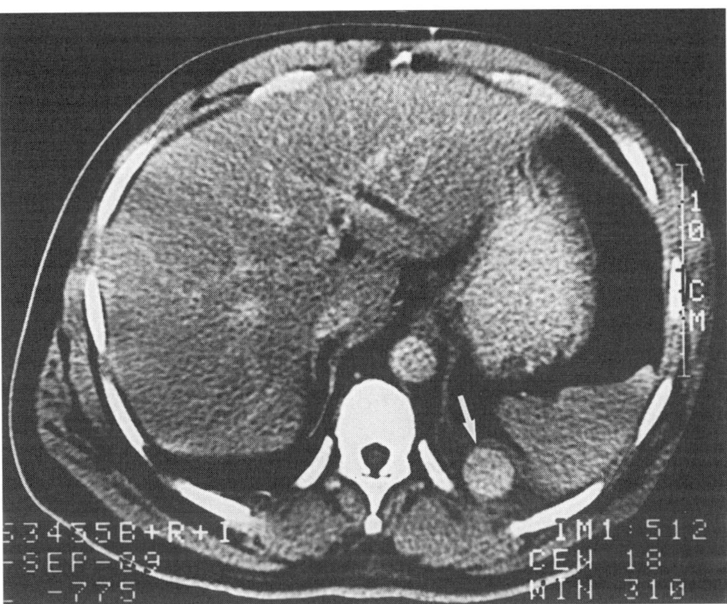

Figure 3. Postoperative computer tomography scan of the abdomen of a patient with a descending thoracic aorta to femoral artery bypass. (A) The white arrow points to the body of the graft, just after crossing the diaphragm posteromedial to the spleen and extraperitoneally.

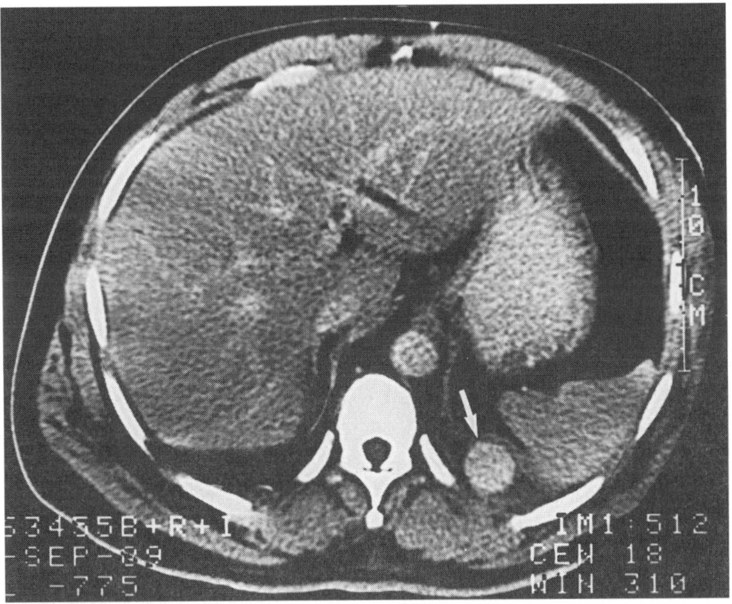

Figure 3B. Postoperative computer tomography scan of the abdomen of a patient with a descending thoracic aorta to femoral artery bypass. (B) The lower section shows the bifurcated protion of the graft (white arrow) posterior to the left kidney. (From Criado,[14] with permission.)

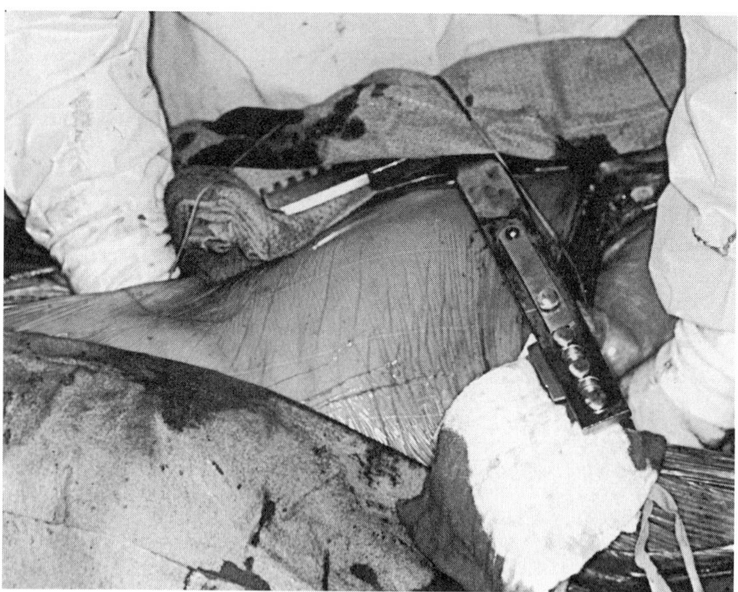

Figure 4. The tunnel from the left pleural space to the left retroperitoneal pelvic area is completed with blunt dissection using one hand from either end. During this maneuver, it is noted that the length of this tunnel is quite short. (The head of the patient is to the right and the feet to the left.)

from the left suprainguinal incision and the other one through the chest, the tunnel is completed and an umbilical tape is left in it to allow graft routing. At this point, the short distance between the posterior left pleural space and the left iliac fossa is noted (Fig. 4). The pleura overlying the distal aorta is incised 8 to 10 cm longitudinally. The descending thoracic aorta is palpated and a soft segment is chosen as distal as possible in the pleural cavity for placement of the proximal anastomosis. The aorta is dissected carefully to avoid intercostal artery injury and widely enough to allow placement of a partially occluding clamp. Circumferential aortic control proximal to the anastomotic site is advisable to allow quick aortic clamping if necessary. After systemic heparinization, a 3- to 4-cm longitudinal aortotomy is performed. A bifurcated Dacron graft is beveled preserving its entire length, and the proximal anastomosis is constructed with continuous 3–0 monofilament polypropylene. When the quality of the aortic wall is in question, an interrupted pledgeted proximal anastomosis is advisable (Fig. 5). Once completed, the graft is clamped and the partial occluding clamp is released to assess hemostasis. Following this, both limbs of the graft are tunneled into the left preperitoneal space with care to avoid kinking or twisting. The left limb of the graft is tunneled under the left inguinal ligament, and the right limb of the graft is tunneled to the right groin. Occasionally, the right limb of the graft requires lengthening which is optimally accomplished by using the redundant segment from the left limb of the graft. The distal anastomoses are then performed in the usual fashion as in a conventional aortofemoral bypass (Fig. 6). Flow is established through the graft and assessed with a continuous wave Doppler probe. When the groins are to be avoided because of the presence of scarring or infection, the tunnels should be appropriately routed to the selected distal anastomotic vessel. If the left groin is to be avoided, the left limb of the graft can be tunneled lateral to the femoral vessels and routed distally to the profunda femoral, superficial femoral, or popliteal artery as required. Obviously, when a bifurcated graft is used to reach the distal femoral vessels, an additional segment of graft has to be anastomosed to each limb of the graft. Alternatively, the left limb of the graft can be tunneled through the obturator canal to the distal profunda, superficial femoral, or popliteal artery avoiding the femoral vessels at the groin level. The same alternatives can be followed when the right groin has to be avoided.

When appropriate, the external iliac arteries can be used for distal anastomosis and for this purpose, the distal incisions are placed parallel and proximal to the inguinal ligament and the external iliac arteries are dissected extraperitoneally. This option, however, is unlikely to be feasible in the presence of retroperitoneal infection. The tunnels are created as previously described. In those situations where the left retrorenal or retroperitoneal spaces are anticipated to be severely scarred or contaminated, the tunnel from the descending thoracic aorta to the lower extremity vessels can be routed anteriorly by dividing the diaphragm anteriorly at the level of the midclavicular line, entering the preperitoneal space posterior to the abdominal wall muscles. A tunnel is then created to the left pelvic preperitoneal space, where further graft routing can be done as described above. An alternative option is to use a straight tube graft from the descending thoracic aorta to the left femoral vessels at any level, and a side graft, jumped to the right groin through a subcutaneous or preperitoneal tunnel. Occasionally, to avoid

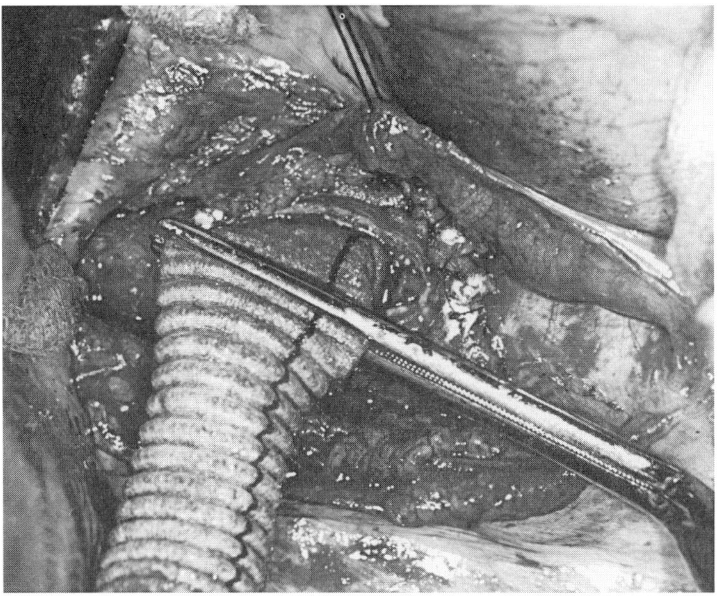

Figure 5. The proximal anastomosis at the level of the descending thoracic aorta is completed with interrupted pledgeted monofilament polypropylene sutures in this case. The proximal anastomosis should be placed as distal as possible in the descending thoracic aorta to minimize graft length requirements. The graft is ready to be tunneled retroperitoneally to the left preperitoneal space. (The head of the patient is to the right and the feet to the left.)

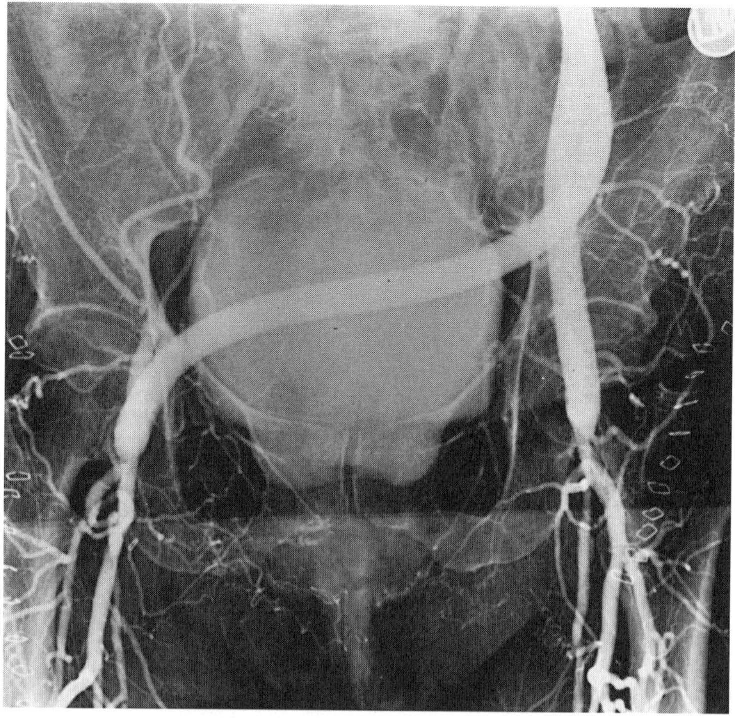

Figure 6. Postoperative angiogram demonstrating the position of the limbs of a descending thoracic aorta to femoral artery bypass anastomosed to the common femoral arteries.

potentially infected areas, a perineal tunnel may be used to cross from the left to the right femoral vessels.

Planning of the bypass should be done individually for each patient, depending on the anatomic areas that need to be circumvented because of scarring or infection and on the availability of adequate distal anastomotic sites. In general, if at all possible, we favor avoiding placement of the body of the graft or anastomosis at any site previously involved with infection, even long after its resolution.

Several techniques of bypass from the descending thoracic aorta to the femoral arteries have been described.[3,14–16] The use of a thoracophrenolaparotomy to expose the descending thoracic aorta is unnecessary and defeats the purpose of avoiding the abdominal aorta when the indication for the procedure is a previously infected infrarenal aortofemoral graft. It would be indicated only when simultaneous exposure of the splanchnic vessel is required. The use of an additional left flank incision to aid in the tunneling is unnecessary when exposure of the left preperitoneal iliac space is gained above the inguinal ligament. It is important to stress that the proximal anastomosis can be safely constructed with a partially occluding clamp. Complete aortic clamping has led to several cases of spinal cord ischemic injury when using this technique.[3] The concerns of long-term renal or mesenteric ischemia following bypass from the descending thoracic aorta to the femoral vessels have not been substantiated. We have not seen a case of progression to renal failure or visceral ischemia in our experience with 32 of these procedures, nor is there any evidence in the literature of these complications arising during long-term follow-up.

In summary, the descending thoracic aorta to femoral artery bypass is an excellent alternative for aortic reconstruction in those situations where the peritoneal cavity or the abdominal aortic segment has to be avoided because of previous infection. The ideal indication for this procedure would be in the presence of proximal aortic graft infection sparing the iliac and femoral vessels. When the infection additionally extends into one or both groins, reconstruction with a bypass from the descending thoracic aorta is also feasible, but much more complicated because of the problems in tunneling the graft to more distal levels. When the infection is confined to one groin, and removal of the entire aortofemoral graft is not necessary, other alternative procedures are more appropriate. Our judgment and the limited experience recorded in the literature suggest that a bypass from the descending thoracic aorta may offer best results in the management of aortic graft infection, when performed in a delayed fashion, following removal of the infected graft and allowing time to clear the infectious process prior to surgery.

References

1. Criado E, Johnson G Jr, Burnham SJ, Buehrer J, Keagy BA. Descending thoracic aorta-to-iliofemoral artery bypass as an alternative to aortoiliac reconstruction. *J Vasc Surg.* 1992;15:550.
2. McCarthy WJ, Mesh CL, McMillan WD, Flinn WR, Pearce WH, Yao JST. Descending thoracic aorta to femoral bypass: 10-year experience with a durable procedure. Presented at the 40th Scientific Meeting of the International Society for Cardiovascular Surgery. Chicago, Illinois; June 10, 1992.
3. Branchereau A, Magnan P-E, Moracchini P, Espinoza H, Mathieu J-P. Use of descending thoracic aorta for lower limb revascularization. *Eur J Vasc Surg.* 1992;6:255–262.
4. Bowes DE, Youkey JR, Pharr WP, Goldstein AM, Benoit CH. Long-term follow-up of descending thoracic aorto-iliac/femoral bypass. *J Cardiovasc Surg.* 1990;31:430–437.
5. Feldhaus RJ, Sterpetti AV, Schultz RD, Peetz DJ Jr. Thoracic aorta-femoral artery bypass: indications, technique, and late results. *Ann Thorac Surg.* 1985;40:588–592.
6. O'Hara PJ, Hertzer NR, Beven EG, Krajewski LP. Surgical management of infected abdominal aortic grafts: review of a 25-year experience. *J Vasc Surg.* 1986;3:725–731.
7. Bandyk DF, Bergamini TM, Kinney EV, Seabrook GR, Towne JB. In situ replacement of vascular prostheses infected by bacterial biofilms. *J Vasc Surg.* 1991;13:575–583.
8. Jacobs MJHM, Reul GJ, Gregoric I, Cooley DA. In situ replacement and extra-anatomic bypass for the treatment of infected abdominal aortic grafts. *Eur J Vasc Surg.* 1991;5:83–86.
9. Walker WE, Cooley DA, Duncan JM, Hallman GL Jr, Ott DA, Reul GJ. The management of aortoduodenal fistula by in situ replacement of the infected abdominal aortic graft. *Ann Surg.* 1987;205:727–732.
10. Reilly LM, Ehrenfeld WK, Stoney RJ. Delayed aortic prosthetic reconstruction after removal of an infected graft. *Am J Surg.* 1984;148:234–239.
11. Reilly LM, Stoney RJ, Goldstone J, Ehrenfeld WK. Improved management of aortic graft infection: the influence of operation sequence and staging. *J Vasc Surg.* 1987;5:421–431.
12. Quinones-Baldrich WJ, Hernandez JJ, Moore WS. Long-term results following surgical management of aortic graft infection. *Arch Surg.* 1991;126:507–511.
13. Costantino MJ. Recurrent aortic graft infection following descending thoracic aorta to femoral artery bypass. *J Cardiovasc Surg.* 1991;32:477–481.
14. Criado E, Keagy BA. Descending thoracic aorta to femoral artery bypass. *Contemp Surg.* 1991;39:15–19.
15. Bowes DE, Keagy BA, Benoit CH, Pharr WF. Descending thoracic aortobifemoral bypass for occluded abdominal aorta: retroperitoneal route without an abdominal incision. *J Cardiovasc Surg.* 1985;26:41–45.
16. McCarthy WJ, Flinn WR, Pearce WH, Yao JST, Bergan JJ. Thoracic aortofemoral bypass. In: Bergan JJ, Yao JST, eds. *Techniques in Arterial Surgery.* Philadelphia: WB Saunders; 1990;363–366.

SECTION VIII

Unusual Cases

A surgeon should be the most capable physician the patient has.

Chapter 24

Unusual Causes and Sites of Graft Infection

T.J. Bunt

Introduction

Although frequently cited as a potential cause of graft infection (GIF), actual specific episodes of documented sepsis leading to subsequent GIF have been noted only by a few authors, with 10 total instances from the roughly 600 published cases.

Graft Infection Due to Sepsis

Szylagyi (1972) noted a *Staphylococcus aureus* GIF following drainage of a large furuncle harboring the same bacteria. Yashar (1978) noted a GIF to follow abdominal wound infection with clinical sepsis after aortic aneurysmorrhaphy. Scobie (1978) noted a GIF to follow urinary tract infection with the same organism. Edwards (1986) noted three *S aureus* infections following prior clinical sepsis. Courmier (1980) noted one GIF to follow acute postoperative appendicitis at original graft placement.[1-5] These instances illustrate the potential for GIFs, but their rarity underscores the reality that most GIFs are caused by local contamination.

Graft Infection Due to Visceral Injury

Visceral injuries with presumed local bacterial contamination of a freshly implanted graft leading to secondary GIF are also rarely reported phenomenon. Iatrogenic injuries of the ureter have been reported by Goldstone (1973) and by Yashar (1978), and aortic reconstruction with concomitant cholecystectomy or gastrostomy by Becker (1976), and three cases by Edwards (1986)[1-7] have all been reported as causes of subsequent GIF. Again, the rarity of these cases underscores other factors as being more important in etiology.

Concomitant Visceral Surgery

The related issue of attempting concomitant visceral surgery while placing an aortic graft has not been resolved, with two vociferous camps periodically publishing either spectral end of the issue.

Ochsner (1960) noted 804 associated procedures performed in 640 patients, rep-

From Bunt, TJ: *Vascular Graft Infections.* Armonk: Futura Publishing Co., Inc.; © 1994.

resenting a combined procedure in 69% of 931 aneurysm patients at Baylor over an 8-year period. The procedures performed included 480 appendectomies, 184 sympathectomies, 51 cholecystectomies, 30 herniorrhaphies, 12 gastric procedures, 11 hiatal herniorrhaphies, 11 enterectomies, 8 colectomies, and an assortment of miscellaneous procedures. They clearly delineated two caveats to such combined procedures: that the patient be stable at conclusion of the primary aortic procedure, and that the retroperitoneum be tightly closed prior to initiation of the secondary procedure. The overall mortality rate was similar; 8.6% (25/291) for primary procedures and 5.5% (37/640) for combined procedures. It was stated that none of the deaths in the combined series were due to complications of the secondary procedure. The conclusions of the authors were that secondary procedure could be safely done, since there was no noted increase in mortality or immediate complications. However, the follow-up is not stated, and there is no specific reference to the development of subsequent graft infections, which is really the primary concern to be addressed.[8]

Stoll (1966) had performed concomitant visceral surgery at the time of aortic grafting, performing eight procedures in six patients, including cholecystectomy, hiatal herniorrhaphy, and abdominoperineal resection. It was stated that there was no increased morbidity, but follow-up was minimal.[9]

Tompkins (1973) reported 22 cases of visceral procedures, including 15 cholecystectomies, 5 appendectomies, 3 gastrostomies, and 2 vagotomies and pyloroplasties. It was stated that no graft infections occurred, but there was no length of follow-up time given and the results appear to be at 30 days at best. Again the salient issue of GIF was not addressed.[10]

Subsequent authors focused on the more limited concept of concomitant cholecystectomy. Ouriel et al. (1983) presented a series from Rochester; 42 patients (4.9%) out of a series of 865 aortic cases were noted to also have cholelithiasis. Eighteen patients underwent combined surgery, aneurysmorrhaphy and cholecystectomy, with development of 1 graft infection at 26 months. That patient had a cholecystectomy at the time of ruptured aneurysmorrhaphy without prior closure of the retroperitoneum. Furthermore, no information was given about the actual pathogen of the secondary GIF to ascertain that there was indeed reasonable causality. Eleven patients did not undergo cholecystectomy, 2 developed acute postoperative cholecystitis (1 fatal) and 7 more developed later symptoms. For acute cholecystitis, it was recommended that the aneurysmorrhaphy be deferred; for chronic combined disease, that both procedures be performed; and for ruptured aneurysmorrhaphy that cholecystectomy could be considered. This last point is peculiar since their data clearly suggest the converse (their only GIF occurred in that situation!).[11,12]

String (1984) noted 50 patients out of a series of 250 aortic cases to have cholelithiasis; 17 had cholecystectomy as a prior surgery, 16 underwent cholecystectomy as a combined procedure, and 17 had cholelithiasis but underwent aortic surgery only. There was no increased mortality to combined surgery; 15 of the 17 who had cholelithiasis but did not have cholecystectomy developed symptomatic disease, and 9 of these came to have subsequent cholecystectomy. They therefore advised concomitant cholecystectomy at the time of aortic surgery in stable patients and after retroperitoneal closure.[13]

Two confusing papers then emanated from Kansas and the Mayo Clinic. Thomas (1984) reported an extensive series; 529 aortic cases in which 86 other procedures in 76 patients were also done. Comparison of results showed equivalent (NSS) mortalities between standard cases (9.6%; 56/521) and combined (17%; 14/76) but an increased mortality if combined procedures were attempted in aortic limb salvage procedures (66% versus 14% $P < .01$). The exact nature of this increased risk category was not well defined. The procedures performed involved 3 cholecystectomies, 6 hernias, 4 splenectomies, 4 nephrectomies, 4 gastrostomies, 3 cases of vagotomy and drainage, 2 oophorectomies, 2 hiatal herniorrhaphies, 2 appendectomies, 3 small bowel resections, and 17 miscellaneous procedures.

This paper confused the issue somewhat by adding an array of concomitant cases that are basically irrelevant to the questions of GIF risk. Thomas concludes the fairly obvious point that adding one more procedure, particularly in the more urgent or complex case, seems to add to morbidity and mortality; but data to determine if these procedures add to GIF risk were not provided in the paper. The mix of urgent, emergency, and elective cases further confuses any meaningful analysis of whether the additional procedure also adds risk.[14]

Bickerstaff (1984) provided a similar data release, dividing 355 aortic aneurysmorrhaphies into 228 standard, 115 with combined vascular procedures and 113 with combined nonvascular procedures. The additional nonvascular operations included 50 cholecystectomies, 8 nephrectomies, 7 splenectomies, 4 appendectomies, 2 colonic cases, and a potpourri of such irrelevant procedures as skin lesions, breast biopsies, and lymph or renal biopsies. Morbidity and mortality rates were 2.6%/12.8% for standard cases, 3.5%/26.1% for aortic plus vascular, and 6.0%/18.5% for aortic plus nonvascular (NSS). The data purport to show an increased morbidity when adding an extra case to aortic aneurysmorrhaphy, but the inclusion of basically irrelevant cases and the lack of correlation between the actual postoperative complications and either the type of extra operation or length of total surgery, leave little room for well-reasoned causality.[15]

Fry et al. (1986) returned to the issue of cholecystectomy, noting 35 (5.1%) of 682 aortic cases to have cholelithiasis. Twelve patients had aortic surgery first, 1 of whom developed subsequent cholecystitis, and 21 had cholecystectomy first, 2 of whom had aortic complications (1 rupture, 1 thrombosis). They therefore conclude that concomitant surgery should not be performed, believing it was rarely indicated and that the risk of GIF did not warrant it.[16]

Discussion

There are two basic issues being considered in these papers. The first is whether or not the additional procedure adds a significant morbidity or mortality to the primary aortic procedure. No one has shown that to be statistically true for elective cases. For more complex, urgent, or complicated situations, there appears to be increased morbidity but the correlation is not direct and causality is difficult to demonstrate. It seems reasonable to state that concomitant additional vascular or nonvascular procedure are reasonably safe if:

1. The patient is currently stable.
2. The patient is not a high medical risk.
3. The additional procedure can be performed quickly and without expectation of major blood loss or other physiologic decompensation.

Conversely, it does not seem reasonable to perform extra procedures in unstable patients, those with high preoperative risk factors, or if there is already gross retroperitoneal or intraperitoneal hemorrhage or soiling (e.g., ruptured aneurysm).

The second issue raised the question as to whether or not performance of the visceral procedure carries an increased risk for subsequent GIF. Theoretically, such GIF might occur from:

1. Direct contamination of the graft by fluids from the opened viscus. This is the basic rationale for secure closure of and packing off of the retroperitoneum prior to the visceral procedure. In the absence of direct visible contamination of these packs, it

is difficult to theorize this route as a cause for concern.

2. Secondary bacteria-positive visceral fluid leaks into the peritoneal cavity with secondary graft contamination (e.g., bile from the gallbladder bed). However, most if not all such leaks are low grade and well localized to the area of origin, forming the not uncommon subhepatic fluid collections seen at follow-up scans.

The statistics quite frankly do not lend any great credence to the myth that a well-done visceral procedure adds risk of GIF. In all the series quoted, only one GIF was encountered, and that was after performance in a situation (ruptured aneurysm) where additional visceral surgery would usually be contraindicated. Furthermore, in the 650 cases of published GIF, only a handful can be traced to prior visceral injury or surgery. Full scale peritoneal leaks (bile ascites) are rare. It is again difficult to theorize graft contamination by this route.

3. Bacteremia from secondary infections related to the visceral procedure. This is a viable and reasonable potential avenue for graft sepsis, but dependent directly on the observation of clinical abscess, cellulitis, leak, sepsis from the visceral procedure. The most likely problems would be anastomotic leaks from bowel (particularly colonic) resections. Since anastomotic leaks are uncommon with noncolonic anastomoses, but are a common enough complication of routine colonic anastomoses, it would seem prudent to avoid colonic surgery and particularly colonic, enteric, or gastric anastomoses. In normal uninflamed tissue it would, however, seem reasonable.

Conversely, it is difficult to appreciate any rationale for incidental appendectomy at the age group vascular surgery is performed in, for incidental Meckel's diverticulectomy, or the necessity for concomitant hiatal herniorrhaphy or ulcer procedure also is quite suspect. There seems little reason to incur even a small and theoretical increased risk for GIF by performing these other procedures concomitantly.

Finally, there is the possibility of avoiding the whole conundrum entirely. If the secondary procedure seems to be necessary and not to be delayed to a subsequent time frame, then one can always entertain alternative reconstructions that effectively separate the implanted graft from the potential complications of the visceral procedure—axillofemoral, thoracofemoral, or retroperitoneal aortic graft placement (with aortic stump ligation and aneurysm exclusion in the case of aneurysm resection). Though not to be generically recommended as a routine case basis, there might be select situations of potential risk where this offers an alternative solution.

A reasonable compromise position regarding concomitant visceral surgery would then seem to be if:

1. this is an elective situation—not for urgent emergency cases, and particularly not with intraperitoneal blood or retroperitoneal suggillation.
2. the patient is stable.
3. the visceral procedure is done only after secure retroperitoneal closure and thorough packing off of a dry retroperitoneal field with clean laparotomy pads.
4. this is restricted to cholecystectomy or upper gastrointestinal procedures (not colonic resection and/or anastomosis, not appendectomy).

Unusual Agents

There have been a smattering of unusual pathogens presented as etiologic causes of recognized graft infections.

Salmonella

Salmonella is a recognized common cause of primary aortic infection and especially of infected aortic aneurysms. Attempts at in situ reconstruction have frequently resulted in secondary Salmonella GIF, with or without GEF.[1] However, a primary Salmonella GIF is rare. We presented (1984) the only case of primary GIF in a man who had Salmonella sepsis-colitis and a prior aortic graft, and developed a GIF during treatment of this.[2]

Fungal

Pasternak (1979) noted a multispecies fungal infection of an axillofemoral graft placed for ischemia in a patient on chemotherapy for chronic lymphocytic leukemia. A disrupted proximal anastomosis 3 weeks postoperatively was repaired in situ, resulting in excision and rerouting of that portion. Graft cultures grew Penicillium, Mycelia sterilia, and Candida parapsilosis species.[3]

Listeriosis

Earnshaw (1991) presented a case of *Listeria monocytogenes* infection of a polytetrafluoroethylene (PTFE) angioaccess graft, presenting as an infected pseudoaneurysm. In situ treatment failed and required graft excision 3 months later.[4]

Histoplasmosis

Miller (1982) noted a case of *Histoplasma capsulatum* GIF 10 years after an aortofemoral grafting was done while the patient was being treated for systemic histoplasmosis and had an infected groin pseudoaneurysm. Resection of the graft and repeat Dacron grafting under ketoconazole prophylaxis was performed uneventfully. Graft cultures and histology both demonstrated Histoplasma.[5]

Tuberculosis

Wright (1977) noted development of a tuberculosis prosthetic GIF in an aortofemoral Dacron graft placed during therapy for renal tuberculosis. Four years later the patient had recurrent renal symptoms and on workup was found to have a large aortic pseudoaneurysm, which on culture and histology (Ziehl-Neelsen stain) showed tuberculosis. Excision and extra-anatomic bypass (EAB) were performed uneventfully.[6]

Yersinia

Verhaegen (1985) noted the development of an infected aortic pseudoaneurysm 2 years after an aortofemoral grafting for claudication. The patient had been treated for a nonspecific colitis for 2 months prior to admission. Six sets of blood cultures taken after admission were all positive for *Yersinia enterocolitica* serotype 3. The patient died prior to laparotomy and was found to have proximal aortic suture line disruption.[7]

Unusual Presentations: Unusual Sites

Many authors briefly mentioned the management of other sites than the common aortic and/or peripheral locations. Many of these involve groin presentations of axillofemoral or cross-femoral grafts, or of femoral patch angioplasties, whose management is little different from other grafts at the same site.

The specific management of patch angioplasties has not been addressed as a separate issue; however, the few case reports would indicate that local therapy is usually successful. This seems reasonable on theoretical grounds, since the foreign body is small, its internal surface becomes well lined with endothelium, and there is no risk for ascending infection with its secondary risks.

Carotid

Najafi (1969) noted an infected Dacron carotid patch angioplasty treated successfully with local measures. Conn (1970) also noted successful local treatment of a Dacron patch angioplasty. Casali (1980) managed an infected axillocarotid and a carotid-subclavian bypass with graft excision without revascularization, with no further problems. Reilly's 1984 series from USF noted five carotid cases whose successful management was not further specified.[1-4]

Little concrete information can be gleaned about the appropriate management of these cases. The carotid infections were all due to *S aureus* and occurred postoperatively; axial grafts were usually excised, while patch angioplasties were successfully managed locally. Presumably there is reendothelialization of the luminal surface of patches within several weeks, which must facilitate clearance of bacteria from the graft matrix. However, the long-term healing is not addressed in any of these sporadic reports—one does not know if occult persistent infection then leads to subsequent thrombosis, recurrent infection, or local stricture.

Axillary

Casali (1980) noted an infected axilloaxillary graft treated successfully with graft excision only.

Szylagyi (1972) noted an infected aortoaxillary graft that presented with an abscess at the axillary anastomosis. Attempted local treatment of this resulted in fatal hemorrhage from the aortic anastomosis.[3,5]

Iliofemoral

Najafi (1969) noted an infected Dacron iliofemoral graft that was successfully managed by excision and in situ grafting. Youmans (1967) noted erosion of a thrombosed iliofemoral graft into adjacent ileum, successfully treated by simple graft excisions.[1,6]

Szylagyi (1972) noted four cases of iliofemoral graft infection. Two were treated with partial excision with recovery in both, and there was one amputation; graft excision alone in one, and graft excision with autologous cross-over femoral reconstruction in one, with fatal myocardial infarction postoperatively.[5]

Thoracic

Najafi (1968) noted fatal exsanguination from infection of a thoracic graft replacement of a thoracic aneurysm for which only local measures were attempted. D'Souza (1987) noted a graft-enteric fistula resulting from erosion of a thoracofemoral graft into the esophagus.[1,7]

Constantino (1991) noted development of infection in a thoraco femoral graft. A graft infection with *Escherichia coli* and graft-enteric erosion (GEE), 1 year following aortofemoral graft had been successfully treated with excision and EAB. Eighteen months later, persistent claudication led to a thoracofemoral tertiary reconstruction, which then became infected with *S aureus* at the site of repeated groin seromas. Excision and repeat axillofemoral grafting was successful until fatal mesenteric ischemia occurred, 1 year later.[8]

Renal

Cerny (1972) noted two cases of thrombosed aortorenal grafts eroding into the duodenum. The first involved the ligated stump of a PTFE graft postnephrectomy for failed bypass, and the second occurred at the site of PTFE patch angioplasty of the aortotomy, postnephrectomy for failed bypass.[9]

Hobson (as quoted in King[10]) noted a GEE from duodenal adhesion to the umbilical tape remnant from renal pedicle ligation at prior nephrectomy.

King (1985) noted a GEE from a woven silk aortorenal bypass originally placed in 1960 and revised and shortened in 1967 for angulation and lengthening. Fifteen years later, the patient presented with erosion of the graft into the duodenum.[10]

Visceral

Youmans (1967) noted a GEE into the stomach from a Dacron aortic superior mesenteric sidelimb of a thoracoiliac graft placed after resection of concomitant thoracic and aortic aneurysms. The graft had been tunneled posterior to the stomach, into which it eroded.[6]

Paaske (1985) noted a similar case in which a Dacron aortomesenteric graft eroded into the duodenum. Criado (1981) noted erosion of one limb of an aortic graft into the appendix. Dachs (1988) noted a highly unusual case of duodenal GEE arising from erosion of a Dacron aortoiliac graft into a concomitant primary duodenal carcinoma.[11–13]

Aortic Thromboendarterectomy

Cordell (1960) presented a case of fatal GEF arising from a primarily closed aortotomy after aortic endarterectomy. Lise (1968) noted a graft-enteric fistula which occurred 4 months postoperatively from duodenal adhesion to a Dacron patch closure of aortotomy for endarterectomy. Sheil (1969) noted four similar cases of GEF from autologous patch closures of endarterectomy aortotomies. Hanning (1986) noted a highly unusual case of acute postoperative bleeding at the groins from acute duodenal erosion and bleeding into the fibrotic tunnel left after resection of an infected aortic graft.[14–17]

References

In this chapter, the references are listed by section, which Dr. Bunt considers the most useful presentation of these references.

Visceral Injuries and/or Surgery

1. Szylagyi DE, Smith RF, Elliott JP, et al. Infection in arterial reconstruction with synthetic grafts. *Ann Surg.* 1972;176:3:321–333.
2. Yashar JJ, Weyman AK, Burnard RJ, et al. Survival and limb salvage in patients with infected arterial prostheses. *Am J Surg.* 1978; 135:4:499–504.
3. Scobie TK, Elder RH, McPhail N. Infected abdominal aortic growth. *Can J Surg.* 1978; 21:6:527–531.
4. Edwards MJ, Richardson JD, Klamer TW. Management of aortic prosthetic infections. *Am J Surg.* 1988;155:2:327–331.
5. Courmier JM, Ward AS, Lagneau P. Infection complicating aortoiliac surgery. *J Cardiovasc Surg.* 1980;21:303–314.
6. Goldstone J, Moore WS. Infection in vascular prostheses: clinical manifestations and surgical management. *Am J Surg.* 1974;128: 225–233.
7. Becker RM, Blundell PE. Infected aortic bifurcation grafts: experience with 14 patients. *Surgery.* 1976;80:5:544–549.
8. Ochsner JL, Cooley DA, DeBakey ME. Associated intra-abdominal lesions encountered during resection of aortic aneurysms. *Dis Colon Rectum.* 1960;3:485–489.
9. Stoll W. Surgery for intraabdominal lesions associated with resection of aortic aneursyms. *Wis Med J.* 1966;65:89.
10. Tompkins WC, Chavez CM, Conn JH, et al. Combining intra-abdominal arterial grafting with gastrointestinal or biliary tract procedures. *Am J Surg.* 1973;5:598–600.
11. Ouriel K, Ricotta JJ, Adams JT, et al. Management of cholelithiasis in patients with abdominal aortic aneurysms. *Ann Surg.* 1983; 198:6:717–719.
12. Ouriel K, Green RM, Ricotta JJ, et al. Acute cholecystitis complicating abdominal aortic aneurysm resection. *J Vasc Surg.* 1984;1:5: 646–648.
13. String SM. Cholelithiasis and aortic reconstruction. *J Vasc Surg.* 1984;1:5:664–669.
14. Thomas JH, McCroskey BL, Iliopoulous JI, et al. Aortoliac reconstruction combined with nonvascular operations. *Am J Surg.* 1983;146: 6:784–787.
15. Bickerstaff LK, Hollier LH, VanPeenen HJ, et al. Abdominal aortic aneurysm repair combined with a second procedure: morbidity and mortality. *Surgery.* 1984;95:4:487–492.
16. Fry WJ, Lindenauer SM. Infection complicating the use of synthetic arterial implants. *Surgery.* 1969;65:539–550.

Unusual Agents

1. Ewart JM, Burke ML, Bunt TJ. Spontaneous abdominal aortic infection: essentials of diagnosis and management. *Am Surg.* 1983;49:1: 37–50.

2. Wooldridge WD, Doerhoff CA, Bunt TJ. Primary salmonella aortic graft infection: first reported case. *Am Surg.* 1983;49:679.
3. Pasternak BM, Samson R, Karp MP. Fungal infection of a vascular prosthesis. *Surgery.* 1979;85:5:586–588.
4. Earnshaw JJ, Wilkins DC. Vascular infection: another hazard of listeriosis. *J Cardiovasc Surg.* 1991;32:475–478.
5. Miller BM, Waterhouse G, Alfodr RH, et al. Histoplasma infection of abdominal aorta aneurysms. *Ann Surg.* 1983;197:1:57–61.
6. Wright RA, Yang F, Moore WS. Tuberculous infection of a vascular prosthesis. *Arch Surg.* 1977;112:1:79–81.
7. Verhaegen J, Dedeyne G, Vansteenbergen W, et al. Rupture of a vascular prosthesis in a patient with *Yersinia entercolitica* bacteremia. *Diag Microbiol Infect Dis.* 1985;3:451–454.

Unusual Sites

1. Najafi H, Javid H, Dye WS, et al. Management of infected arterial implants. *Surg ery.* 1969;65:539–550.
2. Conn JH, Hardy JD, Chavez CM, et al. Infected arterial grafts: experience in 22 cases with emphasis on unusual bacteria and techniques. *Ann Surg.* 1970;171:5:704–710.
3. Casali RE, Tucker ET, Thompson BV, et al. Infected prosthetic grafts. *Arch Surg.* 1980;115:577.
4. Reilly LM, Altman H, Lusby RJ, et al. Late results following surgical management of vascular graft infection. *J Vasc Surg.* 1984;1:1:36–41.
5. Szylagyi DE, Smith RF, Elliott JP, et al. Infection in arterial reconstruction with synthetic grafts. *Ann Surg.* 1972;176:321.
6. Youmans CR, Derrick JR. Gastrointestinal erosion after prosthetic arterial reconstructive surgery. *Am J Surg.* 1967;114:711–715.
7. D'Souza CR, Hebert RJ, Trautman AF, et al. Aortoenteric fistula: case review and a new surgical technique. *Can J Surg.* 1987;30:6:415–417.
8. Constantino MJ. Recurrent aortic graft infection following descending thoracic aorta to femoral artery bypass. *J Cardiovasc Surg.* 1991;32:477–482.
9. Cerny JC, Fry WJ, Gamsie J, et al. Aortoduodenal fistula. *J Urol.* 1972;107:1:12–15.
10. King RM, Sterioff S, Engen DE. Renal artery graft to duodenal fistula: unusual presentation of a recurrent flank abscess. *J Cardiovasc Surg.* 1985;26:509–510.
11. Paaske WP, Hansen HJB. Graft enteric fistula and erosions. *Surg Gynecol Obstet.* 1985;161:161–164.
12. Criado FJ, Classen JN, Wilson TH. Secondary aortoenteric fistulas prosthetic and paraprosthetic. *Ann Surg.* 1981;47:1:313–321.
13. Dachs R, Clement RE, Dziura B, et al. A paraprosthetic- enteric fistula associated with a duodenal tumor. *Ann Vasc Surg.* 1990;4:1:65–68.
14. Cordell AR, Wright RH, Johnston FR. Gastrointestinal hemorrhage after abdominal aortic operation. *Surgery.* 1960;48:6:997–1004.
15. Lise M, Yacoub MH. Aortoduodenal fistula: a complication of abdominal aortic grafts. *J Thorac Cardiovasc Surg.* 1969;10:172–175.
16. Sheil AGR, Reeve TS, Little JM, et al. Aortointestinal fistulas following operations on the abdominal aorta on iliac arteries. *Br J Surg.* 1969;56:11:840–846.
17. Hannig E, Allgayer B, Risch M, et al. Duodenal fistula: a rare complication following the removal of an infected aortic graft: a case report. *Cardiovasc Intervent Radiol.* 1986;9:33–36.

SECTION IX

Peripheral Graft Infections

*God may very well be a surgeon, but one would be wise to
remember that the converse cannot be true.*

Chapter 25

Overview of Peripheral Graft Infections

T.J. Bunt

Introduction

The major focus of the last 30 years' literature on vascular graft infections has been on management of aortic infections with 570 graft infections (GIFs), 490 graft-enteric fistulae (GEFs), and 130 graft-enteric erosions (GEEs) reported on. Similarly, the major focus of the laboratory models, on which GIF management is at least nominally based, has also focused on an aortic model. There are occasional models using the carotid and femoral vessels, but no studies either specifically looking at the clinical peripheral graft or for the longer more subcutaneous grafts represented by axillofemoral or femoropopliteal grafts.

The exact definition of what constitutes a peripheral GIF has also been variably defined in published series, leading to inconsistencies of both technique and results that have then in turn impacted on such evaluable parameters as the reasonableness of the selected management regimen and the veracity or universal applicability of purported results. Defined strictly, a peripheral GIF is an infected noncavitary graft; defined loosely, it may also be the infected portion of an (presumably) otherwise noninfected cavitary graft. The difference is not just one of semantics, since the natural history and, in particular, the relative risks of recrudescent and/or recurrent infection, are quite different. Recognition of this should logically lead to different tenets for management.

We would therefore suggest that the previous set of acronym definitions (GIF, GEE, GEF) be extended to clarify what is being referred to as a *peripheral* infection, by the following definitions.

1. P1 GIF: A true peripheral GIF infection of a graft whose anatomic course is noncavitary with further subdivisions into whether it is: a) autologous; b) synthetic; c) midshaft; or d) perianastomotic. Examples would then be femoropopliteal, axillofemoral, carotid subclavian, popliteal tibial, etc.

2. P2 GIF: extracavitary presentation of an intracavitary graft. Infection of the extracavitary portion (usually inguinal) of a graft whose origin and/or main shaft is intracavitary. Examples would be aortofemoral, iliacofemoral, thoracofemoral, or aortocarotid.

3. P3 GIF: patch angioplasty infections. The rationale for this definition and/or classification is that P2 GIFs may ascend to involve the cavitary portion and/or a major aortic anastomosis, with major risk for clinical sepsis, aortic stump sepsis, GEF-GEE, and aortic pseudoaneurysm—all of which carry significant patient mortality and morbidity. These risks persist even after partial excision of the limb, and are an obvious and not infrequent complication of local and in situ management techniques.

Patch angioplasty infections have been infrequently reported for the carotid, femoral, and aortic positions. They seem to fare well with simple incision and drainage of any overlying abscess; this is perhaps related to the rapid healing of their luminal surface by confluence of endothelial ingrowth. Rupture of the patch and recurrent infection after local management is uncommon. Such cases should *not* be routinely included in a series of P1 GIFs since the routinely positive results for these P3 GIFs skew and obscure the overall management results.

Literature Review

The majority of articles on vascular graft infection over the past 30 years have either focused on aortic graft management or combined the peripheral grafts with more proximal presentations. Fewer than five papers have specifically addressed the concept of management of peripheral infections. We will briefly review the literature first for experience with and lessons learned from managing these infections. These are summarized in Tables 1 and 2.

P2 Graft Infections

Javid (1962) reported the first series of GIFs noting five P2 GIFs presenting at the groin. One patient had the P2 GIF treated locally and died of ascending infection; one

Table 1
Management of P2 GIFs with Local Therapy

Author/year	No. of grafts	Mortality	Amputation	Failure
Carter (1963)	4	1	—	4
Najafi (1963)	1	1	—	1
Conn (1970)	5	2	—	—
Szylagyi (1972)	3	—	—	—
Goldstone (1974)	11	5	—	11
Jamieson (1975)	4	4	—	—
Becker (1976)	9	5	4	4
Crawford (1977)	1	1	1	—
Christenson (1977)	3	—	—	1
Liekweg (1977)	5	—	2	—
Yashar (1978)	1	—	—	—
Almgren (1981)	9	—	—	—
Ghosn (1983)	13	3	3	5
Lorentzen (1985)	31	9	2	13
Seeger (1984)	4	—	—	4
Edwards (1986)	9	1	—	7
Mixter (1989)	8	1	—	1
Calligaro (1990)	5	1	—	1
Perler (1993)	7	1	—	1
Total	133	37 (28%)	12 (9%)	52 (39%)

Table 2
Results of Management of P1 GIFs

Author/year	No. of grafts	Mortality	Amputation	Failure
Excision				
Hoffert (1965)	10	3	8	—
Conn (1970)	4	—	8	—
Szylagyi (1972)	8	—	4	—
Lorentzen (1985)	17	2	7	4
Trout (1985)	1	—	—	—
Yeager (1985)	6	3	2	—
Cherry (1992)				
Bunt (1993)	11	3	4	—
Total	76	9 (12%)	42 (55%)	5 (7%)
EAB				
Szylagyi (1972)	1	1	1	—
Seeger (1984)	1	—	—	—
Lorentzen (1985)	2	—	—	—
Yeager (1985)	5	1	1	—
Cherry (1992)	9	1	2	4
Flinn (1992)	8	1	1	—
Bunt (1993)	11	—	—	—
Total	37	4 (11%)	5 (14%)	4 (11%)
Local				
Carter (1963)	2	—	1	2
Hoffert (1965)	1	1	—	—
Najafi (1969)	4	—	—	—
Conn (1970)	4	3	1	—
Szylagyi (1972)	1	—	—	—
Liekweg (1977)	9	2	5	—
Yashar (1978)	6	—	2	—
Popovsky (1980)	3	—	—	—
Kwaan (1981)	10	—	1	—
Almgren (1981)	9	—	—	3
Lorentzen (1985)	7	1	2	2
Cherry (1992)	11	1	—	2
Mixter (1989)	12	—	—	—
Calligaro (1990)	31	3	4	6
Bunt (1993)	9	—	—	2
Total	119	11 (9%)	16 (13%)	17 (14%)

EAB = extra-anatomic bypass; GIFs = graft infections.

infection was handled by in situ reconstruction with recurrent GIF requiring graft excision; and three patients underwent graft excision and extra-anatomic bypass (EAB) successfully.[1]

Carter (1963) presented the first series advocating local therapy in a paper that has been widely quoted by subsequent authors, despite the fact that the paper's conclusions are simply not consonant with the reported results.[2] He presented six patients with groin presentations from four aortic reconstructions (AR) and two femoropopliteal, all treated with local therapy. There was one mortality with initial therapy but four grafts thrombosed within 8 months of therapy with one further amputation. Since (as will be thoroughly discussed below) one facet of the natural history of an infected graft is to cause graft thrombosis, the actual failure rate of this series was 84% (5/6), hardly stellar results on which to advocate therapy! Regardless, all subsequent proponents of local therapy have quoted Carter, which says little for the thoroughness of current literature review.

In the next 2 decades, there were reports from a number of academic institutions, most detailing their experience with more formal, partial, or complete graft excision. However, within these reports were cases tried locally. Szylagyi (1972) noted three cases all with uneventful courses. Goldstone (1974), however, noted failure in 11 cases, with 1 direct mortality and 4 more mortalities when further surgery was necessary. Jamieson (1975) noted 4 cases, all resulting in mortality. Becker (1976) noted 9 cases, only 1 of which was successful. There were 3 direct mortalities and 2 direct amputations, with 2 additional amputations and 1 mortality with further surgery for the 4 failures of local therapy. Crawford (1977) noted 1 case resulting in both amputation and mortality from a series in which 6 patients treated with graft excision did well. Despite this, he advocated suppression of the local infection with long-term antibiotics for as long as possible. Christenson (1977) noted 3 cases with 1 graft thrombosis. Liekweg (1978) noted 5 cases with 2 amputations. Yashar (1978) noted 1 case with good results.[3–10]

In the past decade, there has been a resurgence of papers extolling the virtues of local therapy for the aortic graft. The improved results of these series undoubtedly derived primarily from a more vigorous debridement and utilization of various mechanisms for more continuous antibiotic-antiseptic delivery to the wound. The first of these was Kwaan and Connolly (1981) who noted five cases, all managed by continuous povidone-iodine irrigation into a colostomy bag closed circulation unit. All five patients had healing of their wounds, and only one graft subsequently thrombosed.

Ghosn (1983), in contrast to these excellent results, published a series of 13 cases in a paper that purported to show that local therapy was preferable to graft excision; however, his results hardly bear witness to his enthusiasm, since there were only 2 positive results in the series. Three patients died and 3 patients underwent amputation during therapy, and on follow-up there were 2 pseudoaneurysms, and 1 recurrent GIF.[11,12]

An extensive experience was presented by Lorentzen et al. (1984) with 31 cases. They recommended a sequential management of the septic groin wound beginning with local therapy and progressing to partial limb resection and thence to total graft excision for respective therapy failures. However, the failure rate for local therapy was 40% (13/31) with 9 mortalities and 2 amputations. Thus, this extensively quoted paper really represented no improvement on conventional therapy.[13]

Almgren (1981) presented nine cases that did well. Seeger (1982) noted four failures in four cases, and Edwards (1988) noted seven failures in nine tries with one mortality and two ascending infections and resultant aortoduodenal fistulae.[14–16]

Three recent papers describe much more promising results with variations on local therapy in large series. Among these are a number of P2 GIFs.

Mixter (1989) presented 21 patients treated with rotational muscle flaps, of which 11 were P2 GIFs. They used mafenide dressings changed B.I.D.-T.I.D., believing that its superior tissue penetration allowed wound sterilization in 5 to 7 days; longer periods of open wounds were felt to predispose to failure by secondary resistant organism colonization. Therefore, rotational muscle flap coverage was usually performed within a week of initial debridement. The results were favorable, with 1 death and 1 delayed healing; that patient died of a stroke at 24 months with healed wounds. There were no thromboses or recurrent infection at a mean follow-up of 36 months (4–102).[17] I would note that 5 of the 10 survivors were followed for less than 2 years and 3 for less than 6 months, which constitutes inadequate follow-up for the conclusion of a complete cure.

Calligaro (1990) summarized 28 patients of which 2 were P2 GIFs. Both of these were said to do well with local therapy alone. The series was used in part to advocate local therapy for P2 GIFs, but the bulk of the experience was with P1 GIFs and 16 of these were of thrombosed grafts.[18]

Perler (1993) presented 19 patients treated with rotational muscle flaps, of which 53 were P2 GIFs. He advocated aggressive and repeated wound debridements and povidone-iodine wound irrigations prior to muscle flap closure; however, 63% underwent flap rotation at initial debridement. There were 2 mortalities, 1 postoperatively and 1 22 months later when ascending infection required excision and EAB, which the patient did not survive. There were 4 additional deaths within 6 months, said to be unrelated to the GIF, and 1 late thrombosis. The follow-up was a mean 39 months (range 8–83).[19]

Additionally, Bandyk (1991) presented 15 carefully selected patients (12 P2 GIF) with chronic graft infections due to *Staphylococcus epidermidis* who were treated by wide excision of the infected bed and fresh in situ replacement with new polytetrafluoroethylene (PTFE) grafts, all without death, amputation, or recurrent infection-thrombosis at a mean follow-up of 21 months (5–50). Four patients died of unrelated causes, 2 of whom at autopsy had no clinical evidence of recurrent infection. On routine duplex follow-up, 3 patients were noted to have recurrent perigraft fluid which were followed; these would have to be classified as failures for a more realistic 25% (3/12) rate.[20]

P1 Graft Infections

The management of truly peripheral grafts (totally extracavitary and/or extra-anatomic) has been less frequently addressed over the years.

Hoffert (1965) first addressed the problem with 12 cases, 8 femoropopliteal and 4 femoral patch angioplasties. The routine management was graft excision without revascularization, which resulted in a 25% mortality and 75% amputation rate. The paper also noted the prevalence of wound problems leading to secondary graft infections, as well as the observation of identical culture of the graft and antecedent pedal septic foci prior to revascularization.[21]

Najafi (1968) noted six cases; four femoropopliteal, one iliofemoral, and one carotid patch angioplasty, all treated locally. The iliofemoral failed and went on to excision and EAB; the other five cases were successful. All femoropopliteal infections were at the midshaft after breakdown of wounds. This led Najafi to outline the basic principles for an attempt at local management: that there be no anastomotic bleeding, that there be no clinical sepsis, and that the infection be well localized.[22] (Table 2).

Conn (1970) underscored the importance of Gram-negative infections in a series of 13 patients, 8 of whom had infected femoropopliteal grafts; 4 treated locally resulted in 3 mortalities and an amputation, while 4 treated by excision without revascularization did not result in mortality but 3 amputations.[23]

Szylagyi (1972) noted 10 femoropopliteal cases; in 8 excision only led to amputation in 4. One case was managed locally and did well, and 1 treated by excision and EAB suffered both amputation and death. Liekweg (1978) noted 9 cases treated locally, resulting in 5 amputations and 2 mortalities. Yashar (1978) noted local therapy in 6 cases to result in 2 amputations. They specifically suggested that any attempt at local therapy be limited to 6 weeks.[3,9,10]

Popovsky (1980) presented 2 axillofemoral and 1 femoral patch angioplasty, all treated locally and successfully with a 3-year follow-up. Kwaan and Connolly (1981) similarly presented 3 axillofemoral and 2 cross-femoral grafts with successful results. Lorentzen's extensive series from Denmark (1985) noted 24 femoropopliteal cases; there were 2 failures, 1 mortality, and 1 amputation in 6 cases with partial excision, and 6 amputations and 1 mortality with excision alone. The best although limited results were in 2 patients undergoing graft excision and revascularization, both of whom did well.[11,13,24]

Almgren (1981) presented 9 cases of femoropopliteal grafts, of which 7 were autologous; all were treated locally with good initial results, but 3 thrombosed within 3 months. The inclusion of autologous grafts inappropriately skews the results. Yeager (1985) noted 11 femoropopliteal cases. There were 3 mortalities and 2 amputations in 6 undergoing excision only. Conversely, graft excision and autologous EAB in 5 patients led to 1 mortality and amputation.[14]

Specific papers that focused on P1 GIF problems then appeared within 5 years of each other, most of them advocating local therapy. The first of these was harshly pessimistic. Kitka (1987) reviewed 32 patients with infrainguinal infection treated variably, and noted a 79% amputation rate and 22% mortality. Eighty-six percent of patients died of ongoing clinical sepsis, with 100% amputation rates in those patients in whom sepsis was present. Forty-two percent (5/12) patients in whom restoration of axial flow was attempted, then died and none achieved limb salvage. The authors concluded that aggressive attempts at limb preservation were associated with unacceptable mortality without the anticipated limb salvage, and therefore suggested that primary amputation was preferable.[25]

Subsequent authors were hardly as maniacally depressive about the morbidity and mortality of P1 GIFs. Mixter (1989) noted eight femoropopliteal and one each cross-femoral or axillofemoral GIFs treated with mafenide dressing changes and early rotational flap closure. There was one failure with recurrent infection requiring excision, but all other grafts healed. There was no mortality or amputation initially, and no recurrences, thromboses, or pseudoaneurysm noted at mean 36 (4–102) month follow-up, with 5 of the 10 achieving 5-year follow-up status.[17]

Calligaro et al. (1990) presented the extensive Montefiore experience with 33 GIFs, 31 of which were P1. They advocated local therapy even for prolonged periods to obtain secondary wound closure without requirement for muscle flaps. When a graft was thrombosed, it was not completely excised but rather a rim of residual graft was left on the artery. Similarly, a short segment of graft might be replaced in situ. They specifically recommended that local therapy not be attempted in the face of either anastomotic hemorrhage or clinical sepsis, but did not believe that Gram-negative bacteria were contraindications. Their mortality rate was 11% (3/28), amputation rate 13% (4/30), and failure 25% (6/25) with 2 infections and 3 late pseudoaneurysms. Although they touted this as optimal therapy, I would note that these mortality and morbidity rates are no better than more conventional excisional therapy and furthermore should not be compared to aortic GIF figures, that 3 late pseudoaneurysms indicated persistent infection, and that 16 grafts were thrombosed at initial therapy, which means only 10 patent grafts were even candidates for revascularization.[18]

Cherry (1992) also advocated aggressive local therapy, detailing the Mayo Clinic experience with 38 patients with femorodistal GIFs. Twenty-eight grafts were treated with either complete (14) or partial (14) excision, with 9 new revascularizations. Five developed new GIFs and 2 died of complications; there were 10 additional amputations. In contrast, 11 patients were treated with local therapy, 5 including local muscle flaps. There was 1 mortality and 1 amputation. On follow-up, there were 2 unrelated late deaths and 2 late (5-year) thromboses. The authors concluded that local treatment in selected patients was successful and achieved a higher rate of limb salvage than that obtained by excisional therapy.[26]

The curious point of this paper is that these were predominantly (35/38) prosthetic grafts despite being purportedly femorodistal grafts. Review of Table 2 in the text reveals that this is a semantic confusion since 14 were above knee, 19 below knee, and only 6 were tibial bypasses. The excision group had a 36% (7/19) amputation rate; those excised and revascularized were said to have a 33% (3/9) amputation rate with 4 failures from reinfections. However, only 2 of the 9 had total graft excision with 3 of the 7 partial excisions failing. Both grafts totally excised were replaced in situ with autologous material, yet both reinfected and led to amputation. Thus, their condemnation of revascularization is unwarranted; what the paper does show is that inadequate control of the infection will reliably lead to further problems. Partial synthetic graft excision led to a 45% failure rate; furthermore, in situ reconstruction should not be done in favor of extra-anatomic placement of a new graft in an noninfected plane.

The validity of this point was subsequently delineated by two successive authors. Flinn (1992) presented 8 patients with perigeniculate infection who were treated by graft excision and revascularization through lateral extra-anatomic approaches to the profunda, popliteal, or tibial vessels. There was 1 mortality, and limb salvage was obtained in 6 of 7 survivors. Also, Bunt (1993) detailed the management of 33 P1 GIFs. In 11, the psychosocial condition of the patient predicated against revascularization and graft excision alone was performed with 4 concomitant or delayed amputations. Nine patients were initially treated locally; 7 autologous vein grafts responded successfully whereas 2 synthetic grafts did not. Fifteen patients were treated with total graft excision and extra-anatomic reconstructions, all successfully without mortality or amputation.[27,28]

Finally, the most recent series was by Perler (1993), who presented the Johns Hopkins experience with rotational muscle flaps in 18 patients, 11 of which were P1 GIFs, including 4 femoropopliteals, 2 cross-femoral, 2 carotid, and 2 axillofemoral grafts. There was no initial mortality, but failure occurred in 2 patients at a mean follow-up of 39 (8/83) months.[19]

Results of Treatment

P2 Graft Infections

The overall treatment of aortic GIFs was summarized in Section VI. It is difficult to accurately assess how many of these 560 GIFs were strictly P2 GIFs and how many were more proximal presentations. Certainly the 133 attempts at local, 15 attempts at in situ , and 106 attempts at partial excision all represent attempts to manage P2 GIFs (Table 3).

Partial Excision

Partial excision of the extracavitary infected portion of the graft has been attempted 106 times with a 19% (20/106) immediate mortality and 44% (47/106) failure rate. The modality meets all the requirements of the tenets for GIF management, based on broad interpretation of the first principle (Table 4). The difficulty with the modality is however twofold:

1. Inability to conclusively determine either preoperatively or intraoperatively that the proximal *uninvolved* end is indeed noninfected.
2. A real potential for recurrent infection of what actually may have been a noninfected proximal graft by ascending infection—either up the poorly disobliterated old graft tract, or potentially by lymphatic contamination of the new seroma-hematoma left at the retroperitoneal graft.

Failure of this therapy has the real and frequently reported propensity for recur-

Table 3
Summary of Literature for the Results of Aortic Graft Infection Management

Type of treatment	No. of pts.	Mortality	Amputation	Recurrent GIFs
None	8	7	—	1
Local	133	37 (28%)	12 (9%)	39
In situ	15	—	—	—
Partial	106	20 (19%)	9 (8%)	47 (44%)
Excise	73	24 (33%)	24 (33%)	—
EAB	238	59 (25%)	32 (13%)	—
Total	573			

EAB = total graft excision and extraanatomic bypass; GIF = graft infection.

rent aortic shaft sepsis with subsequent pseudoaneurysm and/or graft-enteric fistula, especially if reinfection is not clinically recognized. Even if it is diagnosed, the higher level of infection then requires more formal total graft excision with EAB. The second procedure performed in a now sicker possibly septic patient, carries a higher mortality rate and incidentally skews the overall mortality statistics for EAB.

In Situ

In situ replacement intrinsically violates principle 1 as based on an understanding of the laboratory models. A new graft placed in the old infected field is in fact a reliable method for producing a GIF. Even the most recent laboratory studies showed 30% to 80% reinfection rates for in situ grafts with essentially no difference in the rate of infection between Dacron and PTFE; the mode of presentation is different. (See Section II.)

Antibiotic impregnation has been studied by Bandyk, Greco, and Moore (Section III) and in the laboratory significantly decreases the rate of reinfection of in situ-implanted grafts. This additional technology may well make in situ grafting a more reasonable modality.

In our opinion, in situ reconstruction can be reasonable only if:

a. the offending bacteria is of low virulence
b. there is no clinical sepsis
c. there has been complete debridement of the infected tissue field, leaving fresh native tissue to envelop the newly implanted graft
d. an antibiotic impregnated graft is used.

Local Treatment

Local therapy has been tried 133 times with 28% (37/133) mortality and 29% (39/133) failure rate. As has been the purpose of this chapter, it is important when evaluat-

Table 4
Tenets of the Management of Graft Infection

1. Excision of the graft as a foreign body whose presence potentiates the infection
2. Wide debridement of all devitalized and infected tissues to provide a suitable environment in which healing may occur
3. Broad spectrum or culture: directed antibiotics to control local infections spread and prevent systemic sepsis
4. Revascularization of the distal bed

EAB = total graft excision and extra-anatomic bypass; GIF = graft infection.

ing papers on local therapy to specifically differentiate between the aortic (P2) and other groin presentations (P1), so that the mortality and complication rates are being compared with other modalities for aortic GIF. Put in this light, a 28% mortality is reasonable, but no better than the current gold standard (excision-EAB) series. The failure rate is of course disturbing, but hardly unexpected since it parallels that of the laboratory model.

Local therapy clearly does not follow principle 1; failure is usually reported only as clinically recognized early recurrent infection, acute hemorrhage-pseudoaneurysm, or acute graft thrombosis. What is not generally figured into its proponents' assessment is the long-term durability of the modality. In this regard, a healed wound does not indicate a sterilized graft. In the laboratory, graft-matrix bacteria can be uniformly demonstrated, and culture positivity persists in clinically *healed* grafts in 30% of cases. The natural history of the occultly infected graft is to cause ascending problems, pseudoaneurysm, or graft thrombosis. These may not occur for many years, so that follow-ups of less than 3 years are probably inadequate for the claim of demonstrated *cure.*

However, this modality in more recent series seems to have smaller (5% to 10%) mortality and amputation rates than conventional therapy, so that the concept of providing a live patient with a limb despite possible continued occult graft sepsis, must be considered a positive attribute of the modality.

Finally, there is the concept of cost; local therapy entails prolonged intensive care and hospital stays with multiple debridements and (for some) the major costs of rotational flap coverage. This aspect has not been specifically tabulated or addressed in the current literature.

Summary

Clearly, there cannot be one uniform approach to the P2 GIF; each modality has its attractions and its rationales. A complete assessment is needed of all morbidity-mortality-economic costs of all modalities, using as evaluable parameters the in-house initial mortality-complication-amputation rates as well as hospital, system, and physician costs. A 5-year assessment of ongoing morbidity and mortality, including graft thrombosis, pseudoaneurysm formation, recurrent infection, and the total economic costs of all these secondary problems is also necessary. Only then can there be a fair and complete comparison of each modality.

P1 Graft Infections

The natural history and therefore best treatment of the peripheral GIF depends on whether it is autologous or synthetic, whether it is a midshaft or perianastomotic infection, and what distal vessels there are for reconstruction. Unfortunately, most series mix these details together into a polyglot mixture of treatment results, which blurs the possible differential benefit of any one modality for any one clinical situation.

Autologous grafts are essentially intact grafts running through an infected field represented by the acute postoperative wound infection. One essentially never sees a chronic or delayed onset autologous infection. The natural history of such exposed grafts is dessication and frank rupture unless they are restored to a tissue ingrowth-support environment in which nutrient vasovasorum connections may be reestablished.

It is clear, therefore, that such grafts will respond equally well to marsupialization under the extant wound edges or to coverage with local rotational flaps. The earlier this is done, the more likely the improved local environment achieved by such tissue coverage will result in both graft salvage and wound healing. Results of any therapy resulting in restoration of normal physiology could therefore be expected to be excellent.

Synthetic grafts may present as a midshaft or a perianastomotic problem and, in turn, each of these may be acute or chronic in their timing. A midshaft infection is handled as Trout outlined it in Section VI and the results should be excellent. A perianastomotic GIF, however, entails the additional risk of hemorrhage, a risk which must be specifically assessed and accounted for on an individual basis when advocating nonexcisional therapy.

Although theoretically the peripheral GIF should follow the same guidelines as a central infection—e.g., inability to delineate that the remainder of the graft is not currently infected, and/or the possibility of iatrogenic nosocomial contamination of the previously uninfected portion by operative manipulation of the segment in the face of infection elsewhere—, there is a salient difference between P1 and P2 grafts handled in this manner. A P1 graft can recur only as a local GIF with perhaps local pseudoaneurysm or hemorrhage; these may make limb salvage more difficult, but should not commonly threaten the patient's life. This cannot be stated for P2 GIFs, in which ascending infection to the aortic shaft portends risk of dire catastrophe for the patients. It is this major difference in natural history that allows us to more freely recommend trials of local, flap, in situ, or partial excisional therapy for P1 GIFs. Literature review of management of P1 GIFs is summarized in Tables 1 and 2; this does not include all reported cases, since not all can be clearly differentiated as to what was being treated and the method of treatment.

Primary Amputation

Despite the poor experience related by Kitka et al., this modality should be reserved for patients deemed to be inappropriate psychosocial candidates for revascularization. Occasionally, there may be a medically compromised patient with an unrelenting or advanced (usually Gram-nega-

tive or mixed culture) infection and subsequent life-threatening sepsis, who is best served by immediate amputation. In that situation, we would not perform emergency limb amputation, with its recognized excessive mortality, but would instead perform temporizing physiologic amputation. In our hands, this significantly reduces mortality.[29-31]

Excision

Excision of the graft alone has carried a predictably high rate of amputation—55% (44/76)—even though many of these were already thrombosed grafts. The peripheral nature of these grafts does not allow collateral circulation to compensate for the acute loss of axial revascularization. With the current facility in extended and distal revascularization, excision alone should be restricted to thrombosed grafts, or infected grafts in patients believed now to be unacceptable psychosocial candidates for revascularization.

Excision and Extra-Anatomic Bypass

Excision of the graft with EAB reconstruction was rarely attempted until the past several years, when series by Flinn and by Bunt noted excellent results with this modality based on increased familiarity with unusual (especially lateral) approaches to popliteal and tibial vessels. The method clearly fulfills all the basic tenets of GIF management; its limited use simply parallels the related slow development of tibial bypasses, profunda and popliteal-distal femoral arteries as inflow sites, and the realization that the lateral leg was as favorable a conduit site as the routinely used medial leg.

The literature experience is indeed small, but demonstrates respectable overall 11% (4/37) mortality and 14% (5/37) amputation rates. With appropriate distal bypass under extensive cardiopulmonary monitoring, this can be zero, as it was in the 15 patients we reported.[28]

Summary

The choice for therapy of a vascular graft infection should follow as logically as possible from a complete and thorough understanding of the underlying pathophysiology as supported by the available laboratory and/or clinical models. Therapy should seek to expeditiously correct as completely as possible the life and limb threat represented by the infection, without further compromising the patient with injudicious (either overly or inadequately aggressive) treatment.

The eventual choice of therapy would also logically evaluate and respectively weigh the various parameters of the clinical equation, including consideration of the patients's age, compromising medical conditions, psychosocial capability for both ambulation and cognition, and the current and/or eventual status of the underlying occlusive disease that was the initial indication for revascularization. The choice of therapy cannot be a de rigueur application of one modality to all situations, or even to one site and type of infection; all of the individualizing variables must be weighed and placed within the equation.

References

1. Javid H, Julian OC, Dye WS, et al. Complications of aortic abdominal grafts. *Arch Surg.* 1962;85:142–161.
2. Carter SL, Cohen A, Whelan JJ. Clinical experience with management of the infected Dacron graft. *Ann Surg.* 1963;158:249–255.
3. Szylagyi DE, Smith RF, Elliott JP, et al. Infection in arterial reconstruction with synthetic grafts. *Ann Surg.* 1972:176:321–333.
4. Goldstone JL, Moore WS. Infection in vascular prostheses: clinical manifestations and surgical management. *Am J Surg.* 1974;128:225–233.
5. Jamieson CG, Deweese RA, Rob CG. Infected arterial grafts. *Ann Surg.* 1975;181:6:850–852.
6. Becker RM, Blundell PE. Infected aortic bifurcation grafts: experience with 14 patients. *Surgery.* 1976;80:5:544–550.
7. Crawford ES, Manning LG, Kelly TF. "Redo" surgery after operations for aneurysm and occlusion of the abdominal aorta. *Surgery.* 1977;81:1:41–52.
8. Christenson J, Eklof B. Synthetic arterial grafts II: infectious complications. *Scand J Thorac Cardiovasc Surg.* 1977;11:43–50.
9. Liekweg WG Jr, Greenfield LJ. Vascular prosthetic infections: collected experience and results of treatment. *Surgery.* 1977;81:335–342.
10. Yashar JJ, Weyman AK, Burnard RJ, et al. Survival and limb salvage in patients with infected arterial prostheses. *Am J Surg.* 1978;135:499–504.
11. Kwaan JHM, Connolly JE. Successful management of prosthetic graft infection with continuous povidone-iodine irrigation. *Arch Surg.* 1981;116:716–720.
12. Ghosn PB, Rabbat AG, Trudel J. Why remove an infected aortofemoral graft? *Can J Surg.* 1983;26:330–331.
13. Lorentzen JE, Nielson OM, Arendrup H, et al. Vascular graft infections: an analysis of 62 infections in 2411 consecutively implanted synthetic grafts. *Surgery.* 1985;98:81–86.
14. Almgren B, Ericksson I. Local antibiotic irrigation in the treatment of arterial graft infections. *Acta Chir Scand.* 1981;147:33–36.
15. Seeger JM, Wheeler JR, Gregory RT, et al. Autogenous graft replacement of infected prosthetic grafts in the femoral position. *Surgery.* 1983;93:39–45.
16. Edwards WH Jr, Martin RS III, Jenkins JM, et al. Primary graft infections. *J Vasc Surg.* 1987;6:235–239.
17. Mixter RC, Turnipseed WD, Smith R, et al. Rotational muscle flaps: a new technique for covering infected vascular grafts. *J Vasc Surg.* 1989;9:472–478.
18. Calligaro KD, Veith FJ, Gupta SK, et al. A modified method of management of prosthetic graft infections involving an anastomosis to the common femoral artery. *J Vasc Surg.* 1990;11:485–492.
19. Perler BA, Vanderkolk CA, Dufresne CA, et al. Can infected prosthetic grafts be salvaged with rotational muscle flaps? *Surgery.* 1981;110:30–34.
20. Bandyk DF, Bergamini TM, Kinney EV, et al. In situ replacement of vascular prostheses infected by bacterial biofilms. *J Vasc Surg.* 1991;13:575–585.
21. Hoffert PW, Gensler S, Haimovici H. Infec-

tion complicating arterial grafts: personal experience with 12 cases and review of the literature. *Arch Surg.* 1965;90:427–435.

22. Najafi H, Javid H, Dye WS, et al. Management of infected arterial implants. *Surgery.* 1969;65:539–550.

23. Conn JH, Hardy JD, Chavez CM, et al. Infected arterial grafts: experience in 22 cases with emphasis on unusual bacteria and techniques. *Ann Surg.* 1970;171:704–714.

24. Popovsky J, Singer S. Infected prosthetic grafts: local therapy with graft preservation. *Arch Surg.* 1980;115:203–205.

25. Kitka MJ, Goodson SF, Bishara RA, et al. Mortality and limb loss with infected infrainguinal bypass grafts. *J Vasc Surg.* 1987;5:4: 566–571.

26. Cherry KJ, Roland CF, Pairolero PC, et al. Infected femorodistal bypass: is graft removal mandatory? *J Vasc Surg.* 1992;15:2: 295–299.

27. Baxter BT, Mesh CC, McGee GS, et al. Limb-threatening ischemia complicated by perigenicular infection. *J Surg Res.* 1993;54:2: 103–107.

28. Bunt TJ. Vascular graft infections: a personal experience with 55 graft infections. *Cardiovasc Surg.* 1993;1:5:489–494.

29. Bunt TJ. Physiologic amputation for acute pedal sepsis. *Am Surg.* 1990;56:9:520–523.

30. Bunt TJ. Physiologic amputation. AORN December 1991;30.

31. Bunt TJ, Bynoe RP, Haynes JL. Lower extremity amputation: a low mortality operation. *Am Surg.* 1984;50:11:581–585.

Chapter 26

Graft Infections Following Infrainguinal Arterial Surgery

K.E. McIntyre, Jr.
S. Berman

Introduction

Infection in infrainguinal bypass grafts is fortunately an infrequent event, even though it occurs more commonly than with aortic grafts. When these graft infections occur in limbs which depend upon perfusion from the infected conduit, the patient and managing surgeons must often confront the possibility of the therapeutic dilemma of sacrificing the limb in order to preserve the life. Since many patients with infrainguinal bypass infections have significant cardiovascular disease, have had multiple vascular reconstructions, and often lack suitable autogenous tissue for revascularization, successful management with resulting limb salvage is often complex and may involve extensive debridement, creative extra-anatomic revascularization, and wound reconstruction. This chapter will review these concepts in detail with particular emphasis on routes of extra-anatomic bypass for revascularization, groin wound management, and the current recommendations for in situ treatment of infected grafts.

Epidemiology

Vascular graft infections, in general, occur infrequently and sporadically. Usually, a significant amount of time has elapsed between graft implantation and infection presentation. Grafts constructed of prosthetic materials are more commonly complicated by infection than autogenous grafts. In the aortic position where prosthetic grafts are used routinely, graft infections occur on the order of less than 1% to 3% in most reviews.[1-6] Infrainguinal bypass grafts in contrast show an infection incidence more dependent upon graft composition; infection occurs less commonly with autogenous vein grafts (an incidence less than 1%) than with prosthetic grafts (incidence 2% to 12%).[2,7-10]

Other factors, in addition to graft composition, have been identified which influence the risk of graft infection.[11] Graft location can contribute to infection risk. It is surprising how infrequently infections arise in groin incisions despite proximity to the perineum and the contamination inherent to this area, particularly in obese patients.

Rubin et al. have suggested that groin lymphatics may play a role in bypass graft contamination particularly in the presence of distal extremity infection.[12] In their canine study of prosthetic grafts placed in ischemic limbs and inoculated with pathogenic bacteria, careful ligation of lymphatics was associated with a significantly lower incidence of graft infection than with either lymphatic transection or preservation.

Prophylactic antibiotics have been associated with a reduction in graft infection rates. By using prophylactic antibiotics, Goldstone and Moore demonstrated a significant decrease in the incidence of graft infections from 4.1% to 1.5%.[1] Multiple operations can also influence infection risk as demonstrated in a prospective study by Durham et al.[13] They showed that a significant correlation exists between the number of prior operative procedures, positive arterial wall cultures, and subsequent graft infections.

The influence ascribed to the pathogenicity of the causative organisms is reflected by the timing of clinical presentation of the infection. Early infections (less than 4 months) are generally caused by virulent strains such as *Staphylococcus aureus*. Late infections are attributed to more indolent pathogens such as *Staphylococcus epidermidis* and Gram-negative bacteria.[11,14] Additional contributing factors to risk relate to the general health and well being of the patient. As would be expected, those with poor nutritional status or impaired immune systems are at increased risk for bypass infection.[15,16] This point is amplified in the results of one series where diabetes occurred as the significant risk factor in 69% of patients with infrainguinal graft infections.[17]

Since graft infections often begin as a simple wound complication, incisional techniques have been identified as factors which may increase risk for later infection. In addition to systemic factors such as steroid use and/or presence of diabetes, Wengrovitz and associates found a correlation between wound complications and continu-

ous incisions in their series of 163 patients undergoing infrainguinal bypass grafting.[18] Other authors have examined types of incisions and closing techniques as important determinants of wound complications. In separate reports, Delaria et al. and Utley et al. stressed the importance of making a vertical incision through the skin and subcutaneous tissue to avoid producing a devascularized flap when harvesting the saphenous vein.[19,20] Saphenous vein mapping with duplex scanning has been shown by Ruoff et al. to be a useful adjunct in avoiding this potential complication by more accurately directing the incisions to be made.[21] Finally, in a randomized prospective study of 113 patients undergoing saphenous vein harvesting during aortocoronary bypass procedures, Angelini et al. demonstrated no wound complications in those patients who underwent continuous subcuticular closure, compared with to those who underwent skin closure with metal staples and nonabsorbable mattress sutures.[22]

Bacteriology

Early reports of vascular graft infections indicated *S aureus* as the principal pathogen. Many of these reports antedated the routine use of antibiotic prophylaxis in vascular surgery. In the frequently cited reports of Szilagyi et al. in 1972 and Liekweg and Greenfield in 1977, *S aureus* was responsible for 33% and 50% of graft infections, respectively.[2,4] Subsequent to the routine use of perioperative intravenous antibiotics effective against Gram-positive organisms, the bacteriology of vascular graft infections began to change. In more recent reports, *S aureus* accounted for the majority of early infections and was usually related to a wound complication. Because patients with early infections are often hospitalized either from the initial vascular procedure or for subsequent wound care, it is not uncommon to recover Gram-negative organisms such as *Pseudomonas*, *Proteus*, *Serratia*, and

Enterobacter. Nosocomial colonization may explain the appearance of these Gram-negative graft infections in the early postoperative period. Infection caused by *S aureus* or other coagulase-positive *Staphylococcus* species is usually not subtle. These bacteria can produce hemolytic lysins and invade perigraft tissue. *Pseudomonas* infections are likewise quite aggressive due to the production of the destructive enzymes elastase, and alkaline protease and may result in graft or anastomotic disruption[23] (Fig. 1). The propensity to dissolve autogenous tissue was demonstrated in early studies by Bricker, Beall, and Debakey.[24] Although autogenous vein grafts demonstrated a higher patency in their canine model of graft infection, 10% of the animals developed hemorrhage secondary to vein graft necrosis and rupture at the site of inoculation with *S aureus.* Graft infections heralded by significant hemorrhage should be suspected of harboring one of these virulent organisms.

Late graft infections are typically less dramatic in their presentation because of the indolent nature of the causative organisms. The most common organism responsible for late appearing graft infections is coagulase-negative *Staphylococcus* species, especially *S epidermidis.*[11,25,26] Due to the pathogenicity of these organisms, late graft infections are difficult to diagnose, often presenting as nonhealing sinus tracks, anastomotic aneurysms, or simply graft occlusion. In a prospective study, Macbeth et al. demonstrated a relationship between positive arterial wall cultures obtained at the time of elective bypass surgery and later graft infection.[26] *S epidermidis* was the isolated organism in 75% of positive cultures in that study. Bandyk et al. contributed immensely to our understanding of the occult nature of infections caused by coagulase-negative *Staphylococcus* species and developed methods to identify the inciting microorganism.[25,27,28] The ability of coagulase-negative *Staphylococcus* species to produce mucin and exopolysaccharide may enhance

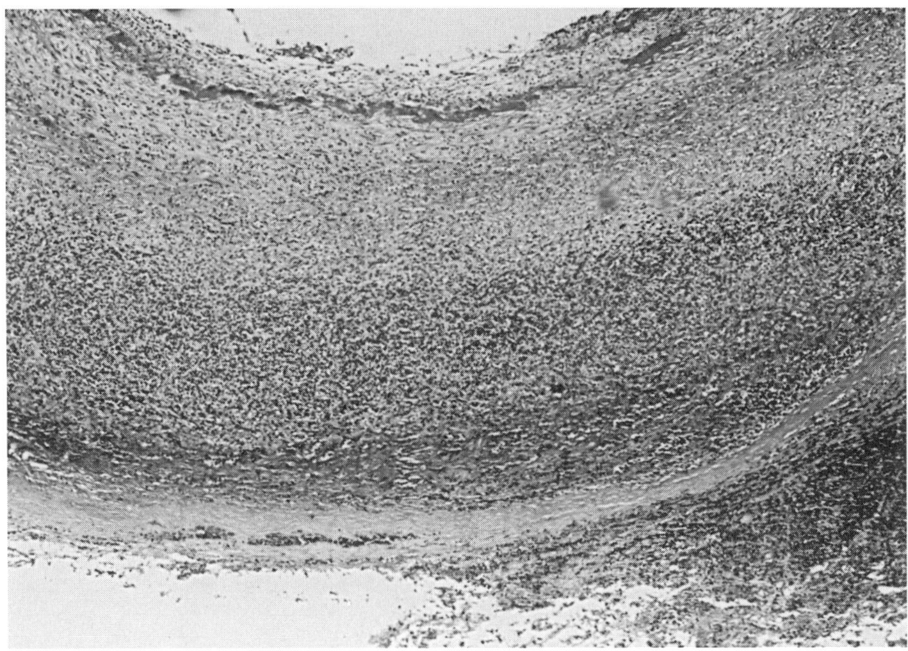

Figure 1. Excised portion of infected vein graft demonstrating organisms and inflammatory cellular infiltrate within the vein graft wall (hematoxylin and eosin, original magnification, 300 ×).

their ability to adhere to vascular grafts and may protect them from the action of antibiotics and leukocytes.[29] With an in vitro model using bacterial adherence to prosthetic grafts, Schmitt et al. showed a significant increase in adherence with mucin- producing in *S epidermidis* compared to a non-mucin-producing strain.[30] This mucin matrix has been designated as a bacterial biofilm and has been implicated as an important factor in the virulence of an otherwise nonpathogenic member of our skin microflora. Infections caused by bacteria which produce bacterial biofilms characteristically demonstrate a chronic perigraft inflammation, graft nonincorporation with sterile exudate, and a pathologic interaction between the graft and the artery at the anastomosis.[11] These attributes have been demonstrated both clinically and experimentally.[28,31]

Bergamini et al. demonstrated an enhanced ability to identify *S epidermidis* in an animal model of late graft infection with bacterial biofilms. Their study was on the recovery rate of *S epidermidis* of late graft infection with bacterial biofilms in an animal model. In their study, the recovery rate of *S epidermidis* was 30% using agar alone, compared to 75% using broth media ($P <$ 0.001) and 83% when mechanical disruption of the biofilm by tissue grinding or sonication was added to broth-media techniques ($P < 0.001$).[27] The clinical application of these culture techniques has improved our ability to identify and treat late infections with culture-specific antibiotic therapy.

Clinical Manifestations

Early infrainguinal graft infections usually occur as a consequence of postoperative wound complications. In their exhaustive review of 3347 cases, Szilagyi et al. developed a classification system for wound complications following vascular surgical procedures.[2] Their scheme was based upon the depth of involvement of the infectious process: grade I infections involved only the dermis; grade II infections involved the dermis and subcutaneous tissue, without involving the graft; grade III infections involved not only the overlying tissue but the graft as well. In their review, all grade I and II infections healed with local treatment and antibiotics. Grade III infections, however, were more complicated, representing a threat to both life and limb. This classification of wound complications has been modified recently by Johnson et al. and by Samson et al.[10,32] In Johnson's version, a fourth category has been added to distinguish wounds with either erythema or seroma formation, but without separation of the wound edges (class 1). Also apparent in this classification scheme is a distinction between wounds that are not grossly infected (classes 1 and 2) from those with overt infections (classes 3 and 4).

A further modification of Szilagyi's wound classification has been described by Samson et al. and applied to the management of peripheral arterial prosthetic grafts.[32] Their schema identifies five categories of wounds: group I infections are confined to the dermis; group II infections involve the subcutaneous tissue but not the graft; group III infections involve the body of the graft but not an anastomosis; group IV infections surround an anastomosis but are not associated with either bacteremia or anastomotic bleeding; group V infections involve an anastomosis and are associated with either septicemia or anastomotic bleeding. The advantage of this classification is that it permits identification of minor infections (groups I, II), which were treated successfully by wound excision alone in 34 cases, and distinguishes major infections which may be amenable to graft salvage (groups III, IV) from those which will require complete graft removal (group V).[32]

Late infrainguinal graft infections may present as an anastomotic pseudoaneurysm, a chronic draining sinus, generalized sepsis, or an acute graft occlusion. Pseudoaneurysms result from degeneration at the graft and/or artery anastomosis and are caused most commonly by technical errors and less commonly by infections or mechanical defects in grafts and sutures. In their review of 45 femoral pseudoaneurysms occurring with prosthetic vascular grafts without other clinical evidence of infection, Seabrook et al. documented infection with positive bacterial isolates in 27 (60%) specimens.[25] By using the sensitive microbiologic techniques alluded to above, occult infection may be demonstrated as a common factor in pseudoaneurysm development. Persistent wound cellulitis associated with a sinus tract may be a manifestation of a late graft infection caused by low-virulence organisms such as *S epidermidis* as described previously. A chronic draining sinus was the most common clinical manifestation in Goldstone and Moore's review of 27 graft infections occurring in 14 patients (52%).[1] This presentation also accounted for 9.2% of infected prosthetic grafts in Liekweg and Greenfield's report of 153 cases.[4] Late-appearing graft infections may exhibit only systemic signs of infection such as fever, chills and generalized malaise, as opposed to local signs related to the graft. This mode of presentation accounted for 12% and 18.5% of patients reported by Liekwig and Goldstone, respectively.[4,1] Graft occlusion, the other frequent clinical manifestation of late graft infection, occurred in 4.6% and 30% of patients respectively in these series.[4,1] Less commonly, however, other notable sequelae of late graft infections included septic embolization and hemorrhage.[4,1]

Diagnosis

Confirming the diagnosis of infrainguinal graft infection can usually be accomplished based upon operative findings at the time of exploration to treat the presenting complication. However, it is advantageous to diagnose graft infection preoperatively so that the surgeon can carefully plan the operative procedure. Indirect evidence of a graft infection may be obtained by a number of imaging modalities. Arteriography can identify anastomotic pseudoaneurysm, which may be the only manifestation of the infection. Although documentation of a pseudoaneurysm does not guarantee an infectious etiology, arteriography is helpful in planning the surgical intervention by providing anatomic information which may be essential in achieving complete debridement of the infected tissue while maintaining distal perfusion and/or planning revascularization should graft removal become necessary. Computed tomography (CT) may provide presumptive evidence of a graft infection by demonstrating a pseudoaneurysm or a perigraft fluid collection. Normally, the small amount of perigraft fluid which is present postoperatively would be expected to be absorbed within a few weeks of the graft procedure. Computed tomography-directed aspiration and culture can furnish organism-specific data for such collections and establish an infectious etiology. In this regard, CT is more applicable for abdominal grafts. In the case of infrainguinal grafts, in our experience, aspiration of perigraft fluid collections is best accomplished by ultrasound imaging using the duplex scanner. A more recent imaging modality applied to diagnose vascular graft infections is indium 111 labeled white blood cell scanning. This technique relies upon the accumulation of indium 111 labeled leukocytes at the site of infection. Chung et al. reported a series of 41 patients suspected of having vascular graft infections who underwent indium 111 labeled white blood cell scanning.[33] Despite the prior treatment of 23 patients with antibiotics, a sensitivity of 100% and a specificity of 85% was achieved in diagnosing vascular graft infection in this series.

The definitive diagnosis of vascular graft infection is usually achieved during exploration. The finding of gross purulence involving the graft and associated with perigraft tissue necrosis or anastomotic disruption makes the diagnosis clinically apparent while usually yielding positive bacteriology. A more difficult task is determining whether or not infection is present with more subtle cases of pseudoaneurysm, chronic sinuses, and graft thrombosis. In these situations, more diligent methods including culture of arterial walls, broth culture, and graft sonication have been useful adjuncts in obtaining a microbiologic diagnosis.[25–27]

Management

The treatment of an infected infrainguinal graft in which limb viability is dependent upon the patency of the bypass represents one of the most challenging clinical problems for vascular surgeons. Management options for this complex problem have evolved over the last 3 decades. Because of the relatively infrequent occurrence of graft infections, the early reports of management options varied diversely. In Szilagyi's experience, treatment of infected femoropopliteal bypasses included graft excision, segmental replacement, graft excision and artery ligation, graft site drainage and irrigation, and secondary wound closure.[2] The heterogeneity of treatment alternatives is reflected in the published series of Goldstone and Moore, Fry and Lindenauer, and Conn et al.[1,34,35] As more experience with the natural history and treatment of infected grafts accumulated, some general principles of management evolved. Two fundamental principles of the earliest reports emphasized: 1) the use of adjunctive intravenous antibiotics, and 2) the necessity for aggressive intervention in the care of patients with infected bypass grafts.

The basic principles of management reflect this evolution of treatment. Modalities applied to meet the objectives of eliminating the infection, preserving the extremity, and minimizing mortality may include debridement of grossly infected, necrotic perigraft tissue, procurement of specimens for bacte-

riology, partial or complete removal of nonviable autogenous graft or unincorporated prosthetic graft material, wound coverage with healthy, well-vascularized tissue, and revascularization to provide continued extremity perfusion. These components represent a continuum of treatment from relatively simple to complex and will be described in detail individually.

Debridement

As with infections elsewhere, removal of grossly infected nonviable tissue is the initial mandatory step in management of infrainguinal graft infections. If the infection is limited to the dermis and subcutaneous tissue and spares the underlying graft, wound excision with aggressive debridement may be the only intervention required. Criteria have been established that define the appropriate situation in which wound excision in combination with antibiotics will likely eradicate the infection without having to remove the graft, thus decreasing the likelihood of limb loss. This treatment approach which leaves the bypass in place has also been referred to as in situ treatment, graft preservation, or local therapy. Necessary criteria include a patent graft, a limited area of infection, absence of anastomotic involvement, and absence of signs of septicemia or embolization.[8] When these criteria are stringently applied, this approach has achieved acceptable results in many of the reported series of graft infections.[1,32] In the earliest reports of Szilagyi et al., all 17 infrainguinal bypasses with grade I or II infections healed without graft removal.[1] Of the 10 infrainguinal grafts classified as grade III infections, only one did not involve an anastomosis, and that graft was successfully treated with drainage and irrigation. In a more recent review of vascular graft infections, 25 of 34 major infections (Samson class III, IV, V) developed in infrainguinal grafts.[32] Ten of 11 patients originally treated with wound excision and antibiotics had their infection clear without the need for graft removal during a mean follow-up of 4 years. One patient required graft removal for an infected thrombosed graft after the original course of local therapy. The results of these two series which span 33 years demonstrate the effectiveness of aggressive debridement and appropriate antibiotics in managing infrainguinal infections with graft preservation when the specific inclusion criteria for that therapy are carefully applied.

The fundamental cornerstone of local therapy is thorough debridement of all nonviable tissue. This should be done only in the operating room with appropriate anesthesia, because only under these optimal conditions can the extent and depth of the infection be adequately evaluated. Wide debridement of all nonviable tissue should be accompanied by copious irrigation with a dilute solution containing antibiotics. At the time of wound excision, tissue specimens should be obtained for Gram stain and cultures including both agar and broth techniques. After sufficient debridement and irrigation, the wounds should be packed and treated using wet-to-dry dressing changes with either normal saline or dilute saline containing antibiotics at intervals of 4 to 6 hours. As the wound forms healthy granulation tissue, secondary intention healing occurs. Adjunctive measures to achieve wound closure for larger wounds will be discussed in a separate section. The most important component of local therapy with wound excision is diligent daily surveillance by the responsible surgeon. Failure of the wound to improve, deepening of the infection to expose the graft, emergence of sepsis or graft thrombosis, or progression to anastomotic involvement mandate more aggressive intervention.

Graft Excision

The presence of a thrombosed graft, anastomotic involvement, systemic sepsis, or septic emboli indicate the necessity for graft removal (either partial or complete) to accomplish extirpation of the infection. This section will outline the role of graft removal in the management of infrainguinal bypass infections.

Partial Graft Removal

Limited removal of the infected graft can be performed when the graft is thrombosed, the limb is viable, and the infection is localized to either the shaft of the graft or the distal anastomosis.[8] This approach avoids dissection of the proximal anastomosis and possible obliteration of the inflow artery or important collaterals in removing the proximal graft segment.[32] Partial graft removal can be accomplished by exposing the graft through an incision remote from the infected site. In the case of an infection at a distal anastomosis, an incision in the distal thigh or proximal calf is made. For infection in the body of the graft, a more proximal incision in the mid to upper thigh may be necessary. If upon making a more proximal incision, there is no purulence or perigraft fluid and the graft is well incorporated, a section of graft is removed for culture and the uninfected proximal portion of the graft is covered with surrounding tissue. This wound is then closed obliterating the graft tunnel. The infected portion of graft is then excised and removed through the distal wound. If the artery at the site of the distal anastomosis is patent, arterial continuity is maintained using a vein patch closure after graft excision. Alternatively, proximal and distal ligation of an obliterated outflow artery may be performed. The wound is treated with dressing changes and allowed to granulate. In Samson's review of prosthetic graft infections, 19 patients were initially treated with partial graft removal.[32] Seven of these patients ultimately required total graft removal; however, of the 12 patients treated with partial graft removal only, significant salvage of a portion of the extremity was attributed to preservation of the graft on the common femoral artery and undisturbed flow through the profunda femoris artery in 5 patients.

Other authors have, however, expressed concern with partial graft excision. In 1981, Johansen and Zorn reported four amputation infections attributed to infected retained prosthetic material from previous failed femoro-distal bypasses.[36] In all four cases, recovery and healing of the amputation site required complete excision of the infected prosthetic graft. Based on this experience, Johansen and Zorn recommend complete excision of failed prosthetic grafts at the time of amputation.

Partial graft removal is a reasonable option provided the criteria described are strictly followed. The key to avoiding the complication of persistent graft infection is the rigorous evaluation of the graft at the proximal incision site and, particularly, the microbiologic evaluation of the excised section of graft. This should include not only Gram stain and routine culture, but also broth culture and even physical disruption of the graft segment by sonication or tissue grinding if *S epidermidis* is suspected. If the evaluation reveals subclinical infection in the incorporated graft, complete excision of the remaining segment is warranted. Persistence of the graft infection, emergence of sepsis, or progression to anastomotic involvement when partial graft excision has been implemented will require reassessment and further intervention.

Complete Graft Excision

The most common method of treatment for infected infrainguinal bypass grafts is complete excision of the graft. Total excision may be combined with immediate revascularization if the limb is threatened, or observation and subsequent revascularization should threatening ischemia develop. Complete graft excision should be performed when any of the following indications occur: involvement of the proximal anastomosis in the infectious process, presence of an infected thrombosed graft in a nonviable limb, presence of systemic sepsis, or evidence of distal emboli.[8] Furthermore, when local therapy fails or when graft cultures from the retained portion of a partial graft excision are positive, total graft excision is warranted.

Complete graft excision is accomplished by detaching the graft from the proximal and distal anastomoses. Arterial continuity at these sites is maintained by closure with patches from either autogenous vein or from endarterectomized segments of the occluded ipsilateral superficial femoral artery. Multiple counter incisions may be required to remove an incorporated length of graft between the proximal and distal anastomoses. One option is to use an arterial ring stripper on the outside of the graft to separate it from the surrounding tissues. Regardless of the method used to excise the graft from the leg, the residual graft tunnel should be adequately drained with closed suction drains. The proximal and distal wounds are treated as outlined in the local care treatment regimen, including wide debridement of nonviable tissue, irrigation, and daily dressing changes. Decisions regarding revascularization are dependent upon the viability of the limb after graft removal, the availability of a suitable outflow artery in the distal circulation, and the general condition of the patient.

Because total graft excision is the most common method used to treat infrainguinal graft infections, there has been an abundant experience reported. In one of the earliest reports of graft infections, Szilagyi used complete graft excision in 8 of 10 patients (80%) with infrainguinal vascular graft infections.[2] Four patients in this group recovered without further intervention; however, four patients required amputation. In the extensive review of Liekweg and Greenfield, 55 infrainguinal graft infections were summarized.[4] Thirty-four patients (62%) were treated by complete graft excision. One patient subsequently required revascularization, 13 patients underwent further amputation, but 19 patients needed no further treatment. Total graft removal was also successfully applied to 3 of 4 (75%) infrainguinal bypass infections reported by Yeager et al. in a series of 25 vascular graft infections.[37] A successful outcome was achieved in two Dacron and one umbilical vein femoropopliteal bypasses. In the fourth case, an umbilical vein femoropopliteal graft was treated with partial graft removal and resulted in nonhealing wounds, although the patient ultimately expired from pulmonary embolism. In a more recent review, Samson et al. performed complete graft removal in 11 patients (32%).[32] Only one patient's limb remained viable without further arterial reconstructive procedures. Three patients in this group had successful revascularization with an extra-anatomic graft and four patients required subsequent amputations. There was one death and two patients who had previously undergone amputations required graft removal only.

Currently, there seems to be a changing role for complete graft excision in the treatment of infrainguinal graft infections. In the reports sited previously, the majority of grafts removed were prosthetic, since infection occurring in an autogenous vein graft is an infrequent event relative to graft infections overall.[8] In more recent reports, there is an evident trend attempting graft salvage rather than proceeding to immediate graft excision. In the review of Calligaro et al., 10 of 11 (91%) patients with infected, patent infrainguinal grafts constructed of either autogenous vein or expanded polytetrafluoroethylene (ePTFE) were successfully treated with wound debridement and antibiotics.[38] In contrast, only 2 of 5 patients with Dacron grafts (40%) were successfully managed with graft salvage. As in previous reports, infection associated with a thrombosed graft (1 Dacron, 5 ePTFE, 1 vein), anastomotic bleeding (5 Dacron, 3 ePTFE, 1 vein), or sepsis (3 Dacron) were managed with immediate total graft excision. The authors concluded that infected ePTFE grafts

may be more suited to in situ treatment with intravenous antibiotics due in part to differences in physical characteristics.[39,40] With the increasing use of ePTFE grafts in the infrainguinal position and recent data suggesting that ePTFE may be more resistant to infection and/or more easily sterilized once infection is established, complete graft excision is finding more limited application than the early experiences with infrainguinal graft infections reported in the 1970s and early 1980s.

Revascularization

Infections occurring in an occluded infrainguinal bypass in a viable extremity can be managed by graft excision without concern for limb loss as long as important collaterals are not compromised during the graft removal. The same cannot be said when the infected graft is patent and the limb's viability is dependent on continued patency of the conduit. When graft removal is required to eradicate the infection, a decision must be made as to the timing and method of revascularization. When a limb requires graft patency for viability, graft removal without revascularization has been demonstrated to result in a significant rate of limb loss.[1,2,4,7] Ideally, such revascularization should be accomplished with either autogenous artery or vein.

Revascularization with an autogenous graft can be routed via extra-anatomic paths, but may also be performed in the same field as the excised infected graft. The ipsilateral occluded superficial femoral artery can be endarterectomized (eversion endarterectomy) and used for a short bypass in the absence of autogenous vein.[41] Moreover, pieces of autogenous vein including segments from the arm, can be combined with endarterectomized artery to form a composite autogenous graft to replace infected distal bypasses. The experimental data of Moore et al. established the use of autogenous tissue for arterial reconstruction in infected fields.[42] In this canine model, 11 of 12 autografts and 10 of 12 allografts used to replace infected femoral arteries were sterile 3 months after implantation. In contrast, 7 of 8 Dacron grafts were found to be infected at the same time interval. Ouriel et al. have cautioned that the ability of an exposed vein graft to heal may be dependent upon bacteriologic factors.[17] In their series of 16 patients with exposed vein grafts, Gram-negative infections were uniformly associated with vein graft disruptions as well as secondary infections of in situ replacement grafts. These data suggest that autogenous reconstruction within the infected field is most successful when the infection is caused by low virulence Gram-positive bacteria.

Unfortunately, with infrainguinal bypass graft infections, autogenous material for revascularization is often not present since most prosthetic grafts have been implanted in patients without suitable saphenous veins. In this setting, alternatives for revascularization are limited to prosthetic materials (commonly ePTFE) or allograft veins. Snyder et al. reported the use of fresh venous allografts to successfully revascularize 6 patients with infected bypass grafts.[43] In a subsequent report from the same institution, cryopreserved venous allografts were used in an additional 5 patients.[44] Revascularization and eradication of the infection was accomplished in 10 of 11 patients. If a prosthetic conduit is the only alternative for revascularization, an extra-anatomic route for the new bypass graft is preferred to avoid contaminated or potentially contaminated fields.

Common Extra-Anatomic Bypass Routes

The extra-anatomic bypass achieves restoration of circulation while avoiding sites of infection. The route of an extra-anatomic bypass is limited only by available inflow and outflow vessels, as well as a sterile path for the graft which does not compromise the luminal configuration with kinks or twists. Common inflow arteries that serve as origins for infrainguinal extra-anatomic revascularization are the aorta, axillary, ipsilateral and contralateral iliac, common femoral, profunda femoris, and distal superficial femoral. Available outflow vessels include the distal profunda femoris, popliteal, and tibial arteries. The standard surgical approaches to the infrainguinal inflow and outflow vessels are familiar to vascular surgeons. The less well-known exposure for the obturatory bypass, the lateral approach to the profunda femoris artery, and the lateral approach to the popliteal artery will be described below.

Obturator Bypass Use of the obturator foramen as a route for an arterial bypass to avoid an infected groin was first described by Shaw and Baue in 1963.[45] This technique is most applicable to bypass an infectious process localized to the groin, for example, an infected aortofemoral graft limb or an infected femoral pseudoaneurysm. However, obturatory bypass can also be used to replace part or all of an infected femoropopliteal bypass since access to the proximal popliteal artery is also possible with this approach.[46,47]

With the obturator bypass, the aorta, iliac artery (common or external) or uninfected proximal graft limb serves as the source of inflow. If necessary, even the contralateral iliac artery can be used to provide inflow when coursing a bypass graft through the obturator foramen. Adequate patient preparation for an obturator bypass includes preoperative arteriography to delineate inflow and outflow vessels. A critical preoperative assessment is confirmation that the infectious process does not involve either the proximal operative field in the pelvis or the planned route of the bypass in the posteromedial thigh. This information can usually be provided by preoperative CT scanning through the pelvis and thigh. The obturatory bypass graft originates from the pelvic vessels and traverses through the obturator foramen along the course of the obturator neurovascular bundle. A thorough understanding of the anatomy of the pelvis and upper thigh is a prerequisite to successful completion of the bypass and avoidance of hemorrhagic or neurological complications.

Access to the pelvis can be gained by either a transperitoneal or retroperitoneal approach. The obturator foramen is located by first identifying the obturator nerve. This nerve usually bisects the angle between the external and internal iliac arteries (Fig. 2A). To avoid bleeding complications, familiarity with the variability in the origin of the obturatory artery and vein is essential.[47] The most common configuration of these vessels occurs with the obturator artery originating as an anterior branch of the internal iliac artery. Alternatively, this artery can originate from the inferior epigastric artery, or share an origin from both the internal iliac and inferior epigastric arteries (Figure 2B,C). A venous anomaly that can compli-

cate access to the obturator foramen is a communicating vein between the external iliac and obturator veins (Fig. 2B). The obturator foramen is identified by palpation just inferior to the superior pubic ramus, superior to the inferior pubic ramus, and by the course of the obturator nerve. The fascia covering the foramen is punctured using a long blunt hemostat. The obturator neurovascular bundle exits through the lateral aspect of the foramen into the medial thigh between the adductor longus and brevis muscles (Fig. 3). This is the usual plane entered when only the groin is to be bypassed since the middle and distal superficial femoral artery can easily be accessed between these two muscles. By using a medial thigh incision, bimanual palpation allows safe passage of a clamp through the obturator foramen. The graft can then be passed through the tunnel created by the clamp. This approach also allows anastomosis be-

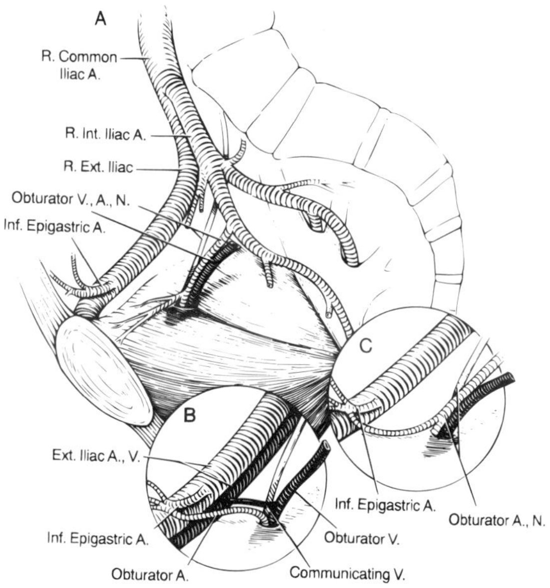

Figure 2. Sagittal view of the pelvis demonstrating the relationship of the obturator nerve to the bifurcation of the common iliac artery into external and internal branches. Most commonly, the obturator artery originates from the anterior portion of the hypogastric artery (A). Alternatively, the obturator artery may originate from the inferior epigastric artery (inset B) or share a common origin from both the hypogastric and the inferior epigastric arteries (inset C). Frequently, a communicating vein exists between the external iliac and obturator veins (inset B).

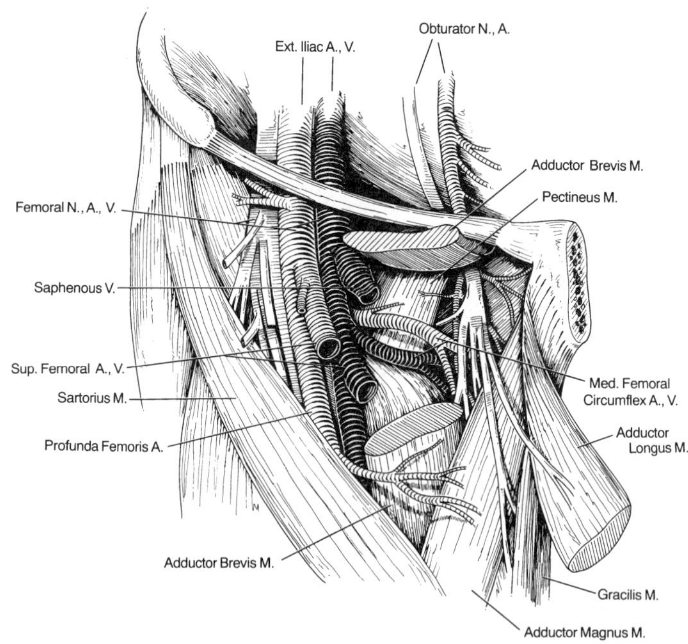

Figure 3. Dissection of the anteromedial thigh demonstrating the course of the obturator neurovascular bundle as it exits the pelvis and enters the thigh between the adductor brevis and pectineus muscles. Infection within the femoral triangle can be avoided by coursing a graft through the obturator foramen.

tween an obturator bypass and an uninfected portion of a prior medially placed popliteal or tibial bypass.[46] Should access to the popliteal artery be necessary for outflow, the medial thigh incision is extended to allow exposure of the popliteal artery deep to the adductor magnus muscle. Exposure of the distal profunda femoris can be obtained through deeper dissection towards the femur in the intermuscular plane between the adductor longus and the adductor brevis muscles.

The obturator bypass offers a durable alternative in the treatment of vascular infections localized to the groin. Bypass through the obturator foramen results in a shorter graft than conduits originating from the axillary artery. As such, late closures are less common as documented by Tilson et al.[48]

Lateral Approach to the Profunda Femoris Artery In patients who lack a patent, accessible common femoral or superficial femoral artery for use as inflow or outflow for bypass surgery, the profunda femoris artery provides a suitable alternative for revascularization. Patients with infected infrainguinal bypass grafts who require total graft excision to treat the infection may fit into this category. In this situation, the profunda may serve as inflow for a bypass to the popliteal or tibial vessels. Nunez et al. successfully used the profunda femoris as an inflow source in five patients who required graft excision and revascularization for limb salvage.[49]

Knowledge of the anatomic variability and relationships of the profunda femoris artery are essential for successful use of this vessel in extra-anatomic revascularizations. The profunda originates as the posterolateral branch of the common femoral artery bifurcation in the groin. It then gives rise to the medial and lateral femoral circumflex branches, either at the bifurcation of the common femoral or within a few centimeters of its course. As the profunda courses distally, it gives off perforating branches to muscles in the thigh. The sartorius muscle serves as a useful landmark in dissection of the profunda femoris. The medial approach is the usual method of controlling the profunda during groin dissections for aorto-femoral or infrainguinal reconstructions. When avoidance of the groin is part of the surgical objective due to the infectious process, direct exposure of the profunda can be achieved with a lateral approach, which refers to the relationship of the dissection to the sartorius muscle.

Exposure of the profunda by the lateral approach begins with an incision placed obliquely in the midanterior thigh along the lateral border of the sartorius muscle. Medial retraction of the sartorius and the underlying superficial femoral neurovascular bundle avoids injury to these structures (Fig. 4). The fibroconnective tissue membrane between the adductor magnus and

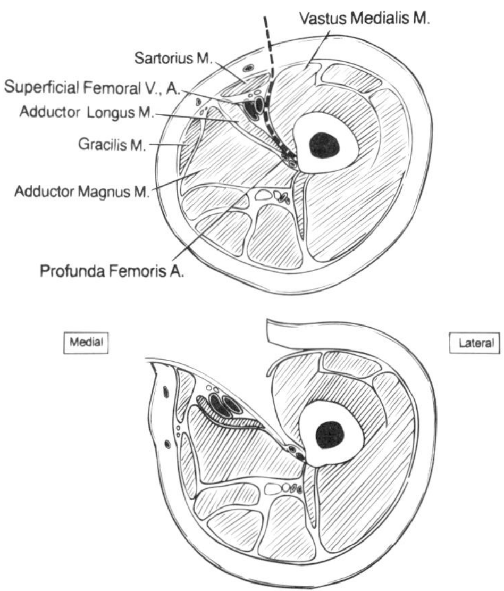

Figure 4. Cross-section of the mid-thigh illustrating the lateral approach to the profunda femoris artery. A longitudinal incision placed on the anterior thigh exposes the sartorius muscle. The dissection then proceeds lateral to the sartorius and the femoral neurovascular bundle.

the vastus medialis is seen in the depth of the wound and incised longitudinally exposing the profunda femoris. As exposure of more distal portions of the profunda are required, a more medially placed incision on the distal thigh will be necessary since the vessel traverses deep to the vastus medialis at this level and exposure through a lateral approach, though feasible, would require difficult retraction on the bulkier portion of this muscle. In the five patients in which the profunda was used as the inflow source for a distal bypass in a limb-salvage situation, Nunez and associates reported an amputation rate of 20%, a patency rate for popliteal bypasses of 50% at 18 months, and a patency rate for infrapopliteal bypasses of 100% at 12 months.[49]

Lateral Approach to the Popliteal Artery Another useful technique which provides access to the popliteal artery while avoiding contaminated fields on the medial aspect of the thigh is the lateral approach to the popliteal artery. In the setting of an infected infrainguinal graft, this procedure can provide exposure of the above knee popliteal to serve as inflow or the below knee popliteal to serve as inflow or outflow for revascularization. The methods to expose the above knee and below knee popliteal artery in these two positions from the lateral approach were originally described by Henry and by Elkin and Kelly, respectively.[50,51]

In an excellent review of this exposure, Veith et al. described in detail the specific steps in the exposure of the below knee and above knee popliteal artery from the lateral approach.[52] Lateral exposure of the above knee popliteal artery is begun with an incision placed longitudinally between the iliotibial tract and the biceps tendon just above the knee joint (Fig. 5). By entering through the intermuscular septum in the depth of the incision, the popliteal space is entered. This exposure permits dissection of the popliteal artery from the neurovascular bundle with care taken to avoid injury to the common peroneal nerve which lies superolater-

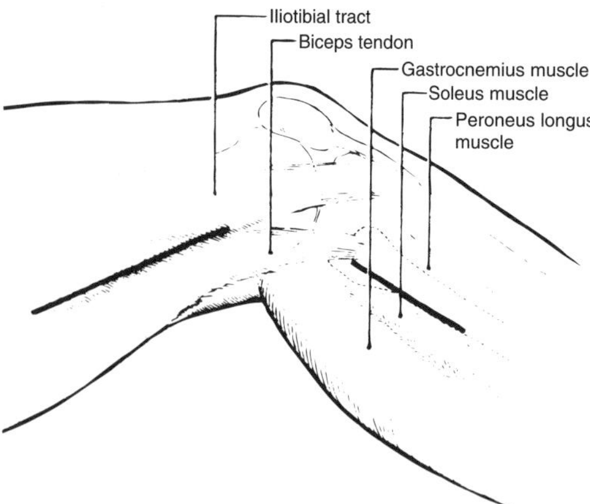

Figure 5. Incision in the lateral aspect of the thigh and calf to gain access to above knee and below knee popliteal artery, respectively (from Veith,[52] with permission).

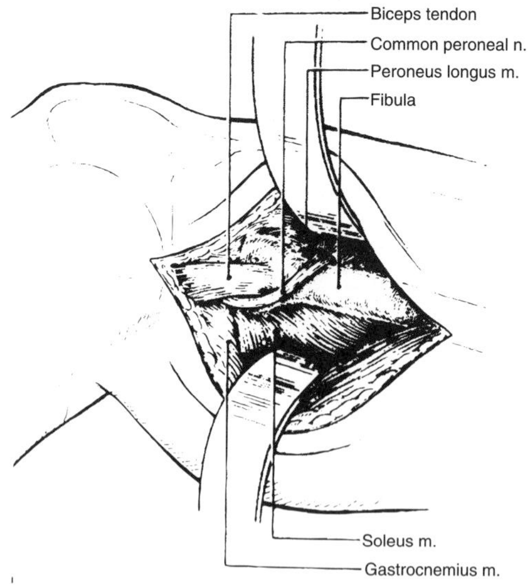

Figure 6. Lateral exposure of below knee popliteal artery and its distal branches before removal of the upper portion of the fibula (from Veith,[52] with permission).

ally in the bundle (Fig. 8). Lateral exposure of the below knee popliteal artery is initiated with an incision over the head and proximal fibula. After dividing subcutaneous tissue and fibromuscular attachments to the fibula, the common peroneal nerve is dissected free as it courses over the fibular neck so that it can be retracted and protected from injury (Fig. 6). Ligamentous attachments to the proximal quarter of the fibula are divided as well as the biceps femoris tendon. When the anterior, lateral, and inferior portion of the fibula are adequately cleared, a 4- to 5-centimeter segment of the bone is mobilized with bone shears. Once the bone is divided, excision of the proximal fibula is accomplished by dividing the medial soft tissue attachments under direct vision. With the proximal fibula removed, the distal popliteal, anterior tibial, and tibioperoneal trunk arteries are easily dissected from the investing tissue, nerves, and veins of the neurovascular bundle (Fig. 7).

In their review of 21 patients who underwent the lateral approach, Veith et al. used the above knee popliteal artery as inflow in 5 patients and as outflow in 6 patients, the below knee popliteal as outflow in 4 patients and the below knee popliteal

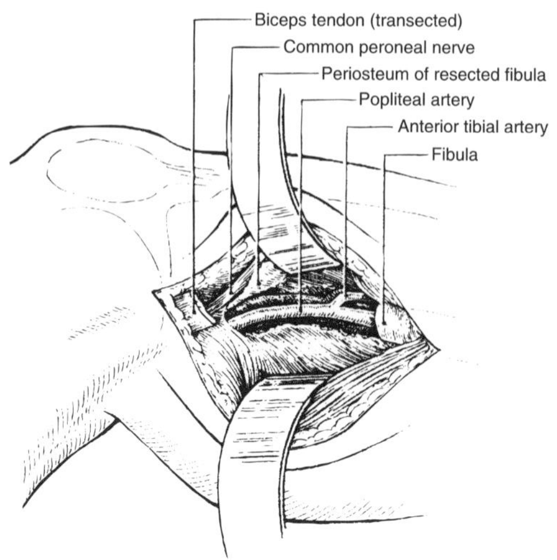

Figure 7. Lateral exposure of the upper quarter of the fibula after its resection. Note the position of the common peroneal nerve, which must be protected from injury (from Veith,[52] with permission).

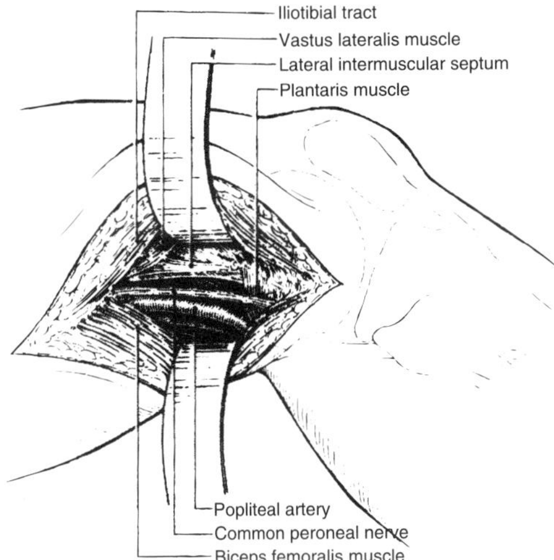

Figure 8. Lateral exposure of above knee popliteal artery (from Veith,[52] with permission).

as inflow in 6 patients. Patients did not develop a subsequent graft infection even though 80% required revascularization using the lateral approach as treatment for prior graft infections. Though no patency statistics were reported, the authors commented that it was comparable to primary bypasses using the standard medial approach. These results indicate that the lateral exposure of the above and below knee popliteal arteries is another useful technique for managing infrainguinal bypass infections.[52]

Primary Amputation Patients with infected infrainguinal grafts who present with a thrombosed graft and inadequate distal vessels for reconstruction usually require amputation as a primary procedure. As a corollary, patients with a necrotizing infection or septic focus in the foot or distal leg should undergo a primary guillotine amputation prior to definitive amputation. McIntyre et al. reported a significant decrease in the rate of below knee stump infection from 22% to 2% when guillotine amputation was performed prior to the definitive below knee procedure.[53] The fate of the infected bypass graft in patients undergoing a pri-

mary amputation remains a point of contention. Similar to the report of Johansen and Zorn, Rubin et al. reported seven episodes of delayed stump healing and recurrent graft sepsis in eight patients who initially underwent partial graft excision and subsequently required complete graft excision.[36,54] In contrast, four patients who underwent complete graft excision experienced primary amputation healing without recurrent sepsis or mortality. With these studies in mind, current recommendations for the management of an infected infrainguinal bypass in a patient requiring amputation are similar to those for partial graft excision.[8] The graft is exposed in a clean field proximal to the site of amputation. If the graft is grossly infected, complete graft removal is performed. If the graft is well incorporated, a segment of graft is removed and cultured. The remaining distal graft is removed at the time of amputation. Positive cultures of the excised proximal graft segment mandate complete graft removal. At the time of primary amputation, delayed wound closure is used to prevent stump healing problems precipitated by removal of the infected distal portion of the graft.

Wound Closure

Once adequate debridement of the infected wound has been performed, daily dressing changes continue until the wound begins to granulate. Granulation will occur provided the wound is kept clean with low bacterial counts ($<10^5$ colony forming units (CFU) per gram of tissue), and daily wet-to-dry dressings provide some degree of mechanical debridement while preventing dessication. As shown by Ouriel et al., granulation tissue will form over exposed autogenous vein grafts in the absence of Gram-negative infections.[16] Adequate debridement often results in inadequate soft tissue coverage of prosthetic grafts. Granulation tissue usually does not form over portions of exposed prosthetic grafts, and therefore requires coverage with vascularized soft tissue to achieve wound healing. One unique approach to this problem has been described by Mendes et al.[55] Omentum was transposed beneath the inguinal ligament to obliterate the dead space and provide a surface for skin coverage in a patient with a vascular graft infection in the groin who had failed local muscle flaps. More commonly applied adjunctive procedures to facilitate wound closure in large granulating wounds or wounds without adequate autogenous soft tissue to cover exposed graft material include skin grafts and rotational muscle flaps.

Skin Grafts

Once wound excision and daily dressing changes have resulted in a granulating wound, split thickness skin grafting can be used to expedite wound closure. Standard techniques for split thickness skin grafting are applied to harvest a graft between 0.010 and 0.020 inches in thickness. Successful grafting will occur in wounds with bacterial counts of less than 10^5 CFU per gram of tissue. Skin grafts can be applied to wounds as an alternative to closure by secondary intention if the wound is of a generous size after treatment by excision. Furthermore, in deeper wounds with exposed autogenous graft material, healing can be expedited using a skin graft, once these wounds are covered with granulation tissue. Finally, in large wounds with exposed prosthetic graft material which require rotational muscle flaps for coverage, skin grafts can be directly applied to the muscle to facilitate healing.

Rotational Muscle Flaps

Early reports of the management of vascular graft infection were not only characterized by significant morbidity and mortality, but were also associated with high costs and prolonged hospitalization for management of open wounds. As criteria have evolved for specific management of the infected graft, likewise techniques have developed to manage the resulting complex wound problems. Rotational muscle flaps, or myoplasties, require the mobilization of local vascularized bulky tissue to cover prosthetic grafts in open wounds. Based upon successful eradication of osteomyelitis through debridement, antibiotics, and coverage of devitalized bone with muscle flaps, this technique has been applied both experimentally and clinically to infected vascular grafts.[56] In an animal model of ePTFE carotid grafts inoculated with *S aureus* at implantation, lower bacterial counts and fewer episodes of anastomotic hemorrhage were achieved in dogs treated with antibiotics and muscle flap coverage when compared with either treatment alone.[57] In one of the earlier clinical reports of the application of these techniques to vascular graft infection treatment, Mixter et al. described the successful use of myoplasties in 20 out of 21 patients.[58] They used myoplasties in patients with patent exposed grafts after wide debridement resulted in a wound with bacterial counts of less than 10^5 CFU per gram of tissue. Familiarity with the more common techniques of myoplasty in the lower extremity is essential for the surgeon who manages patients with infected infrainguinal grafts.

Rectus Femoris

Use of the rectus femoris muscle is a common approach to provide vascularized soft tissue coverage in the proximal leg. The rectus femoris muscle originates from the anterior inferior iliac spine and inserts into the quadriceps tendon. The technique has been described thoroughly in the paper by Mixter et al.[56] The advantages of the rectus femoris myoplasty are the large size of the muscle and its mobility based upon a single vascular pedicle from the lateral circumflex femoral branch of the profunda femoris ar-

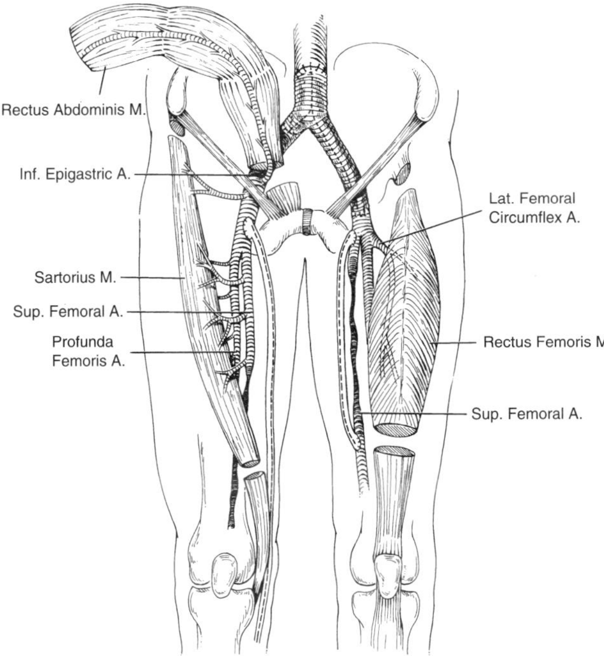

Figure 9. Regional muscle coverage of groin prostheses. Note the blood supply of the rectus abdominis from the inferior epigastric artery pedicle, of the rectus femoris from the lateral circumflex femoral pedicle, and of the sartorius from segmental branches of the superficial femoral (adapted from Mixter,[58] with permission).

tery (Fig. 9). This permits detachment of the muscle from its insertion in the quadriceps tendon and rotation of the length of the muscle belly to provide coverage in the groin. An alternative approach is to detach the origin from the anterior inferior iliac spine and rotate the muscle on its longitudinal axis into the groin wound. This has been used successfully to provide coverage for exposed prosthetic graft material limited to small wounds in the groin and circumvents the need for a large dissection in the thigh (Fig. 10). Disadvantages in using this muscle are the potential for inadequate blood supply secondary to occlusive disease in the profunda femoris and the potential for a functional defect in the extremity after mobilization of the muscle. The rectus femoris muscle, if available, is an excellent choice for myoplasty coverage of exposed prosthetic grafts in the groin or thigh.

Rectus Abdominis

Another technique to provide coverage for exposed prosthetic grafts uses the rectus abdominis muscle.[59] Similar to the rectus femoris, the rectus abdominis is a bulky muscle which can be mobilized based upon a single vascular pedicle, specifically the inferior epigastric artery. Unfortunately, this muscle may not be available because of discontinuity of its blood supply. This can result from previous abdominal surgery particularly transverse or oblique incisions which divide the inferior epigastric artery. More commonly in patients with peripheral vascular disease, iliofemoral occlusive disease often affects the origin of the inferior epigastric artery as well. Confirmation of patency and continuity of the inferior epigastric artery is necessary before proceeding with a rectus abdominis muscle flap. If

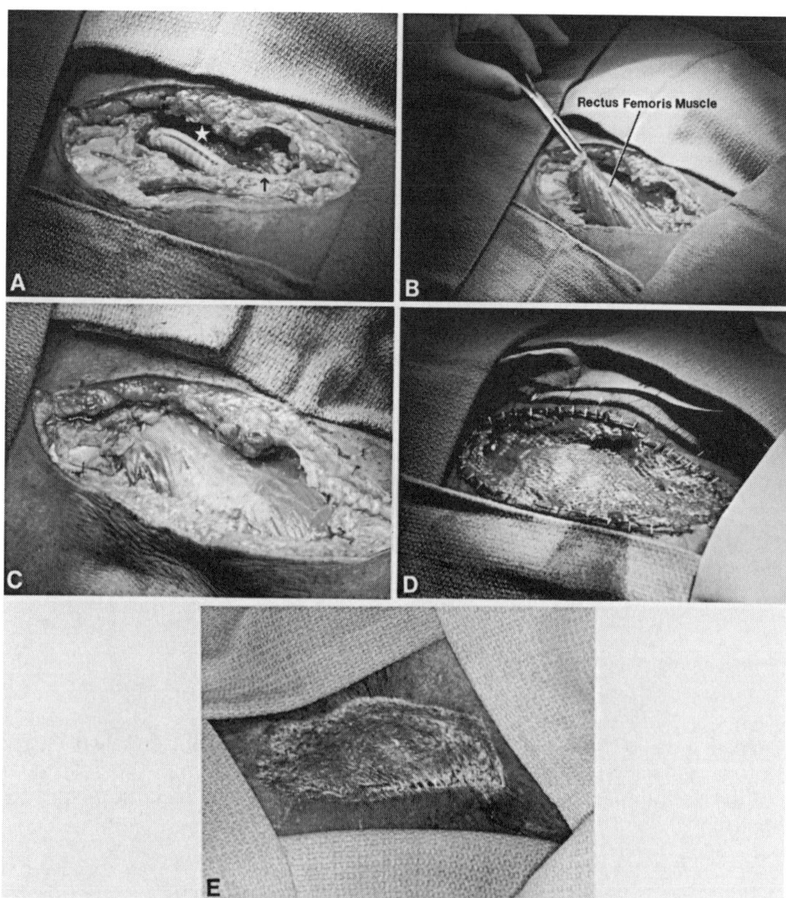

Figure 10. Use of the proximal rectus femoris for soft tissue coverage of an exposed vascular prostheses in the groin. (A) Debridment of necrotic skin and subcutaneous tissue results in an exposed limb of an aortofemoral graft (star) and the femoropopliteal graft (arrow). (B) The rectus femoris muscle is detached from its origin and rotated along its longitudinal axis from lateral to medial. (C) The rectus femoris is sutured into the open wound with interrupted sutures. (D) Apearance after application of a split-thickness skin graft. (E) Wound appearance at follow-up 30 days postdischarge.

its blood supply is intact, the muscle is detached from its origin at the costal margins and dissected from the fascial envelope of the rectus sheath. This can be done through a transverse abdominal skin incision by raising proximal and distal subcutaneous flaps. The proximal mobilized muscle can then be rotated down to the groin or proximal thigh based upon the inferior epigastric artery pedicle (Fig. 9). This flap is generally mobile enough that the contralateral groin can be covered if the ipsilateral rectus flap is not available. Though the dissection of the rectus abdominis flap is more complex, it remains a practical alternative to cover exposed prosthetic grafts in the thigh or groin.

Sartorius

The sartorius muscle is the most popular local muscle used for myoplasty to provide coverage in the upper leg.[60] The usefulness of the sartorius muscle transfer is derived from its proximity to the areas most commonly involved in the infectious process and its relative simplicity of use. The major disadvantages limiting its usefulness are its relative limited muscle bulk and segmental blood supply from the superficial femoral artery which often restricts its mobility. However, the sartorius can be used to cover small wounds in the proximal thigh by detachment of the origin from the anterior superior iliac spine or small wounds in the distal thigh by detachment from its insertion on the medial condyle of the tibia (Fig. 9).

Antibiotic Therapy

From the earliest reports of infectious complications of vascular grafts, parenteral antibiotics have been a mainstay in therapy as well as prevention. However, the duration and route of antibiotic treatment to eradicate infection and prevent recurrence particularly in prosthetic grafts has not been extensively studied. Most authors would agree that a short-term course of high-dose culture-specific intravenous antibiotics is an appropriate component of treatment of vascular graft infections. In an effort to prevent prosthetic graft infections, separate reports by Williams and Fisher and Ernst et al., suggested that this approach was suitable when positive cultures were obtained from aortic aneurysms and their contents.[61,62] MacBeth et al. reported that positive arterial wall cultures correlated with later prosthetic graft infections and prompted an investigation of arterial wall cultures and duration of antibiotic treatment in eliminating graft infection.[26] In a follow-up study by Malone et al., a significant difference in the incidence of arterial wall disruption or hemorrhage was demonstrated between patients with positive arterial wall cultures versus those with negative cultures (7 of 13 versus 0 of 16, $P < 0.005$).[63] Moreover, in the group with positive arterial wall cultures followed up to 76 months, patients treated with long-term culture-specific antibiotics (intravenous for 6 weeks followed by oral for 6 months) had significantly lower episodes of arterial wall

disruption or hemorrhage compared with those treated with short-term antibiotics (intravenous for 7 to 10 days) (0 of 6 versus 7 of 7, $P < 0.005$). Though the data available are limited to date, long-term culture-specific antibiotics are warranted to extirpate the infection and reduce or prevent catastrophic complications when intraoperative arterial wall cultures are positive. In the absence of positive arterial wall cultures at the time of surgical intervention to treat the infection, a short course of high-dose culture-specific intravenous antibiotics is warranted.

Results and Complications

The outcome for treatment of infrainguinal graft infections in numerous series has been referred to throughout this chapter. Piotrowski and Bernhard have compiled the results of reported series which contained enough descriptive information to identify the type of graft material, location of the infection, treatment, and outcome.[6] In their review of 13 reports of 52 infrainguinal graft infections managed with local therapy, the mortality rate was 8%, the amputation rate 10%, and the rate of successful treatment 77%. In 11 reports of graft excision without revascularization comprising 96 patients, mortality occurred in 15%, amputation in 59%, and successful outcome in 29%. No specific review of graft excision and revascularization was reported; however, recent series by Samson et al. and Yeager et al. reveal an amputation rate of 0% to 63%, mortality rates from 0% to 13%, and successful treatment outcome in 25% to 100% of patients with infrainguinal graft infections treated in this manner. This review demonstrates the ominous potential of an infectious complication of infrainguinal revascularization procedures.

Summary

Infection occurring in an infrainguinal bypass graft is an infrequent but potentially devastating complication. The management of an infected infrainguinal graft requires multimodality therapy if the infection is to be eliminated and the limb is to be salvaged. Superficial infection can be successfully treated with debridement and antibiotics. More extensive infections with anastomotic involvement, systemic sepsis, bleeding, or embolization require complete graft removal and revascularization or amputation depending upon the state of the limb and the patency of distal vessels. Partial graft excision can be used successfully, but only in carefully selected cases. Culture-specific antibiotics based upon intensive methods of microbiologic investigation including arterial wall culture and graft sonication are a basic component of all treatment regimens, though the exact duration of antibiotic treatment has not been definitively determined. Adequate wound debridement often results in large wounds which require adjunctive measures including skin grafts to expedite closure or rotational muscle flaps to insure coverage of exposed prosthetic material. Despite these efforts, infection of an infrainguinal bypass continues to be associated with significant mortality and limb loss. Paramount in minimizing the devastation of this complication is prevention, which may be enhanced by the use of prophylactic antibiotics, reduction of patient risk factors, and, in the future, infection-resistant graft material.[64]

References

1. Goldstone J, Moore WS. Infection in vascular prostheses: clinical manifestations and surgical management. *Am J Surg.* 1974;128: 225–233.
2. Szilagyi DE, Smith RF, Elliott JP, Vrandecic MP. Infection in arterial reconstruction with synthetic grafts. *Ann Surg.* 1972;176:321–333.
3. Lorentzen JE, Nielson OM, Arendrup H, et al. Vascular graft infection: an analysis of 62 graft infections in 2411 consecutively implanted synthetic vascular grafts. *J Vasc Surg.* 1985;98:81–86.
4. Liekweg WG Jr, Greenfield LJ. Vascular prosthetic infections: collected experience and results of treatment. *Surgery.* 1977;81: 335–342.
5. O'Hara PJ, Hertzer NR, Beven EG, et al. Surgical management of infected abdominal aortic grafts: review of a 25-year experience. *J Vasc Surg.* 1986;3:725–731.
6. Piotrowski JJ, Bernhard VM. Management of vascular graft infections. In: Bernhard VM, Towne JB, eds. *Complications in Vascular Surgery.* St. Louis: Quality Medical Publishing, Inc; 1991:235–258.
7. Hoffert PW, Gensler S, Haimovici H. Infection complicating arterial grafts. *Arch Surg.* 1965;90:427–435.
8. Durham JR, Rubin JR, Malone JM. Management of infected infrainguinal bypass grafts. In: Bergan JJ, Yao JST, eds. *Reoperative Arterial Surgery.* Philadelphia: WB Saunders; 1986:359–373.
9. Edwards WH Jr, Martin RS III, Jenkins JM, et al. Primary graft infections. *J Vasc Surg.* 1987;6:235–239.
10. Johnson JA, Cogbill TH, Strutt PJ, et al. Wound complications after infrainguinal bypass: classification, predisposing factors, and management. *Arch Surg.* 1988;123:859–862.
11. Bandyk DF. Vascular graft infections: epidemiology, microbiology, pathogenesis, and prevention. In: Bernhard VM, Towne JB, eds. *Complications in Vascular Surgery.* St. Louis: Quality Medical Publishing, Inc., 1991: 223–34.
12. Durham JR, Malone JM, Bernhard VM. The impact of multiple operations on the importance of arterial wall cultures. *J Vasc Surg.* 1987;5:160–169.
13. Rubin JR, Malone JM, Goldstone J. The role of the lymphatic system in acute arterial prosthetic graft infections. *J Vasc Surg.* 1985; 2:92–98.
14. Lindenauer SM, Fry WJ, Schuab G, et al. The use of antibiotics in the prevention of vascular graft infection. *Surgery.* 1967;62:487–492.
15. Casey J, Flinn WR, Yao JST, et al. Correlation of immune and nutritional status with wound complications in patients undergoing vascular operations. *Surgery.* 1983;93: 822–827.
16. McIntyre KE Jr. Wound complications following vascular reconstruction. In: Bernhard VM, Towne JB, eds. *Complications in Vascular Surgery.* St Louis: Quality Medical Publishing, Inc; 1991:291–300.
17. Ouriel K, Geary KJ, Green RM, DeWeese JA. Fate of the exposed saphenous vein graft. *Am J Surg.* 1990;160:148–150.
18. Wengrovitz M, Atnip RG, Gifford RRM, et al. Wound complications of autogenous sub-

cutaneous infrainguinal arterial bypass surgery: predisposing factors and management. *J Vasc Surg.* 1990;11:156–163.

19. DeLaria GA, Hunter JA, Goldin MD, et al. Leg wound complication associated with coronary revascularization. *J Thorac Cardiovasc Surg.* 1981;81:403–407.

20. Utley JR, Thomason ME, Wallace DJ, et al. Preoperative correlates of impaired wound healing after saphenous vein excision. *J Thorac Cardiovasc Surg.* 1989;98:147–149.

21. Ruoff BA, Cranely JJ, Hannan LA, et al. Real-time duplex ultrasound mapping of the greater saphenous vein before in situ infrainguinal revascularization. *J Vasc Surg.* 1987;6:107–113.

22. Angelini GD, Butchart EG, Armistead SH, et al. Comparative study of leg wound skin closure in coronary artery bypass operations. *Thorax.* 1984;39:942–945.

23. Geary KJ, Tomkiewicz ZM, Harrison HN, et al. Differential effects of Gram-negative and Gram-positive infection on autogenous and prosthetic grafts. *J Vasc Surg.* 1990;11:339–347.

24. Bricker DL, Beall AC Jr, DeBakey ME. The differential response to infection of autogenous vein versus Dacron arterial prosthesis. *Chest.* 1970;58:566–570.

25. Seabrook GR, Schmitt DD, Bandyk DF, et al. Anastomotic femoral pseudoaneurysm: an investigation of occult infection as an etiologic factor. *J Vasc Surg.* 1990;11:629–634.

26. MacBeth GA, Rubin JR, McIntyre KE Jr, et al. The relevance of arterial wall microbiology to the treatment of prosthetic graft infections: graft infection versus arterial infection. *J Vasc Surg.* 1984;1:750–756.

27. Bergamini TM, Bandyk DF, Govostis D, et al. Identification of *Staphylococcus epidermidis* vascular graft infections: a comparison of culture techniques. *J Vasc Surg.* 1989;9:665–670.

28. Bandyk DF, Berni GA, Thiele BL, Towne JB. Aortofemoral graft infection due to *Staphylococcus epidermidis. Arch Surg.* 1984;119:102–108.

29. Dougherty SH, Simmons RL. Infections in bionic man: the pathobiology of infection in prosthetic devices: Parts I and II. *Curr Probl Surg.* 1982;19:1–314.

30. Schmitt DD, Bandyk DF, Pequet AJ, et al. Mucin production by *Staphylococcus epidermidis:* a virulence factor promoting adherence to vascular grafts. *Arch Surg.* 1986;121:89–95.

31. Tollefson DF, Bandyk DF, Kaebnick HW, et al. Surface biofilm disruption: enhanced recovery of microorganisms from vascular prostheses. *Arch Surg.* 1986;122:38–43.

32. Samson RH, Veith FJ, Janko GS, et al. A modified classification and approach to the management of infections involving peripheral arterial prosthetic grafts. *J Vasc Surg.* 1988;8:147–153.

33. Chung CJ, Hicklin OA, Payan JM, Gordon L. Indium-111-leukocyte scan in detection of synthetic vascular graft infection: the effect of antibiotic treatment. *J Nucl Med.* 1991;32:13–15.

34. Fry WJ, Lindenauer SM. Infection complicating the use of plastic arterial implants. *Arch Surg.* 1967;94:600–609.

35. Conn JH, Hardy JD, Chavez CM, Fain WR. Infected arterial grafts: experience with 22 cases with emphasis on unusual bacteria and techniques. *Ann Surg.* 1970;171:704–714.

36. Johansen K, Zorn R. Amputation stump infection in patients with retained thrombosed prosthetic grafts. *Am Surg.* 1981;47:228–231.

37. Yeager RA, McConnell DB, Sasaki TM, Vetto RM. Aortic and peripheral prosthetic graft infection: differential management and causes of mortality. *Am J Surg.* 1985;150:36–43.

38. Calligaro KD, Westcott CJ, Buckley RM, et al. Infrainguinal anastomotic arterial graft infections treated by selected graft preservation. *Ann Surg.* 1992;216:74–79.

39. Moore WS, Malone JM, Keown K. Prosthetic arterial graft material: influence on neointimal healing and bacteremic infectability. *Arch Surg.* 1980;115:1379–1383.

40. Stone KS, Walshaw R, Sugiyama GT, et al. Polytetrafluoroethylene versus autogenous vein grafts for vascular reconstruction in contaminated wounds. *Am J Surg.* 1984;147:692–695.

41. Harrison JH, Jordan WD, Perez AR. Eversion endarterectomy surgery. *Surgery.* 1967;61:26–30.

42. Moore WS, Swanson RJ, Campagna G, Bean B. The use of fresh tissue arterial substitutes in infected fields. *J Surg Res.* 1975;18:229–333.

43. Snyder SO, Wheeler JR, Gregory RT, et al. Freshly harvested cadaveric venous homografts as arterial conduits in infected fields. *Surgery.* 1987;101:283–291.

44. Masuda EM, Snyder SO Jr, Wheeler JR, et al. Nine-year experience with the use of venous homografts in infected fields. *J Vasc Surg.* 1993;17:237–238.

45. Shaw RS, Baue AE. Management of sepsis complicating arterial reconstructive surgery. *Surgery.* 1963;53:75–86.

46. DePalma RG, Hubay CA. Arterial bypass via

the obturator foramen: an alternative in complicated vascular problems. *Am J Surg.* 1968; 115:3238.

47. DePalma RG. Obturator foramen bypass grafts in groin sepsis. In: Ernst CB, Stanley JC, eds. *Current Therapy in Vascular Surgery, 2nd ed.* Philadelphia: BC Decker, Inc; 1991: 353–356.

48. Tilson MD, Sweeney T, Gusberg RJ, et al. Obturator canal bypass grafts for septic lesions of the femoral artery. *Arch Surg.* 1979; 114:1031–1033.

49. Nunez AA, Veith FJ, Collier P, et al. Direct approaches to the distal portions of the deep femoral artery for limb salvage bypasses. *J Vasc Surg.* 1988;8:576–581.

50. Henry AK. *Extensile Exposure, 2nd ed.* New York: Churchill Livingstone; 1957:218–223.

51. Elkin DC, Kelly RP. Arteriovenous aneurysm: exposure of the tibial and peroneal vessels by resection of the fibula. *Ann Surg.* 1945;122:529–545.

52. Veith FJ, Ascer E, Gupta SK, Wengerter KR. Lateral approach to the popliteal artery. *J Vasc Surg.* 1987;6:119–123.

53. McIntyre KE Jr, Bailey SA, Malone JM, Goldstone J. The nonsalvagable infected lower extremity: A new look at guillotine amputation. Arch Surg 1984;119:450–453.

54. Rubin JR, Yao JST, Thompson RG, Bergan JJ. Management of infection of major amputation stumps following failed femorodistal grafts. *Surgery.* 1985;98:810–815.

55. Mendes D, Kahn M, Ibrahim IM, et al. Omental protection of autogenous arterial reconstruction following femoral prosthetic graft infection. *J Vasc Surg.* 1985;2:603–606.

56. Ger R. Muscle transposition for treatment and prevention of chronic post-traumatic osteomyelitis of the tibia. *J Bone Joint Surg.* 1977; 59A:784–791.

57. Dacey LJ, Miett TOC, Huntsman WT, et al. Efficacy of muscle flaps in the treatment of prosthetic vascular graft infections. *J Surg Res.* 1988;44:566–572.

58. Mixter RC, Turnipseed WD, Smith DJ Jr, et al. Rotational muscle flaps: a new technique for covering infected vascular grafts. *J Vasc Surg.* 1989;9:472–478.

59. Perler BA, Vander Kolk CA, Dufresne CA, Williams GM. Can infected prosthetic grafts be salvaged with rotational muscle flaps? *Surgery.* 1991;110:30–34.

60. Perler BA. Use of muscle flaps in the treatment of prosthetic graft infection. In: Veith FJ, ed. *Current Critical Problems in Vascular Surgery, Vol 3.* St. Louis: Quality Medical Publishing, Inc; 1991:380–386.

61. Williams RD, Fisher FW. Aneurysms contents as a source of graft infection. *Arch Surg.* 1977;112:415–416.

62. Ernst CB, Campbell HC Jr, Daugherty ME, et al. Incidence and significance of intraoperative bacterial cultures during abdominal aortic aneurysmectomy. *Ann Surg.* 1977;185: 626–633.

63. Malone JM, Lalka SG, McIntyre KE Jr, et al. The necessity for long-term antibiotic therapy with positive arterial wall cultures. *J Vasc Surg.* 1988;8:262–267.

64. Shenk JS, Ney AL, Tsukayama DT, et al. Tobramycin-adhesive in preventing and treating PTFE vascular graft infections. *J Surg Res.* 1989;47:487–492.

Chapter 27

Amputation and Graft Infection

M.C. Hutton
J.R. Rubin

Introduction

Amputation is an operation that dates back to the Neanderthal man in neolithic times. It was perfected through the ages, primarily in the battlefields, where it was performed as a life-saving procedure. With the evolution of antimicrobial therapy, advances in surgical technique, anesthesia, critical care management, today's surgeon is armed with a variety of therapeutic alternatives to primary amputation. Despite these advances, there are limits to limb salvageability and major lower extremity amputation is still frequently required.

Many factors, alone or in combination, may contribute to the final decision to proceed to amputation as the therapeutic option of choice. The individual's rehabilitation potential must be considered. Patients who are chronically nonambulatory, patients with fixed contractures of the hip and/or knee, as well as patients who have already experienced irreversible motor and/or sensory loss, massive soft tissue, muscle, neurologic and/or osseous destruction have limited rehabilitation potential and are probably not candidates for limb salvage heroics. In addition, amputation is often recommended for patients with a severely limited life expectancy as well as those who, due to their multiple medical problems, would not be appropriate candidates for arterial reconstruction. Lastly, amputation may be the procedure of choice in patients with severely dysvascular limbs and who are not felt to have potential for long-term limb salvage due to a lack of a suitable recipient artery or the absence of a suitable bypass conduit. In selected patients, primary amputation may be preferable to secondary or tertiary arterial bypass attempts, when the latter has a low probability of success. This is an important issue in ambulatory individuals since amputation level and primary healing have both been shown to be adversely effected by multiple failed arterial bypasses.[1]

Once the decision has been made to proceed with lower extremity amputation, multiple wound healing factors must be considered prior to performing this operation, if the surgeon anticipates primary uncomplicated wound healing in these patients.

The most common local complications of major lower extremity amputation include delay or failure of wound healing and stump infection. Both of these complications frequently mandate amputation at a higher level, which decreases the likelihood of an early return to independent ambulation and also increases the risk of associated mortality. The surgeon must therefore be concerned with appropriate amputation level selection and potential sources of primary and secondary infection.

Level of Amputation

Amputation level and the patient's overall medical status will affect his or her potential for rehabilitation. Knee preservation is preferable in the patient with strong potential for restoration of bipedal ambulation, while this is unimportant and probably contraindicated in the nonambulatory patient. If it is generally felt by the surgeon, rehabilitation specialist, and prosthetist that the patient might benefit from knee preservation, we routinely use Doppler ultrasonography and transcutaneous oximetry to evaluate wound healing potential. In the presence of a patent arterial bypass graft, which would be ligated at the time of amputation, this information will not be meaningful. In addition, the presence of a significant inflow or outflow arterial lesion may significantly affect distal wound healing and the repair of this lesion might be indicated prior to the selection of the amputation level.

The selection of a below knee as opposed to an above knee amputation level is made on the basis of: 1) absence of local skin, deep soft tissue, or osseous infection at the proposed below knee amputation site; 2) low thigh systolic pressure greater than or equal to 70 mm Hg; and 3) amputation site transcutaneous oxygen pressure greater than or equal to 20 mm Hg.[1-3] Obviously, if a functional graft is to be removed or ligated, or if arterial reconstruction is planned, the blood flow measurements should ideally not be performed until all intervention is completed.

Wound Debridement and Guillotine Amputation

When faced with a dysvascular, nonsalvageable limb and concomitant infection, which may be limb or life threatening, we normally recommend aggressive wound debridement, toe, partial foot or ankle guillotine amputations to control sepsis. Systemic antibiotic therapy is an important concomitant treatment modality for reducing cellulitis and controlling sepsis, prior to definitive amputation. Guillotine amputation, followed by definitive interval amputation, has been found to reduce the incidence of residual limb infection (3%) when compared to single stage procedures (22%) in infected limbs.[4,5] The incidence of postoperative infection in below or above knee amputations should be extremely low if the septic dysvascular limb is treated with aggressive debridement, open amputation, and systemic antibiotic therapy. Interval amputation is generally performed within 5 days of the initial procedure or when the patient is stabilized.[6]

Graft Management

Specific complications related to retained prosthetic graft material in the amputation stump have been recognized by a variety of authors[1,2,7] (Fig. 1).

Existing bypass grafts in dysvascular limbs may be stratified into: 1) clean versus infected grafts; 2) patent versus thrombosed grafts; 3) autogenous versus prosthetic conduits; and, 4) inflow versus outflow bypasses. The handling of a bypass graft at the time of amputation will vary depending upon multiple coexisting conditions.

In general, infected bypass grafts require the same treatment consideration at the time of amputation as they would if amputation was not being considered. Complete removal of all infected graft materials is required. If the infected bypass is prosthetic, we recommend complete graft re-

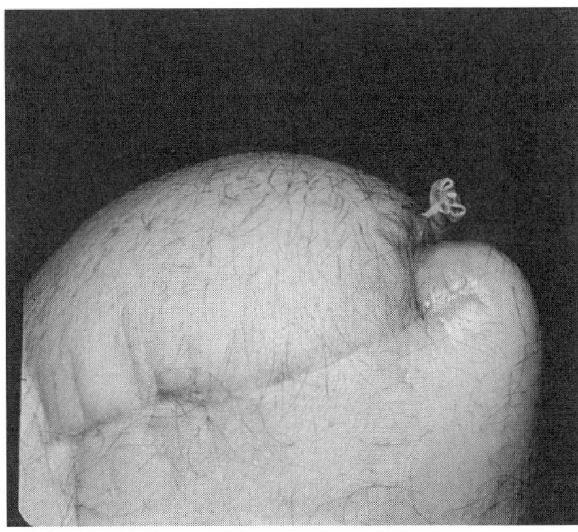

Figure 1. Above knee amputation stump with an extruding prosthetic graft.

moval. When the graft is removed, a femoral artery patch angioplasty is often required. We routinely use autogenous material for the patch, and are generally able to identify and use a portion of vein or an endarterectomized arterial segment for this purpose. Frequently there is a moderate amount of graft incorporation despite the infection and skin incisions that will facilitate prosthetic removal (Fig. 2).

If the infected graft is autogenous vein,

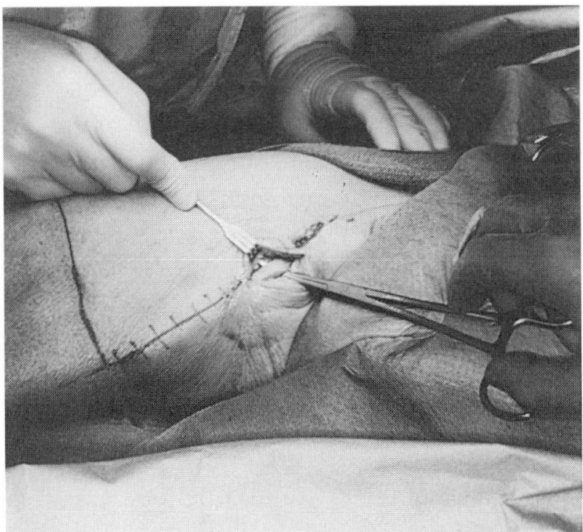

Figure 2. Skip incisions required for an incorporated graft removal.

the extent of the infection will determine to what level the graft will need to be removed. In this case, we will normally remove all infected vein through the amputation incision. If necessary, the vein may be detached through a more proximal incision and the infected segment may be pulled out from the amputation wound.

The handling of clean autogenous bypasses does not require special attention. Simply performing high-suture ligation of the graft and allowing it to retract into the substance of the stump is adequate. If in fact the graft is thrombosed, we generally obtain cultures of the thrombus and graft wall at the time of amputation as a precautionary step.

Based on several prior studies by our group, we recommend complete removal of all nonfunctional prosthetic bypass material.[1,2,6–8] This is concomitant with major lower extremity amputation. This is based on our finding of an increased rate of delayed wound healing, secondary stump infection, operative stump revision, and mortality when residual nonfunctional prosthetic graft material was retained, as opposed to complete removal at the time of amputation.[1,2,7] As previously described, grafts are detached from the femoral artery and are entirely removed through the open operative amputation stump (Fig. 3). Multiple skip incisions are frequently required to aid in dissecting the incorporated graft from its bed. Autogenous femoral artery patch angioplasty is performed if it is believed that primary closure will cause a significant stenosis from the site of the graft detachment.

Functional uninfected graft removal is not recommended at the time of major lower extremity amputation. There has been no documentation of an increased risk of subsequent graft infection when amputation is performed in an extremity with a patent bypass and wound healing, especially of the below knee amputation, which may be seriously compromised if a functioning graft is removed.

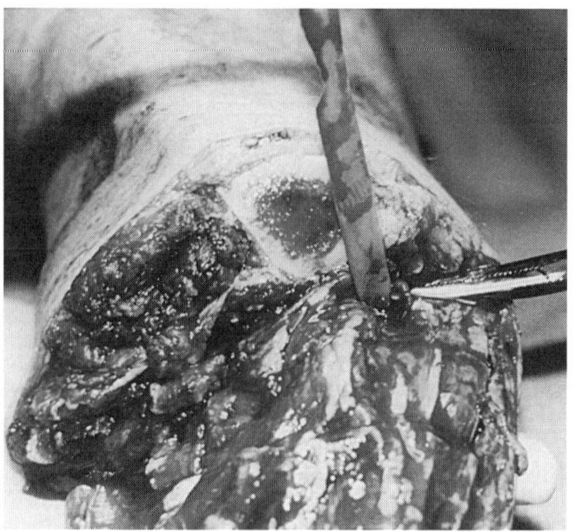

Figure 3. Graft removal through a distal amputation stump.

However, if a functional prosthetic femoral below knee popliteal or femoral-tibial graft is to be exposed and divided during amputation, complete graft removal is recommended since it will no longer be functional subsequent to the amputation.

Generally we do not recommend any manipulation of an inflow bypass graft during amputation, unless there is evidence of graft infection. In this case, graft management preempts amputation and standard principles of management apply.

Summary

Aggressive limb infection management including local debridement, partial foot and ankle guillotine amputation, combined with intravenous antibiotic therapy helps to reduce the incidence of secondary graft infection complications following interval amputation. In addition, appropriate graft handling during amputation has been shown to reduce major complications such as delayed wound healing and secondary stump infection which both result in amputation revision at generally a higher level, and the complication-related mortality rate which is increased as expected in patients requiring further operations.

References

1. Rubin JR, Marmen C, Rhodes RS. Management of failed prosthetic grafts at the time of major lower extremity amputation. *J Vasc Surg.* 1988;7:5:673–676.
2. Rubin JR, Yao JST, Thompson RG, Bergan JJ. Management of infection of major amputation stumps after failed femorodistal grafts. *Surgery.* 1985;98:4:810–815.
3. Thompson, RG. Performance of major amputations for severe ischemia. In: Bergan JJ, Yao, JST, eds. *Gangrene and Severe Ischemia of the Lower Extremities.* New York: Grune and Stratton Inc; 1978; 407–417.
4. McIntyre KE, Bailey ST, Malone JM, Goldstone J. Guillotine amputation in the treatment of nonsalvageable lower extremity infections. *Arch Surg.* 1984;119:450–453.
5. McIntyre KE. Control of infection in the diabetic foot: the rate of microbiology, immunopathology, antibiotics, and guillotine amputation. *J Vasc Surg.* 1985;5:787–790.
6. Rubin JR, Folsom D. The management of lower extremity graft infections. *Semin Vasc Surg.* 1990;3:2:114–121.
7. Johansen K, Zain R. Amputation stump infection in patients with retained thrombosed prosthetic vascular grafts. *Am Surg.* 1981:47: 228–233.
8. Durham JR, Rubin JR, Malone JM. Management of infected infrainguinal bypass grafts. In: Bergan JJ, Yao JST, eds. *Reoperative Arterial Surgery.* Orlando: Grune and Stratton, Inc; 1986;359–373.

Index